Core Curriculum for

TRANSPLANT
NURSES

SECOND EDITION

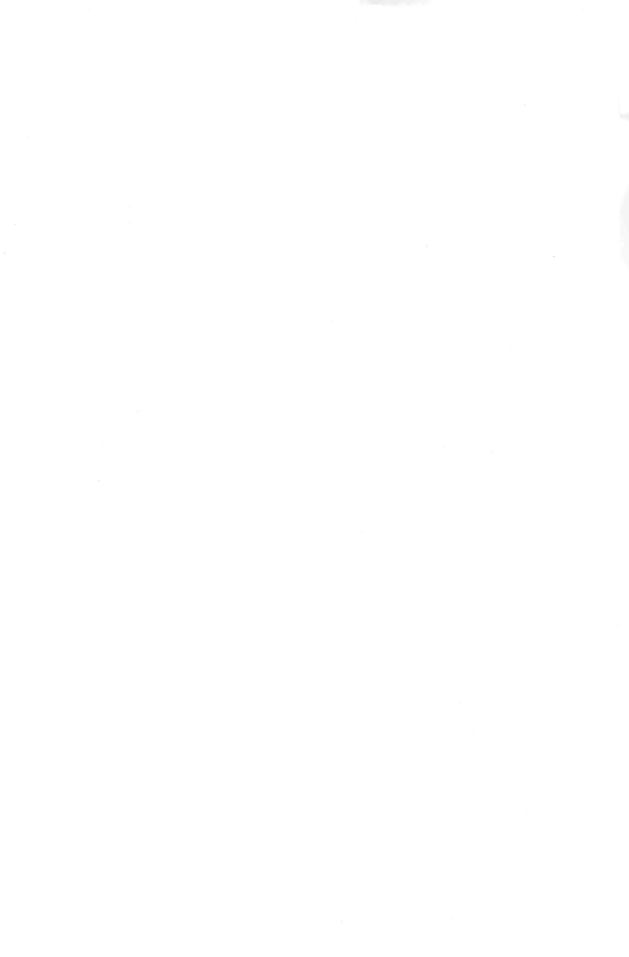

Core Curriculum for

TRANSPLANT
NURSES

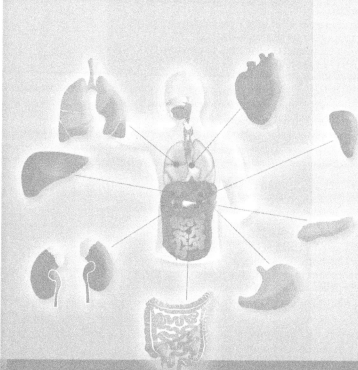

SECOND EDITION

EDITED BY:

Sandra A. Cupples, RN, PhD, FAAN, CAPT, NC, USN RET
Formerly, Heart Transplant Coordinator
Washington Hospital Center
Washington, District of Columbia

Stacee Lerret, RN, PhD, CPNP-AC/PC, CCTC
Assistant Professor, Medical College of Wisconsin
Pediatric Nurse Practitioner, Children's
Hospital of Wisconsin
Milwaukee, Wisconsin

Vicki McCalmont, RN, MS, ANP-BC, CNS, CCTC
Professor, San Diego State University
Heart Transplant Nurse Practitioner
Sharp Healthcare
San Diego, California
Cardiac Nurse Practitioner
Sharp Grossmont Hospital
La Mesa, California

Linda Ohler, RN, MSN, CCTC, FAAN
Quality and Regulatory Manager
Editor Progress in Transplantation
Transplant Quality Consultant
George Washington University Transplant Institute
Washington, District of Columbia

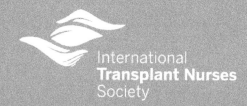

. Wolters Kluwer

Philadelphia • Baltimore • New York • London
Buenos Aires • Hong Kong • Sydney • Tokyo

International
Transplant Nurses
Society

Acquisitions Editor: Nicole Dernoski
Product Development Editor: Maria M. McAvey
Production Project Manager: Marian Bellus
Design Coordinator: Holly Reid McLaughlin
Manufacturing Coordinator: Kathleen Brown
Marketing Manager: Linda Wetmore
Prepress Vendor: SPi Global

Second edition

Library of Congress Cataloging-in-Publication Data
Names: Cupples, Sandra A. (Sandra Ann), editor. | Lerret, Stacee, editor. |McCalmont, Vicki, editor. | Ohler, Linda, editor. | International Transplant Nurses Society, issuing body.
Title: Core curriculum for transplant nurses / edited by Sandra Cupples, Stacee Lerret, Vicki McCalmont, Linda Ohler ; International Transplant Nurses Society.
Description: 2nd edition. | Philadelphia : Wolters Kluwer, [2017] | Includes bibliographical references and index.
Identifiers: LCCN 2016015693 | ISBN 9781451195309
Subjects: | MESH: Organ Transplantation—nursing | Tissue Transplantation—nursing | Perioperative Nursing—methods | Curriculum | Outlines
Classification: LCC RD120.7 | NLM WO 18.2 | DDC 617.9/540231—dc23 LC record available at https://lccn.loc.gov/2016015693

The self-less transplant nurses around the world, who are inspired to care and whose critical thinking and professional skills optimize outcomes of this complex patient population.
Transplant recipients and their families, who remind us about love, life, and commitment.
And organ donors and their families who create an enduring legacy of life.

Sandra A. Cupples
Stacee Lerret
Vicki McCalmont
Linda Ohler

To my children (Cindy, Tim, Meredith, Keith, and Jacqueline) and grandchildren (Andrew, Jillian, Alexei, Bradley, and Sloan) for their incredible encouragement and support; to my co-editors (Stacee, Vicki, and Linda) without whom this book never would have been possible; to each chapter author and reviewer for so generously sharing their time, knowledge, and expertise; to the memory of my parents who instilled in me a love of life-long learning and to Clancy who helped me keep things in perspective.

Sandra A. Cupples

To my husband, Aaron, for his deeply appreciated love and support and to my children (Brendon and Trista) for their love and understanding that this project was very near and dear to my heart.

Vicki McCalmont

To my husband, Brian—you have been an unending source of support and encouragement in every step of my academic and professional journey. I thank you for being there for me then, now, and, most importantly, for all our tomorrows to come. To my three children, Keegan, Amelia, and Nolan—you inspire me to give the very best of myself to children and families every day at my job. I thank you for the gift of being your mother and am truly grateful for the lessons of love, joy, and compassion you teach me every day.

Stacee Lerret

To my husband, Richard Knight, for his endless support and to my dog, Riley, who sat beside me as I wrote, edited, and revised. To my daughter, Pam, and her family, Zack and Alex, who patiently waited for a visit and to my mom who at 92 cheered me on while asking why I do these things!

Linda Ohler

Kim Ansley, MSW, LSW
Transplant Social Worker
The Ohio State University Wexner Medical
    Center
Columbus, Ohio

Debra Bernardina, RN, BSN, CCTC
Liver Transplant Coordinator
Duke Transplant Center
Durham, North Carolina

Robert A. Bray, PhD
Co-Director, Histocompatibility and Molecular
    Immunogenetics Laboratory
Emory University
Atlanta, Georgia

Karýn Ryan Canales, RN, BSN, CCTC
Senior Heart Transplant Clinical Coordinator
Ochsner Cardiomyopathy and Heart Transplant
New Orleans, Louisiana

Kevin C. Carney, MSN, CRNP, CCTC
Nurse Practitioner
Lung Transplant Program
Hospital of the University of Pennsylvania
Philadelphia, Pennsylvania

Cynthia Cassidy, RN, BSN, CCTC
Senior Clinical Heart Transplant Coordinator
Section of Heart Failure, Heart Transplantation
    and Mechanical Circulatory Support
Ochsner Medical Center
New Orleans, Louisiana

Suzanne R. Chillcott, RN, BSN
Mechanical Circulatory Support Lead
Sharp Memorial Hospital
San Diego, California

Samira Scalso de Almeida, RN, MS
Transplant Coordinator Outpatient Care
Hospital Albert Einstein
Organ and Tissue Transplant Study Group
GEDOTT-Escola Paulista de Enfermagem-EPE/
    UNIFESP
São Paulo, Brazil

Maria DeAngelis, MScN, NP
Pediatric Nurse Practitioner
Liver and Intestinal Transplant Program
Transplant Centre
The Hospital for Sick Children
Toronto, Ontario, Canada

Carolyn J. Driscoll, RN, PhD, FNP-C
Nurse Practitioner
Hepatology Section
Division of Gastroenterology, Hepatology,
    and Nutrition
Virginia Commonwealth University Health
    System
Richmond, Virginia

Debra Dumas-Hicks, RN, BS, CCTC, CCTN
Senior Clinical Post Heart Transplant
    Coordinator
Cardiomyopathy and Heart Transplant Section
Ochsner Medical Center
New Orleans, Louisiana

Christopher R. Ensor, PharmD, BCPS
Assistant Professor of Pharmacy and Medicine
Associate Member, Starzl Transplantation
    Institute
Clinical Faculty, Thoracic Transplantation
University of Pittsburgh
Pittsburgh, Pennsylvania

Wendy Escobedo, RN, MSN, PHN, CCTN
Renal Services Manager
Dialysis and Transplantation
St. Joseph Hospital
Orange, California

Linda A. Evans, RN, PhD
Nursing Program Director
Center for Nursing Excellence
Brigham and Women's Hospital
Boston, Massachusetts

Fawn Fitzmorris, RN, CCTC
Senior Heart Transplant Clinical Coordinator
Ochsner Multi-Organ Transplant Institute
New Orleans, Louisiana

Maureen P. Flattery, RN, MS, ANP-BC, CCTC
Heart Transplant Coordinator
Pauley Heart Center
Virginia Commonwealth University Health
    System
Richmond, Virginia

Leslie Gallagher, RN, MS, ANP-BC
Advanced Practice Nurse
Transplant Surgery
Hume-Lee Transplant Program
Virginia Commonwealth University
    Health System
Richmond, Virginia

Judy Gierlach, RN, BSN, CCTC
Clinical Transplant Coordinator
University of Rochester Medical Center
Rochester, New York

Leslie Hazard, RN, MS, ANP-BC, CNS
Nurse Practitioner
Sharp Memorial Hospital Heart Transplant/
    Mechanical Circulatory Support
San Diego, California

J. Eric Hobson, MSN, CRNP
Senior Nurse Practitioner
Lung Transplant
Hospital of the University of Pennsylvania
Philadelphia, Pennsylvania

Michelle James, RN, MS, APRN-CNS, CCTN
Transplant Clinical Director
Solid Organ Transplant Department
University of Minnesota Health
Minneapolis, Minnesota

**T. Nicole Kelley, MS, ACNP, CCRN,
CPSN, CANS, RNFA**
Plastic and Reconstructive Surgery Service
R. A. Cowley Shock Trauma Center
University of Maryland Medical System
Baltimore, Maryland

Kay Kendall, MSW, LISW-S, ACSW, CCTSW
Social Worker, Heart Transplant and Mechanical
    Circulatory Support Team
Cleveland Clinic
Cleveland, Ohio

Beverly Kosmach-Park, RN, DNP, FAAN
Clinical Nurse Specialist
Department of Transplant Surgery
Children's Hospital of Pittsburgh
Pittsburgh, Pennsylvania

Stacee Lerret, RN, PhD, CPNP-AC/PC, CCTC
Assistant Professor, Medical College of
    Wisconsin
Pediatric Nurse Practitioner, Children's Hospital
    of Wisconsin
Milwaukee, Wisconsin

Vicki McCalmont, RN, MS, ANP-BC, CNS, CCTC
Professor, San Diego State University
Heart Transplant Nurse Practitioner
Sharp Healthcare
San Diego, California
Cardiac Nurse Practitioner
Sharp Grossmont Hospital
La Mesa, California

Karina Dal Sasso Mendes, RN, PhD
Specialist Nurse
General and Specialized Nursing
    Department
University of São Paulo at Ribeirão Preto
    College of Nursing
Pan American Health Organization/World
    Health Organization
Collaborating Centre for Nursing Research
    Development
São Paulo, Brazil

Luciana Carvalho Moura, RN, MS, MBA(c)
Nurse Program Transplant Coordinator
Organ and Tissue Transplant Study Group,
    GEDOTT, Escola Paulista de Enfermagem,
    EPE/UNIFESP
Hospital Albert Einstein
São Paulo, Brazil

Linda Ohler, RN, MSN, CCTC, FAAN
Quality and Regulatory Manager
Editor Progress in Transplantation
Transplant Quality Consultant
George Washington University Transplant
    Institute
Washington, District of Columbia

Kristi Ortiz, RN, MS, ANP-BC, CNS
Nurse Practitioner
Sharp Memorial Heart Transplant/Mechanical
    Circulatory Support
San Diego, California

Darla K. Phillips, RN, MSN, CCTC
Clinical Operations Director
Duke Transplant Center
Durham, North Carolina

Dianne LaPointe Rudow, ANP-BC, DNP, CCTC
Associate Professor
Department of Health Evidence and Policy
    Director
Zweig Family Center for Living Donation
    Recanati/Miller Transplant Institute
The Mount Sinai Medical Center
New York, New York

Cynthia L. Russell, RN, PhD, FAAN
Professor
School of Nursing and Health Studies
University of Missouri–Kansas City
Kansas City, Missouri

Margaret J. Schaeffer, RN, MS, MSHA, NE-BC
Transplant Administrator
Hume-Lee Transplant Program
Virginia Commonwealth University Health
    System
Richmond, Virginia

Ashley H. Seawright, DNP, ACNP-BC
Lead NP for Transplant, Hepatology, Endocrine
    and Urology
Instructor
Division of Abdominal Transplant and
    Hepatobiliary Surgery
Department of Surgery
University of Mississippi Medical Center
Jackson, Mississippi

Melissa Skillman, MSW, LISW-S
Transplant Social Worker
The Ohio State University Wexner Medical
    Center
Columbus, Ohio

Gail Stendahl, RN, DNP, CPNP-AC/PC, CCTC
Heart Transplant Coordinator
Children's Hospital of Wisconsin
Milwaukee, Wisconsin

Angela Velleca, RN, BSN, CCTC
Clinical Lead Cardiothoracic Transplant
    Coordinator
Comprehensive Transplant Center
Cedars-Sinai Advanced Health Sciences Pavilion
Los Angeles, California

Rebecca P. Winsett, RN, PhD
Nurse Scientist
St. Mary's Medical Center
Evansville, Indiana

Caron Burch, RN, MSN, FNP, CCTC
Heart and Lung Transplant, MCS and
ECMO Programs
University of California San Francisco
Medical Center
San Francisco, California

Marian B. Charlton, RN, SRN, CCTC
Chief Kidney Transplant Coordinator
New York Presbyterian Hospital
Weill Cornell Medical College
Kidney and Pancreas Transplant Program
New York, New York

**Sandra A. Cupples, RN, PhD, FAAN,
CAPT, NC, USN RET**
Formerly, Heart Transplant Coordinator
Washington Hospital Center
Washington, District of Columbia

Wendy Escobedo, RN, MSN, PHN, CCTN
Manager Renal Services
Dialysis and Transplantation
St. Joseph Hospital
Orange, California

Tonya Elliott, RN, MSN
Assist Device and Thoracic Transplant
Coordinator
Inova Transplant Center at Inova Fairfax
Hospital
Falls Church, Virginia

Deborah Ann Hoch, DNP, ACNP-BC, CCRN
Clinical Instructor, Tufts University School of
Medicine
Maine Medical Center Division of Nephrology
and Transplantation
Portland, Maine

Haley Hoy, PhD, ACNP
Associate Dean, Graduate Programs
University of Alabama Huntsville College of
Nursing
Lung Transplant Coordinator/Nurse Practitioner
Vanderbilt Medical Center
Nashville, Tennessee

Eddie Roy Island Jr, MD
Associate Director for Pediatric Transplantation
Georgetown Transplant Institute
Washington, District of Columbia

Annette M. Jackson, PhD, D(ABHI)
Associate Professor of Medicine
Director, Immunogenetics Laboratory
Johns Hopkins University School of Medicine
Baltimore, Maryland

Michelle James, RN, MS, APRN-CNS, CCTN
Clinical Director
Solid Organ Transplant Department
University of Minnesota Health
Minneapolis, Minnesota

Jon Kobashigawa, MD
DSL/Thomas D. Gordon Professor of Medicine,
Cedars-Sinai Heart Institute
Associate Director, Cedars-Sinai Heart Institute
Director, Advanced Heart Disease Section,
Cedars-Sinai Heart Institute
Director, Heart Transplant Program, Cedars-Sinai
Heart Institute
Los Angeles, California

Maricar F. Malinis, MD, FACP
Assistant Professor of Medicine
Section of Infectious Diseases
Yale School of Medicine
New Haven, Connecticut

Megan Maltby, MSW
Clinical Social Worker III
Virginia Commonwealth University Medical
Center
Richmond, Virginia

Paul J. Mather, MD, FACC, FACP
The Lubert Family Professor of Cardiology
Director
Advanced Heart Failure and Cardiac Transplant
Center at the Jefferson Heart Institute
Sidney Kimmel Medical College of Thomas
Jefferson University
Philadelphia, Pennsylvania

Vicki McCalmont, RN, MS, ANP-BC, CNS, CCTC
Professor, San Diego State University
Heart Transplant Nurse Practitioner
Sharp Healthcare
San Diego, California
Cardiac Nurse Practitioner
Sharp Grossmont Hospital
La Mesa, California

Jerome Menendez, DNP, FNP-C
Transplant Manager
Carolinas HealthCare System
Charlotte, North Carolina

Linda Ohler, RN, MSN, CCTC, FAAN
Quality and Regulatory Manager
Editor Progress in Transplantation
Transplant Quality Consultant
George Washington University Transplant
    Institute
Washington, District of Columbia

Jignesh Patel, MD, PhD
Co-Medical Director
Heart Transplant Program
Cedars-Sinai Heart Institute
Associate Clinical Professor
David Geffen School of Medicine at the
    University of California
Los Angeles, California

Michael Petty, RN, PhD, APRN-CNS, CCNS
Cardiothoracic Clinical Nurse Specialist
University of Minnesota Medical Center
Minneapolis, Minnesota

Bohdan Pomahac, MD
Director of Plastic Surgery Transplantation
Director of BWH Burn Center
Division of Plastic Surgery
Brigham and Women's Hospital
Boston, Massachusetts

Nancy Radke, RN, MSN, CCTC
Senior Pancreas Transplant Coordinator
University of Wisconsin Hospital and Clinics
Transplant Program
Madison, Wisconsin

Linda Anne Ridge, RN, BA, CCTC
Senior Liver Transplant Coordinator
Division of Transplant Surgery
University of Maryland Medical Center
Baltimore, Maryland

Eduardo D. Rodriguez, MD, DDS
Chair, Department of Plastic Surgery
Director, Institute of Reconstructive Plastic
    Surgery

Helen L. Kimmel
Professor of Reconstructive Plastic Surgery
New York University
Langone Medical Center
New York, New York

Anne Sanford, RN, BSN, CCTC, CPHQ
Quality Manager
Cedars-Sinai Medical Center
Comprehensive Transplant Center
Los Angeles, California

Kathy Schwab, RN, CCTC
Transplant Integrity and Compliance
    Coordinator
Mayo Clinic
Rochester, Minnesota

Eric M. Tichy, PharmD, BCPS, FCCP, FAST
Manager, Clinical Pharmacy Services
Director, PGY2 Residency Transplantation
Yale-New Haven Hospital
New Haven, Connecticut

Professional licensure indicates that a clinician has met the basic requirements of a generalist within a field of practice. Certification, however, provides validation that a nurse has obtained requisite knowledge and expertise within a specialized area. With both education and practice requirements, certification assures the public that a specialist meets consistent standards of quality established by a professional association.

Certification has become a key measure of professional competencies in nursing. The Institute of Medicine (IOM) has issued several reports on patient safety in its *Quality Chasm* series. In its evaluation of education for health care professionals, the IOM states that professional organizations that grant certification to clinicians are ensuring that those individuals have met the highest professional standards within a given area of specialization.[1]

Recognizing the value and importance of certification for the highly specialized field of transplant nursing, the American Board of Transplant Certification, in collaboration with the International Transplant Nurses Society (ITNS), developed a standardized credentialing examination for transplant nurses: the Certified Clinical Transplant Nurse (CCTN) examination.

The purpose of the *Core Curriculum for Transplant Nurses* is to articulate the knowledge base relative to the art and science of transplant nursing practice—and thus serve as a comprehensive resource for all transplant clinicians and particularly for nurses preparing for the CCTN examination. The text uses the CCTN examination blueprint as a basis for determining relevant content. Information is presented in an embellished outline format so that the text can be used as an easy reference guide.

Information pertinent to the pre- and posttransplant care of each type of abdominal, thoracic, and vascular composite allograft transplant recipient is presented in seven organ-specific chapters. Other chapters address key elements that are common to all types of solid organ transplantation: the evaluation process, immunology, pharmacology, psychosocial aspects of transplantation, patient education, infectious and noninfectious complications, and quality assurance/process improvement. Four chapters focus on professional issues in transplantation, care of living donors, pediatric transplantation, and the care of patients with mechanical circulatory assist devices. More than 200 sample test questions are included to assist readers with evaluating their comprehension of the material presented. Over 200 tables and figures complement the text and provide additional information in a concise, at-a-glance format.

Transplant patients are one of the most complex and challenging of all patient populations. Recognizing the value of certification and committed to enhancing both patient safety and quality care, we and ITNS hope that this text will not only contribute to a nurse's success on the CCTN examination but also serve as a comprehensive resource for transplant nurses around the globe.

We wish to thank ITNS for providing us with this opportunity and to extend our sincere gratitude to our expert contributors and reviewers. Without their willingness to share their knowledge, expertise, time, and talents, this book would not have been possible.

Sandra A. Cupples, RN, PhD, FAAN, CAPT, NC, USN RET
Vicki McCalmont, RN, MS, ANP-BC, CNS, CCTC
Stacee Lerret, RN, PhD, CPNP-AC/PC, CCTC
Linda Ohler, RN, MSN, CCTC, FAAN

---

[1]Institute of Medicine: *Patient Safety: Achieving a New Standard of Care.* Washington, DC: National Academies Press.

Contents

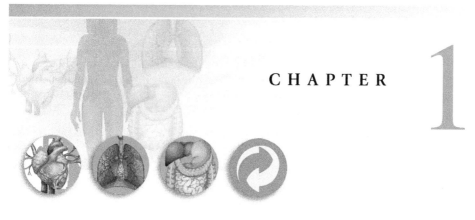

CHAPTER 1

Solid Organ Transplantation: The Evaluation Process

Maureen P. Flattery, RN, MS, ANP-BC, CCTC
Judy Gierlach, RN, BSN, CCTC

 I. GENERAL EVALUATION

A. Introduction
1. Solid organ transplantation (SOT) is a viable treatment option for end-stage disease. Posttransplant care requires adherence with a complex medical regimen for a successful outcome.
2. In addition, the immunosuppressant regimen can exacerbate pre-existing conditions that can adversely affect both quality of life and survival.

B. Purpose of transplant evaluation process
1. Many patients referred for transplantation have one or more chronic illnesses that might affect their candidacy for transplantation.
   a. Therefore, it is paramount that patients be thoroughly evaluated to determine the appropriateness of proceeding with transplantation.
   b. Additionally, the transplant evaluation may reveal problems amenable to interventions other than transplantation.

C. This chapter outlines the evaluation process for SOT and describes
1. General procedures for all organs as well as organ-specific requirements
2. Waiting list criteria for specific organs

D. Coordination of the transplant evaluation and patient education
1. The role of the transplant coordinator includes overseeing the transplant process and providing education to patients and their families/members of their support system.
   a. Often, the coordinator is the first contact that the patient may have with the transplant team.
      i. The transplant coordinator presents an overview of the transplant evaluation process and discusses the role of the interdisciplinary transplant team so that patients and family members will know to whom they should address particular questions as they proceed through the evaluation process.

        ii. Patients and families should be given detailed information about each test and consult so they know what to expect and how to prepare.

   b. Information may be obtained over the phone, prior to the patient's initial appointment, for example:

        i. Past medical history

        ii. Payer or insurance information

        iii. Current medications

   c. During the assessment process, the coordinator consults with the patient and family to provide education concerning the evaluation and transplant process.

   d. This education should include information about

        i. Names and roles of members of the interdisciplinary transplant team

        ii. Organ-specific United Network for Organ Sharing (UNOS) listing criteria

        iii. Transplant center-specific survival statistics as reported by the Scientific Registry for Transplant Recipients[1]

        iv. What the patient should expect during the evaluation process

        v. The timeline for transplant team decision making regarding whether or not the patient meets eligibility criteria for placement on the UNOS waiting list

        vi. Issues concerning the waiting period for transplant

           • Estimated time to await an organ

           • Availability of hospital-based support groups or educational forums

        vii. The organ allocation process

        viii. What to expect after transplantation

           • Hospitalization

           • Medications (particularly immunosuppressants)

           • Postdischarge follow-up and self-care management

           • Financial responsibility including insurance coverage, out-of-pocket costs for medications, clinic visits, and testing co-payment

   e. The stress of the situation may interfere with the ability of patients and members of their support system to understand and/or retain information. Members of the interdisciplinary transplant team should frequently assess the patient's and their support persons' understanding and expect to repeat information throughout the evaluation process. Refer to the chapter on patient education for more detailed information on this topic.

  2. General evaluation process

   a. All patients referred for organ transplantation will undergo a general evaluation process prior to more specific and invasive testing.

   b. This process begins with a thorough history and physical examination of the patient.

   c. Following this, baseline lab work and consultations will be performed as outlined below.

E. Lab work

  1. Patients referred for SOT undergo a battery of lab tests to

   a. Determine if the patient meets physiological eligibility criteria for transplantation.

   b. Identify any comorbid conditions.

  2. General lab work typically includes basic metabolic panel, hepatic panel, lipid profile, complete blood cell count, thyroid panel, rapid plasma reagin (RPR),

urinalysis, and estimated glomerular filtration rate (extrarenal transplant candidates only).
3. In addition, transplant-specific lab work is performed. This includes the following:
   a. **ABO blood typing**. It is a UNOS requirement that prospective recipients have blood typing performed on two separate occasions.[2]
      i. Both results should be recorded in the medical record.
      ii. At the time of listing, a second member of the transplant team will confirm the blood type in the UNOS UNet system.
      iii. Currently, neither Australia nor Canada has a written policy for blood type confirmation.
      iv. Information regarding Eurotransplant is available at www.eurotransplant.org.[3]
   b. **Panel reactive antibody (PRA).**
      i. In order to determine the likelihood of hyperacute rejection following SOT, the serum of a prospective recipient is tested for the presence of circulating antibodies reactive against human leukocyte antigens (HLA).
         - Different techniques can be utilized, but currently, most SOT programs use solid-phase immunoassays, composed of solubilized HLA molecules bound to polystyrene beads and performed on a fluoroanalyzer (Luminex).[4]
         - Other techniques used include enzyme-linked immunosorbent assay (ELISA), complement- dependent cytotoxicity (CDC), and flow cytometry.[5]
         - This result is generally expressed as a percent of panel reactivity (% PRA) between 0% and 99%. This percentage represents the proportion of the population to which the person being tested will react because of preformed antibodies.
      ii. Additionally, transplant programs may choose to determine the calculated PRA (cPRA).
         - This calculation specifically looks at antigens deemed unacceptable and determines risk. A cPRA calculator can be accessed online.[6]
         - Each program determines which antigens are considered unacceptable for a particular transplant candidate based on the degree of risk the program is willing to assume.
         - Before a candidate with a cPRA score >98% receives offers in allocation classifications per UNOS guidelines updated with the new kidney allocation, the transplant program's HLA laboratory director and the candidate's transplant physician or surgeon must review and sign a written approval of the unacceptable antigens listed for that candidate. A member of the transplant team must document this approval in the candidate's medical record.
         - Antigens may be considered unacceptable based on the level of HLA-specific antibody binding, which is expressed as the mean fluorescence intensity (MFI) of the reporter signal.[4]
      iii. A prospective crossmatch may be performed at the time of transplantation based on center- and organ-specific determination of risk of hyperacute rejection.
      iv. Additionally, specific therapies may be attempted to desensitize the recipient prior to transplantation. This, too, is center and organ specific.

c. **HLA typing**. HLA is the term that describes six separate polymorphic genetic loci clustered together in a single area of the human genome and expressed on the lymphocyte that can predict rejection.[4]

i. HLA is assessed preoperatively and is used in the allocation of deceased donor kidneys and pancreata. HLA typing is required by UNOS when listing patients as kidney, kidney/pancreas, and pancreas transplant candidates.[7]

ii. Eurotransplant requirements: "Every potential transplant recipient should be HLA typed on two different occasions using two different samples. Every recipient and every organ donor must be typed for HLA-A, -B, -DR, HLA-C, and –DQ."[8]

iii. In other organs, it is considered useful information to predict rejection and is a necessary step in determining crossmatch positivity but may not be performed until the time of transplant.

iv. The increased use of molecular testing to determine HLA can lead to confusion in the setting of recent blood transfusions.

- The sensitivity of this method can identify antigens from the transfusion and obscure the HLA.
- For that reason, it is best to avoid HLA testing within 72 hours of a blood transfusion.[4]

d. **Virology screening**. Virology screening is performed to determine a patient's suitability for transplantation and posttransplant infection risk. As a result of their immunosuppressive status, organ transplant recipients are at greater risk for developing more severe viral infections than healthy individuals. Assessment includes

i. Human immunodeficiency virus (HIV). The initial test for HIV is done by enzyme immunoassay.

- Equivocal or positive results are confirmed by Western blot.
- Currently, most centers consider the presence of HIV a contraindication to transplantation.
- However, with the advent of highly active antiretroviral therapy to treat HIV and the improved survival of HIV-infected individuals, some centers are performing transplants on patients who are HIV positive.[9]
- There are case reports of HIV-positive patients receiving both heart and lung transplants; however, the practice is currently limited to a few centers.[10,11]

ii. Hepatitis screening. Hepatitis screening is performed both to determine previous exposure to hepatitis and the need for further testing or treatment for those who may have been infected in the past.

- Chronic hepatitis B or C infection is an indication for liver transplantation.
- However, any active hepatitis infection is typically a contraindication to the transplantation of other solid organs.
- Initial hepatitis screening consists of the convalescent battery (Table 1-1).
- To determine candidacy, further testing will be necessary if initial hepatitis B results are positive (Table 1-2).
- Patients may need to be referred to a hepatologist to determine appropriate treatment prior to listing for extrahepatic transplantation.

TABLE 1-1 **Convalescent Hepatitis Battery for Screening**

Test	Positive Results Indicate
Anti-HCV (Hepatitis C antibody)	Exposure to hepatitis C
HBsAg (Hepatitis B surface antigen)	Infection with hepatitis B
HBsAb (Hepatitis B surface antibody)	Immunity to hepatitis B
HBcAb IgG (Hepatitis B core antibody)	Previous hepatitis B infection/exposure

iii. Herpes virus screening.
- The herpes family of viruses are the most common disease-causing viral pathogens in the transplant population.[12]
- Knowledge of a patient's previous exposure and immune status may direct the acceptance of donor organs as well as determine the need for prophylactic therapy.

iv. Cytomegalovirus (CMV) screening. CMV is a member of the Betaherpesvirinae family.
- Approximately 80% of adults are exposed to CMV during the first two decades of life either as an asymptomatic infection or as a benign infectious mononucleosis-like syndrome.[13]
- At the time of infection, cell-mediated immune responses develop but do not completely eradicate the virus.
- CMV establishes latency and may therefore reactivate later in life.
- Historically, up to 85% of SOT recipients who are CMV seronegative and receive an organ from a CMV-seropositive donor develop CMV disease.[14]
- CMV status is established by testing the patient's blood for the presence of CMV antibodies, specifically immunoglobulin G (IgG).
- The CMV status of the recipient and donor will determine the need for, and the length of, prophylactic therapy.[15]

v. Epstein-Barr virus (EBV) screening. EBV is a member of the Gammaherpesvirinae family and is acquired in adolescence or early adulthood.
- EBV is responsible for the infectious mononucleosis syndrome.
- EBV is classified as a group 1 carcinogen and is strongly associated with Burkitt's lymphoma, nasopharyngeal carcinoma, Hodgkin's disease, and immunosuppression-related lymphoproliferative disease.[16]

TABLE 1-2 **Hepatitis B Surface Antigen Positive (HBsAg+): Further Testing**[*]

Hepatitis B e antigen (HBeAg)

Hepatitis B e antibody (HBeAb)

Hepatitis B virus DNA (HBV DNA)

Hepatitis B core antibody IgM (HBcAb IgM) = acute hepatitis B or reactivation of virus

[*]Suggest referral to a hepatologist for further assessment and management of hepatitis.

- Posttransplant lymphoproliferative disease can affect both graft and patient survival.
- EBV status is established by testing the patient's blood for the presence of EBV antibodies, specifically IgG.

   vi. Herpes simplex type 1 (HSV1) screening. HSV is an Alphaherpesvirinae, which is also acquired in childhood or young adulthood.

- Impairment of the immune response as a result of immunosuppression predisposes transplant recipients to reactivation infection.
- HSV status is established by testing the patient's blood for the presence of HSV antibodies, specifically IgG.

e. Toxoplasma screening. *Toxoplasma gondii* is a coccidian parasite of the cat population for which humans are intermediate hosts.[17]

   i. Although a large proportion of the population is infected by *Toxoplasma gondii*, toxoplasmosis is an uncommon disease.

   ii. In immunocompromised individuals, however, toxoplasmosis can be life threatening.

   iii. Toxoplasma-negative patients who receive an organ from a donor with prior exposure are at high risk for developing toxoplasmosis after transplantation.

   iv. Patients with prior exposure to *Toxoplasma gondii* are at risk for developing an active infection after transplant.

   v. Toxoplasma status is established by testing the recipient's blood for the presence of Toxoplasma antibodies, specifically IgG.

f. Tuberculosis (TB) testing. All patients should be tested for TB.

   i. The most commonly performed test is the purified protein derivative (PPD), an intradermal skin test.

   ii. Those patients with a prior TB exposure or those who have been vaccinated with bacille Calmette-Guérin (BCG) may have a positive PPD test. Therefore

- A chest radiograph is indicated.
- A QuantiFERON Gold test may be indicated.
- Consultation by an infectious disease physician is recommended to determine need for treatment in the event of a positive test.

   iii. Patients who are extremely ill may be anergic, meaning they cannot respond appropriately to immune stimuli.

- Therefore, it is best to apply a control test at the same time as the PPD to determine response.
- *Candida* and mumps are two commonly used PPD controls because most people have been exposed to these two organisms.

g. Cancer screening. Transplant recipients are at increased risk of developing cancer because of their immunosuppressive regimen.

   i. Any undetected, pre-existing cancer, in the setting of immunosuppressive medications, may become untreatable and lead to the recipient's death.

   ii. Patients should be screened based on

- Past medical history (e.g., history of colon polyps, family history of cancer)
- History of exposure to carcinogens

- Age- and gender-appropriate screening as outlined by the American Cancer Society.[18] This includes
  - Cervical cancer screening for women older than 21 (younger if sexually active), mammography for women older than 40, and colonoscopy for men and women older than 50
  - Prostate-specific antigen (PSA) blood test and digital rectal examination for men over 50

iii. All candidates should have a chest radiograph performed, although this is a poor method for detecting lung cancer.

h. Osteoporosis screening. All postmenopausal women, as well as all candidates with a smoking history, chronic corticosteroid use, or cholestatic liver disease, should be assessed for osteopenia or osteoporosis by bone densitometry.

   i. SOT recipients are at increased risk of developing bone loss as a result of the immunosuppressive regimen.[19]

   ii. All abnormal findings should be treated appropriately.

F. Psychosocial evaluation

1. This is an integral part of the pretransplant evaluation process.
2. The purpose is to assess a patient's
   a. Appropriateness for transplantation
   b. Ability to give informed consent
   c. Past adherence history
   d. Ability to adhere to the complex postoperative regimen
   e. Social support structure[20]
3. Patients are screened for any current and/or past history of substance abuse. Additional laboratory screening may be required to determine if the patient is currently smoking or using illegal drugs or alcohol.
4. This evaluation is performed by a social worker with input from a psychologist or psychiatrist. Some centers require a psychologist to perform a separate mental health evaluation.
5. See the chapter on Psychosocial Issues in Transplantation for additional information on this topic.

G. Financial evaluation

1. Pre-, peri-, and postoperative transplant care is expensive. Therefore, private or public insurance is a requisite.
2. Private insurance
   a. Third-party payors may have their own transplant eligibility criteria and may refer patients to their designated transplant centers of excellence.
3. Public insurance
   a. In the United States, Medicare (the federally funded program that provides medical insurance for the elderly and disabled) funds transplants only at transplant programs that have been approved by the Centers for Medicare and Medicaid Services (CMS).
   b. Medicaid is a state program; requirements and provisions vary from state to state.
4. Requirements in countries other than the United States will vary depending on each country's payment system.
5. The purpose of the financial evaluation is to determine if the patient has access to sufficient financial resources to facilitate a positive outcome following transplantation.

H. Nutritional evaluation
1. All patients referred for SOT should undergo a nutritional assessment with a registered dietitian.
   a. This is especially important for patients who are either overweight or underweight or who may have impaired digestion.
      i. Obesity is considered a comorbidity and, if severe, may be a contraindication to transplantation.[21-24]
      ii. Cachexia can adversely affect surgical outcome; cachectic patients may require nutritional intervention in the form of supplements or enteral or parenteral nutrition.[21-23]
2. This evaluation also includes educating the patient about risks for posttransplant disorders such as immunosuppressant-induced hyperlipidemia or diabetes mellitus (DM) and the need for a heart healthy diet.
3. The increasing prevalence of nonalcoholic fatty liver disease as an indication for liver transplantation means many patients have features of metabolic syndrome that results in the development of DM.[25]

I. Surgical evaluation

In addition to determining if transplantation is the appropriate procedure for the patient, it must also be determined if the transplant is surgically feasible.
1. Patients may be poor surgical candidates for a variety of reasons such as contraindications identified by pretransplant testing and consultations, as well as anatomic barriers to transplantation, most notably from previous surgeries.
2. The transplanting surgeon must determine if the intended procedure can be done safely.

J. Consultations

In addition to determining if the planned transplant is the appropriate procedure for a patient, tests and consultations are performed to identify perioperative risks that may preclude a successful, long-term outcome. This includes
1. Cardiac evaluation. All patients, regardless of age, should have an electrocardiogram.
   a. More extensive testing should be done based on the patient's medical history and age.[26]
   b. An echocardiogram should be performed on any patient for extracardiac transplantation who complains of shortness of breath or who has a murmur noted on physical examination.
   c. Patients who are currently smoking or those with a history of coronary artery disease, hypertension, diabetes, or smoking will require a cardiac stress test to evaluate myocardial perfusion.
      i. Exercise stress testing is the most accurate; however, many patients with end-stage organ disease are unable to walk on a treadmill.
      ii. In those cases, adenosine, dipyridamole, or dobutamine stress testing is appropriate.
   d. Patients with a positive stress test should be referred to a cardiologist for further evaluation, including cardiac catheterization.
2. Pulmonary evaluation
   a. All patients referred for transplantation should have a chest radiograph and oxygen saturation evaluated by pulse oximetry.
   b. In addition, patients with a smoking history or a history of chronic obstructive lung disease should undergo pulmonary function testing.
   c. Any patient with abnormal findings should be referred to a pulmonologist for further evaluation.

      d. Most organ transplant programs require a period of smoking cessation before listing patients who are currently smoking or who have a recent smoking history. Smoking cessation is confirmed by random urine cotinine testing.

      e. Effects of smoking in specific transplant populations

         i. Heart transplant recipients with a smoking history have an increased risk of developing coronary atherosclerosis, graft dysfunction, and loss after transplantation.[26]

         ii. Cigarette smoking has been implicated in a number of adverse outcomes in liver transplant recipients including cardiovascular mortality and an increased incidence of hepatic artery thrombosis.[27]

         iii. Kidney transplant recipients who smoke are at increased risk for cardiovascular events, renal fibrosis, rejection, and malignancy.[27]

  3. Vascular evaluation

      a. All patients with a history of diabetes, coronary artery disease, claudication, or cerebrovascular accident should undergo Doppler imaging and ankle-brachial index testing.

         i. This should include at least bilateral lower extremity and bilateral carotid artery imaging.

         ii. Abnormal results may indicate the need for angiography and/or referral to a vascular surgeon.

  4. Patients referred for specific types of SOT may require additional consultations with medical specialists based on clinical findings, test results, and comorbid conditions.

II. ORGAN-SPECIFIC EVALUATION

This section pertains to additional tests necessary to evaluate patients referred for specific types of organ transplant procedures. Heart, lung, heart/lung, liver, liver/kidney, kidney, kidney/pancreas, pancreas, and intestinal transplantation will be discussed in detail.

  A. **Heart transplantation**

    1. Cardiac transplantation is indicated for patients with end-stage heart failure and advanced congestive heart failure (New York Heart Association Class III to IV) for whom there are no other medical or surgical options to improve quality of life and survival.

    2. The primary indication for heart transplantation has shifted away from an equal distribution between ischemic and nonischemic cardiomyopathy. Currently, the majority (54%) of patients who receive a heart transplant have a diagnosis of nonischemic cardiomyopathy.[28]

    3. Nonischemic cardiomyopathy includes the diagnoses of

      a. Dilated cardiomyopathy

         i. Idiopathic cardiomyopathy

         ii. Peripartum cardiomyopathy

         iii. Cardiomyopathy associated with valvular disease or congenital heart disease

      b. Restrictive cardiomyopathies, such as certain infiltrative diseases (amyloidosis, sarcoidosis)

      c. Hypertrophic cardiomyopathy

    4. Patients referred for cardiac transplantation will have a thorough evaluation of cardiac function and anatomy to determine if another procedure, such as coronary artery bypass grafting or valve repair/replacement will relieve symptoms and improve quality of life. Patients will also undergo testing to determine the severity of their illness and the urgency for transplantation. These tests include

a. Cardiac catheterization: Patients referred for cardiac transplantation will require both a right and left heart catheterization.
   i. Right heart catheterization is performed to determine right heart function and degree of pulmonary hypertension.
      • Severe, fixed pulmonary hypertension (typically pulmonary vascular resistance >5 Wood units or transpulmonary gradient >20) is a contraindication to heart transplantation; therefore, those patients with pulmonary hypertension may require additional therapy to determine if the hypertension can be reversed.
      • This may include the use of vasodilators, such as oxygen, nitric oxide, nitroglycerin, milrinone (Primacor), nesiritide (Natrecor), or prostaglandin (Flolan) during the catheterization procedure.
      • Oral pulmonary hypertension therapy may be initiated with the intention to re-evaluate the patient's hemodynamic parameters to determine if there has been an improvement.[29]
      • Once a patient is listed for heart transplantation, right heart pressures should be re-evaluated at regular intervals to detect changes in the patient's condition as well as to direct therapy.
   ii. Coronary angiography, or left heart catheterization, is performed to determine if there are any lesions amenable to intervention that would relieve the patient's symptoms and obviate the need for transplantation. Angiography need not be repeated unless changes in the patient's symptoms warrant additional investigation.
b. Cardiopulmonary exercise testing (CPET) with direct measurement of ventilatory gas exchange provides the most reliable determination of functional capacity in patients with congestive heart failure.[30]
   i. The test is performed by exercising the patient on either a treadmill or bicycle ergometer using a standard protocol of increasing workload.
   ii. During exercise, the patient will breathe through a mouthpiece, which allows for the continuous measurement of gas exchange to determine the patient's aerobic capacity.
   iii. CPET is used to assess progression of disease and determine timing for transplantation as well as to provide an exercise prescription for cardiopulmonary rehabilitation.
c. Computerized tomography (CT) scanning of the chest may be performed to identify thoracic anatomic abnormalities, especially in patients who have had previous surgery.
d. Cardiac magnetic resonance imaging (MRI) or positron emission tomography scan: Patients who are being considered for revascularization or ventricular aneurysmectomy may require more extensive testing to determine myocardial viability. Both tests are limited by the patient's suitability for the procedure (presence of MRI contraindications such as a pacemaker, stent, metal implants in the body) and availability of scanners.

5. Waiting list criteria for cardiac transplantation vary from country to country.
   a. These criteria play an instrumental role in organ allocation, regardless of location.
   b. Policies for allocation of donor hearts are reviewed by a committee of transplant specialists on a regular basis to ensure equitable distribution. The goal of these policies is to provide suitable donor hearts to individuals with the greatest need and the greatest chance of survival.

    c. Allocation systems are frequently reviewed and revised in order to ensure that the systems are just and make judicious use of a scarce national resource.

    d. In the United States and Canada, hearts are allocated based on severity of disease as well as medical urgency. Table 1-3 outlines the information required at the time of listing and Table 1-4 outlines medical urgency categories.

6. For additional information, see the chapter on Heart Transplantation

B. **Lung transplantation**

1. Lung transplantation is indicated for patients with end-stage pulmonary disease who are sick enough to need a transplant but well enough to survive a transplant.

2. The most common indications for lung transplantation are non α-1 antitrypsin disease, chronic obstructive pulmonary disease (COPD), interstitial lung disease, bronchiectasis associated with cystic fibrosis, pulmonary hypertension, and COPD associated with α-1 antitrypsin disease.[33]

3. As with heart transplantation, there are patients who may benefit from a procedure other than lung transplantation.

    a. Some patients with emphysema may be suitable candidates for lung volume reduction surgery.[34] The decision to perform this surgery is based on the results of pulmonary function testing, functional capacity as determined by a 6-minute walk test, quantitative ventilation perfusion scan, and oxygen requirements. Unfortunately, few patients qualify for lung volume reduction surgery.

    b. There is no alternative surgical therapy for patients with end-stage lung disease caused by pulmonary fibrosis, cystic fibrosis, pulmonary hypertension, or connective tissue disorders.

4. Patients referred for lung transplantation will undergo additional testing. This includes[35]

    a. CT scan: CT scanning (with contrast) is performed to define the anatomy of the thorax and identify any barriers to surgery. Additionally, it may help define the pulmonary pathology.

TABLE 1-3 UNOS Listing Criteria for Heart Transplant Candidates[31]

Demographic information
- Date of birth
- Ethnicity
- Gender
- State or province of residence

ABO blood typing (confirmed by second person in UNet system)

Height and weight

Diagnosis

Medical urgency

Need for prospective crossmatch

Donor information:
- Height and weight range
- Age range
- Distance willing to travel to procure organ

TABLE 1-4 Medical Urgency for Heart Transplantation[31,32]

United States	Canada	Medical Urgency
7		*Adult and Pediatric*: On hold, not currently accumulating time on the waitlist
2	1	*Adult*: Waiting at home; does not meet any other criteria *Pediatric*: Waiting at home; does not meet status 1A or 1B criteria

	2	*Adult*: Hospitalized patient or patient on outpatient inotropic therapy not meeting other criteria
		    Cyanotic congenital heart defect; resting oxygen saturation 65%–75% or prolonged desaturation
		    Fontan palliation with protein-losing enteropathy or plastic bronchitis
		    Multiple organ candidates (other than heart-lung)
		Pediatric: At home with CPAP/BIPAP
		    Failure to thrive <5th percentile; CCHD with resting saturation 65%–75% or prolonged desaturation
		    Fontan palliation with protein-losing enteropathy or plastic bronchitis; multiple organ transplant candidates
		    Hospitalized not meeting other criteria

2	2	In hospital, stable, and on oral medications
2	1	Waiting at home; doesn't meet any other criteria

1B		*Adult*: VAD or IV inotropes in hospital or at home
		    TAH at home
		Pediatric: Infusion of one or more inotropic agents but does not quality for pediatric status 1A
		    Less than 1 y of age at the time of the candidate's initial registration and has a diagnosis of hypertrophic or restrictive cardiomyopathy

1A		*Adult*: In ICU on high-dose inotropic therapy with hemodynamic monitoring
		    On intra-aortic balloon pump, on mechanical ventilation, or in hospital with TAH or VAD using 30 d "1A status time"
		    VAD malfunction or significant device-related complications such as thromboembolism and device infection
		Pediatric: Continuous mechanical ventilation and admitted to the hospital
		    Assistance of an intra-aortic balloon pump and admitted to the hospital
		    Ductal dependent pulmonary or systemic circulation, with ductal patency maintained by stent or prostaglandin infusion and admitted to the hospital
		    Congenital heart disease requiring infusion of multiple inotropes or a high dose of a single inotrope and admitted to the hospital
		    Assistance of a mechanical circulatory assist device.

	3	*Adult*: VAD not meeting Status 4 criteria
		    Patients on inotropes in hospital, not meeting above criteria
		    Heart/Lung recipient candidates
		    Cyanotic congenital heart disease with resting saturation <65%
		    Congenital heart disease—arterial-shunt-dependent
		    Adult-sized complex congenital heart disease with increasing dysrhythmic or systemic ventricular decline
		Pediatric: VAD not meeting Status 4 criteria including outpatient VAD
		    Less than 6 months of age with congenital heart disease
		    Cyanotic congenital heart disease with resting saturation <65%
		    Congenital heart disease—arterial shunt dependent (i.e., Norwood)
		    Patients on inotropes in hospital, not meeting above criteria
		    Inpatient with CPAP/BIPAP support for HF management
		    Heart/Lung recipient candidates

	3.5	*Adult*: High-dose or multiple inotropes in hospital; non-VAD candidates; acute refractory ventricular arrhythmias *Pediatric*: Hospitalized with VAD; <6 mo of age on prostaglandin for congenital heart disease On high-dose or multiple inotropes and NOT a VAD candidate; acute refractory ventricular arrhythmias

TABLE 1-4 **Medical Urgency for Heart Transplantation**[31,32] **(*Continued*)**

United States	Canada	Medical Urgency
	4	*Adult*: Ventilated with high-dose single or multiple inotropes +/- mechanical support (ECMO); VAD malfunction or complication; life-threatening arrhythmia
		Pediatric: VAD in patient <8 kg; ventilated +/- mechanical support; VAD malfunction or complication
	4S	*Adult*: High PRA (>80%) or PRA > 20% with three prior positive crossmatches, assuming negative virtual or actual donor/recipient-specific crossmatch
		Pediatric: High PRA (>80%) or three prior positive crossmatches, assuming negative virtual or actual donor/recipient-specific crossmatch

CPAP/BIPAP, continuous positive airway pressure /bilevel positive airway pressure; CCHD, cyanotic congenital heart disease; VAD, ventricular assist device; TAH, total artificial heart; ICU, intensive care unit; ECMO, extracorporeal membrane oxygenation; PRA, panel reactive antibody.

    b. Ventilation/perfusion (V/Q) scan: V/Q scanning is performed to determine each lung's function in the event that a single lung transplant is the intended surgery.
       i. The percent of ventilation by each lung is determined as well as the perfusion to each lung.
       ii. A significant mismatch or inequality will help determine which lung to replace.
    c. Six-minute walk test: A 6-minute walk test is performed to determine degree of functional impairment as well as the patient's rehabilitation potential.
       i. The patient is asked to walk for 6 minutes at his or her own pace.
       ii. The patient is allowed to stop as often as needed. The distance is then determined at the end of the 6 minutes.
       iii. Oxygen saturation is monitored and degree of dyspnea is evaluated at intervals during the 6 minutes.
    d. Arterial blood gas: The results of an arterial blood gas may be useful in determining the need for supplemental oxygen, progression of disease, and overall prognosis.
    e. Continuous pH testing: Severe gastric reflux disease can contribute to infectious complications in the transplanted lung. Continuous ambulatory monitoring may be performed to determine the need for either medical or surgical intervention to correct reflux.
  5. In 2005, UNOS implemented the Lung Allocation Score (LAS) as an attempt to allocate donor organs more equitably. Prior to this system, organs were allocated by seniority on the waiting list. The LAS algorithm attempts to assign urgency to patients listed for transplant. Refer to Table 1-5 for the variables required for listing. Each candidate's LAS is updated every 6 months.

C. Simultaneous heart/lung transplantation
  1. Simultaneous heart/lung transplantation is indicated for either patients with concurrent end-stage heart and lung disease or those with severe, fixed pulmonary hypertension.
  2. The procedure is most commonly performed in adult candidates with congenital cardiac anomalies who have developed pulmonary hypertension as a result of long-standing cyanosis or shunting (Eisenmenger syndrome). Additional indications for heart/lung transplantation include idiopathic pulmonary artery hypertension, sarcoidosis with both pulmonary and cardiac manifestations, cystic fibrosis, and acquired heart disease.[33]

TABLE 1-5 Lung Transplantation: Criteria for United Network for Organ Sharing Listing and Lung Allocation Score[36]

Demographics
- Date of birth
- Height and weight
- Gender
- Ethnicity
- State or province of residence

Donor information
- Desired height range
- Desired age range
- Distance willing to travel to procure organ
- Requested organs: right, left, either, and both lungs

Diagnosis
- Diabetes (yes/no, insulin dependent, unknown)
- Assisted ventilation (yes/no, continuous vs. intermittent, BIPAP, or CPAP)
- Requires supplemental oxygen (yes/no and amount)
- Current partial pressure carbon dioxide (PCO_2)
- Highest PCO_2
- Lowest PCO_2
- Percent predicted forced vital capacity

Most recent heart catheterization results (date)
- Pulmonary artery systolic pressure (mm Hg)
- Pulmonary artery pressure mean (mm Hg)
- Pulmonary capillary wedge pressure (mm Hg)

Six-minute walk distance (feet) (date)

Serum creatinine (mg/dL) (date)

3. The number of centers performing simultaneous heart/lung transplantation has significantly decreased in the last decade. This decline has been related to an increase in the use of bilateral lung transplantation for some indications as well as increasing competition for organs. Currently, less than one hundred heart/lung transplants are performed every year worldwide.[33]

4. The evaluation process includes those procedures outlined in the sections above on heart and lung transplantation.

5. Candidates for heart/lung transplantation are listed for both heart and lung transplantation. The listing center must provide the same information as outlined in the sections on heart and lung transplantation.

D. **Liver transplantation**

1. Liver transplantation is indicated for patients with severe, acute, or advanced chronic liver failure unamenable to medical therapy.

   a. Occasionally, liver transplantation is performed as a curative measure for certain metabolic disorders, which do not directly provoke liver failure (e.g., primary hyperoxaluria, familial amyloidosis, polyneuropathy).

   b. The more common etiologies for liver disease and complications of acute and chronic liver failure are listed in Table 1-6.

2. The nature of the disease and the degree of failure will determine the elements included in the evaluation as well as the urgency of the timing for evaluation.[37]

TABLE 1-6 Common Etiologies for and Complications of Acute and Chronic Liver Disease/Failure

Etiologies for Chronic Liver Disease/Failure

Alcoholic cirrhosis

α-1 antitrypsin deficiency

Autoimmune hepatitis

Biliary atresia

Budd-Chiari syndrome

Hemochromatosis

Metabolic disorders

Nonalcoholic steatohepatitis

Primary biliary cirrhosis

Primary sclerosing cholangitis

Viral hepatitis

Wilson's disease

Complications of Chronic Liver Disease/Failure

Ascites

Encephalopathy

Hepatocellular carcinoma

Refractory variceal hemorrhage

Synthetic dysfunction

Chronic gastrointestinal blood loss due to portal hypertensive gastropathy

Etiologies of Acute Liver Failure

Autoimmune hepatitis

Toxin/drug induced

Wilson's disease

Viral hepatitis

3. In addition to the general transplant evaluation, the following tests are typically performed:
   a. Lab work. Additional blood tests are performed to evaluate the etiology of the chronic liver disease (Table 1-7).
      i. In addition, patients at risk for the development of cancer are tested for α-fetoprotein (AFP), a tumor marker for hepatocellular carcinoma (HCC), and carbohydrate antigen (CA) 19-9, a tumor marker for cholangiocarcinoma.
         • Cholangiocarcinoma under special pretransplant treatment guidelines can be an indication for liver transplantation.
      ii. Additional evaluation may be warranted depending upon the etiology of liver failure (e.g., hypercoagulation screening for patients with Budd-Chiari syndrome).
   b. Pathologic assessment. A liver biopsy is not routinely performed; however, in some cases, it may be warranted for
      i. Identification or staging of HCC
      ii. Identification of the underlying liver disorder
   c. Abdominal imaging. An abdominal ultrasound with Doppler imaging is performed to assess the patency of the portal vein and to exclude HCC.

TABLE 1-7 Additional Lab Work for Chronic Liver Diseases

- Viral hepatitis:
  - Hepatitis B surface antigen (HBsAg)
  - Hepatitis B DNA viral load quantitative
  - Hepatitis C virus antibody (anti-HCV)
  - Hepatitis C virus viral load quantitative
  - Hepatitis C virus genotype
- Autoimmune hepatitis: immunoglobulins, antinuclear antibody, and antismooth muscle antibody
- Primary biliary cirrhosis—anti-mitochondrial antibody
- Wilson's disease—ceruloplasmin and 24-h urine for copper
- Hemochromatosis—C282Y and ferritin
- α-1 antitrypsin disease—α-1 antitrypsin level
- Budd-Chiari syndrome—hypercoagulation screen
- Hepatocellular carcinoma—α-fetoprotein
- Cholangiocarcinoma—CA19-9

    i. Focal liver lesions suggestive of HCC may be identified and require further imaging.

- Patients with HCC who have stage T2 lesions and meet UNOS criteria (per UNOS Policy 9.3.G.) will be listed at their calculated MELD.[38] This is often referred to as "an exception" or "exception points." In order for the candidate to maintain an HCC-approved exception, an updated MELD exception application must be submitted every 3 months. At the time of the second extension, the candidate will be assigned a MELD score equivalent to a 35% risk of 3-month mortality (28). For each subsequent extension, the candidate will receive additional MELD points equivalent to a 10% point increase in the candidate's mortality risk every 3 months with the MELD being capped at 34.
- Prior to applying for an exception, the candidate must undergo a thorough assessment that includes all of the following:
  - Evaluation of the number and size of tumors using a dynamic contrast-enhanced abdominal/pelvic CT or MRI.
  - A chest CT or MRI to rule out any extrahepatic spread or macrovascular involvement.
  - An indication that the candidate is not eligible for resection.
  - α-Fetoprotein level.

    ii. For patients with primary or secondary sclerosing cholangitis, endoscopic retrograde cholangiopancreaticography or magnetic resonance cholangiopancreaticography may be warranted for further visualization of the biliary tree.

    iii. If thromboses are identified in vessels, angiography may be necessary to determine the adequacy of these vessels for surgical anastamoses.

d. Gastrointestinal evaluation. Upper endoscopy is routinely done to survey for esophageal varices due to portal hypertension and provide therapeutic intervention if necessary.

    i. This test can prove beneficial for screening for peptic ulcer disease, *Helicobacter pylori,* and Barrett's esophagus.

    ii. Prior to listing, patients with inflammatory bowel disease, hepatocellular cancer, or cholangiocarcinoma require colonoscopy screening with biopsy to rule out dysplasia.

    e. Alcohol screening. Alcohol ingestion can worsen liver function. It is imperative that all candidates for liver transplantation remain abstinent.
       i. Protocols for assessment of abstinence vary from center to center.
      ii. Most centers require a 6-month period of abstinence prior to listing, if possible.
     iii. Alcohol-related cirrhosis and acute alcoholic hepatitis remain an indication for transplantation.[37]
     iv. Some centers require that patients with alcohol-related liver disease participate in a formal rehabilitation program or an Alcoholics Anonymous program. Patients are evaluated for their ability to benefit from this type of therapy, depending on degree of illness.
      v. Centers may also require the patient sign a behavioral contract indicating that they will abstain from alcohol and undergo random toxicology screening to confirm ongoing abstinence.

4. Additional evaluation. Patients with liver failure may also have concurrent dysfunction of other organ systems, most notably the renal and pulmonary systems, as a direct result of chronic liver failure.
    a. Both hepatopulmonary syndrome (HPS) and hepatorenal syndrome (HRS) are reversible with transplantation and are not contraindications to liver transplantation.
    b. HPS
       i. HPS is associated with increased mortality and liver transplant is the only available treatment option.[39]
      ii. The evaluation for HPS includes the following:
         • Standing and supine arterial blood gas analyses are performed on room air and with 100% oxygen.
         • A macroaggregated albumin scan is performed to assess for a shunt.
         • Bubble echocardiography may be performed to assess for the presence of a right-to-left atrial shunt.
         • The following tests are typically required to exclude alternate causes for arterial desaturation[39]:
            ○ A chest radiograph and/or CT scan
            ○ Pulmonary function tests
     iii. Specific MELD exception: Candidates with all of the following will receive a MELD score of 22 and then will receive a MELD score equivalent to a 10% point increase in the risk of 3-month mortality every 3 months that the PaO_2 remains under 60 mm Hg:
         • Evidence of portal hypertension
         • Evidence of a shunt
         • PaO_2 <60 mm Hg on room air
         • No significant clinical evidence of underlying primary pulmonary disease[38]
    c. HRS
       i. A nephrology consult is indicated for assessment of the potential need for dialysis as a bridge to transplantation.

5. Ongoing assessment. Because waiting times can be prolonged for liver transplant candidates, ongoing assessment is required.
    a. All candidates require surveillance for HCC with a minimum of an ultrasound every 3 to 12 months depending upon the underlying diagnosis. Some centers use CT or MRI scan for surveillance.[38]

b. If the candidate is at risk for cholangiocarcinoma, a CA19-9 should also be performed periodically.

c. Based on the transplant candidate's MELD score, a total bilirubin, creatinine, international normalized ratio (INR), and sodium are required at differing intervals in order for the candidate to remain active on the transplant waiting list.

d. Surveillance and therapeutic endoscopies are performed as indicated.

e. Review of other organ systems and updating of tests are done as indicated by the patient's clinical status.

6. Organ allocation. Equitable allocation of organs remains problematic. Systems have been devised in order to allocate the organs justly, with an attempt to give organs to those patients with the greatest need and the greatest chance of survival.

a. Different countries have different systems that are based not only on specific criteria but also on sharing agreements.

b. In the United States, the status system for nonacute liver failure was changed to a scoring system in 2002.

   i. The model for end-stage liver disease/pediatric model for end-stage liver disease (MELD/PELD) score determines how urgently a patient will require liver transplantation within the next 3 months.

      - MELD Score is for candidates 12 years of age or older
      - PELD Score is for candidates <12 years of age

   ii. This calculation is based upon total bilirubin, creatinine, international normalized ratio (INR), sodium (NA), and etiology of disease.

   iii. Scores range from 6 (less ill) to 40 (gravely ill).

   iv. Scores must be updated at regular intervals (Table 1-8).

TABLE 1-8 Model for End-Stage Liver Disease/Pediatric Model for End-Stage Liver Disease

MELD: $0.957 \times \log_e$ (creatinine mg/dL) + $0.378 \times \log_e$ (bilirubin mg/dL) + $1.120 \times \log_e$ (INR) + 0.643

Laboratory values <1.0 will be set to 1.0 when calculating a candidate's MELD score.

The following candidates will receive a creatinine value of 4.0 mg/dL:

- Candidates with a creatinine value >4.0 mg/dL
- Candidates who received two or more dialysis treatments within the prior 7 d
- Candidates who received 24 h of continuous venovenous hemodialysis (CVVHD) within the prior 7 d

The maximum MELD score is 40. The MELD score derived from this calculation will be rounded to the tenth decimal place and then multiplied by 10.

For candidates with an initial MELD score >11, the MELD score is then recalculated as follows:

MELD = MELD(i) + 1.32*(137-Na) − [0.033*MELD(i)*(137-Na)]

Sodium values <125 mmol/L will be set to 125, and values >137 mmol/L will be set at 137.

PELD: [0.436(age <1 y)] − $0.678 \times \log_e$ (albumin g/dL) + $0.480 \times \log_e$ (total bilirubin mg/dL) + $1.87 \times \log_e$ (INR) +0.067 [growth failure (<2 standard deviations present)]

MELD Score	Frequency of Recalculation
>25	Every 7 d
19–24	Every 30 d
11–18	Every 90 d
<10	Yearly

From Organ Procurement and Transplantation Network. *Policy 9. Allocation of Livers and Liver-Intestines.* Available at http://optn.transplant.hrsa.gov/resources/by-organ/liver-intestine. Accessed January 29, 2016.

E. **Simultaneous liver/kidney transplantation**

1. The number of simultaneous liver/kidney (SLK) transplant procedures has increased in the last few years.[40]
2. SLK transplant is indicated for patients with
   a. End-stage renal disease (acute HRS excluded) with cirrhosis
   b. Liver failure with chronic kidney diseases and a GFR <30 mL/min
   c. Acute kidney injury or HRS with a creatinine ≥ 2.0 mg/dL and dialysis for >8 weeks
   d. Chronic kidney disease and liver failure with a renal biopsy demonstrating >30% glomerulosclerosis or fibrosis.[40]

F. **Kidney transplantation**

1. Kidney transplantation is indicated for patients with end-stage renal disease (ESRD).
2. Early referral has been shown to improve transplant outcomes.
3. Discussion of and preparation for transplant assessment ideally begin early in the workup of ESRD, even prior to dialysis.
4. Pre-emptive transplantation may also be offered.
5. In addition to the general transplant evaluation, the following tests are performed[41]:
   a. Laboratory evaluation. Further testing is done to assess other metabolic parameters and organ systems (Table 1-9).
      i. Specific urine tests are performed. Urine volume, protein, microscopy, and culture and sensitivity are assessed to establish a preoperative baseline.
      ii. Any patient with a history of grafts or shunt thrombosis should be screened for hypercoagulability, including testing for
         • Activated protein C resistance
         • Factor V and prothrombin gene mutations
         • Anticardiolipin lupus anticoagulant
         • Protein C and S
         • Antithrombin III
         • Homocysteine levels
   b. Abdominal imaging.
      i. Ultrasound to assess the kidneys

TABLE 1-9 **Additional Lab Tests for Kidney, Kidney/Pancreas, and Pancreas Assessment**

Electrolytes including calcium, magnesium, phosphorus

Fasting blood glucose and hemoglobin A1c (HgbA1c)

Pancreatic profile: amylase and lipase

Lipid profile

International normalized ratio/prothrombin time (INR/PT)

Urinalysis/culture and sensitivity

24-h urine for protein

Creatinine clearance

From Abramowicz D, Cochat P, Claas FH, et al. European renal best practice guideline on kidney donor and recipient evaluation and perioperative care. *Nephrol Dial Transplant.* 2015;30(11):1790–1797.

TABLE 1-10 Urological Assessment

Uroflowmetry and residual urine
Pressure flow urodynamic studies
Video urodynamics
Retrograde pyelogram
Cystoscopy
Ureteroscopy

    ii. CT scanning may be necessary to further delineate anatomic abnormalities.

    iii. In some cases, renal vessel angiography is indicated.

    iv. Patients with a history of bladder dysfunction or urinary tract disease may require a kidney-ureter-bladder (KUB) radiograph as well as a voiding cystourethrogram.

- These patients should be referred to a urologist to determine if existing, uncorrected urinary tract disease may lead to posttransplant morbidity.[42,43]
- Table 1-10 lists other tests, which may be performed to further evaluate urological function.

    v. Men, especially those over age 50, who exhibit symptoms of urinary retention or who have an enlarged prostate by digital rectal examination may require a transrectal biopsy of the prostate to rule out malignancy.

6. Organ Procurement and Transplantation Network (OPTN) Policies
   a. Waiting Time Policy.[44]
      i. Candidates registered at age 18 years or older: Waiting time is based on the earliest of the following:
         - Registration date with a measured or calculated creatinine clearance or glomerular filtration rate (GFR) < or equal to 20 mL/min
         - The date after registration that the candidate's measured or calculated creatinine clearance or GFR becomes < or equal to 20 mL/min
         - The date that the candidate began regularly administered dialysis as an ESRD patient in a hospital-based, independent non–hospital-based, or home setting
      ii. Candidates registered prior to age 18: The candidate's waiting time is based on the earlier of the following:
         - The date that the candidate was registered on the UNOS waiting list regardless of clinical criteria
         - The date that the candidate began regularly administered dialysis as an ESRD patient in a hospital-based, independent non–hospital-based, or home setting.
   b. Estimated Posttransplant Survival (EPTS) Score
      i. Each candidate on the kidney waiting list after turning 18 years old receives an EPTS score. This score represents the percentage of kidney candidates in the nation with a longer expected posttransplant survival time.
      ii. The EPTS score is based on all of the following:
         - Candidate's time on dialysis
         - Whether or not the candidate currently has a diagnosis of diabetes
         - Whether or not the candidate has received any prior SOT
         - The candidate's age

    c. Kidney Donor Profile Index (KDPI)
       i. Kidneys from deceased donors are classified according to the KDPI.
      ii. A donor's KDPI score is derived from the Kidney Donor Risk Index, which takes the following donor characteristics into consideration:

- Age
- Ethnicity
- Creatinine (mg/dL)
- History of hypertension
- History of diabetes
- Cause of death
- Height
- Weight
- Donor type (donation after cardiac death [DCD] donor or non-DCD donor)
- HCV status

    d. Allocation of deceased donor kidneys is a complicated algorithm that takes into consideration blood type, tissue type, degree of sensitization, donor's KDPI score, and the candidate's EPTS score. With the increased use of perfusion devices, kidneys can remain outside of the body for longer periods of time. Therefore, it is possible to allocate kidneys across greater distances than other solid organs.

7. Kidney Paired Donation
    a. Kidney paired donation (KPD) is a potential transplant option for those candidates who have a living donor who is willing and medically suitable to donate a kidney but who is incompatible with the intended recipient.
    b. In the United States, the KPD Pilot Program is part of the OPTN, which registers and tracks all donors and recipients participating in the KPD program.
    c. The following individuals are eligible to join the KPD program:
       i. Recipients who are eligible for a kidney transplant, are under the care of a US transplant center, and have a living donor who is willing and medically able to donate a kidney
      ii. Donors who are willing to participate in the KPD program and undergo extensive medical and psychological evaluations to determine if they are eligible to donate a kidney
     iii. Nondirected ("altruistic" or "Good Samaritan") donors: those individuals who are interested in donating a kidney to a person who they do not know
    d. See the chapter on the Care of Living Donors for additional information.

G. **Pancreas transplantation or simultaneous kidney/pancreas transplantation**

1. Pancreas transplantation is indicated for patients with labile type 1 or type 2 diabetes mellitus, or to halt or prevent secondary complications of DM. If the patient also has ESRD, a simultaneous kidney/pancreas (K/P) transplant is indicated.
2. The evaluation process for pancreas transplantation or simultaneous K/P is similar to the evaluation process for patients undergoing isolated kidney transplantation.
3. Patients referred for K/P and pancreas transplantation have DM, which increases the risk of postoperative morbidity and mortality associated with their
    a. Higher rates of cardiovascular and peripheral vascular disease. It is essential that these patients undergo careful and extensive evaluation, as outlined in the sections on cardiovascular and vascular evaluation.[26]

b. The more aggressive immunosuppressive strategies used in simultaneous K/P exposes the patient to increased risk of bacterial, fungal, and viral infections. Preoperative evaluation by infectious disease or other specialists may be indicated to determine postoperative risk as well as for management of existing problems.[45]

4. Diabetic gastroparesis in itself is not a contraindication to transplantation.
   a. Gastroparesis should be evaluated in order to effectively manage it in the peri- and postoperative phase.
   b. The diagnosis of gastroparesis is often based on symptomatology; however, a gastric-emptying study may be necessary.

5. Patients referred for pancreas transplantation who are not on dialysis require the same renal assessment as patients referred for extrarenal transplantation.

6. Candidates who remain on the waiting list for prolonged periods will require reassessment of their cardiac and vascular status at 1- to 2- year intervals.[26,35]

H. **Intestinal and multivisceral transplantation.**

1. Intestinal transplantation is a recognized therapy for both children and adults with life-threatening complications from intestinal failure.

2. Candidate selection and early referral are important factors for successful outcomes.[46]

3. The assessment process is key to candidate selection and helps to determine if ongoing medical therapies are sufficient or if transplantation is warranted.[46,47]

4. Depending upon the underlying disease process and other coexisting organ failure, three transplant options exist for candidates with intestinal failure:
   a. Isolated intestinal transplant
   b. Liver/small bowel transplant
   c. Multivisceral transplant

5. Two broad classifications of intestinal failure exist: structural and functional failure (Table 1-11).
   a. Structural problems are the result of massive surgical resection or anatomical loss.
   b. Functional problems, which can affect both children and adults, are characterized by disease processes that impair gut motility or absorption.[47,48]

TABLE 1-11 Structural and Functional Causes of Intestinal Failure

Structural	Functional
Adult	*Adult*
• Crohn's disease	• Radiation damage
• Ischemia	• Pseudo-obstruction
• Familial adenomatous polyposis	
• Trauma	
Pediatric	*Pediatric*
• Necrotizing enterocolitis	• Hirschsprung disease
• Gastroschisis	• Microvillus inclusion disease
• Malformation/volvulus	• Pseudo-obstruction
• Atresia and stenosis	
• Trauma	

TABLE 1-12 **Lab Tests for Intestinal/Multivisceral Assessment**

Electrolytes including calcium, magnesium, and phosphorus

Blood urea nitrogen and creatinine

Complete blood cell count

International normalized ratio/partial thromboplastin time (INR/PTT)

Liver function: bilirubin total and direct, albumin, INR

Liver enzymes: aspartate transaminase, alanine transaminase, and alkaline phosphatase

Viral serology

Urinalysis and microscopy

Blood cultures (if sepsis is a concern)

6. Intestinal transplantation is typically warranted in the setting of organ failure in conjunction with one or more life-threatening complications or failure of parenteral nutritional therapy. These complications include
   a. Loss of vascular access preventing fluid and nutritional maintenance
   b. Frequent episodes of severe sepsis or dehydration
   c. Presence of or impending liver failure[47]
7. In addition to the general transplant evaluation, the following tests and consults are obtained:
   a. Lab work to obtain baseline parameters of nutritional state and renal and hepatic function (Table 1-12).
   b. Abdominal imaging of the intestinal tract to detect structural or functional abnormalities.
      i. If motility issues are a concern, gastric-emptying studies and other motility testing may be warranted.
      ii. Visualization of the gastrointestinal tract with upper endoscopy and/or colonoscopy may be required.
      iii. Refer to Table 1-13 for a list of potential additional tests.
   c. Liver evaluation. If the patient has liver dysfunction, a thorough evaluation of liver function is required to ascertain the need for simultaneous liver transplantation.
      i. An examination of the patient may reveal hepatomegaly, splenomegaly, or stigmata of chronic liver disease, which may be suggestive of hepatic dysfunction.

TABLE 1-13 **Imaging and Diagnostic Evaluation for Intestinal/Multivisceral Transplant**

- Upper gastrointestinal series
- Small bowel follow-through
- Barium enema
- Upper endoscopy
- Colonoscopy
- Gastric-emptying study
- Esophageal motility and pH studies
- Abdominal computerized tomography
- Abdominal ultrasound and portal vein Doppler study
- Doppler ultrasound of vessels

TABLE 1-14 Nutritional Assessment

Thorough History
- Nutrition history
- Height and weight including recent weight loss or gain
- Oral or enteral intake and formula
- TPN and formula
- Elimination patterns/stormy output
- Diet and eating history
- Medication history
- Eating behaviors/aversions

Diagnostics
- Calorie counts
- Fecal fat measurement
- Bone density measurement
- Serial anthropometries

  ii. An abdominal ultrasound and portal vein Doppler study may assist in further diagnosis.

  iii. A liver biopsy may be necessary to determine the degree of fibrosis or presence of cirrhosis.

 d. Consultation with a dietician for nutritional assessment and ongoing management (Table 1-14).

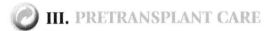

III. PRETRANSPLANT CARE

A. Vaccinations

 1. Adult candidates

  a. Should be vaccinated for hepatitis A and hepatitis B, *S. pneumoniae*, tetanus, varicella, and herpes zoster.

  b. Annual influenza vaccines are recommended for most transplant candidates during the waiting period.[49]

  c. The meningitis vaccine should also be considered for candidates enrolled in colleges or universities.[50,51]

 2. Children awaiting organ transplantation should receive age-appropriate vaccinations.

 3. Family members, close contacts, and health care workers should be vaccinated against influenza annually.[47,50,51]

B. Periodic re-evaluation during the waiting period

 1. Candidates are closely followed by their respective transplant centers with physical examinations, tests, and consults. The specific types of tests are determined by organ-specific waitlist management requirements and the patient's diagnosis, severity of illness, clinical status, and comorbidities.

 2. The frequency of re-evaluation is determined by the severity of the patient's illness as well as comorbidities such as obesity, diabetes, and pulmonary disease.

 3. In addition, transplant candidates undergo routine, age-appropriate health screening, such as annual prostate specific antigen for men over the age of 50 and mammograms and gynecologic examinations for women.

4. **Heart transplant candidates**
   a. Heart transplant candidates with left ventricular assist devices are followed according to the transplant center's protocol.
   b. The following tests are repeated as necessary by most transplant centers to re-evaluate the candidate's health status and determine the need for any changes in therapy or listing status:[28]
      i. Right heart catheterization to evaluate pulmonary pressures
      ii. Echocardiogram or MUGA to evaluate ejection fraction and ventricular contractility
      iii. Cardiopulmonary exercise test with
         • Peak oxygen consumption (MVO_2)
         • Minute ventilation/carbon dioxide production relationship (VE/VCO_2 slope)
      iv. End-organ function is monitored by serial tests including serum creatinine and hepatic parameters including aspartate aminotransferase, alanine transaminase, bilirubin, and albumin. A decline in renal or hepatic function may indicate the need to consider additional therapy (inotropic therapy or ventricular assist device) or a change in the patient's status on the transplant list.
      v. PRA for sensitized patients or those who may require a prospective crossmatch at the time of transplant.
      vi. See chapter on Heart Transplantation for additional information.
5. **Lung transplant candidates**
   a. Candidates for lung transplantation are usually required to participate in a pulmonary rehabilitation program several times a week. Each center may have different requirements for follow-up based on diagnosis, severity of illness, and comorbidities.[34]
   b. The Lung Allocation Score (LAS) requires updated information every 6 months in order to determine appropriate organ allocation. This includes
      i. Forced vital capacity
      ii. Six-minute walk distance
      iii. Serum creatinine
      iv. Changes to any other required variables (see Table 1-5)
6. **Liver transplant candidates**
   a. Periodic re-evaluation tests are program specific and may include the following:
      i. Patients with known HCC: every 3 months.
         • Imaging studies
         • AFP
         • This testing is required by UNOS for patients with HCC to continue to receive MELD exception points.
      ii. Cirrhotic patients should have abdominal imaging every 6 months with ultrasound, CT scan, or MRI.
      iii. Annual cardiovascular testing (typically, a dobutamine stress echocardiogram).
      iv. AFP to evaluate for hepatocellular carcinoma (every 3 months).
      v. Complete blood cell count, CMP, PT, INR, and NA based on MELD score (every 3 months as part of waitlist management).
7. **Kidney and kidney/pancreas transplant candidates**
   a. Follow-up lab tests are obtained on a regular basis from the patient's dialysis center.

      b. High-risk kidney transplant candidates, defined as those with comorbid conditions such as diabetes, coronary heart disease, obesity, or advanced age, require closer follow-up.[52]

      c. Tests used by the majority of kidney transplant centers in managing candidate risk factors include[52]

         i. Assessment of cardiac risk by one or more of the following:

            • Dobutamine echocardiogram

            • Coronary angiography

            • Exercise thallium test

            • Nuclear perfusion scan

         ii. Monthly (or more frequent) PRAs for candidates who are sensitized

8. Intestinal and multivisceral transplant candidates

      a. Patients require ongoing assessment for complications of intestinal failure and malnutrition.

      b. Periodic re-evaluation typically includes

         i. Abdominal imaging for the development of HCC

         ii. Endoscopy for changes in or the development of varices

         iii. Lab tests for changes in end-organ function.

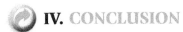

IV. CONCLUSION

A. The success of SOT is based on the appropriate referral and thorough evaluation of potential transplant candidates.

B. This chapter outlines the typical evaluation process for each type of SOT. However, this information is general. Individual transplant programs may have additional evaluation policies or procedures.

REFERENCES

1. Scientific Registry of Transplant Recipients. Available at www.srtr.org. Accessed September 26, 2014.
2. United Network for Organ Sharing. Organ Blood Typing Policy. Available at www.unos.org/policies. Accessed September 12, 2014.
3. Eurotransplant. Blood Typing Policy. Available at http://www.eurotransplant.org. Accessed September 12, 2014.
4. Tait BD, Susal C, Gebel HM, et al. Consensus guidelines on the testing and clinical management issues associated with HLA and non-HLA antibodies in transplantation. *Transplantation.* 2013;95:19–47.
5. Fuggle SV, Martin S. Tools for human leukocyte antigen antibody detection and their application to transplanting sensitized patients. *Transplantation.* 2008;86:384–390.
6. OPTN: Organ Procurement and Transplantation Network cPRA Calculator. Available at http://optn.transplant.hrsa.gov/resources. Accessed September 12, 2014.
7. OPTN: Waitlist Registration. Available at http://optn.transplant.hrsa.gov/ContentDocuments/OPTN_Policies.pdf. Accessed June 5, 2015.
8. Eurotransplant Manual, Version 3.0, March 17, 2015. Available at www.eurotransplant.org/cms/mediaobject.php?file=chapter10_histocompatibility6.pdf. Accessed June 21, 2015.
9. Roland ME, Stock PG. Review of SOT in HIV infected patients. *Transplantation.* 2003;75:425–429.
10. Uriel N, Nahumi N, Colombo PC, et al. Advanced heart failure in patients infected with human immunodeficiency virus: is there equal access to care? *J Heart Lung Transplant.* 2014;33:924–930.
11. Kern RM, Seethamraju H, Blanc PD, et al. The feasibility of lung transplantation in HIV-seropositive patients. *Ann Am Thorac Soc.* 2014;11:882–889.
12. Carratala J, Montejo M, Perez-Romero P. Infections caused by herpes viruses other than cytomegalovirus in solid organ transplant recipients. *Enferm Infecc Microbio Clin.* 2012;30(suppl 2):63–69.
13. Razonable RR, Humar A. Cytomegalovirus in solid organ transplantation. *Am J Transplant.* 2013;13(suppl 4):93–106.

14. Preiksaitis JK, Sandu J, Strautman M. The risk of transfusion acquired CMV infection in seronegative solid-organ transplant recipients receiving non-WBC-reduced blood components not screened for CMV antibody (1984 to 1996): experience at a single Canadian center. *Transfusion.* 2002;42:396–402.

15. Roman A, Manito N, Campistol JM, et al. The impact of the prevention strategies on the indirect effects of CMV infection in solid organ transplant recipients. *Transplant Rev.* 2014;28:84–91.

16. Crawford DH. Biology and disease associations of Epstein-Barr virus. *Philos Trans R Soc Lond B Biol Sci.* 2001;356:461–473.

17. Lumbrebas C, Aguado JM. Toxoplasmosis after solid organ transplantation. In: RA Bowden, P Ljungman, CV Paya, eds. *Transplant Infections.* 2nd ed. Philadelphia, PA: Lippincott Williams & Wilkins; 2003:541.

18. American Cancer Society. Cancer Detection Guidelines. Available at http://www.cancer.org/docroot/PED/content/PED_2_3X_ACS_Cancer_Detection_Guidelines_36.asp/. Accessed September 15, 2014.

19. Yu TM, Lin CL, Chang SN, et al. Osteoporosis and fractures after solid organ transplantation: a nationwide population-based cohort study. *Mayo Clin Proc.* 2014;89:888–895.

20. Maldonado JR, Dubois HC, David EE, et al. The Stanford Integrated Psychosocial Assessment for Transplantation (SIPAT): a new tool for the psychosocial evaluation of pre-transplant candidates. *Psychosomatics.* 2012; 53:123–132.

21. Chamogeorgakis T, Mason DP, Murthy SC, et al. Impact of nutritional state on lung transplant outcomes. *J Heart Lung Transplant.* 2013;32:693–700.

22. Amarelli C, Buonocore M, Romano G, et al. Nutritional issues in heart transplant candidates and recipients. *Front Biosci (Elite Ed).* 2012;4:662–668.

23. Hade AM, Shine AM, Kennedy NP, et al. Both under-nutrition and obesity increase morbidity following liver transplantation. *Ir Med J.* 2003;96:140–142.

24. Singh D, Lawen J, Alkhudair W. Does pretransplant obesity affect the outcome in kidney transplant recipients? *Transplant Proc.* 2005;37:717–720.

25. Kuo HT, Sampaio MS, Ye X, et al. Risk factors for new-onset diabetes mellitus in adult liver transplant recipients, an analysis of the Organ Procurement and Transplant Network/United Network for Organ Sharing database. *Transplantation.* 2010;89:1134–1140.

26. Lentine KL, Costa SP, Weir MR, et al. Cardiac disease evaluation and management among kidney and liver transplantation candidates: a scientific statement from the American Heart Association and the American College of Cardiology Foundation: endorsed by the American Society of Transplant Surgeons, American Society of Transplantation, and National Kidney Foundation. *Circulation.* 2012;126:617–663.

27. Corbett C, Armstrong MJ, Neuberger J. Tobacco smoking and solid organ transplantation. *Transplantation.* 2012;94:979–987.

28. Lund LH, Edwards LB, Kucheryavaya AY, et al. The Registry of the International Society for Heart and Lung Transplantation: thirtieth official adult heart transplant report—2013; focus theme: age. *J Heart Lung Transplant.* 2013;32:951–964.

29. Mehra MR, Kobashigawa J, Starling R, et al. Listing criteria for heart transplantation: International Society for Heart and Lung Transplantation guidelines for the care of cardiac transplant candidates-2006. *J Heart Lung Transplant.* 2006;25:1024–1042.

30. Kato TS, Collado E, Khawaja T, et al. Value of peak exercise oxygen consumption combined with B-type natriuretic peptide levels for optimal timing of cardiac transplantation. *Circ Heart Fail.* 2013;6:6–14.

31. UNOS Heart Allocation. Available at http://optn.transplant.hrsa.gov/ContentDocuments/OPTN_Policies.pdf. Accessed May 8, 2015.

32. Canadian Heart Allocation. Available at http://www.lhsc.on.ca/Patients_Families_Visitors/MOTP/Organ_and_Tissue_Donation/algorithmheartallocation.pdf. Accessed May 8, 2015.

33. Yusen RD, Christie JD, Edwards LB, et al. The Registry of the International Society for Heart and Lung Transplantation: thirtieth adult lung and heart-lung transplant report—2013; focus theme: age. *J Heart Lung Transplant.* 2013;32:965–978.

34. Kaplan RM, Sun Q, Naunheim KS, et al. Long-term follow-up of high-risk patients in the National Emphysema Treatment Trial. *Ann Thorac Surg.* 2014;98(5):1782–1789. doi: 10.1016/j.athoracsur.2014.06.031.

35. Orens JB, Estenne M, Arcasoy S, et al. International guidelines for the selection of lung transplant candidates: 2006 update—a consensus report from the Pulmonary Scientific Council of the International Society for Heart and Lung Transplantation. *J Heart Lung Transplant.* 2006;25:745–755.

36. Lung Allocation Score (Policy 10). Available at http://optn.transplant.hrsa.gov/ContentDocuments/OPTN_Policies.pdf. Accessed October 4, 2014.

37. Martin P, DiMartini A, Feng S, et al. Evaluation for liver transplantation in adults: 2013 practice guideline by the American Association for the Study of Liver Disease and the American Society of transplantation. *Hepatology.* 2014;59:1144–1165.

38. Organ Procurement and Transplantation Network. *Policy 9: Allocation of Livers and Liver-Intestines.* Available at http://optn.transplant.hrsa.gov/resources/by-organ/liver-intestine. Accessed January 29, 2016.

39. Koch DG, Fallon MB. Hepatopulmonary syndrome. *Clin Liver Dis.* 2014;18:407–420.

40. Nadim MK, Sung RS, Davis CL, et al. Simultaneous liver-kidney transplantation summit: current state and future directions. *Am J Transplant.* 2012;12:2901–2908.

41. Bunnapradist S, Danovitch GM. Evaluation of adult kidney transplant candidates. *Am J Kidney Dis.* 2007;50:890–898.

42. Abramowicz D, Cochat P, Claas FH, et al. European renal best practice guideline on kidney donor and recipient evaluation and perioperative care. *Nephrol Dial Transplant.* 2015;30(11):1790–1797.

43. Power RE, Hickey DP, Little DM. Urological evaluation prior to renal transplantation. *Transplant Proc.* 2004;36:2962–2967.

44. Organ Procurement and Transplantation Network. Policy 8: Allocation of Kidneys. Available at http://optn.transplant.hrsa.gov/resources/by-organ/kidney-pancreas. Accessed May 25, 2015.

45. UpToDate. Benefits and Complications Associated with Kidney-pancreas Transplantation in Diabetes Mellitus. Available at http://www.uptodate.com/contents/benefits-and-complications-associated-with-kidney-pancreas-transplantation-in-diabetes-mellitus. Accessed July 5, 2015.

46. UpToDate. Overview of Intestinal and Multivisceral Transplantation. Available at http://www.uptodate.com/contents/overview-of-intestinal-and-multivisceral-transplantation. Accessed October 1, 2014.

47. Robinson J. Intestinal transplantation: the evaluation process. *Prog Transplant.* 2005;15:43–53.

48. Palocaren MS. An overview of intestine and multivisceral transplantation. *Crit Care Nurs Clin North Am.* 2011;23:457–469.

49. UpToDate. Immunizations in Solid Organ Transplant Candidates and Recipients. Available at http://www.uptodate.com/contents/immunizations-in-solid-organ-transplant-candidates-and-recipients. Accessed June 5, 2015.

50. Danzinger-Isakov L, Kumar D; AST Infectious Diseases Community of Practice. Guidelines for vaccination of solid organ transplant candidates and recipients. *Am J Transplant.* 2009;9(suppl 4):S258–S262.

51. CDC Immunization Schedule. Available at http://www.cdc.gov/vaccines/schedules/easy-to-read/adult.html. Accessed September 16, 2014.

52. Bunnapradist S, Danovitch GM. Evaluation of adult kidney transplant candidates. *Am J Kidney Dis.* 2007;50:890–898.

SELF-ASSESSMENT QUESTIONS

1. The purpose for evaluating patients for solid organ transplantation includes which of the following?
   a. To determine if there are other options for managing the current disease
   b. To determine if there are comorbidities that would contraindicate transplantation
   c. To evaluate the patient's ability to comply with long-term posttransplant follow-up requirements
   d. a and b only
   e. All of the above

2. Most patients will have an intradermal skin test for tuberculosis. However, some patients may be anergic due to the severity of their illness. In such cases, the patient will have controls placed. The two most commonly used skin test controls are:
   a. Bacillus Calmette-Guérin (BCG) and human T-lymphotrophic virus-1 (HTLV-1).
   b. Candida and mumps.
   c. Measles and influenza.
   d. Mumps and BCG.

3. HIV testing is done by enzyme immunoassay at many centers. Equivocal or positive results are confirmed by which of the following methods?
   a. Enzyme-linked immunosorbent assay (ELISA)
   b. Complement-dependent cytotoxic assay
   c. Flow cytometry
   d. Western blot

4. There are no surgical alternatives other than lung transplantation for which of the following diseases?
   a. Pulmonary hypertension
   b. Cystic fibrosis
   c. Pulmonary fibrosis
   d. Emphysema
   e. a, b, and c only
   f. All of the above

5. A ventilation/perfusion (V/Q) scan is ordered for patients being considered for lung transplantation to determine
   a. The lung with the best ventilation and perfusion.
   b. A mismatch between ventilation and perfusion.
   c. Which lung to replace.
   d. The difference in lung function between right and left lungs.
   e. b and c only
   f. All of the above

6. Simultaneous liver/kidney transplantation is indicated if the patient has the following:
   a. End-stage renal disease (acute HRS excluded) with cirrhosis
   b. Liver failure with chronic kidney disease and GFR <30 mL/min and acute kidney injury or HRS with creatinine ≥ 2.0 mg/dL
   c. Dialysis for >8 weeks or liver failure with CKD and renal biopsy demonstrating >30% glomerulosclerosis or >30% fibrosis
   d. a and b only
   e. All of the above

7. Patients referred for transplantation are evaluated by a social worker and/or psychologist in order to:
   a. Assess the patient's ability to give informed consent.
   b. Assess the patient's social support network.
   c. Determine if the patient likes the transplant team.
   d. Determine if the patient has the money to pay for a transplant.
   e. a and b only

8. The Lung Allocation Score requires updates every 6 months on which of the following tests?
   a. Forced vital capacity (FVC)
   b. Serum creatinine
   c. 6-minute walk
   d. a and c only
   e. All of the above

9. High-risk kidney transplant candidates include which of the following?
   a. Those of advanced age
   b. Obese individuals
   c. Patients with diabetes as a comorbidity
   d. Patients with coronary disease
   e. b and c only
   f. All of the above

10. Tests most commonly used to evaluate potential heart candidates include which of the following?
    a. MUGA or ECHO to determine ejection fraction
    b. MVO_2 to determine functional capacity
    c. Left heart catheterization to determine pulmonary pressures
    d. Right heart catheterization to determine pulmonary pressures
    e. a, b, and c
    f. a, b, and d

CHAPTER 2

Basics in Transplant Immunology

Linda Ohler, RN, MSN, CCTC, FAAN

Robert A. Bray, PhD

 I. INTRODUCTION TO THE HUMAN IMMUNE SYSTEM

A. **Functions of the immune system**

1. The human body is challenged daily by millions of exogenous and endogenous threats that could cause us physiological harm unless our bodies are able to defend themselves.

   a. The key characteristic of the immune system is that it defends us by its ability to distinguish self from nonself.

   b. To fight off these daily threats, humans possess a complex system of defense called the immune system (Figure 2-1).

      i. The immune system consists of highly mobile and complex cellular and soluble antibodies and chemokines/cytokines that are located throughout the body.

      ii. This complex system is comprised of cells and proteins spread throughout the body providing rapid defense against infection.

         • These cells are categorized as "lymphocytes" and include neutrophils, monocytes, T cells, B cells, and natural killer (NK). These are all found in the white blood cells (WBC).

         • Major proteins include antibodies, chemokines, cytokines, and complement proteins.

         • Cells located throughout the body detect foreign or nonself molecules (antigens), and when identified, immune cells are recruited to provide protection against invaders via complex immune reactions.

      iii. Throughout life, the immune system will adapt and respond to a variety of complex immune reactions or life experiences: illness, infection, pregnancy, drug exposure, or transfusions (Figure 2-2).

         • The immune system creates antibodies in response to these events that cause a reaction if/when the event recurs.

         • Over time, the lymphocytes of immune system learn to adapt and recognize self (our own tissue) versus foreign invaders (nonself).

Immune System

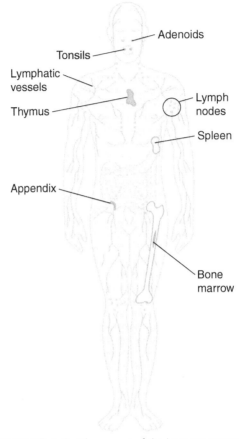

FIGURE 2-1   The organs of the immune system.

- T cells are either cytotoxic or helper cells. The T-cytotoxic cells quickly kill any signs of foreign invaders or infection, and the T-helper cells work with the B cells perform their functions.
- B cells produce immunoglobulins or antibodies that turn into memory cells. These memory cells identify past infections and activate a rapid response if the infection returns. They are highly specialized cells that are able to detect self versus nonself and selectively activate only when the nonself threat is detected.
- For example, vaccines are given to stimulate the T-helper cells and B cells to produce antibodies against a virus. If the body detected the virus, the immune system quickly responds to kill the virus before it can mount a significant illness.
- In transplant, the new grafted organ is detected as a foreign invader (nonself), and immediately the body attempts to stimulate a response to kill it. Immunosuppressive medications are given to adapt the lymphocytes of the immune system and tolerate the new graft.

c. In transplant, another component of this self-recognition process is accomplished at the molecular level through a group of proteins called human leukocyte antigens (HLAs) or tissue molecules.

TYPE III IMMUNE REACTION (IMMUNE COMPLEX HYPERSENSITIVITY)

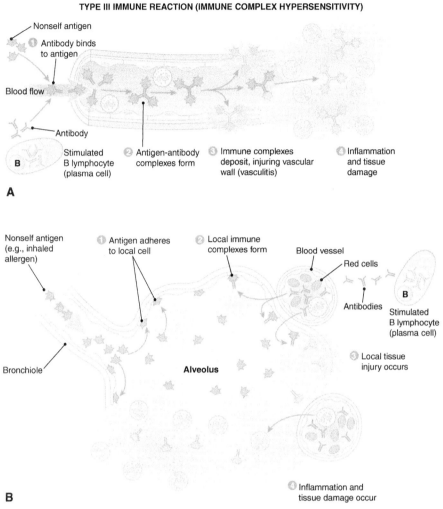

FIGURE 2-2 Type III immune reaction: immune complex hypersensitivity. Antigen and antibody bind together to create an immune complex. **A.** Systemic immune complex reaction. In systemic autoimmune reactions, immune complexes cause vasculitis and widespread tissue damage. **B.** Local immune complex reaction. In local autoimmune reactions, immune complexes form and cause damage to transplanted organ (e.g., antigen-antibody reaction with rejection).

2. The immune system provides protection by several different mechanisms designed to recognize and destroy invaders while maintaining a balance to avoid unnecessary destruction of self.[1-6]
   a. *Surveillance*: Direct recognition of foreign antigens present on membranes of cells or microorganisms and indirect recognition of antigens presented by HLA molecules.
   b. *Defense*: There are nonspecific and specific mechanisms that destroy foreign intruders and protective memory that targets particular foreign intruders to which there has been previous exposure.
   c. *Homeostasis*: The capacity of maintaining a balance between the protection of self and destruction of nonself.

3. In transplantation, we focus on two components of an immune response associated with rejection of a transplanted organ: humoral and cellular immune responses.
   a. The humoral immune reaction involves the production of soluble proteins (immunoglobulins), also referred to as antibodies, that bind and damage the transplanted organ. Antibodies are secreted by specialized B cells called plasma cells.
   b. The cellular immune reaction involves interactions or communication signals between cells such as lymphocytes and antigen-presenting cells (APCs).
      i. APCs are cells such as dendritic cells, monocytes, and macrophages.
      ii. APCs alert cytotoxic T lymphocytes of nonself antigens such as the following:
         - Donor kidney, liver, heart, lung, intestines, or vascularized composite tissue allotransplant (VCA).
         - These cytotoxic T cells evoke cellular reactions such as rejection.
      iii. Thus, when we transplant a new organ into a patient, the immune response is alerted to react against what it has determined to be nonself.
      iv. To protect the new organ from being rejected, we immediately begin to suppress the immune system with immunosuppressive medications (see Figure 2-3). See chapter on Transplant Pharmacology for additional information.
      v. Many transplant programs start the process of suppressing the immune system with induction therapy.[7]
      vi. Induction therapy is the administration of an immunosuppressive agent, such as antithymocyte globulin, prior to implantation of the new organ. Induction therapy often continues for several doses during the immediate posttransplant period.
      vii. The goals of induction therapy are to delete or suppress lymphocytes and decrease the impact of an immune response that would immediately recognize the new organ as nonself.
      viii. There are many factors that can influence our ability to suppress the immune system enough to prevent recognition of the new organ.
         - First, the physician will select a graft that is ABO compatible without any unacceptable preformed antibodies to the recipient to prevent a hyperacute rejection immune response.
         - Next, the physician will select an immunosuppression regimen that will suppress the intensity of the immune response and minimize any toxic adverse effects to the recipient. Refer to the pharmacology chapter for immunosuppression strategies.
      ix. The communication system among cells is quite complex.
         - When cells are destroyed, cellular communication sends an alert to the bone marrow to increase production of those cells being destroyed by medication therapies.
      x. Our principle challenge is to manage the transplant recipient in balancing the suppression of the immune system enough to prevent rejection, but not too much to increase the patient's risk of developing an infection or malignancy.
         - Morbidity and mortality risks due to infection are greater than the risk of graft loss due to rejection.
         - Thus, we need to learn how to balance the immune system between infection and rejection.

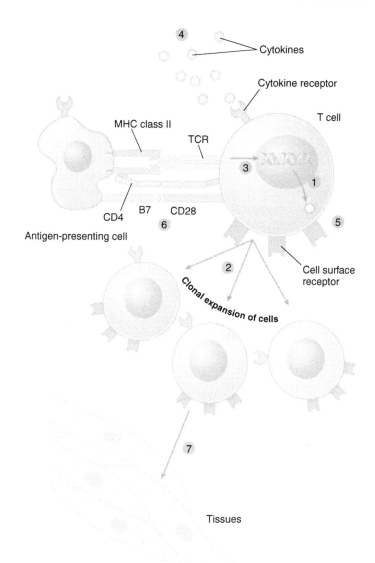

FIGURE 2-3 Overview of mechanisms of pharmacologic immunosuppression. The molecular mechanisms by which immune cells are activated and function provide eight major points for pharmacologic intervention by immunosuppressive agents. Blockade of T-cell activation can be accomplished by (*1*) inhibition of gene expression, (*2*) selective attack on clonally expanding lymphocyte populations, (*3*) inhibition of intracellular signaling, (*4*) neutralization of cytokines and cytokine receptors required for T-cell stimulation, (*5*) selective depletion of T cells (or other immune cells), (*6*) inhibition of costimulation by antigen-presenting cells, and (*7*) inhibition of lymphocyte-target cell interactions. Suppression of innate immune cells and complement activation may also block the initiation of immune responses (not shown).

xi.   This chapter is designed to provide readers with a basic understanding of how the immune system functions and how we attempt to manipulate it in transplantation.

B.   **Types of transplants**

1. Autotransplantation is transplantation of self-tissue.
   a. An example would be the removal of bone marrow from an individual prior to potentially toxic chemotherapy, followed by reinfusion of the marrow back into the same individual following the medical intervention.

b. Another common example is for an individual to donate blood for himself/herself prior to an elective surgery.
   i. This blood is then autotransfused into the same patient if needed during the procedure.
   ii. These transplanted tissues are not foreign; therefore, there is no risk for an immune response or antibody production.

2. Iso- or syngeneic transplantation refers to the transplantation of tissue or organs between genetically identical individuals, such as identical twins. Because all tissues and their proteins are genetically identical, this type of transplantation does not activate an immune response.

3. Allotransplantation occurs between genetically different individuals where the donor antigens will be seen as foreign (nonself) by the recipient and will trigger an immune response.
   a. Allotransplantation is the type of transplant we will be discussing throughout this chapter.
   b. Whether the donor is living or deceased, solid organ transplants between genetically dissimilar individuals are termed allogeneic transplants.
      i. Allograft simply refers to a transplanted organ from an individual of the same species.
      ii. While the term allograft could refer to a bone marrow or stem cell transplant, in this chapter, we will focus on solid organ transplantation.
      iii. Currently in allogeneic organ transplantation, morbidity and mortality result mainly from infections that develop from the need to suppress the immune response to decrease the risk of rejection.

4. Xenotransplantation involves transplantation between biologically different species and, at this time, poses the greatest risk for rejection. In this instance, the organ is referred to as a xenograft.
   a. This procedure is being studied by researchers as an option to help alleviate the human organ shortage.
   b. The use of animal organs, mostly pigs or baboons, has been very controversial for a number of reasons.
      i. While risks of rejection pose a great challenge in xenotransplantation, the risks of infections that are common in animals are of equal concern if transmitted to humans.
      ii. Recent reports of genetically engineered pigs are promising to resolve the rejection issue.[8,9]
      iii. While this research continues with transplantation among various species of animals and demonstrates some promise, clinical trials with humans are not currently being done.

II. ANTIGEN RECOGNITION MECHANISM OF THE IMMUNE SYSTEM

A. The major histocompatibility complex (MHC)
   1. The system that is responsible for initiating and regulating immune mechanisms is known as the major histocompatibility complex.
   2. The human MHC is located on the short arm of chromosome.[6]
   3. In humans, the MHC also referred to as the human leukocyte antigen (HLA) system.

a. HLA antigens are proteins that reside on the surface of nearly all cells in the body and define the immunologic identity of an individual.
b. HLA molecules are responsible for presenting foreign proteins to the immune system.
c. After recognition of the foreign antigens, the immune system initiates a specific cascade of responses to destroy the foreign tissue identified.
d. With the development of clinical transplantation, this system has been closely studied and analyzed over the last six decades.

4. Human leukocyte antigens/proteins act as a genetic identification label.
   a. The antigens are determined genetically by multiple loci (HLA-A, HLA-B, HLA-C, HLA-DR, HLA-DQ, and HLA-DP) and are inherited as a unit or haplotype: one from each parent.
   b. Each individual possesses two haplotypes derived hereditarily from the biological parents. One set comes from the biological father and one set from the biological mother of an individual.
   c. The diversity of HLA antigens results in an immense number of different haplotypes; thus, the probability of finding a perfect HLA match within a population is often quite low.
      i. Within a family, the probability that a sibling will be a "perfect match" to another sibling is 1:4 or a 25% chance.[10,11]
      ii. Outside an individual's immediate family, the chance of finding an identical HLA match within the general population is 1: 50,000.[11]
   d. HLA antigens are not found on mature erythrocytes; this accounts for not considering HLA antigens for blood transfusions.
      i. In addition, the rhesus (Rh) antigens are not present on lymphocytes or tissue cells, explaining why they are not taken into account for organ transplantation.
      ii. As ABO antigens are present on all cells, we ensure that the blood types are compatible between donors and recipients, but we need not be concerned with whether the Rh is positive or negative.
      iii. Nevertheless, recent clinical protocols have been implemented to allow transplantation between ABO-incompatible donors and recipients.[12]
   e. HLA antigens are divided into two different classes, class I and class II.[1-6]
      i. Class I contains three main loci that we consider in solid organ transplantation, HLA-A, HLA-B, and HLA-C, while class II consists of multiple loci that code for HLA-DRB1, HLA-DRB3, HLA-DRB4, HLA-DRB5, HLA-DQ, and HLA-DP. Each of these loci produces individual HLA molecules or antigens.
         • Class I HLA antigens are expressed on the surface membranes of all nucleated cells of the human body.
         • Class II HLA antigens are expressed on B cells and APCs as well as on other cells of the immune system when these cells become activated.
         • Both class I and class II antigens trigger humoral and cellular immune responses through the presentation of small foreign peptides on the surface antigen-presenting cells to the immune system.
      ii. If a potential recipient possesses specific antibodies against a donor's HLA antigens, she/he most likely will be excluded from consideration

for transplantation with that donor due to the likelihood of rejecting the transplanted organ.

- If HLA antibodies are identified in the patient's serum, they have been "sensitized" toward foreign HLA antigens.
- The presence of preformed anti-HLA antibodies in transplant recipients leads to a higher incidence and risk of rejection.[13,14]
- Sensitization to HLA antigens can occur following exposure to foreign tissue, during sensitizing events such as pregnancy, transfusions, or previous transplantation.[12,13]
- Hence, screening for anti-HLA antibodies and identifying the HLA antigens of the individual through tissue typing is important for finding compatible organ transplant recipients/donor pairs, reducing rejection, and avoiding the potential for graft loss.
- A complete HLA immune profile of the recipient can influence the allocation of more compatible organs for that individual, ultimately impacting the long-term success of the transplant.

B. **Tissue typing**

1. In years past, tissue typing was done with serology testing and often required 6 to 8 tubes of fresh blood.
2. Today, this test can be performed using DNA technology and can be accomplished with a small amount of blood, a hair follicle, or a swab from mucous membrane such as the buccal epithelium.
3. HLA tissue typing identifies an individual's antigens at each of the major loci.
4. For the majority of thoracic and liver transplant recipients, HLA matching is not considered in donor selection.[13,14]
   a. With thoracic transplantation, concerns regarding ischemic time mandate a retrospective review of force a review of donor and recipient HLA.
   b. With a 4- to 5-hour window of cold ischemic time, the ability to match organs on HLA compatibility has not been feasible.
5. Our ability to identify specific antigens to which an individual would be reactive has contributed to improved outcomes in transplantation of all solid organs.

C. Calculated panel of reactive antibodies (CPRA)[15]

1. The number of HLA antigens to which a patient is sensitized or makes antibody toward is reflected in the calculated panel of reactive antibodies (CPRA). The CPRA is a calculation that tells a clinician the likelihood of finding an organ donor to which a patient will not make HLA antibodies.
   a. Preformed donor-specific HLA antibodies (DSA), which are specific for the donor HLA mismatches, put a newly transplanted organ at risk for rejection.
      i. Transplanting sensitized patients with DSA without initiating desensitization protocols puts the individual at risk for a hyperacute rejection and subsequent destruction of the organ.
2. HLA antibody testing and CPRA calculations are performed on potential candidates for solid organ transplantation.[15-17]
   a. Test results are reported as a percentage and serve as an index of probabilities of finding a compatible donor.
   b. Testing for HLA antibody is performed using solid phase immunoassays. Serum from a potential candidate is mixed with beads that are coated with purified HLA antigens. HLA antibody bound to a bead is detected with a

fluorescence reagent and is reported as the median fluorescence intensity (MFI) for each positive bead.

   c. If the candidate does not possess antibodies against any HLA antigens, the test result is reported as negative.

   d. If, however, the candidate reacts against some or many HLA antigens, a CPRA is reported.[15]

      i. Here is where probabilities and the risk thresholds for a given transplant center enter the equation.

      ii. The PRA reported is a calculated PRA (CPRA). That is, once the HLA specificity has been determined, one can calculate the frequency with which that antigen (or antigens) occurs in the population of potential donors. This is done by using HLA-typing data from previous donors.

      iii. For example, if the patient has an antibody against A2, the CPRA will be approximately 48%. That means that 48% of the donors in the pool of previously typed organ donors had an A2 antigen.[17,18]

      iv. If we add an antibody against other HLA antigens, the CPRA will increase based on the frequency with which these antigens occur in the donor database. For example:

        A2 = 48%
        A2, B7 = 59%
        A2, B7, C7 = 77%
        A2, B7, C7, DR7 = 83%
        A2, B7, C7, DQ7, DQ2 = 88%

      v. When reporting the CPRA, centers may decide not to include all HLA antibodies, depending on the strength of the antibody. Some centers enter all HLA antibodies independent of strength, while other centers enter only the strongest HLA antibodies that would yield a positive crossmatch. This decision is dependent on the center's ability to remove donor-specific HLA antibodies perioperatively and reduce the risk of rejection posttransplant.

   e. It has been reported that individuals requiring support from a ventricular assist device (VAD) have developed HLA antibodies within a few weeks after device implantation due to the transfusions they receive during this surgical procedure.[19]

      i. All patients who have a VAD placement have their CPRA tested according to the transplant center's protocol.

      ii. This could be monthly, and in the case of patients on VADs, it may be performed more frequently

   f. CPRA retesting may also be warranted after a proinflammatory event such as infection, surgery, or vaccination.

D. HLA antibody specificities[20]

  1. Immunology laboratories are able to identify HLA antigens to which an individual has developed preformed antibodies.

  2. In addition to calculating a CPRA value, clinicians list the specific HLA antibodies as "unacceptable HLA antigens" in the organ allocation computer system at the United Network for Organ Sharing (UNOS).

   a. When a deceased donor becomes available, the donor's HLA is entered into the system.

   b. If a candidate has a specific antibody against this donor's HLA, the recipient is excluded from the match run.

E. Crossmatch[18,20]

1. This test is performed prospectively prior to kidney transplantation.
2. Liver, heart, and lung candidates may also have a retrospective crossmatch performed.
3. However, a candidate with preformed donor-specific HLA antibodies is going to require a prospective crossmatch due to the likelihood of a positive reaction with the donor.
4. A crossmatch is performed by mixing donor lymphocytes (isolated from blood, spleen, or lymph nodes) with serum (which may contain antibodies) from the potential recipient.
5. If the recipient has antibodies against donor antigens, the recipient antibodies will bind to the donor cells.
6. Detection of the bound antibody may be via a cytotoxicity assay or, more commonly, using flow cytometry.
7. In the cytotoxicity assay, cell death is the readout, whereas flow cytometry uses a fluorescent reagent and the readout is increased fluorescence intensity above a negative control serum.
   a. For either assay, a positive crossmatch would demonstrate donor-specific HLA antibody (DSA) and may be a contraindication to transplantation or signal the need for the use of antibody reduction protocols (i.e., plasmapheresis) and more aggressive immunosuppression.[12,21]
   b. DSA are HLA antibodies specific for donor HLA mismatches. A PRA provides us with the percentage of HLA antibodies an individual has, but does not indicate the presence of DSA.[22]
   c. Knowing specifically which anti-HLA antibodies a patient has allows us to avoid transplanting our patients with a donor that possesses those antigens. The PRA tells us how revved up the immune system is, but the DSA identifies the specific antigens to avoid reactivity.
   d. Protocols have been developed whereby recipients are treated preoperatively with plasmapheresis, intravenous immunoglobulins (IVIG), and rituximab to decrease the levels of HLA antibodies and, hence, reduce the risks associated with transplanting highly sensitized patients.[21,23]
   e. Long-term graft survival results of transplants performed in the setting of DSA are not comparable to the long-term survival results of transplants performed in the absence of DSA. However, given the morbidity and mortality associated with long-term dialysis, many centers have adopted this type of "desensitization" strategy to help highly sensitized candidates receive a transplant.[23]
8. Given the improved specificity of solid phase HLA antibody testing, a virtual crossmatch may be requested.
   a. A virtual crossmatch compares the HLA antibody specificities of the recipient with the HLA type of the prospective donor. This process is done by qualified HLA lab personnel.
      i. The virtual crossmatch is considered compatible when none of the recipient's antibodies, as determined in the solid phase assay, were directed against the donor's HLA antigens.
      ii. The virtual crossmatch is considered incompatible when any of the recipient's antibodies directed against the donor's HLA antigens results in an elevated MFI. There is no universally accepted MFI cutoff. Each transplant program determines their own MFI cutoff.[24]

III. IMPACT OF BRAIN DEATH ON DECEASED DONOR ALLOGRAFT OUTCOMES[25]

A. When an organ is transplanted between two genetically different individuals, an immense number of foreign cells and antigens are exposed to the recipient's immune system.

B. Circumstances surrounding the donor before, during, and after organ procurement activate the expression of antigens on the cell membranes of the organ, thereby increasing the immune reactions associated with organ transplantation.[25]

C. Brain death and cell ischemia reinforce antigen expression through extensive and massive cytokine release, while tissue reperfusion injury results in an antigen response and triggering of the host immune system.[25]

D. The combination of HLA antigen differences between the donor and recipient and the physiologic impact of cell ischemia and reperfusion injury may create a strong immune response and contribute significantly to the risk of rejection.[25]

E. This is the reason we see more optimal results in living donor, HLA-matched kidneys and well HLA-matched deceased donor kidneys.
   1. In the first group, the cell ischemia is less.
   2. In the second group, the allogeneic difference is smaller.

 IV. BUILDING UP THE IMMUNE RESPONSE: REJECTION

A. The immune response is a cascade of various reactions activated after the immune system of the host has identified "foreign" cells.[2,4,5]

B. Although the timing is not really clear, there are essential steps that occur within the immune system to mount the best possible defense.

C. Rejection is an immunologic response involving the HLA recognition of exposed antigens on the donor endothelial cells by recipient-derived lymphocytes or circulating antibodies.

D. T-cell activation occurs through costimulatory effect on the T-helper cells by APCs.[26]
   1. This step is essential for proliferation of T cells and B cells (Figure 2-4).

E. Types of rejection[27]:
   1. The rate and timing of rejection after transplantation depends entirely on the underlying effector mechanism.
   2. In order to devise methods to prevent rejection, it is necessary to understand the underlying mechanism as well as the time frame in which rejection can occur.
      a. Hyperacute rejection occurs minutes to a few hours after recirculation of the vascularized organ.
         i. It occurs in patients who have preexisting antibodies against the transplanted graft, based on earlier exposure to HLA antigens of the same type as the donor's antigens.

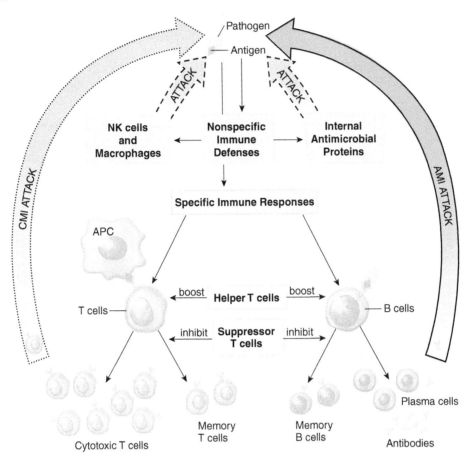

FIGURE 2-4 Summary of immune responses. Nonspecific immune defenses (*dashed arrows*) protect the body from all types of pathogens. Specific immune responses include the recognition of specific antigens by B and T cells. Activation of B cells produces an antibody-mediated immune (AMI) response (*solid arrow*), and activation of T cells leads to a cell-mediated immune (CMI) response (*dotted arrow*). In transplant, the graft replaces the pathogen in this immune response figure.

     ii. Anti-HLA antigens can occur in patients with numerous blood transfusions, multiple pregnancies, and previous organ transplants.

     iii. ABO incompatibility and xenotransplantation also lead to hyperacute rejection, due to natural antibodies in our immune system against the ABO type and other animal species.

     iv. In most cases, hyperacute rejection can be avoided by a prospective crossmatch and identification of donor-specific HLA antibody.

  b. Acute rejection occurs after a few days to a few weeks, and the underlying mechanism is based on primary activation of the T cells. Antibody-mediated rejection or AMR occurs in patients with known HLA sensitization.

     i. When a recipient has preformed DSA to antigens of the graft, a secondary, more rapid activation of T cells and B cells takes place and causes a faster rejection process.

  c. Chronic rejection occurs after months and even years and is based on a slow buildup of the immune reaction.

     i. Chronic rejection remains the greatest challenge in long-term graft survival.

      ii. A relationship between pretransplant DSA and chronic rejection has been identified.

      iii. De novo DSA has been reported to develop in the posttransplant period.[22]

      iv. Both pre- and posttransplant DSA are considered risk factors for the development of AMR.[22]

V. DECREASING THE RISK OF REJECTION

A. Downregulation of the host immune system after allotransplantation is necessary to guarantee successful patient and graft outcomes.

B. However, the function of the immune system should stay intact at a level to maintain protection against infections and malignancies.

C. The greatest challenge in immunosuppressive therapy is to find the ideal balance, considering three key factors:
   1. Immunosuppression must be
      a. Sufficient to protect the graft against immunogenic response, but be
         i. Low enough to maintain protection against infection
         ii. Low enough to maintain protection against malignancy

D. Finding methods for monitoring total immune function would be ideal.
   1. This process would allow us to determine if we are oversuppressing or undersuppressing the function of the immune system.
   2. A blood test called ImmuKnow has been used by some transplant programs to monitor total immune function with varied outcomes reported.[28]
   3. Researchers are continuing to study ways to monitor immune function to decrease the risk of overimmunosuppressing patients.[28]
   4. Trough levels of drugs only tell us the safety of a medication.
   5. We need to be able to determine the total impact of immunosuppression on immune function.
   6. Testing immune function prior to transplantation could provide a baseline for determining the impact of immunosuppression.

E. See the chapter on Transplant Pharmacology for additional information.

VI. IMMUNOSUPPRESSION THERAPY

A. Over the last 30 years, the number of immunosuppressive drugs available to combat rejection has steadily increased, with the greatest surge occurring in the last 5 years.

B. Most immunosuppressive drugs, with the exception of prednisone, interfere with T-cell and B-cell function and proliferation.

C. Immunosuppressive therapy is designed to reduce the intensity of the immune response to the grafted organ.

D. All immunosuppressive therapy regimens are based on a combination of agents to maintain a balance between efficacy in avoiding allograft rejection and safety in order to prevent various side effects, acutely and long term (Figure 2-5).

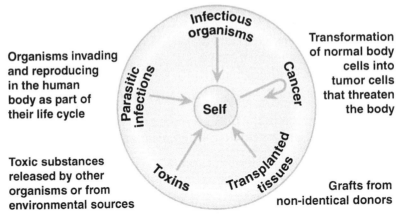

Infectious organisms taking advantage of breaches in the body's barriers

Transformation of normal body cells into tumor cells that threaten the body

Organisms invading and reproducing in the human body as part of their life cycle

Toxic substances released by other organisms or from environmental sources

Grafts from non-identical donors

FIGURE 2-5 The immune defense system. The immune system defends the body against invading microorganisms, as well as toxins in the environment. This includes protection against infectious organisms, parasitic infections, toxins, and cancerous cells. Unfortunately, cells of transplanted tissues are recognized as "nonself" or invaders. For this reason, immunosuppressive drugs are needed to keep the body's immune system from rejecting a transplant.

E. One difficulty with immunosuppressive drugs is the wide variability in patient response to the same regimen.
   1. Finding a balance between therapeutic and toxic doses is very individual, thus making immunosuppression unique in its setting.
   2. Tailoring the immunosuppressive regimen to the individual transplant recipient is the most ideal approach.

F. See chapter on Transplant Pharmacology for additional information.

 VII. FUTURE PERSPECTIVES: CHIMERISM AND TOLERANCE

A. **Chimerism**
   1. Chimerism is the presence of both donor and recipient hematopoietic cells in transplant recipients.
      a. This was first noted in liver transplant patients who stopped their immunosuppressive agents unbeknownst to the medical team.
      b. Research in these patients showed that many had detectable donor cells in their blood and/or tissues. These donor cells coexisted with recipient cells and were no longer recognized as foreign.
      c. The evidence indicated that a greater number of donor hematopoietic cells present in the liver graft migrated to the host thymus and, as such, were seen as acceptable by the developing host immune system under the unique condition of immune suppression.
      d. After stopping the immunosuppressive medications, this particular graft was no longer recognizable by the immune system of the host.
      e. A case report from Australia describes the development of a chimeric state in a 9-year-old girl with acute liver failure who received a liver transplant from a 12-year-old boy. Seventeen months later, she was reported to be chimeric and required no further immunosuppression therapy. Her HLA and ABO blood type had changed to that of her donor.[29]

      f. Cases such as that in the Australian report are those we need to study. This will help us determine how to create an immune-tolerant or chimeric state for our patients.

B. **Tolerance**[30,31]

1. Research into solutions to prevent chronic rejection without the need for immunosuppressive drugs is tending to focus more and more on the induction of tolerance of the host to the donor graft.[30,31]
2. Functional or clinical tolerance is seen as long-term survival of primary grafts in the absence of or with very low doses of immunosuppressive drugs, where the graft is tolerated by the host.
3. Immunologic tolerance is seen as the absence of detectable immune response, or T-cell hyporesponsiveness, to specific donor alloantigens in an immunosuppressive-free regimen.
4. How to induce such tolerance is a difficult task.
5. Tolerance can be created in neonates because the adaptive immune system has not gained exposure to sensitizing events that would lead to the formation of memory responses. Therefore, the neonate immune system can be modulated to accept foreign cells.
   a. This form of "learned" immune tolerance is also known as central tolerance. Central tolerance discriminates self from nonself.[3,32]
6. However, in transplantation, peripheral tolerance is the goal, and the mechanisms to induce this are currently being studied.
   a. Peripheral tolerance prevents overreactivity of the immune response to external stimuli, such as donor antigens.[3]
   b. Induction of transplant tolerance improves graft outcomes (see Figure 2-5).
7. Various protocols have already been investigated and implemented, such as stem cell transplantation of donor cells together with the donor organ.

VIII. CONCLUSION

A. An overview of the normal functions of an intact immune system shows how complex this system really is.

B. It is a proof that selective actions undertaken to block certain mechanisms within the system can ultimately affect many other systems.

C. Organ transplantation has created a specific domain in immunology, flirting with all basic principles of resistance against foreign intruders of the human body.

D. The main goal of organ transplantation focuses on the lifesaving treatment of patients with end-organ damage while preserving a high quality of life, long term.

E. The desire to preserve optimal organ function after allotransplantation drives the work of all clinical professionals working in the field of organ transplantation.

F. Transplant nurses:

1. Play a key role in identifying barriers to medication adherence and implementing evidence-based interventions to overcome these barriers. See the International Transplant Nurses Society Pocket Guide: Interventions to Common Medication Adherence barriers.[33]

2. Ensure safe delivery of immunosuppressive medications.
3. Collaborate with the interdisciplinary team to plan for effective, efficient, and safe care in the complex medical regimen in transplantation.

G. Knowledge of the immune system guides our understanding of the importance of immunosuppression and its effect on long-term outcomes in organ transplantation.

REFERENCES

1. Rote N. Mechanisms of self defense. In: Huether S, MCCance K, eds. *Understanding Pathophysiology*. 5th ed. St. Louis, MO: Elsevier/Mosby; 2012.
2. Kirk AD. Immunosuppression without immunosuppression? How to be a tolerant individual in a dangerous world. *Transpl Infect Dis*. 1999;1(1):65–75.
3. George JF. Immunology in relation to cardiac transplantation. In: Kirklin JK, ed. *Heart Transplantation*. New York, NY: Churchill Livingstone; 2002:14–29, 37–48.
4. Martinez O, Rosen HR. Basic concepts in transplant immunology. *Liver Transpl*. 2005;11(4):370–381.
5. Hale D. Basic transplant immunology. *Surg Clin North Am*. 2006;86(5):1103–1125.
6. Kumbala D, Zhang R. Essential concept of transplant immunology for clinical practice. *World J Transplant*. 2013;3(4):113–118.
7. Wiseman AC. Induction therapy in renal transplantation: why? What agent? What dose? We may never know. *Clin J Am Soc Nephrol*. 2015;10(6):923–925.
8. Fishman JA, Scobie L, Takeuchi Y. Xenotransplantation-associated infectious risk: a WHO consultation. *Xenotransplantation*. 2012;19(2):72–81.
9. Cooper DK. The case for xenotransplantation. *Clin Transplant*. 2015;29(4):288–293.
10. Rajalingam R, et al. Major histocompatibility complex. In: Xiang Li, Jevnikar A, eds. *Transplant Immunology*. West Sussex, UK: John Wiley and Sons Publishing; 2015.
11. Kessinger A, Sharp JG. Circulating hematopoietic stem cell transplantation. In: Lanza RP, ed. *Handbook of Stem Cells Book*. Vol. 2. St. Louis, MO: Elsevier; 2004.
12. Montgomery JR, Berger JC, Warren DS, et al. Outcomes of ABO incompatible transplantation in the United States. *Transplantation*. 2012;93(6):603–609.
13. Picascia A, Sabia C, Grimaldi V, et al. Lights and shadows of anti-HLA antibodies detected by solid phase assay. *Immunol Lett*. 2014;162:181–187.
14. Opelz G, Wujciak T, Dohler B, et al. HLA compatibility and organ transplant survival. Collaborative Transplant Study. *Rev Immunogenet*. 1999;1(3):334–342.
15. Organ Procurement and Transplantation Network. Explanation of CPRA for professionals. Available at https://www.unos.org/wp-content/uploads/unos/CPRA_Professionals.pdf?b2d5de. Accessed October 24, 2015.
16. Leffell MS, Kim D, Vega RM, et al. Red blood cell transfusions and the risk of allosensitization in patients awaiting primary kidney transplantation. *Transplantation*. 2014;97(5):525–533.
17. Barbari A, Abbas S, Jaafar M. Approach to kidney transplant in sensitized potential transplant recipients. *Exp Clin Transplant*. 2012;10(5):419–427.
18. Baxter-Lowe LA, Cecka M, Kamoun J, et al. Center defined unacceptable HLA antigens facilitate transplants for sensitized patients in multicenter kidney exchange program. *Am J Transplant*. 2014;13(7):1592–1598.
19. Askar M, Hsich E, Reville P, et al. HLA and MICA allosensitization patterns among patients supported by left ventricular assist devices. *J Heart Lung Transplant*. 2013;32(12):1241–1248.
20. O'Leary JG, Demetris AJ, Friedman LS et al. The role of donor specific alloantibodies in liver transplantation. *Am J Transplant*. 2014;14(4):779–787.
21. Jordan S, Choi J, Vo A. Kidney transplantation in highly sensitized patients. *Br Med Bull*. 2015;114(1):354–362.
22. Pietroni V, Toscano A, Citterio F, Donor specific antibody in transplantation: where are we? *Int Trends Immunity*. 2015;1(4):1–7.
23. Montgomery RA, Lonze BE, King KE et al. Desensitization in HLA incompatible kidney recipients and survival. *N Engl J Med*. 2013;368(10):318–326.
24. Kobashigawa J, Mehra M, West L, et al. Report from a consensus conference on the sensitized patient awaiting heart transplantation. *J Heart Lung Transplant*. 2009;28:213–225.
25. Dziodzio T, Biebl M, Pratschke J. Impact of brain death on ischemia/reperfusion injury in liver transplantation. *Curr Opin Organ Transplant*. 2014;19(2):108–114.
26. Chen L, Flies DB. Molecular mechanisms of T Cell Co stimulation and co-inhibition. *Nat Rev Immunol*. 2013;13:227–232.

27. Malhotra P. Immunology of transplant rejection. *Medscape 2013*. Available at http://emedicine.medscape.com/article/432209-overview#a5. Accessed September 13, 2015.
28. Kobashigawa JA, Kiyosaki KK, Patel JK et al. Benefit of immune monitoring in heart transplant patients using ATP production in activated lymphocytes. *J Heart Lung Transplant*. 2010;29(5):504–508.
29. Alexander S, Smith N, Hu M, et al. Chimerism and tolerance in a recipient of a deceased donor liver transplant. *N Engl J Med*. 2008;358:369–374.
30. Leventhal JR, Elliott MJ, Yolcu ES, et al. Immune reconstitution/immunocompetence in recipients of kidney plus hematopoietic stem/facilitating cell transplants. *Transplantation*. 2015;99(22):288–298.
31. Kawai T, Sachs D, Sprangers B, et al. Long term results in recipients of combined HLA mismatched kidney and bone marrow transplantation without maintenance immunosuppression. *Am J Transplant*. 2014;14(7):1599–1611.
32. Alpdogan O, Van den Brink MR. Immune tolerance and transplantation. *Semin Oncol*. 2013;39(6):629–642.
33. International Transplant Nurses Society. Pocket Guide: Interventions to Common Medication Adherence Barriers. Available at http://www.itns.org/patienteducation.html. Accessed October 28, 2015.

SELF-ASSESSMENT QUESTIONS

1. An example of autotransplantation is:
   a. transplanting the organs from one species to another.
   b. transplanting organs from one human to another human.
   c. transplanting a kidney from one identical twin to another.
   d. transfusing a pint of a patient's blood back into the same patient.

2. Examples of antigen-presenting cells include:
   a. macrophages, monocytes, and erythrocytes.
   b. dendritic cells, macrophages, and monocytes.
   c. erythrocytes, lymphocytes, and platelets.
   d. mitochondria, macrocytes, and thrombocytes.

3. The test that identifies HLA antigens to which a patient is sensitized or makes antibody toward is called:
   a. final crossmatch.
   b. tissue typing.
   c. calculated panel of reactive antibodies (CPRA).
   d. molecular chimerism.

4. Desensitizing protocols have been implemented at many transplant programs and include which of the following interventions to decrease patient antibody titers?
   a. Plasmapheresis
   b. IVIG
   c. Rituximab
   d. All the above

5. Antibody-mediated rejection (AMR) may occur several months after transplantation and may be the result of:
   a. development of de novo donor-specific antibodies.
   b. overimmunosuppression.
   c. a lack of antibodies.
   d. inability to suppress the T-helper cell.

6. The goals of induction therapy include which of the following:
   a. To decrease the amount of immunosuppression needed during the life of the new organ
   b. To increase the patient's quality of life after transplantation
   c. To suppress the lymphocytes and prevent an immediate recognition of the new organ
   d. To stimulate an immune response and prevent the development of an infection

7. The first dose of induction therapy often is given in the operating room. A common drug used as induction therapy is called:
   a. tacrolimus.
   b. mycophenolate mofetil.
   c. sirolimus.
   d. thymoglobulin.

8. In searching for a perfect 6 antigen match kidney, what is the likelihood of finding that perfect match with a sibling?
   a. 100%
   b. 75%
   c. 50%
   d. 25%

9. Which of the following statements is TRUE about ABO compatibility factors when accepting an organ for a candidate?
   a. Rh factor is not considered because Rh is not found on lymphocytes.
   b. Rh factor must be considered since the Rh factor resides on all tissues of the body.

10. Preformed antibodies develop as a result of which of the following?
   a. Pregnancies
   b. Blood transfusions
   c. Previous transplants
   d. All the above

CHAPTER

3

Education for Transplant Patients and Caregivers

Debra Bernardina, RN, BSN, CCTC
Darla K. Phillips, RN, MSN, CCTC

I. INTRODUCTION

   A. Patient education is a key element of transplant nursing.[1]

   B. Patient education provides the foundation that enables patients to better achieve optimal health before and after organ transplantation.

   C. The role of the transplant coordinator is to design patient education to meet the learning needs of the patient, taking into consideration the patient's developmental level, readiness to learn, cultural values, and beliefs.[1]

   D. Caregivers play a vital role in the care of the transplant patient and must be engaged in patient education throughout the transplant continuum.

II. LEARNING THEORY MODELS FOR TRANSPLANTATION

   A. Educational models
      1. Guide the interdisciplinary transplant team to plan, design, and implement appropriate educational interventions based on the patient's individual needs.
      2. Support the nursing process in determining if the patient is ready to move to the next phase of learning.

   B. Health belief model (HBM)
      1. The HBM is one educational model to explain, predict, and influence patient health-related behavior.
      2. This model
         a. States that patients will not act to improve health unless they[2]
            i. Believe they are susceptible to the poor health condition in question.
            ii. Believe the condition, if contracted, would seriously affect their life.
            iii. Believe the benefits of actions to improve health outweigh the barriers.
            iv. Possess confidence that they can perform the action.

b. Identifies motivation for adherence by examining six aspects related to health care decisions to modify behavior[2,3]:
  i. Patient's perception of severity of illness
  ii. Patient's perception of illness susceptibility and its consequences
  iii. Value of treatment benefits including a cost/benefit analysis
  iv. Barriers to treatment
  v. Physical and emotional cost of treatment
  vi. External influence that stimulates action toward treatment of illness
c. Targets missing information to ultimately motivate the patient for change to improve health.

III. LEARNING NEEDS

A. Learning needs in each phase of the transplant continuum may differ as patient's and caregiver's previous experiences, learning needs, and changes in health are incorporated into their current perceptions and understanding of the patient's overall health condition. Per the Centers for Medicare and Medicaid, the transplant phases of care are
  1. Pretransplant phase: extends from evaluating the patient and placing the patient on the transplant program's waiting list to the preoperative preparation
  2. Transplant phase: extends from the preoperative preparation until the patient is awake and alert following surgery
  3. Discharge phase: extends from when the patient is awake and alert following surgery through posttransplant clinical management and follow-up.[4]

B. The educational content of the each phase is dependent upon:
  1. The patient's stage of and adjustment to illness.[5]
    a. Educational strategies that were effective for a previous stage of the disease process may not be effective for the current stage.[5]
    b. Acute organ failure may limit the time available to teach the patient or caregiver and the unknown or unpredictable course of the disease process is stressful for patients and caregivers.
    c. A recently diagnosed patient may not be able to fully comprehend the effect and implications of end-stage organ disease, whereas a patient who has had end-stage organ disease since childhood may have anticipated transplant in his or her future.
  2. The organ to be transplanted.
    a. Each organ has unique indications, surgical procedures, outcomes, and complications.
  3. Requirements established by the transplant center.
    a. Each transplant center defines eligibility criteria, including behavioral expectations.
    b. In order to meet regulatory requirements, all patients must be informed of specific aspects of transplantation (see Table 3-1).
  4. Patient and caregiver readiness to learn
    a. Personal perceptions, experiences, and motivations impact readiness to learn.

IV. ASSESSMENT OF READINESS TO LEARN

A. Motivation to learn
  1. Determine patient's expectation for improving health
  2. Identify patient's motivation for improving health
  3. Focus on the patient's strengths and recognize accomplishments

B. Learning style: Ask patients:
1. How they like to learn
2. To identify and describe past learning experiences that were positive
3. To identify and describe past learning experiences that were negative

C. Barriers to learning
1. Insufficient time to teach or learn
2. Cognitive dysfunction that may be due to[5]
   a. Effects of medications
   b. Effects of disease process
   c. Intellectual ability
3. Physical disability, for example:
   a. Hearing loss
   b. Visual changes or loss
   c. Lack of dexterity to perform tasks
4. Fatigue or pain
5. Anxiety
6. Cultural factors related to[6]
   a. Perception of illness
   b. Language differences
   c. Religious beliefs
   d. Social order of the family
   e. Communication behaviors
   f. Expression of pain
   g. Folk health beliefs
7. Low-health literacy
   a. Health literacy is the ability to read, comprehend, and use medical information to make decisions.[7]
   b. Commonly associated with lower-socioeconomic levels.[8]
8. Disruptive environment

 V. STRATEGIES FOR EFFECTIVE PATIENT EDUCATION

A. Provide environment conducive to learning
1. Create non-threatening, respectful, and psychologically safe environment in which patients and caregivers can
   a. Communicate openly and ask questions about complex and personal health care issues.
   b. Gain confidence as they learn information and try new skills.
2. Encourage active participation on the part of patients and caregivers.
3. Reinforce education through evaluation of the patient's learning. This can be accomplished with written or verbal questions or through discussions.
4. Acknowledge the large amount of information to learn; reassure patients and caregivers that learning occurs over time.
5. Recognize and be sensitive to the patients' right to choose treatment options that are best for them.[5]

B. Include caregivers in patient education[7,9,10]
1. Advantages include, but are not limited to, the following:
   a. Educates those individuals who will be providing care to the patient throughout the transplant continuum.
   b. Allows patient and caregiver to mutually prepare for evaluation and formulate questions.[7]

      c. Enables caregivers to ask questions the patient may not think of.

      d. Allows patient and caregiver to learn expectations regarding life after transplant early on in the transplant process.[10,11]

C. Prior to the first transplant appointment:

    1. Provide educational information for the patient and caregiver.

      a. Instruct patient and caregiver to bring these materials to the evaluation conference.

D. Establish a buddy system.

    1. Reduces anxiety by allowing a patient and caregiver to speak with someone who has experienced the transplant evaluation process[10]

E. Use a structured approach to patient teaching.

    1. Establish day-to-day learning expectations.

      a. This has been shown to increase engagement on the part of patients and caregivers and between nurses and patients.[9]

    2. Increase consistency of information delivered to patients through the use of a checklist of topics to discuss with patients and caregivers.[11]

    3. Encourage patients to evaluate educational sessions after participating in structured classes.[12]

F. Relate information to familiar aspects of patient's daily life. For example:

    1. Describe lifting restrictions by comparing 5 pounds to a familiar object such as a gallon of milk

    2. Provide a visual illustration when explaining medical details to patients when possible. For example, when describing cirrhosis, compare the smooth surface of an apple to a healthy liver and the rough, bumpy surface of an orange to a cirrhotic liver.

G. Adjust teaching methods to accommodate for learning style, and health literacy[3]

    1. Focus on core skills for success.

    2. Use chronological or step-by-step timeline.

    3. Provide a small amount of information at a time.

    4. Emphasize the most important topics by placing them at the beginning or end of an educational session.

    5. Limit medical terminology and explain unfamiliar concepts.[8]

    6. Have patient restate information taught (teach back).

H. Engage all members of the interdisciplinary team[9]

    1. Patient education is an important component of the role of each member of the interdisciplinary team.

    2. The educational plan should provide time for patients and caregivers to meet each member of the team.

VI. STYLES AND FORMATS FOR EDUCATIONAL SESSIONS

A. One-to-one teaching format

    1. Advantages

      a. Preferred format in both pretransplant and transplant phase.[13]

      b. Ability to adjust speed and content to the learners.

      c. Brief topics may be reviewed daily during hospitalization.

        i. Helps to avoid "information overload" in the days immediately prior to discharge which overwhelms patients.[11]

B. Verbal information
   1. Easily provided during any encounter.
   2. Least preferred in a group setting.[13]

C. Written information[2]
   1. Provide material that is at the fifth to eighth grade reading level.
   2. Organize key messages so they are easy to find.
   3. Include pictures and words that create imagery and enhance retention of material.
   4. Develop content to be easily transferred to other formats including the Internet.[10]
   5. Advantage: Provides opportunity to reinforce verbal instructions.

D. DVD/video
   1. Second most preferred teaching format, pretransplant and transplant phase
      a. DVDs: Most preferred teaching format in posttransplant phase[13]
      b. Advantages:
         i.   Patient determines time for learning.
         ii. May be distributed in any phase of care.
         iii. Allows patients to review and re-learn content relevant to their interest.
         iv. Serves as a resource for caregivers who could not attend clinic sessions.

E. Group class
   1. Least preferred teaching format in posttransplant phase.[13]
   2. Advantage: patients may learn from experience of others.
   3. Disadvantage: some patients may not want to share experiences in a forum with other patients.
      a. Offer such patients alternate learning environments.

F. Demonstration
   1. Advantage: Provides patients and caregiver guided practice experience with equipment or skills required for home care.
   2. As applicable, plan teaching so that there are at least three nurse-supervised practice sessions.

G. Telephone or in-person follow-up after appointments[7]
   1. Advantages:
      a. Provides opportunity to
         i.   Summarize the plan of care
         ii. Reinforce learning specific to patient's current health or situation
         iii. Reinforce patient's understanding of the next steps he or she is responsible for in the plan of care
      b. Allows patients' time to reflect on their recent appointment and identify additional questions

H. Internet resources[14]
   1. Advantages:
      a. May be included as a reference to supplement written materials provided to patients.
      b. May be accessed independently by the patient or caregiver for information on demand.
      c. Patient education material on a transplant center Internet site may be less expensive for transplant centers to maintain.
   2. Disadvantage: Must be updated more frequently than other formats
   3. Instruct patients to review the website sponsor:
      a. Government, non-profit, or commercial sources have different missions, purposes, goals, and intended audiences.

I.   Summary

1. No single intervention or strategy is a guarantee of successful or satisfactory educational outcomes for patients or caregivers.[15]
2. The combination of a DVD format with in-person instruction is very beneficial for learning.[7]
3. Multiple content formats are important to meet the needs of all learners and caregivers.[10]
4. Learners retain:
   a. 10% of what they read
   b. 20% of what they hear
   c. 30% of what they see
   d. 50% of what they see and hear
   e. 70% of what they see, hear, and say and
   f. 90% of what they say and do[16]

 VII. EDUCATION ACROSS THE TRANSPLANT CONTINUUM

A.   Pretransplant phase (Table 3-1)

1. Education begins at the time of the referral.
   a. Phone interviews provide an opportunity for education prior to the patient's arrival.
   b. Materials may be sent prior to the evaluation to prepare the patient and caregivers for the evaluation process.
2. Key considerations for education during the pretransplant phase
   a. Advise patients to maintain a journal of questions between clinic visits. The journal also may be used to record and monitor physiologic trends.
   b. A recent study of lung transplant patients noted that approximately 50% of candidates are focused on getting listed and topics pertinent to the pretransplant phase and 72% of candidates were interested in how to sustain their transplant.[10] Many patients reported feeling overwhelmed with too much information (pretransplant, transplant, posttransplant education all given in one setting) at one time and preferred learning about self-care pertinent to each stage of the transplant process that they are currently in.
   c. When assessing a patient's knowledge or understanding of a particular topic, use open-ended interviewing techniques rather than questions that can be answered with a "Yes" or "No."
3. Initial assessment
   a. Patient's understanding of the illness
      i.   Tell me why your doctor referred you to the transplant center.
      ii. Tell me about your organ disease or your health problems.
      iii. Tell me what caused your organ disease.
      iv. Tell me about the medicines you take and why you take them.
   b. Patient's knowledge about transplant process
      i.   What have you already learned about transplantation?
      ii. Tell me about someone you know who has had a transplant.
      iii. Tell me about any research you have done, including using the Internet.
   c. Patient's quality of life[10]
      i.   How would you describe your quality of life today?
      ii. Describe how transplantation would affect your quality of life.
      iii. What goals would you like to achieve following transplantation?
         • Goals may be related to work or school, family events, or personal achievements.

- Explore goals with patient and create the vision that transplant is a step toward these goals and not the goal itself.

4. Informed consent[4]
   a. Transplant programs must have policies and procedures that delineate
      i. Who is responsible for discussing the informed consent process with the patient
      ii. Where discussions concerning the informed consent are *documented* in the medical record
      iii. The methods used by the program to ensure and document patient understanding
      iv. When the discussion will take place
   b. Transplant centers must implement written transplant patient informed consent policies that inform each patient of
      i. The evaluation process
      ii. The surgical procedure
      iii. Alternative treatments
      iv. Potential medical or psychosocial risks
      v. National and transplant center–specific outcomes[17]
      vi. Organ donor risk factors that could affect the success of the graft or the health of the patient
      vii. His or her right to refuse transplantation
      viii. Medicare Part B coverage for immunosuppressive medications (see Table 3-1)
   c. As part of the evaluation process, transplant programs must inform and provide each patient it evaluates with information and written materials explaining all of the following options[18]:
      i. Listing at multiple transplant hospitals
      ii. Transferring primary waiting time
      iii. Transferring their care to a different transplant hospital without losing accrued waiting time.
   d. Each transplant program must document that it fulfilled these requirements and maintain this documentation.[18]
      i. Per Appendix B of UNOS bylaws, transplant programs must provide patients a written summary of the program coverage plan. This is given to the patient at the time of listing and with any changes in the program or personnel.[19]
      ii. UNOS requires that all transplant programs have transplant surgeon(s) and physician(s) available 365 days a year, 24 hours a day, and 7 days a week for program coverage. Any deviation must be approved by the OPTN/UNOS Membership and Professional Standards Committee (MPSC).
      iii. A patient or family member may contact UNOS about organ allocation and transplant data at any time.

5. Transplant evaluation process
   a. Purpose of the evaluation
      i. To assess health and to determine if transplantation is the optimal treatment for the patient's disease
      ii. To identify physical, psychosocial, and financial barriers to successful transplantation
   b. Consultation by and role of interdisciplinary team members
      i. Medical physician
         - Directs the medical management of disease process and determines medical suitability for transplantation

TABLE 3-1 Education Topics for Pre-transplant Patients and Caregivers

Subject	Required Content
The evaluation process	Results of physical examination, labs, and diagnostic testing
	Patient selection criteria and suitability for transplant
	Relevance of psychosocial issues to transplant success
	Financial responsibilities for transplant
	Requirement to follow a strict medical regimen
	Outcome of the evaluation

The surgical procedure
• Discussion should occur:
  – On several occasions prior to the transplant surgery
  – Prior to placement of the patient on the waiting list
	Detailed discussion of surgical procedure

	Anesthesia risk
	Risk related to the use of blood or blood products
	Other potential risks
	Expected postsurgical course
	Benefits and risk of transplant surgery relative to other alternatives
Alternative treatment to transplant	Options for alternative treatment
Potential medical risks of transplantation	Wound infection
	Pneumonia
	Blood clot formation
	Organ rejection, failure, or retransplant
	Lifetime immunosuppression therapy
	Arrhythmias and cardiovascular collapse
	Multiorgan failure
	Death
Potential psychosocial risk of transplantation	Depression
	Posttraumatic stress disorder
	Generalized anxiety
	Anxiety regarding dependence on others
	Feelings of guilt
	Future health problems may not be covered by insurer
	Alternative financial resources
	Future attempt to obtain medical, life, or disability may be jeopardized
National and transplant center–specific outcomes from most recent SRTR center–specific report. • Discussions should occur prior to date of placement on the waiting list • Transplant programs should communicate any updated information to patients when follow-up discussions occur prior to the transplant surgery	Expected 1-year patient and graft survival rates
	Observed 1-year patient and graft survival rates
	How these rates compare to national averages
	Whether the latest reported rates in the SRTR center–specific report comply with Medicare's outcome requirements
	If center does not meet outcomes, Medicare B will not pay for immunosuppression medications.
	Provided website www.srtr.org and https://optn.transplant.hrsa.gov

(*continued*)

TABLE 3-1 Education Topics for Pre-transplant Patients and Caregivers (*Continued*)

Subject	Required Content
Organ donor risk factors that could affect the success of the graft or the health of the patient	Possibility of graft failure and/or other health risks related to the health status of the organ donor, including: • Medical and social history and age of donor • Condition of the organ(s) • Risk of disease transmission including: 　– Human immunodeficiency virus 　– Hepatitis B virus and hepatitis C virus 　– Cancer 　– Malaria • Disease may not be detectable at time of donor recovery Note: After an organ offer is made for a patient, the transplant program must discuss with the patient the possible risks associated with transplantation of that specific organ. The discussion of risks should include any issues that could affect the success of the organ transplant (the condition of the organ) and any issues that could potentially place the health of the patient at risk (e.g., known increased-risk behaviors in the donor's background)
Right to refuse transplantation	Advise patient of right to withdraw consent for transplant or that he or she understands this right
Medicare B coverage of immunosuppressive drugs	Transplant must be performed at a Medicare-approved facility for Medicare B to pay for immunosuppressive medications
United Network for Organ Sharing (UNOS)	
Multiple listing and transfer of time between transplant centers	Right to be listed at more than one transplant center and the ability to transfer accumulated wait time between transplant centers
Program coverage plan	Coverage plan for medical and surgical provider
Increased risk donor	Advise patient at time of organ offer of increased risk donor
Other Relevant Topics	
Role of the interdisciplinary team members	
Information for how to talk to others about living donation	

  ii. Transplant surgeon
    • Determines if transplantation is the best option based on medical evaluation, surgical risks, and potential complications
  iii. Transplant coordinator
    • Provides education about evaluation process, listing for transplant, and patient responsibilities before and after transplant
    • Synthesizes information from interdisciplinary team members and physical assessments for presentation at selection committee meeting
  iv. Licensed social worker
    • Evaluates patient's social support system, ability to cope with the stress of transplantation and potential for adhering to pre- and posttransplant medical regimen.

- Identifies resources for patients and caregivers to promote healthy adjustment to illness and future recovery
  v. Registered dietitian
    - Assesses nutritional status based on medical information
    - May provide nutritional education to manage disease complications, optimize weight, and enhance overall nutritional status
  vi. Financial coordinator
    - Reviews transplant benefits provided by private and/or public insurers
    - Discusses costs associated with transplantation, including medications required after transplantation
    - Identifies financial responsibilities for the patient for costs not covered by insurance
    - In concert with social worker, provides information regarding fundraising options or access to insurance or disability programs
  vii. Transplant pharmacist
    - Reviews patient medications, makes recommendation to minimize drug–drug and/or food–drug interactions, and optimizes ongoing medical therapy
    - In concert with other members of the interdisciplinary team, educates patients regarding posttransplant medications
  viii. Other medical consultations may be required based on recommendations from transplant team members, such as
    - Psychologist
    - Anesthesiologist
    - Infectious disease specialist
    - Cardiologist
- c. Diagnostic testing
  i. Transplant programs define organ-specific protocols for diagnostic studies to validate end-organ disease and determine the overall health status of a patient to safely undergo organ transplantation.
  ii. May identify previously unknown disease or physiologic states.
  iii. Age- and gender-specific health maintenance testing must be current with national guidelines for disease prevention and detection and may be completed at the transplant center or by a local care provider.
    - Mammogram
    - Papanicolaou test
    - Bone densitometry
    - Colonoscopy
    - Skin assessment
    - Assessment of dentition
  iv. Examples of common diagnostic tests performed during a transplant evaluation include
    - Radiologic imaging
      ○ Chest radiograph
      ○ Computed tomography (CT) scan
      ○ Magnetic resonance imaging (MRI)
      ○ Bone densitometry
    - Cardiac studies and imaging
      ○ Electrocardiogram
      ○ Echocardiogram

- ○ Cardiac stress testing
- ○ Cardiac MRI
- ○ CT angiography
- ○ Right and/or left cardiac catheterization
- • Pulmonary testing
  - ○ Pulmonary function tests
  - ○ Bronchoscopy
  - ○ Arterial blood gas
  - ○ 6-Minute walk test
  - ○ Ventilation–perfusion (V–Q) scan
- • Gastrointestinal (GI) studies
  - ○ Esophagogastroduodenoscopy (EGD)
  - ○ Colonoscopy
  - ○ Swallow assessment
  - ○ GI motility studies
  - ○ pH manometry
- • Laboratory assessment
  - ○ Complete blood count.
  - ○ Comprehensive metabolic panel.
  - ○ Coagulation profile.
  - ○ Viral blood studies to determine previous exposures as well as current immunity.
  - ○ Disease screening studies to confirm or eliminate disease. Examples include prostate specific antigen, alpha-fetoprotein, alpha-1 antitrypsin levels, copper, hemoglobin A1C, brain natriuretic peptide, creatine kinase.
- • Biopsies—performed based on patient's history and physical examination to
  - ○ Confirm presence or etiology of disease.
  - ○ Determine if abnormalities are malignant (a potential contraindication to transplantation).

6. Risks associated with transplantation
   a. Death
      i. On the waiting list
      ii. During the transplant surgery
      iii. Following transplantation
   b. Organ rejection
      i. The immune system recognizes the transplant organ as "foreign" and causes rejection.
      ii. Rejection can occur at any time after implantation of the organ(s).
      iii. Need for lifetime immunosuppression.
   c. Organ failure
      i. Primary nonfunction may require immediate relisting and retransplantation.
      ii. Delayed graft function may require supportive care and can increase length of the transplant hospital stay.
   d. Retransplantation
      i. May be indicated in cases of primary graft dysfunction, severe allograft dysfunction, advanced chronic rejection, vasculopathy, infection or return of end stage disease that is not amenable to medical or surgical therapies.[20–23]

    ii. Every transplant program determines indications for retransplantation and evaluates each candidate on a case-by-case basis. See your program criteria for more information.

  e. Infection

    i. Risk is higher due to immunosuppressed state after transplantation.

    ii. Risk of donor-transmitted disease.

- Unknown disease of donor when organ was recovered.
- Detection depends on
  - Specific tests done by the Organ Procurement Organization (OPO) coordinator during the donor evaluation process.
  - Viral incubation period: Early in the disease process, some viral diseases may not be detectable in the donor's blood at the time of the donor evaluation.
  - Advanced nucleic acid testing may reduce risk of disease transmission by detecting early-stage infections during the "window period" before antibody seroconversion is documented.[24]
- Diseases that may be undetected at the time of the donor evaluation include, but are not limited to[24-26]
  - Human immunodeficiency virus (HIV)
  - Hepatitis B or C
  - Malignancy (including melanoma)
  - Gonorrhea
  - Syphilis
  - Trichomonas
  - Chlamydia
  - Rabies

    iii. Potential sites of postoperative infection:

- Wound
- Blood stream
- Lungs
- Bladder
- Chest or abdominal cavity

  f. Cardiovascular complications

    i. Stroke

    ii. Blood clots

- Prevention may require use of sequential compression devices.
- Sequelae can affect heart, lungs, and brain.

    iii. Patients undergoing general anesthesia are at risk for complications such as myocardial infarction, dysrhythmias, and cardiac collapse.

  g. Medication side effects

    i. Both immunosuppressive and antimicrobial agents have known side effects that the transplant team monitors closely.

    ii. Patients are educated about common side effects:

- Hyperglycemia
- Hypertension
- Kidney dysfunction
- Digestive problems
- Headaches
- Tremors
- Nerve damage
- Weight gain

   iii. The transplant team may change medications based on the patient's report of side effects and monitoring of lab values.
h. General surgical risks associated with any type of surgery
   i.   Anesthesia
   ii. Nerve damage (temporary or permanent)
   iii. Bleeding
      * May require a return to the operating room to control
      * May require the use of blood and/or blood products
i. Psychosocial risks (see Table 3-1)
7. Selection criteria and evaluation outcome
   a. Information from the physical, psychosocial, and financial evaluations is reviewed by interdisciplinary transplant team to determine if the patient meets established medical and psychosocial eligibility criteria for transplantation.
   b. Eligibility is determined by selection criteria defined by each organ transplant program. Criteria differ from center to center but may include
      i.   Inclusion criteria
      ii. Exclusion criteria
      iii. Absolute or relative contraindications.
   c. Patients are informed of the following potential evaluation outcomes:
      i.   The patient met eligibility criteria and is approved as a candidate.
      ii. The patient is approved as a candidate with conditions, such as
         * Weight loss
         * Better control of diabetes or other chronic diseases
         * Approval from insurance
         * Completion of smoking, drug and/or alcohol cessation program
      iii. The transplant team is unable to make a determination at this time and further evaluation is required.
      iv. The patient does not meet selection criteria and will not be placed on the waiting list.
8. Organ allocation[18]
   a. Organ donation and transplantation processes in the United States are coordinated by the United Network for Organ Sharing (UNOS).
   b. The national waiting list is maintained 24 hours a day and 365 days per year to ensure timely allocation of organs per national allocation policies
   c. Candidates are listed in the UNOS candidate database (UNet).
      i.   Information about the candidate (blood type, height, weight, and other clinical variables) is entered into UNet.
   d. The OPO enters medical and other information about the potential donor into the UNOS donor database (DonorNet).
   e. The computerized UNOS system matches candidates to potential donors and generates a prioritized list of potential recipients that are ranked per organ-specific OPTN allocation policies.
   f. The transplant center is notified of their patients who appear on the ranked list; the on-call team considers the organ offer in terms of donor factors (e.g., age, organ quality), recipient factors (e.g., recipient's condition and availability) and logistical factors (e.g., potential ischemic time during transport of organ).

g. If the donor is identified as Public Health Service (PHS) increased risk donor, the patient is notified at the time of the organ offer and must consent to proceed with transplantation.
   i. The patient may refuse the organ offer without affecting his or her status on the national waitlist.
9. Waitlist management
   a. Patients and the interdisciplinary transplant team are responsible for waitlist management.
   b. Patient responsibilities:
      i. Notify the transplant team of any changes in their
         * Health status (including admissions to hospitals other than the transplant center)
         * Health insurance
         * Contact information (address, phone numbers)
         * Availability to come to the transplant center
            ○ Patients are instructed that unavailability must be discussed in advance with the transplant team and that their unavailability may result in a potential loss of an organ offer
      ii. Obtain required diagnostic studies, bloodwork, or consultations while waiting for transplantation to ensure they remain viable candidates for transplant.
         * This includes organ-specific lab or other tests that may be required in order for the patient to remain active on the waiting list.[27]
         * Examples: tests to calculate the Lung Allocation Score (LAS) or the Model for End Stage Liver Disease (MELD) score.
         * Failure to complete required testing may result in a change in candidate's priority on the waitlist.[18]
      iii. Patients must attend transplant clinic appointments on a schedule determined by the severity of their end-organ disease or program protocol.
      iv. In addition to the transplant team, patients should have a primary care provider to attend to and assist with their health maintenance and acute health needs.
   c. Transplant coordinator responsibilities
      i. Identify the requirements for candidates to maintain active status on the UNOS waitlist in accordance to the organ-specific allocation system
      ii. Monitor physical and emotional health of candidates during the waiting time.[28]
      iii. Arrange studies, labs or consultations for waitlist management
      iv. Educate candidates about any changes in their waitlist status and rationale for additional tests or procedures studies.[28]
         * Failure to complete required testing, may result in a change in the candidate's priority on the waitlist.
      v. Identify resources for patient and caregiver support including:
         * Social worker
         * Registered dietician
         * Financial coordinator
         * Support groups including one-on-one interaction with a previous transplant recipient willing to share experiences.
10. Living donation
    a. Kidney, liver, and lung programs may perform living donor surgery.

b. Transplant professionals may provide information to candidates about how to speak to others about being a living organ donor.[7,29]

c. See the chapter on Care of Living Donors for additional information

11. Examples of patient and caregiver concerns while on the waiting list include[29,30]

a. Deteriorating physical health

b. Psychological concerns:
   i. Fear of dying before an organ becomes available
   ii. Depression
   iii. Anxiety

c. Financial concerns:
   i. Loss of employment
   ii. Insurance coverage[28]

d. Other healthcare providers
   i. Lack of education, information and support from various healthcare providers.[30]
   ii. Contradiction among providers regarding information relevant to the patient's health status.[31]

e. Caregiver burdens
   i. Fatigue[32,33]
   ii. Depression[34]

B. Transplant phase

1. Education pertaining to the transplant phase:
   a. Begins during evaluation in order to prepare the patient and caregivers about the hospitalization
   b. Continues throughout the hospitalization with the goal of preparing the patient and caregivers for discharge and assuming self-care

2. Key considerations for education during the transplant phase:
   a. Include caregivers in all aspects of transplant education.
   b. When assessing readiness for learning, consider learner's physiologic and psychological state for potential barriers to learning (e.g., effects of medications, pain, and anxiety).
   c. Develop a structured education plan that outlines day-to-day expectations for patient learning or activity.
      i. A structured plan increases patient and caregiver engagement and creates uniformity in the delivery of content.[9]
   d. Adapt teaching methods to the learner's literacy skills or disability.
   e. Focus educational topics on the minimal knowledge required for the patient and caregiver provide safe care from discharge to the first posttransplant clinic visit.
   f. Utilize educational checklists which are advantageous because they
      i. Reduce the variability in the information that is provided by different members of the interdisciplinary transplant team.
      ii. Facilitate the learner's understanding of the goals of transplant education.[11]
   g. Ensure that all members of the interdisciplinary team participate in the education plan.
   h. Teach the most important topics at the beginning or the end of the education session.
   i. Provide written instructions with simple terminology including clear, concise pictures.

    j. Link instructions for patient actions at home to activities of daily living like bathing, meals, and waking and sleeping times.

    k. Provide demonstration for skills needs to be performed at home; provide opportunities for patients and caregivers to give a return demonstration.

    l. Providing an excessive amount of information at one time may overwhelm learners and reduce the amount of information they can recall. Therefore, schedule educational sessions throughout the hospitalization to prevent overloading patients and caregivers with too much information on the day of discharge.[11]

3. General educational topics:
   a. Surgical procedure and progression of postoperative recovery
   b. Potential postoperative complications
   c. Medications and medication management
   d. Daily home monitoring and activity
   e. Nutrition and food safety
   f. Psychosocial concerns
   g. Lifestyle changes
   h. Communication with the transplant team
   i. Health maintenance after transplantation

4. Discussion points for general educational topics (*Note*: Detailed information is patient- and organ-specific)
   a. Surgical procedure and progression of postoperative recovery
      i. Placement of the organ in the patient's body, site, and size of incision
      ii. Whether or not native organ will be removed
      iii. Length of time in the operating room dependent on the procedure(s) to be completed
      iv. Periodic updates from operating room staff
      v. Possible need for use of blood products during the operation
      vi. Immediate recovery period after the operation (organ and patient specific)
         - Intensive monitoring in the postoperative period
            ○ Vital signs
            ○ Intake and output
            ○ Cardiac monitoring
            ○ Mechanical ventilation
            ○ Management of surgical wound(s)
            ○ Surgical drains (e.g., chest tubes, Jackson-Pratt [JP] drains)
            ○ Invasive lines, tubes, and catheters (e.g., intravenous line, arterial line, nasogastric tubes, Swan–Ganz pulmonary artery catheter, Foley urinary catheter)
         - Pain assessment
            ○ Source and type of pain
            ○ Use of pain scale to rate severity of pain[35]
            ○ Types of pain medications available
            ○ Alternative forms of pain management[36]
         - Pain management strategies
            ○ Take pain medication 45 minutes to 1 hour prior to activity such as ambulation or activities of daily living
            ○ Specify the pain scale score at which pain medication is needed to facilitate ambulating, breathing, and sleeping comfortably.
         - Routine postoperative activities

○ Pulmonary toilet
○ Early ambulation and sitting in chair
○ Sequential compression devices
○ Splinting of incision during pulmonary toilet and other activity
- Fluid and nutritional needs
  ○ Needs will be assessed throughout the recovery trajectory.
  ○ Oral intake will be resumed as the team determines the patient is ready for liquids; patient will be slowly progressed to a solid diet.
  ○ Potential need for additional nutrition resources in the form of enteral nutrition or oral supplements due to their pretransplant cachexia or posttransplant complications.
- Length of stay
  ○ Varies according to organ(s) transplanted, postoperative complications, and recovery.
- Monitoring for rejection
  ○ Daily laboratory work including immunosuppression lab values.
  ○ Radiographic studies,
  ○ Invasive testing (based on organ transplanted) may include biopsy, bronchoscopy, and ileoscopy.
- Monitoring for infection
  ○ Daily laboratory work
  ○ Cultures
  ○ Clinical manifestations of infection including:
    ▪ Fever
    ▪ Pain, redness, swelling, and purulent discharge at the incision
    ▪ Nausea/vomiting/diarrhea

b. Potential postoperative complications
  i. Primary graft nonfunction
    - Possible need for relisting for another transplant
      ○ Potential that team will determine patient is not a candidate for retransplantation
    - Ongoing care while waiting for that organ to become available
    - Potential need for palliative or end-of-life care
  ii. Delayed graft function
    - Supportive therapies available to maintain optimal patient status until graft function improves (organ specific)
      ○ Dialysis
      ○ Ventilator support
      ○ Mechanical circulatory assist devices
      ○ Medications (e.g., inotropic agents)
  iii. Bleeding: Management may require
    - Return to the operating room
    - Use of blood and blood products
  iv. Clinical manifestations of rejection (see Table 3-2)[37,38]
  v. Clinical manifestations of infection
c. Medications and medication management
  i. Medications are administered according to organ-specific protocols.
  ii. Some patients may undergo induction immunosuppression at the time of allograft implantation and in the postoperative recovery period.

TABLE 3-2 **Signs and Symptoms of Infection**

- Fever (over 37.8°C)
- Persistent chills or "hot flushes"
- Cough (persistent or production of colored sputum)
- Changes in urination (increased frequency, burning, pain, hematuria)
- Shortness of breath
- Persistent fatigue
- Anorexia/weight loss
- Nausea, vomiting, or diarrhea lasting more than 24 h

- Joint pain or muscle ache
- Swollen glands
- Persistent or severe sore throat
- Persistent "head cold" symptoms such as nasal discharge, sinus pain, and/or headache
- Skin rash or lesions
- Persistent headache, with or without alteration in level of consciousness
- Vaginal discharge or burning
- Redness, swelling, pain, odor, or discharge at wound, drain, or stoma site

Cupples S, Ohler L. *Transplant Nursing Secrets*. Philadelphia, PA: Hanley & Belfus, 2003; Randolph S, Scholz K. Self care guidelines: finding common ground. *J Transpl Coord*. 1999;9(3):156–160.

   iii. Patient response to immunosuppression medications is monitored closely.
- Adjustments to dosing of immunosuppression are patient-specific and can be based on therapeutic drug levels and individual patient's response to the medications.

   iv. Side effects of immunosuppressants and antimicrobial agents to prevent or treat infection are monitored closely.
- The patient's treatment plan may be altered based on the ability to tolerate medications.
- See section on Medication Side Effects above.

   v. Decisions regarding antimicrobial agents are based on both donor- and recipient-specific information.
- Cytomegalovirus (CMV) prophylaxis is determined by the recipient and donor CMV IgG status at the time of transplantation. This determines the need for and duration of prophylaxis.
- Anti-bacterial and anti-fungal medications may be given to prevent Pneumocystis pneumonia (PCP), thrush, and other infections that are of concern for a specific patient.

   vi. Patient-specific medication education is provided by the transplant pharmacist and the transplant coordinator.[39] Topics include
- Right medication:
  - Name of each medication (including brand name and generic name)
  - Purpose of each medication
  - Potential side effects the patient and caregivers should monitor
- Right dose:
  - The patient should understand the dose of each medication and how to identify different strengths of the same medication
  - Dose of medications can change, sometimes on a daily basis. This may be in response to a specific lab value, such as a drug level, or due to patient's side effects.

- Right time
  - Taking medications at the same time every day is very important.
  - Critical-dose drugs such as tacrolimus, cyclosporine, sirolimus, and everolimus must be taken at specific time intervals to allow for therapeutic drug monitoring.
  - This is of particular importance on the days that the patient is having a serum drug level drawn.
  - Patients must understand when they are to take their immunosuppressant medications prior to a serum blood draw: the night before the blood draw or the morning of the blood draw. The timing will depend on whether these immunosuppressant medications are taken once daily or every 12 hours.
  - Patients should understand what to do if they miss a dose of medication, or they are unable to take medication due to nausea/vomiting or have prolonged diarrhea.
  - Utilizing a structured approach to taking medications may be helpful to patients and their families. This may include
    - Use of a medication box with day and hour subdivisions. The box may be pre-loaded by the pharmacist at the time of discharge with the patient and caregivers participating to ensure accuracy of the medications at the appropriate times.
    - A written medication roster identifying pictures, times and doses of each medication.
    - A written list of acceptable over-the-counter medications as applicable.
    - Setting alarms on devices such as watches and smart phones as reminders for dosing times.
    - Scheduling medication times around other activities of daily living such as meals and bedtime may assist a patient with remaining on schedule.
- Right way:
  - Patients should know how to take each medication; for example, whether or not
    - A tablet can be crushed or a capsule can be opened.
    - The medication should be taken with or without food.
  - Drug–drug and drug–food interactions.
    - Interactions with over-the-counter drugs or supplements.
    - Interactions with foods, such as grapefruit, which increase serum levels of certain immunosuppression medications
- Other
  - Patients should notify the transplant team before starting any new medication prescribed by another provider.
  - Patients should avoid non-steroidal medications as these may increase risk of renal toxicity after transplant.
  - Patients should not take over the counter medications (unless previously approved by the transplant team), dietary or herbal supplements or Chinese medications.
  - Instructions on the correct storage of medications (e.g., medications should not be kept in the kitchen or bathroom).

d. Daily home monitoring and activity
  i. Vital signs should be monitored and recorded daily in the early posttransplant phase. This may include

- Temperature
- Blood pressure
- Weight
  - Same scale, same time of day
  - Weights on home scale may differ slightly from weight on clinic scale
- Spirometry (lung transplant)
- Intake and output provide
  - Demonstration and return demonstration on correct way to measure.
  - Handout with volume of commonly used containers.
  - Container to measure output
- Monitoring should be done at the same time every day
- More frequent monitoring may be required if a patient has clinical manifestations of a potential complication
- Patients should be given specific parameters for which patients should contact the transplant team (e.g., particularly regarding parameters pertaining to temperature, blood pressure, spirometry volume, and weight gain)

ii. Surgical site
- Should be assessed at least daily for
  - Appearance
  - Color (any redness?)
  - Swelling
  - Drainage (type; amount)
  - Odor
  - Signs of wound separation, dehiscence
- The patient should be given instructions about when to call the transplant center with concerns.
- If the patient is discharged with wound care needs, such as packing, the patient or caregiver should give a return demonstration of the proper technique and have supplies in hand at the time of discharge.
- Some patients may require referral to a home health agency to assist with wound care if complex (wound vac).

e. Nutrition and food safety
  i. The dietitian provides education about the general discharge nutrition plan for each patient.
  - General instructions for a healthy diet
  - Specific instructions as indicated, for example:
    - Diabetic diet
    - Limitations regarding fluid intake or consumption of foods high in potassium
    - Enteral feedings with recommendations for formula and length of feeds including additional water supplementation if needed
    - Weight loss or weight gain
  - Additionally, patients are given instructions regarding posttransplant food safety precautions
    - See section on Infection Prevention below

f. Psychosocial concerns
  i. Potential psychosocial concerns related to transplantation[33]
  - Adjustment to medication side effects

- Independence from equipment, medications, and procedures related to the previous end-organ disease
- Changes in self-perception
- Uncertainty regarding the future
- Unrealistic expectations
- Disappointment in the early outcomes of the transplant phase
- Guilt about donor death
- Mood swings
- Whether or not to contact the donor family

    ii. Mental health resources

g. Lifestyle changes

    i. Potential activity restrictions:

- Lifting any item > 5 to 10 pounds
- Soaking in a tub or swimming and using a hot tub.
- Contact sports.
- Driving will be prohibited until the patient is re-assessed by the transplant team.

    ii. Physical activity is encouraged.

- Patients should engage in walking and activities of daily living.
- The physical therapist may give recommendations regarding a posttransplant exercise plan.
- Resumption of more vigorous activity such as running or gym workouts should be discussed first with the transplant team.

    iii. Infection prevention

- Family members and visitors should
  - Wash their hands well before and after contact with the patient.
    - Sanitizing hand gels may be used if soap and water are not immediately available.
  - Cover mouth and nose when coughing and sneezing.
  - Avoid contact with the patient if they are sick.
- Patients should not
  - Share eating utensils or drinking containers with others
  - Clean cat litter, bird cages, or fish tanks
  - Handle animal waste, which can harbor organisms
  - Be in areas with large crowds, particularly if air is being recycled (e.g., in movie theaters, airplanes)
  - Change diapers or care for children who have just received a live vaccine
- Patients should promptly report any exposure to a communicable disease to the transplant team

    iv. Travel

- Patients should not travel extensively immediately after discharge due to
  - The need for close monitoring and follow-up
  - Potential unplanned tests or clinic visits
  - Potential need for readmission to the hospital

h. Communication with the transplant team

    i. Patients and caregivers should have a clear understanding of when and how to contact the transplant team members.

    ii. Non-urgent matters may include
- Medication refills
- Verification of appointment date and time
- Questions following a clinic visit or lab work
- General concerns about diet, activity, and exercise

   iii. Urgent matters may include
- Signs and symptoms of infection (Table 3-2)[37,38]
- Signs and symptoms of rejection (Table 3-3)[37,40-44]
- New drainage from the wound
- Chest pain
- Shortness of breath
- Bleeding: potential sources:
  - Oral (e.g., emesis)
  - Rectal
  - Wound
  - Ostomy
- Signs of stroke: "FAST" Stroke Recognition and Response[45]
  - Facial weakness
  - Arm weakness
  - Speech problems
  - Time to act

   iv. Patients and caregivers should have written information on how to reach the transplant team during business hours, after hours, and on weekends and holidays.

TABLE 3-3 **Summary of Signs of Rejection**

Liver[40]	Kidney[41]	Heart[42]	Lung[43]	Pancreas[44]	Intestine[37]
Elevated liver enzymes	Elevated urea and creatinine	Irregular heartbeat	Shortness of breath	High blood glucose levels	Change in stool output
Tenderness over liver	Decreased urine output	Very fast or very slow heartbeat	Tiredness		Tiredness
Yellow color to eyes or skin	Weight gain	Low blood pressure	Productive cough		Abdominal pain or distention
Dark urine	Pain at site of kidney	Shortness of breath	Change in color of sputum		Nausea and vomiting
Fatigue	Fatigue	Leg swelling	Decrease in spirometry readings		Dusky stoma
Ascites	Leg swelling	Weight gain	Fever		Weight loss
Fever	Fever	Fatigue			Bleeding
		Fever			Fever

Cupples S, Ohler L. *Transplant Nursing Secrets*. Philadelphia, PA: Hanley & Belfus, 2003; Grogan TA. Liver transplantation: issues and nursing care requirements. *Crit Care Nurs Clin North Am*. 2011;23:443–456; Murphy F. The role of the nurse post-renal transplantation. *Br J Nurs*. 2007;16(11):667–675; Wade CR, Reith KK, Sikora JH, et al. Postoperative nursing care of the cardiac transplant recipient. *Crit Care Nurs Q*. 2004;27(1):17–28; Dabbs ADV, Hoffman LA, Iacono AT, et al. Are symptom reports useful for differentiating between acute rejection and pulmonary infection after lung transplantation? *Heart Lung*. 2004;372–380; White SA, Shaw JA, Sutherland DER. Pancreas transplantation. *Lancet*. 2009;373:1808–1817.

v. Patients may be diagnosed with hyperglycemia or post-transplant diabetes during the transplant phase.

- Diabetic education should be provided so the patient and caregiver understand how to measure glucose readings with a glucometer. The patient and caregiver should be able to demonstrate how to utilize the glucometer.
- If insulin is prescribed to the patient, then the patient and caregiver should understand
  - The type of insulin(s) to be used
  - How to administer insulin by injection, and give a return demonstration including drawing up or dialing up the correct dosage, preparing the injection site, and rotation of sites.
  - The patient and caregiver should also be able to state signs and symptoms of hypo- and hyperglycemia.
  - Patients and caregivers should have contact information and parameters for contacting the team managing their glucose control.
- Patients and their caregivers should understand basic signs and symptoms of infection.

C. Posttransplant Phase
1. Posttransplant education
    a. Begins during the transplant admission and continues until graft failure or patient death
    b. Includes topics that range from postoperative recovery to long-term health maintenance
2. Key considerations for education during the posttransplant phase:
    a. The initial discharge event may be overwhelming to patients; call the patient the day after discharge to answer questions and review medications.
    b. Every interaction with a patient and caregiver is an opportunity to teach and reinforce information.
    c. Encourage patient to use a daily log of activity, vital signs, and questions; review the log with the patient at each clinic visit.
    d. Although the frequency of postdischarge clinic visits are organ-specific and change as recovery progresses, these visits provide opportunities to reinforce and review content taught during the transplant phase.
    e. Patients often identify topics of importance as they progress physically and emotionally and are ready to return to their normal activities.
    f. Topics may be repeated when they relate to the patient's recovery or as reminders to patients who are not progressing as expected.
        i. Repeating previously discussed education topics at 3 months posttransplant reinforces concepts at a time when patients are more aware of how a transplant affects their overall health, emotional state and lifestyle.[15]
    g. As patients experience new complications or conditions, timely education allows the patient to integrate new information when it is most meaningful and relates to their health.
3. Goals for patient education in the posttransplant phase
    a. Self-management is the overall goal of patient education after transplantation.[38]
        i. Self-management is a set of skills that patients demonstrate to follow a prescribed therapy, avoid health deterioration, and preserve function.

      ii. Poor self-management may result in poor clinical outcomes including rejection, infection, graft failure, or death.[15]

      iii. Tasks of self-management.

         • Manage illness and symptoms by maintaining a healthy lifestyle and following prescribed therapies.

         • Maintain meaningful role in everyday life.

         • Manage emotions associated with living with chronic illness.

      iv. Transplant nurses promote self-management by

         • Providing explanations about all medications, interventions, or recommendations[15]

         • Teaching skills for monitoring vital signs, medication preparation and obtaining medication refills[46]

4. Key educational topics

  a. Daily self-monitoring

      i. Temperature, blood pressure, heart rate, and weight[47]

      ii. Urine and indwelling drain output if present

      iii. Blood glucose monitoring[47]

      iv. Wound appearance and drainage

  b. Activity

      i. Regular exercise is recommended to maintain a healthy weight and improve cardiovascular health.

      ii. Recreational and athletic activity may improve self-esteem and prevent depression.[48]

      iii. Walking is a generally safe exercise that may be increased gradually over time.[47] Explore patient's options for walking and assist them in developing a plan to gradually increase activity over time. Options may include

         • Treadmill at health club or in home

         • Outside in neighborhood or park

         • Retail malls may be open for walking in early morning

         • School tracks

      iv. Contact sports should be avoided.

      v. Heart transplant patients must perform 10- to 15-minute warm-up activity to increase circulating catecholamine due to the denervated heart's inability to quickly increase rate. A cool down period is also important.

      vi. Patients should discuss engaging in strenuous activities such as weightlifting with their providers.

         • Weightlifting, for example, may lead to incisional hernias.

  c. Medications and medication management

      i. Medication adherence is a key component to maintaining health after transplantation.

      ii. Assess patient's adherence through interviewing to determine patterns of missed medications.

         • Reasons for not taking medications may include

            ○ Forgetfulness

            ○ Fear of side effects such as weight gain

            ○ Frustration with frequency or number of medications

            ○ Belief that medications are no longer needed

- The International Transplant Nurses Society Pocket Guide *Interventions to Common Medication Adherence Barriers* is an evidence-based tool that is useful in identifying barriers to medication adherence and potential solutions to adherence problems (www.itns.org).

   iii. Adherence can also be assessed by

- Review of pharmacy records of prescription refills
- Discussions with caregiver

   iv. Transplant clinicians and providers can promote adherence by

- Fostering positive relationships between patients and healthcare providers
- Providing ongoing reinforcement and support
- Encouraging self-management
- Discontinuing medications when no longer indicated
- Simplifying the medication regimen to align with daily activities and reducing number of times medications are given.
- Providing written materials, audiovisual education and verbal instruction tailored to the patient's health literacy level.[48]

   v. Assess patient's knowledge of medications and provide additional education any time a medication is added or discontinued or there is a change in administration (e.g., dose, time of day).

   vi. Assist the patient in medication self-administration.

- Use medication organizers or reminder devices.
- Link medication administration to daily activity.
- Review and reconcile medications at each visit.[48]

d. Diet

   i. Diet recommendations change over time and are unique to each patient's situation in the early discharge phase.

- Patients may be below their ideal body weight due to pretransplant cachexia or a decreased appetite posttransplant. Therefore, patients may be allowed to have a high calorie, high fat diet initially to promote weight gain.
- Certain dietary restrictions may be required due to renal function or volume status but will usually be removed later in the recovery period.

   ii. Encourage a healthy diet low in fat, sugar and salt and high in fiber.[47]

   iii. Reinforce provider's orders regarding fluid intake.

e. Infection prevention

   i. Hand hygiene: Patients are instructed to

- Wash their hands frequently, as hand-washing is a best practice to prevent infection
- Wash hands with soap and water
- Wash hands
  - Before preparing meals
  - Before and after eating
  - Before and after touching wounds or mucous membranes
  - After using the bathroom
  - After contact with any excretions or secretions, including nasal secretions

- ◦ After contact with animals
- ◦ After changing diapers (note: it is preferable that another individual change diapers rather than the patient)
- ◦ After touching any items that may have come in contact with feces (human or animal)
- ◦ After touching plants and soil
- • Carry antibacterial gel to use when hands are not visibly soiled and when water and soap are not available.

ii. Airborne infections

- • Avoid individuals with known infection
  - ◦ Ask visitors who have had recent infections to postpone visiting
  - ◦ If contact cannot be avoided, the transplant recipient and the ill person should wear surgical masks
- • Avoid crowded areas where close contact is likely including shopping malls and subways especially when community rates of influenza are high.[48]
- • Avoid smoking (tobacco and marijuana) and exposure to tobacco smoke

iii. Dietary precautions

- • Do not eat raw or undercooked meat and seafood.
- • Do not consume raw eggs or eggs that are not thoroughly cooked, including eggs in batter, cookie dough, certain salad dressings and other products.
- • Do not consume unpasteurized foods including:
  - ◦ Milk
  - ◦ Products made from unpasteurized milk (e.g., certain soft cheeses)
  - ◦ Fruit or vegetable juices or ciders
- • Do not eat raw seed sprouts
- • Prevent cross-contamination between raw and cooked foods when preparing food.
- • Wash "bag" lettuce, spinach, and other vegetable products, even though the labeling states that the product does not require re-washing.
- • Monitor local reports of foodborne illness outbreaks

iv. Waterborne infections[48,49]

- • Drinking water from wells may need to be tested for organisms that may place the immunosuppressed patient at risk (e.g., *Cryptosporidium*).
- • Observe local "boil water" advisories.
- • Avoid swallowing water from lakes, rivers, or the ocean.
- • Assess cleanliness of pools, lakes, rivers, and the ocean prior to entering.

v. Animal safety

- • Keep pets immunized and in good health[49,50]
- • Avoid cleaning aquariums, bird cages, and feeders; avoid handling fecal matter especially cat litter where bacteria may become airborne.
  - ◦ If this is unavoidable, recipient should wear gloves (disposable) and a surgical mask.
- • Avoid contact with pets or other animals with diarrhea.

- Avoid stray animals; do not pet stray animals as they may bite and/or scratch.
- Postpone getting new pets until immunosuppression is more stable (6 to 12 months after transplant).
- Follow strict hand hygiene guidelines after contact to help reduce the risk of infection transmission.[49]

vi. Others
- Complete medication for infection prophylaxis or treatment as directed.
- Clean and cover recent cuts or wounds.
- Wear gloves and mask for garden activity or working in dirt.
- Avoid changing diapers of children who were recently vaccinated[51]
  ○ Shedding after vaccination with live virus vaccines may continue for days, weeks or months, depending upon the vaccine given and the health or other individual host factors of the vaccinated person.[51]

vii. Transplant programs may have additional infection prevention guidelines regarding the consumption of tap water, use of water filters, potential exposure to mold spores, use of hot tubs, etc.

f. Psychological care
  i. Psychological health after transplant is as important as physical health.
  ii. Monitor patient for signs of depression and anxiety.
  iii. Differences in perceived expectation versus actual outcome may contribute to patient's psychological health.

g. Health maintenance after transplantation
  i. Obtain all labs tests and other studies to monitor levels of immunosuppression and organ function.
  ii. Obtain all recommended inactivated vaccinations
  - Annual influenza vaccine (not the live vaccine option)
    ○ Note: It is important for caregivers, family members, and co-workers to receive annual influenza vaccinations unless otherwise contraindicated.
  - Pneumococcal vaccine ≥8 weeks after transplant.
  - Hepatitis A and B if not immunized pretransplant.
  - Human papillomavirus (HPV) for pediatric patients prior to sexual activity.[50,52]
  - Transplant recipients may require boosters earlier, due to immunosuppression.
  - Immunosuppressed patients should not receive live-virus vaccines.
    ○ Varicella and herpes zoster vaccines are contraindicated after transplantation.[51,53]
    ○ Avoid contact with family members who have had live virus vaccine within 2 weeks.[51,53]

  iii. Reduce risk of malignancy through recommended screening and healthy lifestyle.
  - Counsel recipients who continue to smoke about the increased risk of lung cancer; provide smoking cessation resources.
  - Breast health
    ○ Monthly self-examination

- ○ Mammograms per provider's assessment or as recommended by the American Cancer Society.[53]
- Papanicolaou test: Regular assessment by gynecologist
- Testicular health
  - ○ Monthly self-examination
- Prostate health
  - ○ Annual prostate screening antigen (PSA)
  - ○ Obtain urology consultation for symptoms of urinary obstruction and recurrent urinary tract infection
- Colonoscopy
  - ○ Complete first screening examination by age 50 or as recommended for history of inflammatory bowel disease or family history of colon cancer.
  - ○ Outcome of the exam determines the follow-up interval.[54]
- Skin care
  - ○ Examination by a health care provider annually.[52,55]
  - ○ Routine self-examination; report any changes immediately
  - ○ Risk of skin cancer
    - ▪ Squamous cell carcinoma increases over time after transplantation.[55]
    - ▪ Skin cancer is the most common malignancy in transplant recipients. The types and prevalence of skin cancers are discussed in the noninfectious diseases chapter.
    - ▪ Sun exposed areas of skin are the predominant location of squamous cell carcinomas
  - ○ Sun precautions:
    - ▪ Reduce exposure to sun
    - ▪ When in the sun encourage the use of sunscreen with an SPF >50, high-UVA absorption, hats, and clothing.[56]
    - ▪ Plan outdoor activities for early or late in the day.
    - ▪ Dental care
    - ▪ Regular visits to the dentist are recommended.
    - ▪ Inform dentist of immunosuppressed status.
    - ▪ Dental prophylaxis may be required depending upon the type of dental procedure. Discuss with transplant team at least a week before appointment.
  - h. Rejection
    - i. Rejection occurs because patient's immune system has recognized foreign tissue.
    - ii. Risk of rejection persists throughout patient's life; risk may be higher after decreases in immunosuppression dose or with changes to other formulations or brands.
    - iii. May evoke fear in recipients and caregivers; explain how recipient is monitored for rejection.
    - iv. Types of rejection
      - Acute cellular
        - ○ Initiated by activation of lymphocytes.
        - ○ May occur within a few days of transplant.
        - ○ More common initially after transplant but may occur at any time.

○ Typically a short-term condition that responds to treatment.
○ Patient will continued to be monitored with clinic visits, lab tests, and possible rebiopsy.[57]
- Chronic rejection
  ○ Leads to vasculopathy in the transplanted organ
  ○ May occur weeks to years after transplantation
  ○ Typically does not respond to therapy given for acute rejection
  ○ May lead to retransplantation[20-23]

v. Diagnosis of rejection
- Clinical manifestations
- History of symptoms
- Physical assessment
- Biopsy:
  ○ Direct assessment of tissue to determine pathophysiological state
  ○ May be performed per protocol or based on patient's symptoms
  ○ Procedure specific to type of organ transplanted

vi. Treatment of rejection
- Determined by type and severity of rejection
- Readmission might be required for IV medications and/or patient monitoring

i. Reactivation of latent viruses
  i. Cytomegalovirus (CMV)
  - Typically managed with posttransplant prophylaxis
  - Potential risk throughout patient's lifetime
  - May reactivate after treatment for severe rejection
  - Requires treatment and surveillance of viral load

  ii. Varicella zoster
  - Lesions typically appear along dermatome
  - Requires anti-viral therapy; may require pain medication to prevent post herpetic neuralgia.

  iii. Herpes simplex virus: Lesions may reappear following transplantation
  iv. See Chapter on Infectious Diseases for additional information

j. Long-term effects of immunosuppression.
  i. Diabetes mellitus (DM).
  - May be induced by immunosuppressive agents.
  - Patients may develop DM as they age.
  - Requires strict management of blood glucose levels to minimize long-term effects.[57,58]

  ii. Hypertension
  - Side effect of certain immunosuppressants
  - Deleterious to kidney function
  - May require antihypertensive agents

  iii. Hyperlipidemia
  - Side effect of medications
  - May be managed with medications,[58,59] dietary changes, and exercise

  iv. Renal dysfunction
  - May develop over time
  - Potential etiology: medications, pre-existing kidney disease, infection, and hypovolemia

- Potential treatment options:
  - Reduction or modification of immunosuppressant dose
  - Renal-sparing diuretic agents
- May progress to renal failure and need for kidney transplantation
  v. Osteopenia or osteoporosis
  - Certain patients may be at higher risk due to pretransplant illness.
  - Immunosuppression may reduce bone mass.
  - Exercise recommended to slow bone loss.
  - May require medication, calcium and vitamin D supplements.[58]
k. Sexual health
  i. Transplant recipients and their partners want information regarding sexual activity.
  ii. Typically may resume sexual activity when they are comfortable in doing so, unless otherwise contraindicated.
  iii. Encourage use of condoms to prevent sexually transmitted diseases.[49]
  iv. Discuss use of oral contraception with provider; may be contraindicated due to risk of thromboembolic events.
  v. Emergency contraception may be considered in certain circumstances.
  vi. Counsel recipients about increased risk of infection with intrauterine devices.[40]
  vii. Sexual dysfunction or changes in libido may be related to medications. Encourage patients to openly communicate their concerns to healthcare providers
  viii. Posttransplant body image changes may affect the recipient.
  ix. Pediatric recipients should receive the HPV and hepatitis B vaccine prior to engaging in sexual activity.[44]
l. Pregnancy after transplantation
  i. Encourage patient to discuss potential pregnancy with transplant team and obstetrician; it is important for patient to understand
    - Timing of pregnancy
    - Risk of medications to fetus
    - Potential risk of rejection
    - Physical effects of pregnancy on recipient
    - Ethical considerations relative to the lifespan of the recipient and ability to care for a child[34]
  ii. Males may father a child after transplantation
  iii. Recommendation: Postpone pregnancy until 1 year after transplant when immunosuppressant doses are likely to be lower[29,40]
  iv. Refer pregnant recipients and males who have fathered a child to the National Transplant Pregnancy Registry: www.giftoflifeinstitute.org
m. Appearance
  i. Transplantation may lead to body image changes associated with medications and sequelae of surgical procedure.
  ii. Weight gain and hair loss may occur with certain medications.
n. Return to work
  i. Timing depends on patient's recovery and type of employment.
  ii. Counsel patient to initially telework or work part-time (e.g., half days) and gradually increase to full-time employment as energy level improves.

  iii. Assess patient's work activities to determine suitability; discuss potential restrictions (e.g., weightlifting; exposure to toxic agents) and required precautions.

  iv. Refer patients to Social Worker or Vocational Rehabilitation if patients should not return to their previous employment.

o. Travel

  i. Patients are typically instructed to avoid traveling away from home during the first few months posttransplant

  ii. Considerations for selection of travel destinations:

- Current health of patient, including any physical limitations
- Risk of infection, including risk of endemic infections in area

  iii. Assist patient in locating health care provider at destination should medical care be required.

  iv. Medications.

- Pack 2- to 3-day supply in carry-on luggage
- Bring more medication than needed in case of unexpected delays; store in original containers[60,61]

  v. Bring

- Basic first-aid kit that includes a thermometer, antiseptic, and medications to treat cuts, bruises, nausea, and diarrhea
- Summary of health history including surgical procedure and current medications

  vi. Consider travel insurance and purchase of a medic alert tag

  vii. Depending on destination, consultation with Travel Clinic to identify potential health hazards and need for specific medications or vaccinations to prevent infection[60]

  viii. The Centers for Disease Control and Prevention has useful travel information for patients and clinicians: www.nc.cdc.gov/travel.

p. Donor–recipient confidentiality

  i. Recipients may be informed of specific donor information if it is critical to recipient informed consent for transplantation. Examples include

- Possible donor-transmitted disease risks
- Organ characteristics or anatomic abnormality that could affect organ function

  ii. The Organ Procurement Organization (OPO) may provide general information about the recipient status to the donor family without permission as this communication is deemed part of organ allocation. Donor families will receive a letter from the OPO within 30 days of the donation. Information that may be provided without recipient permission includes

- Age described in decades (child, teenager, adult)
- General status of health
- Gender[62]

  iii. Information that should *not* be shared without the recipient's permission:

- Religion
- Ethnicity/race
- Specific diagnosis

- Sexual orientation
- Chronic illness unrelated to the donation
- Transplant complication or death of recipient if related to transplant

iv. Potential donor family–recipient communication

- Requires consent from donor family and recipient.
- No specific time requirement before communication may begin.
  - It is preferred to allow the recipient time to recover and the donor family time to grieve.
- Timing depends on individual needs of recipient and donor family.
- OPO facilitates mutually agreed-upon communication.[62]
- This process varies from program to program. See your transplant guidelines for more information.

REFERENCES

1. International Transplant Nurses Society. *Transplant Nursing Scope and Standards of Practice.* 1st ed. Silver Spring, MD: American Nurses Publishing; 2009.
2. Redman BK. *The Practice of Patient Education: A Case Study Approach.* St. Louis, MO: Mosby; 2007.
3. Rankin S, Stallings K, London F. *Patient Education in Health and Illness.* Philadelphia, PA: Mosby; 2005.
4. Center for Medicare and Medicaid Services. *Organ Transplant Interpretive Guidelines. X150: Standard: Informed Consent for Transplant Patients.* Available at https://www.cms.gov/Medicare/Provider-Enrollment-and-Certification/SurveyCertificationGenInfo/downloads/SCLetter08-25.pdf, http://www.cms.gov/Medicare/Provider-Enrollment-and-Certification/GuidanceforLawsAndRegulations/Downloads/SurveyCertLetterInterpretiveGuidance.pdf. Accessed September 7, 2015.
5. Curtis C, Rothstein M, Hong B. Stage-specific educational interventions for patients with end-stage renal disease: psychological and psychiatric considerations. *Prog Transplant.* 2009;19(1):18–24.
6. Chang M, Kelly A. Patient education: addressing cultural diversity and health literacy issues. *Urol Nur.* 2007;27(5):411–417.
7. Wilson R, Brown D, Boothe M, et al. Improving delivery of patient education about kidney transplant in a transplant center. *Prog Transplant.* 2012;22(4):403–412.
8. Gordon E, Wolf M. Health literacy skills of kidney transplant patients. *Prog Transplant.* 2009;19(1):25–34.
9. Frank-Bader M, Beltran K, Dojlidko D. Improving transplant discharge education using a structured teaching approach. *Prog Transplant.* 2011;21(4):332–339.
10. Davis L, Ryszkiewicz E, Schenk E, et al. Lung transplant or bust: patient's recommendations for ideal lung transplant education. *Prog Transplant.* 2014;24(2):132–141.
11. Schaevers V, Schoonis A, Frickx G, et al. Implementing a standardized, evidence-based education program using the patient's electronic file for lung transplant recipients. *Prog Transplant.* 2012;22(3):264–270.
12. Patzer R, Perryman J, Pastan S, et al. Impact of a patient education program on disparities in kidney transplant evaluation. *Clin J Am Soc Nephrol.* 2012;7:648–655.
13. Myers J, Pellino T. Developing new ways to address learning needs of adult abdominal organ transplant recipients. *Prog Transplant.* 2009;19(2):160–166.
14. Possemato K, Geller P. Web resources for transplant candidates, recipients, and donors. *Prog Transplant.* 2007;17(2):161–166.
15. Haspeslagh A, De Bondt K, Kuypers D, et al. Completeness and satisfaction with the education and information received by patients immediately after kidney transplant: a mixed-models study. *Prog Transplant.* 2013;23(1):12–22.
16. Ohler L. Patient education. In: Cupples S, Ohler L, eds. *Transplant Nursing Secrets.* Philadelphia, PA: Hanley & Belfus; 2003:305–311.
17. SRTR Scientific Registry of Transplant Recipients. Available at http://srtr.transplant.hrsa.gov/. Published July 2014. Accessed September 20, 2014.
18. Organ Procurement and Transplantation Network. *Policy 3: Candidate Registrations, Modifications, and Removals.* Available at http://optn.transplant.hrsa.gov/media/1200/optn_policies.pdf#nameddest=Policy_03. Accessed October 12, 2015.
19. UNOS. *Attachment I to Appendix B of UNOS Bylaws.* Available at https://www.unos.org/wp-content/uploads/unos/Appendix_B_AttachI_XIII.pdf June 28–29, 2011. Accessed November 2, 2015.
20. Kawut SM. Lung retransplantation. *Clin Chest Med.* 2011;32(2):367–377. doi: 10.1016/j.ccm.2011.02.013.

21. Yoo PS, Umman V, Rodriguez-Davalos MI, et al. Retransplantation of the liver: review of current literature for decision making and technical considerations. *Transplant Proc.* 2013;45(3):854–859.

22. Lund LH, Edwards LB, Kucheryavaya AY, et al. The registry of the International Society for Heart and Lung Transplantation: thirty-first official adult heart transplant report—2014; focus theme: retransplantation. *J Heart Lung Transplant.* 2014;33(10):996–1008.

23. Huang J, Danovitch G, Pham PT, et al. Kidney retransplantation for BK virus with active viremia without allograft nephrectomy. *J Nephrol.* 2015;28(6):773–777.

24. Fishman JA. New technologies for infectious screening of organ donors. *Transplant Proc.* 2011;46(6):2443–2445.

25. Xiao D, Craig JC, Chapman JR, et al. Donor cancer transmission in kidney transplantation: a systematic review. *Am J Transplant.* 2013;13(10):2645–2652.

26. Zou S, Dodd R, Stamer S, et al. Probability of Viremia with HBV, HCV, HIV, and HTLV among tissue donors in the United States. *N Engl J Med.* 2004:751–759.

27. Ohler L. Waitlist management. *Prog Transplant.* 2007;17:254–256.

28. Ivarsson B, Ekmehag B, Sjoberg T. Heart or lung transplanted patients' retrospective views on information and support while waiting for transplantation. *J Clin Nurs* 2012;22:1620–1628.

29. Rudow D, Hayes R, Rodriguez J, chairs. *Best practices in living kidney donation consensus conference, Executive Summary.* Held in Rosemont, IL on June 5–6, 2014.

30. Naef R, Bournes DA. The lived experience of waiting a parse method study. *Nurs Sci Q.* 2009;22(2):141–153.

31. Denney B, Keinhuis M. Using crisis theory to explain the quality of life of organ transplant patients. *Prog Transplant.* 2011;21(3):182–188.

32. Lynch SH, Lobo ML. Compassion fatigue in family caregivers: a Wilsonian concept analysis. *J Adv Nurs.* 2012;68(9):2125–2134.

33. Rodrigue JR, Dimitri N, Reed A, et al. Quality of life and psychosocial functioning of spouse/partner caregivers before and after liver transplantation. *Clin Transplant.* 2011;25:239–247.

34. Bolkhir A, Loiselle MM, Evon DM, et al. Depression in primary caregivers of patients listed for liver or kidney transplantation. *Prog Transplant.* 2007;17:193–198.

35. Darcy Y. Pain management by the numbers: using rating scales effectively. *Nursing.* 2007;11:14–15.

36. Arneson P. Multimodal approaches to pain management. *Nursing.* 2011;3:60–61.

37. Cupples S, Ohler L. *Transplant Nursing Secrets.* Philadelphia, PA: Hanley & Belfus, 2003.

38. Randolph S, Scholz K. Self care guidelines: finding common ground. *J Transpl Coord.* 1999;9(3):156–160.

39. Maldonado A, Weeks D, Bitterman A, et al. Changing transplant recipient education and inpatient transplant pharmacy practices: a single center perspective. *Am J Health Syst Pharm.* 2013;70:900–904.

40. Grogan TA. Liver transplantation: issues and nursing care requirements. *Crit Care Nurs Clin North Am.* 2011;23:443–456.

41. Murphy F. The role of the nurse post-renal transplantation. *Br J Nurs.* 2007;16(11):667–675.

42. Wade CR, Reith KK, Sikora JH, et al. Postoperative nursing care of the cardiac transplant recipient. *Crit Care Nurs Q.* 2004;27(1):17–28.

43. Dabbs ADV, Hoffman LA, Iacono AT, et al. Are symptom reports useful for differentiating between acute rejection and pulmonary infection after lung transplantation? *Heart Lung.* 2004;372–380.

44. White SA, Shaw JA, Sutherland DER. Pancreas transplantation. *Lancet.* 2009;373:1808–1817.

45. Jin J. Warning signs of a stroke. *JAMA.* 2014;311(16):1704. Page 34.

46. Schmid-Mohler G, Schafer-Keller P, Frei A, et al. A mixed method study to explore patients' perspective of self-management tasks in the early phase after kidney transplant. *Prog Transplant.* 2014;24(1):8–18.

47. Lorig K, Holman H. Self-management education: history, definition, outcomes and mechanisms. *Ann Behav Med.* 2003;26:1–7.

48. Neyhart C. Patient questions about transplantation: a resource guide. *Nephrol Nurs J.* 2009;36(3):279–285.

49. Avery, RK, Michaels, MG; AST Infectious Diseases Community of Practice. Strategies for safe living after solid organ transplantation. *Am J Transplant.* 2013;13(suppl 4):304–210.

50. Danzinger-Isakov, L, Kumar, D; the AST Infectious Diseases Community of Practice. Vaccination in solid organ transplantation. *Am J Transplant.* 2013;13(suppl 4):311–317.

51. Fisher BL. The emerging risks of live virus & virus vectored vaccines: vaccine strain virus infection, shedding & transmission. *National Vaccine Information Center.* 2014:13.

52. Murphy F. Managing post-transplant patients in primary care. *Pract Nursing.* 2011;22(6):292–297.

53. American Cancer Society. *Available at.* Available at http://www.cancer.org/healthy/findcancerearly/cancerscreeningguidelines/american-cancer-society-guidelines-for-the-early-detection-of-cancer. Last revised 10/20/15. Accessed on November 2, 2015.

54. USPSTF Program Office. *Published Recommendations. US Preventive Services Task Force.* Available at http://www.uspreventiveservicestaskforce.org/BrowseRec/Index/browse-recommendations, Published Dec 2014. Accessed on 12/18/2014.

55. Zwald F, Brown M. Skin cancer in solid organ transplant recipients: advanced in therapy and management. *J Am Acad Dermatol.* 2011;65(2):253–263.

56. Ulrich C, Jurgensen JS, Degen A, et al. Prevention of non-melanoma skin cancer in organ transplant patients by regular use of a sunscreen: a 24 months, prospective case-control study. *Br J Dermatol.* 2009;(suppl 3):78–84.

57. Fullwood D, Jones F, Lau-Walker M. Care of patients following liver transplantation. *Nurs Stand.* 2011; 25(49):50–56.

58. Hasley P, Arnold R. Primary care of the transplant patient. *Am J Med.* 2010:123(3):205–212.

59. Monday K. After liver transplant. *Advance for NPs and PAs.* 2012;3(2). Available at http://nurse-practitioners-and-physician-assistants.advanceweb.com/Features/Articles/After-Liver-Transplant.aspx. Accessed August 14, 2014.

60. Nelson C, Kotton D. Immunocompromised travelers. In: Freedman-Brunette, GW, ed. *CDC Health Information for International Travel 2014.* 1st ed. New York, NY: Oxford University Press; 2014:444–555.

61. Roberts M, Wheeler K, Neibeisel M. Medication adherence part three: strategies for improving adherence. *J Am Assoc of Nurse Pract.* 2014;26(5):281–287.

62. Organ Procurement and Transplant Network. *Guidance for Donor and Recipient Information Sharing.* Available at http://optn.transplant.hrsa.gov/ContentDocuments/Guidance_Information-Sharing_HIPAA_2012.pdf. Published February 27, 2012. Accessed November 24, 2014.

SELF-ASSESSMENT QUESTIONS

1. When a patient is notified of an organ offer from a donor identified as PHS increased risk, the patient:
   a. must be told the donor's status at the time of the organ or prior to transplant.
   b. must agree? Consent to proceed with transplantation prior to the surgery.
   c. may refuse the organ and be automatically removed from the candidate waitlist.
   d. a and b.
   e. all of the above.

2. A patient who is preparing for discharge after his first liver transplant. The transplant coordinator provides education about which of the following health maintenance activities to monitor side effects of medications?
   a. Daily blood pressure monitoring.
   b. Daily weight monitoring.
   c. Completing bloodwork as instructed.
   d. Increase physical activity daily.
   e. a and b only.
   f. d only.
   g. a, b, and c.

3. Patient education must meet the learning needs to the patient considering:
   a. patient's developmental level.
   b. readiness to learn.
   c. cultural values and beliefs.
   d. a and b only.
   e. all of the above.

4. The transplant nurse is planning an educational session with a liver transplant candidate and reviews the medical record. The patient is a 44–year-old male with hepatitis C. His medication list includes lactulose. He completed 9th grade and has worked in a factory until 3 months ago when his illness progressed. Factors to consider include:
   a. possible cognitive dysfunction related to liver disease.
   b. if he qualifies for disability.
   c. ability to comprehend patient education materials.
   d. current hepatitis C treatment plan.
   e. a and b.
   f. a and c.
   g. all of the above.

5. Successful patient education design principles include:
   a. a single approach convenient for the transplant nurse.
   b. engagement of multidisciplinary team to teach patients.
   c. teaching critical information on the day of discharge.
   d. relate teaching points to the patient's own experiences.
   e. a and b.
   f. b and d.
   g. all of the above.

6. When teaching the posttransplant patient about immunosuppression all of the following would be included EXCEPT:
   a. transplant patients are more likely to become sick compared to non-transplant patients.
   b. medication may be taken at different times each day.
   c. notify the transplant coordinator if a new medicine if prescribed by the patient's primary care doctor.
   d. some foods and medications may change the metabolism of immunosuppressant drugs.

7. While interviewing a patient who was discharged after his heart transplant last week, he describes his pain as a level 8 out of 10 every day as he is showering and dressing. The best response is:
   a. assure him the pain is related to surgery and will subside over time.
   b. advise him to take a warm shower to relieve the pain.
   c. suggest that he take pain medication at least 1 hour before beginning ADLs.
   d. review his medication list to re-educate him about which medicines alleviate pain.

8. Psychological effects related to transplantation include all of the following EXCEPT:
   a. unrealistic expectations.
   b. guilt related to the donor's death.
   c. certainty that health will be restored.
   d. disappointment with early outcome of transplant.

9. When preparing a patient and their caregiver for discharge about monitoring the surgical wound, it should include:
   a. number of staples, color, and drainage.
   b. color, drainage, and odor.
   c. number of staples, depth of wound, and drainage.
   d. odor, number of staples, and drainage.

10. Patients and caregivers need instruction about invasive monitoring in the post-operative period. Education should include:
    a. invasive intravenous lines.
    b. ventilator.
    c. postoperative drains (chest tubes, JPs, etc.).
    d. Foley catheter and NG tube.
    e. all of the above.

Correct Answers:
1.d 2.g 3.e 4.f 5.f 6.b 7.c 8.c 9.b 10.e

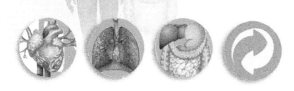

C H A P T E R

4

Transplant Pharmacology

Christopher R. Ensor, PharmD, BCPS
Vicki McCalmont, RN, MS, ANP-BC, CNS, CCTC

 I. INTRODUCTION

A. Overview

1. The use of immunosuppressive agents has evolved over the years, improving transplant opportunities, longevity, and quality of life.

2. Immunosuppressing agents are designed to alter the immune system before, during, and after transplantation. The actions of these agents are specific to immune mechanisms associated with rejection.

   a. Desensitizing agents are used prior to transplantation to reduce/remove circulating antibodies, thereby allowing highly sensitized patients to have a successful transplant.[1,2]

   b. Induction therapy is typically used for patients at high risk for cellular or antibody-mediated acute rejection or patients with impaired renal function that need delayed or calcineurin inhibitor–free immunosuppression maintenance therapy.[3–10]

   c. Maintenance therapy begins at the time of transplant and typically starts with triple therapy and is titrated to the patient's need.

   d. Rejection treatment is targeted to the type of rejection. Antibody-mediated rejection (AMR) and cellular rejection are treated according to the severity of rejection and may range from adjusting the maintenance immunosuppressive regimen, pulse steroids, use of antibodies (polyclonal or monoclonal), plasmapheresis, and intravenous immune globulin (IVIG).[11–20]

3. Risks associated to immunosuppression include rejection, infection, and cancer.

   a. Inadequate immunosuppression places the patient at risk for rejection. Rejection may occur when

      i. Immunosuppressive doses are decreased too rapidly.

      ii. Drug interactions between immunosuppressants and other drugs or foods lower immunosuppressive drug levels.

      iii. Patients are nonadherent with their medications (intentional or unintentional).

b. Overimmunosuppression places the patient at risk for infection and malignancy due to the weakened immune system.

c. Antimicrobial agents are commonly used to prevent or treat infection, for example:

   i. Antifungal agents are typically used to prevent oral candidiasis.

   ii. Antibacterial agents are typically used for *Pneumocystis carinii (jiroveci) pneumonitis* (PCP) or toxoplasmosis (*Toxoplasma gondii*) prophylaxis.

   iii. Antiviral agents are used for prevention or treatment of common posttransplant viral infections, such as

   * Cytomegalovirus (CMV)
   * Herpes simplex virus (HSV)
   * Epstein-Barr virus (EBV)

B. Immunosuppressive agents

1. Target-specific mechanisms of immune activation (Figure 4-1)

2. Have unique pharmacological and toxicity profiles

   a. Used to produce a potent state of immunosuppression

   b. Used in combination to maximize efficacy and minimize short- and long-term toxicity

3. Can be classified under two major categories:

   a. Immunosuppressive antibody therapy may be used for desensitization, induction, or treatment of rejection.[21-23]

      i. Polyclonal antibodies:

      * Used for induction and treatment of acute rejection
      * Rabbit antithymocyte globulin (rATG)
        ○ Thymoglobulin
        ○ ATG-Fresenius
      * Equine antithymocyte globulin
        ○ Atgam

      ii. Antilymphocyte monoclonal antibodies include the following:

      * Alemtuzumab (Campath-1H) is a monoclonal antibody against the CD52 lymphocyte (both T and B cells), anti-CD20 antibodies
      * Rituximab (Rituxan) is a monoclonal antibody that depletes CD20 positive B cells
      * Eculizumab (Soliris) is a monoclonal antibody directed against the C5 fragment in the complement cascade
        ○ Used for desensitization and antibody-mediated rejection

      iii. Protease inhibitors: Bortezomib (Velcade)

      * Used for desensitization and antibody-mediated rejection

      iv. Interleukin-2 (IL-2) receptor antibodies: Basiliximab (Simulect)

      * May be used off-label for induction and antibody-mediated rejection

   b. Maintenance immunosuppression therapy

      i. These agents are classified based on their mechanism of actions into[24-30]

      * Calcineurin inhibitors (CNI)
      * Antiproliferative agents
      * Corticosteroids
      * Proliferation signal inhibitors
      * Costimulation inhibitors

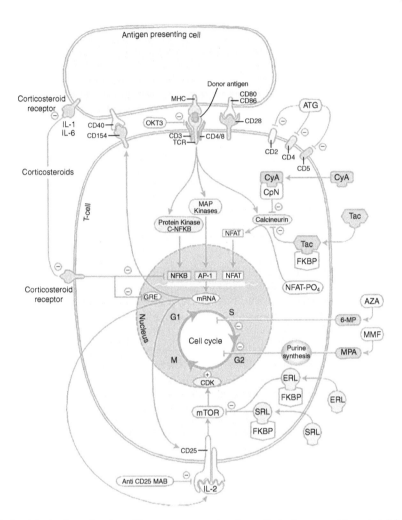

FIGURE 4-1   Mechanism of action of immunosuppressive drugs. Typically, one calcineurin inhibitor, one antiproliferative, or proliferation signal inhibitor, and a corticosteroid are used in combination. Monoclonal and polyclonal antibodies are used to delay the use of a calcineurin inhibitor or to treat rejection. The calcineurin inhibitors, cyclosporine (CsA) and tacrolimus (Tac), bind to cyclophilin (CpN) and FK-binding protein (FKBP), respectively, and then inhibit calcineurin-dependent dephosphorylation of NFAT. Mycophenolic acid (MPA), the active derivative of mycophenolate mofetil (MMF), inhibits inosine monophosphate dehydrogenase–dependent purine biosynthesis. Azathioprine (AZA) is metabolized to 6-mercaptopurine (6-MP), which inhibits cell cycling by providing a "false" purine. Sirolimus (SRL) and everolimus (ERL) bind to FKBP and inhibit molecular target of rapamycin (mTOR), preventing cyclin-dependent kinase (CDK)-mediated cell cycling. Antithymocyte globulins (ATG) bind to T-cell surface antigens (e.g., CD2, CD4, or CD5) enabling lymphocyte opsonization by the reticuloendothelial system (RES). Anti-CD25 monoclonal antibodies (MAB) like basiliximab prevent IL-2 and IL-2 receptor engagement and are not used to treat rejection. Corticosteroids act by binding to corticosteroid receptors, negatively impact glucocorticoid response elements (GRE), and decrease production and action of multiple interleukins. *Abbreviations*: CD, cluster determinant; MHC, major histocompatibility class; MAP, mitogen-activated protein; AP-1, activating protein 1; NFκB, nuclear factor κB; mRNA, messenger ribonucleic acid.

 II. IMMUNOSUPPRESSIVE ANTIBODY THERAPY

　　A.　In the past decade, transplantation across incompatible barriers has become necessary due to the organ shortage and challenges with highly sensitized patients. The use of desensitization protocols using newer antibody agents, plasmapheresis, and IVIG has allowed programs to successfully transplant patients who were deemed not-transplantable in the past. In addition, antibody therapy and/or IVIG have been used as "induction therapy" immediately after transplant in highly sensitized patients or those who need delayed initiation of nephrotoxic immunosuppressant drugs. Induction therapy is considered a form of intense immunosuppression that facilitates early graft acceptance. Lastly, antibody therapy can be used for treatment of severe rejection episodes.

B. Protocols for treatment are evolving as a result of improved technology for the detection of human leukocyte antigen (HLA) antibody and panel-reactive antibody (PRA) testing prior to transplant and donor-specific antibody (DSA) testing after transplant.

　1. PRA and HLA testing prior to transplant identify highly sensitized patients who may benefit from desensitization therapy to reduce their antibody load and prepare them for a successful transplant. Prior to the availability of this testing and subsequent antibody reduction therapy, these patients were never able to get a transplant due to the extremely high risk of hyperacute rejection.[1,2]

　2. Posttransplant, DSA testing monitors the immune response and facilitates the early detection of donor antibodies. This early detection allows for immunosuppressive medication adjustments to prevent AMR.

　　a. Transplant center protocols may include scheduled DSA testing at regular intervals for rejection prevention.

　　b. DSA testing may also be used to

　　　i. Detect suspected acute antibody-mediated rejection and assess severity

　　　ii. Measure antibody presence after a course of treatment for rejection

C. Desensitization therapy

　1. Over the past decade, the advent of desensitization therapy has increased transplant opportunities for patients referred for all types of solid organ transplantation.[1,2]

　　a. Prior to these desensitization protocols, if a transplant candidate had an antibody specific to a potential donor's HLA, that donor was declined due to the risk for hyperacute rejection.

　　b. Desensitization therapies aim to remove circulating antibodies, thereby affording a candidate an opportunity to potentially undergo transplantation with a negative crossmatch.

　　c. Timing of this therapy varies based upon donor availability.

　　　i. While on the transplant waiting list, highly sensitized patients may receive treatment to remove circulating antibodies, thereby increasing the number of acceptable donor offers.

　　　ii. Preoperative or perioperative desensitization is given to candidates with an elevated PRA ≥30%, multiple HLA mismatches, or positive crossmatch with a medically urgent need.[2]

　2. Desensitization agents used (Table 4-1)[13–16]

　　a. Plasmapheresis[17,18]

　　　i. Always done prior to the administration of IVIG or antibody therapy because plasmapheresis removes IVIG and other monoclonal antibodies during the plasma exchange.

　　b. IVIG[16–18]

　　c. Antilymphocyte monoclonal antibodies:

　　　i. Alemtuzumab (Campath-1H) is a monoclonal antibody against the CD52 lymphocyte (both T and B cells), anti-CD20 antibodies.[4,5]

TABLE 4-1 Desensitization/Antirejection therapies

Therapy	Use	Class	Mechanism of Action	Adverse Reactions	Comments
Plasmapheresis	D AMR	Procedure	Removal of circulating antidonor antibodies from peripheral blood	Hypotension, arrhythmias	Takes 1–3 h for a plasma exchange using a dialysis catheter
IVIG	D AMR	Pooled polyclonal antibodies	Repletes immunoglobulins removed by plasmapheresis, reduces allosensitization and ischemic-perfusion reactions through B-cell apoptosis	Infusion reaction Headache	Premedicate with acetaminophen. Given by slow infusion Half life is 3–4 wk May follow plasmapheresis or antibody therapy
Eculizumab (Soliris)	D AMR	Monoclonal antibody	Complement C5 inhibitor to prevent complement-mediated rejection	Infusion reaction, headache, hypertension, leukopenia, infection	Complement is the final step in the AMR pathway. Patients refractory to other monoclonal antibody therapies may respond to eculizumab
Rituximab (Rituxan)	D I AMR	Monoclonal antibody	Binds to CD20 on B cells to deplete circulating B cells	Infusion reaction (fevers, rigors, pain), risk for serious infection, PML, SJS	Premedicate with acetaminophen, antihistamine, and steroids Given by IV infusion, slowly PCP and antiviral prophylaxis may be given up to 12 m postdose
Alemtuzumab (Campath-1H)	AMR	Monoclonal antibody	Binds to CD52 on mature lymphocytes and depletes T and B cells	Infusion reaction, fevers, rash, nausea, hypotension, cytopenia infection: CMV	Premedicate with acetaminophen, antihistamine PCP and antiviral prophylaxis may be given for a minimum of 2 mo postdose
Bortezomib (Velcade)	D AMR	Protease inhibitor	Protease inhibitor. Promotes apoptosis in plasma cells, which generate antibodies	Bone marrow suppression, neuropathy, hypotension, GI toxicity	Premedicate with antiemetics and antidiarrheals Reduce dose if the patient has moderate hepatic dysfunction
Basiliximab (Simulect)	I	Monoclonal antibody	Blocks the IL-2 receptor thus preventing T-cell replication (reducing immune response) and B-cell activation (reducing antibodies)	Infusion reaction, agranulocytosis, edema headache, GI toxicity	Is typically give as IV infusion over 20–30 min Monitor labs: (↑Cr, ↑K, ↓ Phos)

Infusion reactions may include fever, rigors, hypotension, tachycardia, arrhythmias, dyspnea, bronchospasms, wheezing, respiratory failure, rash, or other hypersensitivity reaction such as anaphylaxis. GI toxicity may include nausea, vomiting, dyspepsia, diarrhea, constipation, and abdominal pain.

D, desensitization; AMR, antibody-mediated rejection; I, Induction; IV, intravenous; PCP, *Pneumocystis carinii* pneumonia; CMV, cytomegalovirus; GI, gastrointestinal; IL, interleukin; Cr, Creatinine; K, Potassium; Phos, phosphorus.

Kim M, Martin ST, Townsend RK, et al. Antibody-mediated rejection in kidney transplantation: a review of pathophysiology, diagnosis and treatment options. *Pharmacotherapy*. 2014;34(7):733–744; Hendrikx TK, Klepper M, Ijzermans J, et al. Clinical rejection and persistent immune regulation in kidney transplant patients. *Transpl Immunol*. 2009;21(3):129–135; Colaneri J. An overview of transplant immunosuppression: history, principles, and current practices in kidney transplantation. *Nephrol Nurs J*. 2014;41(6):549–561; Jordan SC, Totoda M, Kahwaii J, et al. Clinical aspects of intravenous immunoglobulin use in solid organ transplant recipients. *Am J Transplant*. 2011;11(2):196–202.

      ii. Rituximab (Rituxan) is a monoclonal antibody that depletes CD20 positive B cells.[8,17]

      iii. Eculizumab (Soliris) is a monoclonal antibody directed against the C5 fragment in the complement cascade.[9–11]

- Used for desensitization and treatment of AMR.
- To date, the results of small studies are controversial with regard to the efficacy of eculizumab in treating refractory AMR.[9,10] Therefore, it is too soon to determine the true benefit in all solid organ transplant recipients without additional data.

  d. Protease inhibitor: bortezomib (Velcade)

    i. Used for desensitization and treatment of AMR[11,12,15]

  e. Interleukin-2 (IL-2) receptor monoclonal antibody: basiliximab (Simulect)[22]

3. Any of the above agents may be used alone or in combination to deplete circulating antibodies, to deplete antibody-producing cells, and to block antibodies from binding to the epithelium (with subsequent rejection), thus protecting the allograft from damage.[13–16]

  a. In addition to desensitization therapy, the above agents may also be used for the treatment of AMR. See Table 4-1 for desensitization and antirejection therapies.[13–16]

  b. Refer to your transplant program protocol for the timing and dosing of the above agents.

D. Induction or acute rejection immunosuppression therapy

1. Induction immunosuppression agents are used immediately posttransplant to neutralize the initial robust T-cell–mediated immune response. These agents reduce the risk of rejection by depleting T cells and/or interrupting T-cell activation and proliferation.

  a. Due to their potent and immediate immunosuppressive effects, induction agents allow for CNI therapy to be postponed in the setting of delayed graft function.

  b. These same agents may also be used to treat acute rejection

2. There are four types of agents used for induction therapy or the treatment of acute rejection:

  a. Polyclonal antibodies

  b. Monoclonal antibodies

  c. Interleukin-2 (IL-2) receptor antibodies

  d. High-dose glucocorticoids

3. Polyclonal antibodies

  a. Polyclonal antibodies are produced by immunizing animals such as rabbits (rabbit antithymocyte globulin [rATG]; Thymoglobulin; rabbit ATG-Fresenius) or horses (Atgam)[17–19] with human lymphoid cells.[22]

  b. General mechanism of action

    i. Polyclonal antilymphocyte globulins are a group of antibodies targeting multiple antigens (CD2, CD3, CD4, CD8, CD11a, and CD18) on the cell membrane of lymphocytes (hence the name "polyclonal")

    ii. These antithymocyte antibodies bind to lymphocytes that display the specific surface antigen and deplete lymphocytes from the circulation for several weeks. This helps to prevent early posttransplant ischemia-reperfusion injury.

iii. In addition, rabbit antithymoglobulin (rATG) has been shown to prevent B-cell proliferation and differentiation, which decreases circulating antibodies and promotes antibody-dependence cell-mediated cytotoxicity.

iv. This lymphopenia is the basis for the immunosuppressive action of polyclonal antibodies.

c. Use in transplantation

   i. In the United States, rATG and Atgam are approved by the Food and Drug Administration (FDA) for the treatment of acute rejection in kidney transplant recipients.

   ii. Both rATG and Atgam are also used off-label as induction therapy agents in nonrenal solid organ transplantation.

   iii. When given intraoperatively, prior to reperfusion, rATG has been shown to reduce the incidence of delayed graft function in both kidney and heart transplant recipients.

d. Specific polyclonal antibody agents:

   i. Antithymocyte globulin—Rabbit (rATG, Thymoglobulin)

   - Dosage and administration—Induction therapy
     - Dose used in clinical trials is usually 1.5 mg/kg/day for 3 to 7 days.

   - Dosage and administration—Treatment of acute rejection
     - Recommended dose: 1.5 mg/kg/day for 7 to 10 days

   ii. ATG-Fresenius

   - Dosage and administration—Induction therapy
     - Dose ranges from 2 to 5 mg/kg body weight given as an infusion over 4 hours. Duration of therapy may last 5 to 14 days.
     - Single shot infusion over 4 hours (4 to 6 mg/kg body weight) for one dose prior to initiation of standard immunosuppression and administration.

   - Dosage and administration—AMR therapy
     - Dose ranges from 3 to 5 mg/kg body weight given as an infusion over 4 hours. Duration of therapy may last 5 to 14 days.

   iii. Lymphocyte immune globulin—Equine (Atgam)

   - Dosage and administration—Induction or AMR therapy
     - Doses range from 10 to 15 mg/kg given over a 4-hour infusion for up to 14 days.
     - Intradermal skin test Instructions for Atgam: 0.1 mL of 1:1,000 dilution (5 µg horse IgG) in 0.9% sodium chloride injected intradermally with a contralateral 0.9% sodium chloride control injection. Monitor patient and skin test area every 15 to 20 minutes for 1 hour. A positive skin test result consists of a local reaction equal to 10 mm with erythema and/or wheal or marked local swelling.

   - The following precautions are recommended to prevent infusion-related adverse effects for all polyclonal antibody agents:
     - Patients receive premedication with corticosteroids, acetaminophen, and an antihistamine 30 to 60 minutes prior to the infusion, this is typically used prior to the first three doses (regardless if used for induction or AMR therapy or the length of treatment).
     - Always administered through a high-flow vein.

⊃ The first dose should be infused over at least 6 hours and subsequent doses should be infused over at least 4 hours. This process should be followed with every course of therapy regardless if used as induction or AMR treatment.

⊃ Assess for anaphylaxis during first three doses as those are the highest risk for adverse effects.

- Consider dose reduction in setting of
  ⊃ Platelet count between 50,000 and 75,000 cells/mm³
  ⊃ White cell count between 2,000 and 3,000 cells/mm³
  ⊃ Consider discontinuing treatment in the setting of
    ▪ Persistent and severe thrombocytopenia (<50,000 cells/mm³)
    ▪ Leukopenia (<2,000 cells/mm³)
- Drug interactions
  ⊃ No formal drug-drug interactions have been reported to date
- Adverse effects of polyclonal antibodies
  ⊃ The most common side effects are infusion-related (fever, chills, headache), leukopenia, and thrombocytopenia.
  ⊃ Other side effects include serum sickness, hypertension, tachycardia, dyspnea, abdominal pain, myalgias, and diarrhea.
- Serious immune–mediated reactions have been reported with the use of polyclonal antibodies ranging from a systemic rash, serum sickness to anaphylaxis with tachycardia, dyspnea, hypotension, or death. The infusion should be immediately stopped and the physician should be notified.
- Some programs have an emergency anaphylaxis kit available for use if suspected anaphylactic reactions occur. These kits may contain the following:
  ⊃ Epinephrine 1:1,000, 3 vials (0.5 mg SQ)
  ⊃ Solucortef 100 mg IV (to be given over 30 seconds)
  ⊃ Diphenhydramine 50 mg IV (give 25 mg over 1 minute)
  ⊃ Albuterol inhaler (give 2 puffs for anaphylaxis)
  ⊃ Prefilled saline syringes
  ⊃ Ambu bag, face mask and oral airway
- Anytime polyclonal therapy is used, the patient may need to be treated with anti-infective prophylaxis (refer to your program protocols) including:
  ⊃ Nystatin swish and swallow 5 mL po or clotrimazole (Mycelex) troche 10 mg QID for antifungal prophylaxis
  ⊃ Acyclovir (Zovirax) 400 mg po every 12 hours (if CMV, *low*-risk category)
  ⊃ Valganciclovir (Valcyte) 900 mg po daily (if CMV, *moderate* or *high* risk)
  ⊃ Trimethoprim/sulfamethoxazole (Bactrim) double strength, 1 tablet once daily, three times a week or weekly depending on your center protocol for pneumocystis prevention.

4. Monoclonal antibodies: alemtuzumab (Campath-1H)
  a. There have been several monoclonal antibodies developed for use in transplantation over the last two decades. Many of these antibodies have been subsequently withdrawn from the worldwide market.

b. Alemtuzumab (Campath-1H)
   i. Alemtuzumab is a humanized monoclonal antibody directed against the CD52 receptor and used for induction therapy in solid organ transplantation.[5]
      - Alemtuzumab is FDA approved only for treating refractory B-cell chronic lymphocytic leukemia and multiple sclerosis and is used off-label for induction therapy in solid organ transplantation by a limited number of transplant centers.
      - Studies in kidney transplant recipients have shown that use of alemtuzumab as induction therapy was superior to rATG and conventional immunosuppression for the prevention of rejection in the first year.[5,6]
   ii. Alemtuzumab—Dosing and administration
      - Give alemtuzumab 30 mg intravenously (IV) or subcutaneously (SC) once at the time of transplantation
      - Must premedicate with a minimum of methylprednisolone 250 mg IV to avoid immunoactivation and immune-mediated infusion reactions
      - Infusion-related side effects of alemtuzumab are common including fever, chills, hypertension, and hypotension. These side effects are reduced when alemtuzumab is administered SC.
   iii. Alemtuzumab—Adverse effects:
      - The side effects of alemtuzumab in solid organ transplant patients are different than the side effects in oncology patients because of the differences in dosage used.
      - Lymphopenia is the basis of alemtuzumab's immunosuppressive action.
      - Therefore, patients receiving alemtuzumab are at increased risk of opportunistic infections, autoimmune disorders, and profound pancytopenia
   iv. Alemtuzumab—Black box warning
      - Alemtuzumab carries a black box warning stating increased risk of severe hematologic toxicities, infusion reactions, infection, and opportunistic infections.
      - Alemtuzumab—Therapeutic drug monitoring
         ○ Complete blood counts and platelet counts should be monitored routinely.
5. Interleukin-2 (IL-2) receptor antibodies: Basiliximab (Simulect)[22]
   a. A nondepleting monoclonal antibody that serves as an interleukin-2 (IL-2) receptor antagonist.
   b. Currently approved as induction therapy to prevent rejection in patients who have a low-to-moderate risk of rejection.
   c. Also a chimeric (murine/human) monoclonal antibody that contains more mouse than human proteins; produced by recombinant DNA technology.
   d. Basiliximab—Mechanism of action
      i. Binds to the alpha subunit of the IL-2 receptor expressed only on activated T cells to inhibit their proliferation without destroying the lymphocyte.
   e. Basiliximab—Dosing and administration
      i. 20 mg given IV over 15 to 30 minutes or IV push on day 0 and day 4 posttransplant.

f. Basiliximab—Drug interactions
 i. No formal drug-drug interactions have been reported to date.
g. Basiliximab—Adverse effects
 i. Basiliximab is well tolerated.
 ii. Occasionally infusion-related side effects such as fever and chills have been reported.
h. Basiliximab—Therapeutic drug monitoring.
 i. Currently, routine therapeutic monitoring of basiliximab is not indicated.
6. Glucocorticoids in high dose: Methylprednisolone (Solu-Medrol); prednisone
a. Discussed under maintenance immunosuppression below

III. MAINTENANCE IMMUNOSUPPRESSION THERAPY

A. Goal
 1. The primary goal of immunosuppressive therapy in solid organ transplantation is to maintain graft tolerance using the least amount of drugs possible.
 2. Triple immunosuppression allows adequate treatment combining three drugs in lower doses to minimize side effects, reduce the risk of allograft rejection or graft dysfunction, and prevent long-term complications such as infection, chronic kidney disease, cancer, or other comorbidities.[24-30]
 3. Currently, the combination of tacrolimus (often referred to as "TAC"), mycophenolate mofetil (MMF), and a corticosteroid is the most frequently used triple immunosuppression regimen for solid organ transplant recipients in the United States across all organ systems.[24-30]

B. Calcineurin inhibitors[31-42]
 1. Quickly became the standard for primary immunosuppression through selective immunosuppressive actions which have dramatically decreased the incidence of acute cellular rejection with minimal toxicities to the bone marrow.
 2. The decision on the initial dose and the time to initiate CNIs is dependent on
  a. Initial allograft function.
  b. Other medical conditions (e.g., presence of active infection or impaired renal function).
  c. Use of concurrent immunosuppressive agents.
  d. Subsequently, the dose of CNI is adjusted to achieve target trough blood concentrations.
 3. Types of CNIs:
  a. Cyclosporine
  b. Tacrolimus
 4. Cyclosporine[31-33,35-37]
  a. Overview
   i. First CNI used in transplantation.
   ii. Introduced in the early 1980s and revolutionized transplant medicine by transforming organ transplantation from an experimental procedure into routine clinical practice.
  b. There are two formulations of cyclosporine:
   i. Nonmodified (Sandimmune).
   ii. Modified, as microemulsion (Neoral, Gengraf).
   iii. There are generic equivalents for both formulations of cyclosporine.
   iv. Most importantly, these formulations are not easily interchangeable.
  c. Cyclosporine—Mechanism of action.[37]

i. CNIs primarily suppress the activation of T lymphocytes and inhibit intracellular gene transcription in the production of the lymphokine IL-2. IL-2 is essential for activation and proliferation of T cells in response to alloantigens.

ii. Cyclosporine
- Inhibits calcineurin by binding to an intracellular protein cyclophilin.
- Reversibly inhibits production of lymphokines such as IL-2 in immunocompetent lymphocytes. This leads to preferential inhibition of T lymphocytes.

d. Cyclosporine—Dosing and administration[32,33,37]
i. Recommended starting oral dose in following recipients:
- Kidney: 3 mg/kg/day in 2 divided doses
- Liver: 4 mg/kg/day in 2 divided doses
- Heart: 3 mg/kg/day in 2 divided doses
- Lung: no dosing recommendations, is used off-label as there are no immunosuppressive medications with FDA approval for lung transplantation.[30]

ii. The IV dose is usually one-third the oral dose and is administered as a continuous infusion, or as an intermittent bolus twice daily with a 4- to 6-hour infusion time per dose.[37]

e. Cyclosporine—Therapeutic drug monitoring
i. The reported therapeutic range for 12-hour trough levels appears to be between 100 and 400 ng/mL.[33]
ii. Trough targets are program, patient, agent, and regimen specific. Generally, the cyclosporine trough target will be highest within the first 6 posttransplant months, tapering to lower target maintenance troughs after 6 to 12 months, depending on rejection pathology.

f. Cyclosporine—Drug interactions (Table 41-2)[37-41]

TABLE 4-2. Drugs that Commonly Interact with Cyclosporine (CsA) and Tacrolimus (TAC)

Increases CsA or TAC Concentrations	Decreases CsA or TAC Concentrations

Antifungal agents
  Clotrimazole, fluconazole, itraconazole, ketoconazole, voriconazole, posaconazole
	Antibiotics
	  Nafcillin, rifabutin, rifampin

Calcium channel blockers
  diltiazem, nicardipine, nifedipine, verapamil
	Antiepileptic agents
	  carbamazepine, phenobarbital, phenytoin

Macrolide antibiotics
  clarithromycin, erythromycin
	Others
	  St. John's wort, octreotide, orlistat, coadministration of electrolytes (potassium/magnesium)

HMG-CoA reductase inhibitors simvastatin, lovastatin	
Others bromocriptine, danazol, fluvoxamine, grapefruit juice, protease inhibitors	

Neoral® [Package Insert]. East Hanover, NJ: Novartis Pharmaceutical Corp.; March 2015. Available at https://www.pharma.us.novartis.com/product/pi/pdf/neoral.pdf. Accessed October 17, 2015; Issa N, Kukla A, Ibrahim HN. Calcineurin inhibitor toxicity: a review and perspective of the evidence. *Am J Nephrol.* 2013;37(6):602–612; Castrogudin JF, Molina E, Vara E. Calcineurin inhibitors in liver transplantation: to be or not to be. *Transplant Proc.* 2011;43(6):2220–2223; Prograf® [Package Insert]. Deerfield, IL: Astellas Pharma U.S., Inc.; May 2015. Available at https://www.astellas.us/docs/prograf.pdf. Accessed October 17, 2015; Patel JK, Kobashigawa JA. Tacrolimus in heart transplant recipients: an overview. *BioDrugs.* 2007;21(3):139–143.

      i. Any drugs that either inhibit or induce cytochrome P-450 3A4 will alter the metabolism of cyclosporine:
- Drugs that inhibit cyclosporine metabolism can lead to higher drug levels and increase the risk for toxicity.
- Drugs that induce cyclosporine metabolism can lead to subtherapeutic cyclosporine drug levels and increase the risk of rejection.

      ii. A list of drugs that commonly interact with cyclosporine and tacrolimus is provided in Table 4-2[37–41]
- Please note that this list is not comprehensive.
- Drugs that are nephrotoxic such as IV tobramycin and non-steroidal anti-inflammatory drugs (NSAIDs) such as ibuprofen may potentiate the nephrotoxic effects of CNI.
  - Concurrent administration of these agents should be avoided unless no other therapeutic options exist.

g. Cyclosporine—Adverse effects

      i. The most common side effects of cyclosporine are as follows[37–41]:
- Hypertension.
- Dyslipidemia.
- Cosmetic (hirsutism, gingival hyperplasia).
- Nephrotoxicity.
- Diabetes mellitus (DM).
- Tremor.
- Rare: seizures, posterior reversible encephalopathy syndrome, hallucination, and migraine.
- As with all immunosuppressive agents, long-term use of cyclosporine is associated with an increased risk of opportunistic infection and malignancy.

5. Tacrolimus (Prograf, Hecoria, Astagraf)[40–44]

a. Overview

      i. A macrolide lactone antibiotic isolated from the fungus *Streptomyces tsukubaensis.*

      ii. Introduced in 1994

      iii. Differs structurally from cyclosporine; more potent than cyclosporine

      iv. Used in solid organ transplantation as part of dual or triple immunosuppressive maintenance regimens to prevent allograft rejection

      v. Initiated at the time of transplantation and usually continued for the life of the allograft

      vi. Most frequently used CNI

b. Tacrolimus—Mechanism of action[40]

      i. Tacrolimus inhibits calcineurin by binding to the intracellular cytosolic protein called FKBP-12 (FK-binding protein).

      ii. Prevents gene transcription and the formation of lymphokines such as IL-2 and gamma interferon.

      iii. The net effect is inhibition of T-cell activation resulting in immunosuppression.

c. Tacrolimus—Dosing and administration[25,29,33,34,40]

    i. Recommended **weight**-based starting oral dose in following types of transplant recipients:
- Adult kidney: 0.2 mg/kg/day in 2 divided doses
- Adult liver: 0.10 to 0.15 mg/kg/day in 2 divided doses
- Adult heart: 0.075 mg/kg/day in 2 divided doses
- Pediatric liver: 0.15 to 0.20 mg/kg/day in 2 divided doses.

    ii. Fixed-dose starting oral dose:
- All organs: **start** around 2 mg/day in divided doses titrating (increasing or decreasing) the dose by 1 to 2 mg/day to achieve target trough
- The typical IV dose is 0.03 to 0.05 mg/kg/day as a continuous infusion. Similar to cyclosporine, the typical infusion dose is 1/3 to 1/5 of the oral dose per day delivered as a continuous infusion.

d. Tacrolimus—Therapeutic drug monitoring[25,29,33,34,40]

    i. Reported therapeutic tacrolimus range for 12-hour trough levels from whole blood typically ranges between 5 and 20 ng/mL.

    ii. Trough targets are organ, time posttransplant, patient, agent, and program specific. Generally, the trough target will be highest within the first 6 posttransplant months, tapering to lower target maintenance troughs after 6 to 12 months depending on rejection pathology.

    iii. The target therapeutic range for CNIs varies depending on
- Type of organ transplanted.
- Functional **status** of the allograft.
- Medical conditions of the patient. (e.g., presence of active infection or impaired renal function)
- Concurrent **immunosuppressive** agents used.

e. Tacrolimus: Drug interactions (see Table 4-2)[37–41]

    i. Any drugs that either inhibit or induce cytochrome P-450 3A4 will alter the metabolism of tacrolimus.
- Drugs that inhibit tacrolimus metabolism can lead to higher drug levels and increase the risk for toxicity.
- Drugs that induce tacrolimus metabolism can lead to subtherapeutic tacrolimus drug levels and increase the risk of rejection.[21,22]

    ii. A list of the drugs that commonly interact with cyclosporine and tacrolimus is provided in Table 4-2.[37–41]

f. Tacrolimus—Adverse effects

    i. Similar to those of cyclosporine

    ii. The most common side effects of tacrolimus are[39–42]
- Hypertension
- Dyslipidemia
- Adrenal insufficiency
- Nephrotoxicity
- DM
- Tremor
- Gastrointestinal (GI), typically diarrhea
- Cosmetic effects: Alopecia
- Rare: Seizures, posterior reversible encephalopathy syndrome (PRES), hallucination, and migraine

    iii. Tacrolimus is more likely to result in DM, hypertension, and neurologic toxicities than cyclosporine.[37,40]

      iv. Tacrolimus is less likely to result in hyperlipidemia and cosmetic problems than cyclosporine.[37,40]

      v. As with all immunosuppressive agents, long-term use of tacrolimus is associated with an increased risk of opportunistic infection and malignancy.[40]

6. CNIs and rejection prophylaxis

   a. Both CNIs provide excellent rejection prophylaxis.

      i. Results of randomized, multicenter trials comparing tacrolimus and cyclosporine have demonstrated tacrolimus to be more effective in preventing acute rejection than cyclosporine in kidney, liver, pancreas, heart and lung transplant recipients.[25,29,33,34,40]

         • However, some analyses have shown no differences in efficacy between cyclosporine and tacrolimus with the current dosing strategies and the use of microemulsion formulation of cyclosporine.

      ii. Recent clinical trials have focused on identifying immunosuppressive regimens that avoid or minimize side effects of CNIs.[44–46]

         • Withdrawing cyclosporine at 3 months posttransplant and initiating sirolimus (Rapamune) in selected patients resulted in the prevention of chronic allograft nephropathy.[45–50]

         • Long-term use of cyclosporine or tacrolimus may be limited by side effects, specifically nephrotoxicity, which is known as calcineurin-induced nephropathy (CIN).[38]

7. Use of CNIs in combination with other immunosuppressants:

   a. Clinical studies have compared the relative safety and efficacy of triple immunosuppressive therapy using tacrolimus, MMF, corticosteroids versus cyclosporine, MMF, and corticosteroids and found the tacrolimus, MMF, and corticosteroid combination was more effective in preventing acute rejection and better tolerated in renal and heart transplant recipients.[42,51]

C. Antiproliferative agents[52–57]

1. Overview

   a. Sometimes referred to as antimetabolites, these agents were first used in transplantation in the early 1960s after the development of azathioprine (AZA), which suppresses T- and B-cell proliferation in all solid organ transplant recipients.

   b. Current use of AZA has declined significantly since the approval of MMF in 1995.

   c. MMF has rapidly replaced AZA as the primary antiproliferative agent used in clinical transplantation.

   d. Enteric-coated mycophenolate sodium (MPS) was developed and approved by the FDA in 2004 to help circumvent the upper GI effects by facilitating release in the small intestine rather than the stomach. This has resulted in less nausea and improved GI-related quality of life compared to MMF.

   e. Both MPS and MMF are converted to mycophenolic acid by esterases in the GI system and other sites including the biliary tree and the liver.

   f. Role in solid organ transplantation

      i. Antiproliferative agents are used in conjunction with other maintenance immunosuppressive agents in solid organ transplantation to prevent graft rejection.

      ii. They are most effective when given at the time of transplantation and are usually continued for the life of the allograft.

2. Current antiproliferative agents
   a. Mycophenolate mofetil (CellCept)
   b. Mycophenolate sodium (Myfortic)
   c. Azathioprine (Imuran)
3. Mycophenolate mofetil and mycophenolate sodium[52-56]
   a. Overview
      i. MMF is utilized in combination with cyclosporine or tacrolimus plus a corticosteroid and recently has been used in combination with proliferation signal inhibitors to avoid CNIs.
      ii. MMF is the most frequently used antiproliferative agent.
      iii. Clinical trials have demonstrated that MMF is superior to either placebo or AZA in prevention of acute rejection in kidney, pancreas, liver, and heart transplantation.[57]
      iv. MMF does not appear to be nephrotoxic or to adversely effect glucose and lipid metabolism.[53]
      v. MMF may cause severe diarrhea that can lead to dehydration and renal insufficiency or acute renal failure.
      vi. MMF has become an integral component of low toxicity regimens that aim to minimize patient exposure to the nephrotoxic effects of CNI and the metabolic complications of corticosteroids.
   b. Mechanism of action
      i. Mycophenolate mofetil and mycophenolate sodium both inhibit inosine 5′ monophosphate dehydrogenase, a key enzyme in purine synthesis.[33]
      ii. Interferes with the de novo pathway of purine synthesis and DNA replication and are most effective against cells undergoing proliferation or differentiation.
      iii. Produces cytostatic effects on B and T cells to arrest the cell cycle in the G1 to S phase.
      iv. Myfortic, an enteric-coated formulation of mycophenolate sodium, may have some theoretical advantages over MMF resulting in less adverse effects.
   c. Mycophenolate mofetil (CellCept)—Dosing and administration[53]
      i. The recommended oral starting dose, given in two divided doses
         • 2 g/day in kidney, liver, pancreas, and lung transplant recipients.
         • 3 g/day in heart transplant recipients.
         • The starting dose in pediatric kidney transplant patients is 1.2 g/m^2.[37]
      ii. The recommended IV dose, given twice daily, is the same as the respective oral dose above.
         • Usually infused over ≥2 hours.
      iii. Dosing adjustment is necessary in patients with renal dysfunction due to accumulation of MMF metabolites.
   d. Mycophenolate sodium (Myfortic)—Dosing and administration[54]
      i. Recommended starting dose is 720 mg twice daily
      ii. If transitioning from MMF to MPS, the equivalent doses are: MMF 500 mg = MPA 360 mg or MMF 1,000 mg = MPA 720 mg.
   e. Therapeutic drug monitoring—MMF (CellCept) and MPS (Myfortic)
      i. Complete blood counts, including platelets, should be monitored frequently during the early posttransplant period, and at least every 3 months thereafter.

ii. Frequent monitoring of white blood cell counts is recommended to monitor for neutropenia.

iii. Both MMF and MPS are metabolized to mycophenolic acid and mycophenolic acid serum levels can be measured.

iv. Clinical utility of mycophenolic acid monitoring:

- Controversial and not currently recommended routinely.
- Most studies were done between 2000 and 2010; results are mixed.
- One small study by Savary and colleagues assessed the utility of monitoring trough mycophenolic acid levels in 56 liver transplant recipients and found that predose monitoring of mycophenolic acid levels on days 3 to 10 posttransplant was applicable in this cohort, conferring protection from ineffective immunosuppression.[58]
- Zuk and Pearson's 2009 systematic review of the extant literature (1996 to 2008) evaluated the relationship between mycophenolic acid levels and rejection in heart transplant recipients and could not find evidence supporting any benefit for assessing mycophenolic acid levels.[59]

f. Drug interactions—MMF (CellCept) and MPS (Myfortic)

i. Antacids with magnesium and aluminum hydroxides or medications that increase gastric pH, such as proton pump inhibitors, can decrease the absorption of MMF. MPS absorption remains preserved.

ii. Drugs that are myelosuppressive, such as valganciclovir (Valcyte), may amplify the bone marrow toxicity of MMF and MPS.[53-57]

g. MMF (CellCept) and MPS (Myfortic)—Adverse effects

i. The most common side effects of MMF and MPS are as follows:

- GI (diarrhea, constipation, nausea, vomiting).
- There are mixed results in the literature regarding which medication (MMF or MPS) has fewer GI side effects.[57,60]
- Many programs try changing patients who have persistent GI adverse effects from MMF to MPS and assessing them for improved tolerance.[61]

ii. Bone marrow suppression (leukopenia, thrombocytopenia, anemia).

iii. Black box warning for birth defects.

- Patients should be advised to talk with providers in planning pregnancies.
- Mycophenolate products carry risks of craniofacial malformations such as cleft palette when given during the first trimester.
- As such, mycophenolate products are typically avoided during pregnancy; though, late-stage use may be acceptable in very select cases (such as refractory acute cellular rejection).[56]

4. Azathioprine (Imuran)[52]

a. Azathioprine—Mechanism of action

i. Azathioprine is a purine analog.[52]

ii. Incorporates into cellular deoxyribonucleic acid (DNA) and ribonucleic acid (RNA) to cause nonsense mutations. These mutations result in misfolded proteins and a decrease in functional cell proliferation.

b. Azathioprine—Dosing and administration[52]

i. The recommended initial oral dose is 1 to 3 mg/kg once daily.

ii. Dose is adjusted to a maintenance dose of 1 to 3 mg/kg/day depending on the patient's tolerance.

    c. Azathioprine—Therapeutic drug monitoring
      i. Complete blood counts, including platelets, should be monitored
         frequently during the early posttransplant period and at least every 3
         months thereafter.
    d. Azathioprine—Drug interactions
      i. Any thiopurine S-methyltransferase enzyme inhibitor may increase
         azathioprine concentration.
      ii. Significant drug interactions have been reported to occur with
         allopurinol, aminosalicylates, and warfarin.[52]
    e. Azathioprine—Adverse effects[52,55]
      i. Bone marrow suppression, resulting in leukopenia, pancytopenia,
         thrombocytopenia, and/or macrocytic anemia, occurs to varying
         degrees in >50% of patients.
      ii. Other side effects include nausea, vomiting, hepatotoxicity, and
         pancreatitis.

D. Corticosteroids
    1. Overview—Role in solid organ transplantation[27,34,44,62–66]
      a. Corticosteroids were the first immunosuppressive drugs used in
        transplantation.
      b. Highly effective; have anchored maintenance immunosuppressive
        regimens since the early 1960s.
      c. Never FDA approved for use in organ transplantation.
      d. Are utilized in organ transplantation for both the treatment of acute organ
        rejection and maintenance immunosuppression.
      e. Typically used as part of a combination immunosuppressive regimen
        including CNIs and an antiproliferative agent.
      f. Used as a first-line agent to treat acute cellular rejection.
      g. Have numerous side effects, especially when used in combination with
        CNIs.
      h. Either directly or in part, the use of corticosteroids has been associated
        with posttransplant:
        i. Hypertension
        ii. Bone loss[67]
        iii. DM[67]
        iv. Increased incidence of infection[67]
      i. The safety profile associated with corticosteroid use, along with the cost
        of therapy for treatment of corticosteroid-associated adverse events, has
        motivated increased efforts to minimize or eliminate corticosteroids as a
        component of immunosuppressive therapies.
      j. Corticosteroid weaning may begin as early as several weeks posttransplant
        to several months after transplantation.
      k. Early corticosteroid withdrawal, or rapid discontinuation, must be
        differentiated from corticosteroid avoidance. This is organ specific:
        i. Renal transplant studies show increased risk for rejection and graft loss
          on steroid free regimens.[65]
        ii. Heart transplant studies report a 60% to 80% success rate with late
          steroid withdrawal.[44]
        iii. Liver transplant studies report success with late steroid withdrawal.[68]
      l. In corticosteroid avoidance, the medication is either administered for a
        very short period of time (up to 7 days) or not administered at all.

2. Corticosteroids—Mechanism of action[67]
   a. The mechanism of action is complex and multifaceted.
   b. Corticosteroids are produced by the adrenal gland and are part of the normal endocrine system of animals and humans.
   c. Corticosteroids have a wide spectrum of effects
      i. Diffuse effects of corticosteroids on the body reflect the fact that most mammalian tissues have glucocorticoid receptors within the cell cytoplasm that serve as targets for the effects of corticosteroids.
      ii. Bind to receptors where they alter RNA and DNA synthesis.
      iii. Inhibit secretion of interleukin-1 (IL-1) from macrophages and interleukin-2 (IL-2) secretion from T cells.
      iv. Inhibit the generation of cytotoxic T cells.
3. Corticosteroids—Dosing and administration
   a. The dose varies depending on
      i. Type of preparation
      ii. Type of transplant
      iii. Timing of transplantation (induction vs. maintenance)
      iv. Indication (prevention or treatment of rejection)
   b. Methylprednisolone is the most frequently used corticosteroid during the early posttransplant period
      i. Used as an induction agent.[25,27,29,33]
      ii. Doses range from 250 to 1,000 mg given intraoperatively with a subsequent tapering regimen.[25,27,29,33]
   c. Prednisone is the most frequently used corticosteroid during the maintenance phase
      i. Doses ranges from 0 to 10 mg/day or may be dosed by weight: 0.5 mg/kg divided in two doses immediately posttransplant and rapidly tapered.
      ii. Initial dosing is based upon organ transplanted and center protocol.
   d. The corticosteroid dose used to treat acute rejection also varies depending on
      i. Type of transplant
      ii. Severity of rejection
      iii. The typical treatment regimen is methylprednisolone 250 to 1,000 mg IV daily for 3 to 5 days.[19,68,69]
4. Corticosteroids—Adverse effects[67]
   a. Corticosteroid side effects depend on the dose and the duration of exposure.
   b. Short courses of a corticosteroid are usually well-tolerated with fewer and milder side effects than longer courses of corticosteroids.
   c. Side effects of corticosteroids are well known, well described, range from mild annoyances to serious, irreversible bodily damages and include the following:
      i. Glucose intolerance, hyperglycemia or worsening diabetes
      ii. Weight gain
      iii. Psychotic disturbances
      iv. Bone growth inhibition in children
      v. Osteoporosis
      vi. Osteonecrosis
      vii. Hypertension
      viii. Hyperlipidemia

      ix.   Glaucoma, cataracts

      x.   Suppression of the hypothalamic- pituitary-adrenal axis

      xi.   Fluid retention

      xii.   Puffiness of and hair growth on the face

      xiii.   Potassium loss

      xiv.   Headache

      xv.   Muscle weakness

      xvi.   Thinning and easy bruising of the skin

      xvii.   Peptic ulceration

      xviii.   Irregular menses

      xix.   Convulsions

E.   **Proliferation Signal Inhibitors**

    1.   Role in solid organ transplantation.[44,45,47–51,66,70–75]

      a. Also known as mammalian target of rapamycin (mTOR) inhibitors which are a key regulatory kinase in the process of cell division.

         i.   The term "mTOR inhibitor" refers to immunosuppressant drugs whose mode of action is closely linked to inhibition of this kinase.

      b. Sirolimus (Rapamune), the first mTOR inhibitor, was approved for use in adult kidney transplant recipients by the FDA in 1999.

         i.   A series of clinical trials demonstrated that, when used in combination with cyclosporine and a corticosteroid, sirolimus produced a significant reduction in the incidence of cellular rejection episodes in the early posttransplant period.[45,47,48]

      c. Everolimus (Zortress, Afinitor) are additional proliferation signal inhibitors that were FDA approved in 2010 for use in kidney transplant recipients.[45,48]

         i.   Everolimus is similar to sirolimus with regard to mechanism of action and side effect profile.[45,48]

         ii.   Everolimus has a black box warning against use in heart transplantation due to a numerically increased risk of mortality seen in clinical trials.

      d. Proliferation signal inhibitors are used in solid organ transplantation as part of a maintenance regimen in conjunction with other maintenance immunosuppressive agents to prevent cellular rejection.

         i.   Proliferation signal inhibitors were initially developed for use with cyclosporine

            • However, this combination increased nephrotoxicity, hemolytic-uremic syndrome, and hypertension.[50,51]

         ii.   Subsequently, sirolimus has been used in combination with tacrolimus to avoid the toxicity of sirolimus/cyclosporine combinations.[50]

         iii.   Additional studies have indicated that sirolimus may potentiate tacrolimus nephrotoxicity, especially at higher doses.[50,74,75]

            • Clinical trials in renal and heart transplantation showed that sirolimus plus tacrolimus produced more renal dysfunction and hypertension than did MMF plus tacrolimus.[73]

            • Other studies are evaluating the withdrawal of CNIs in patients receiving proliferation signal inhibitors.

      e. Proliferation signal inhibitors are used as part of various CNI minimization and withdrawal regimens to

         i.   Improve renal function in renal and other solid organ transplant recipients

    ii. Reduce cardiac allograph vasculopathy and improve survival in heart transplant recipients

- There is some evidence to indicate that late conversion (>1 year post heart transplantation) of CNI to sirolimus is associated with decreased allograft vasculopathy and improved long-term survival over CNI.[74]

    iii. Possible antineoplastic effects in patients with posttransplant cancer or who are at higher risk for cancer.

    iv. Some studies suggest a decreased incidence of recurrent, refractory, or resistant CMV infections.[76]

    v. Early heart transplant data suggest that withdrawing cyclosporine in these patients reduces renal dysfunction and hypertension.[77]

2. Sirolimus (Rapamune)

  a. Sirolimus is a macrolide antibiotic isolated from *Streptomyces hygroscopicus* that is structurally similar to tacrolimus but mechanistically different.[78]

  b. Sirolimus is FDA approved only for use in kidney transplantation

  c. Sirolimus—Mechanism of action.

    i. Modulates the immune response by inhibiting the activity of a regulatory protein critical to the coordination of events required for cells to move from G_1 to the S phase of the cell cycle.

    ii. Sirolimus has potent antiviral and antineoplastic properties

  d. Sirolimus—Dosing and administration.

    i. The recommended loading dose for kidney transplant is 6 mg once followed by a maintenance dose of 2 mg/day when replacing CNI.[77]

- This dose may vary depending on type of organ transplanted

    ii. After withdrawal of the CNI, the sirolimus dose should be adjusted to obtain whole blood trough concentrations between 8 and 16 ng/mL

    iii. The recommended loading dose is 2 mg once followed by maintenance of 1 mg/day when adding to a CNI.

    iv. Note: Must be spaced out by 4 hours away from CNI dose to minimize additive renal damage

    v. Sirolimus has been reported to be associated with impaired wound healing and delay in renal allograft recovery. Therefore, delaying the initiation of sirolimus may be warranted in these clinical situations[78,79]

  e. Sirolimus—Therapeutic drug monitoring

    i. Routine monitoring of sirolimus trough level is recommended.

    ii. Therapeutic target is typically between 4 and 12 ng/mL dependent on concurrent immunosuppression.

    iii. During and following CNI withdrawal, it is recommended that the dose of sirolimus be adjusted to maintain a therapeutic target between 8 and 16 ng/mL.

    iv. Optimally, trough levels should be obtained at least 4 to 5 days after a dose change to ensure that the trough level is at steady state before any further dosing adjustment is made.

  f. Sirolimus—Drug interactions

    i. Metabolized by the CYP3A enzyme system, its drug interaction profile is very similar to that of cyclosporine and tacrolimus.

  g. Sirolimus—Adverse effects.[77-79]

      i. The adverse effects of sirolimus and everolimus are very similar.

      ii. The most common side effects are as follows:

- Hypertension
- Hypercholesterolemia
- Hypertriglyceridemia
- Hyperlipidemia
- Thrombocytopenia
- Anemia
- Diarrhea
- Acne
- Rash

      iii. Both proliferation signal inhibitors (sirolimus and everolimus) have also been associated with pneumonitis.[72]

      iv. Renal dysfunction has been reported with both sirolimus and everolimus.

- Typically this is due to worsening proteinuria.[71]

    h. Sirolimus—Black box warning

      i. Sirolimus has a black box warning against use in liver transplantation due to association with an increased rate of hepatic artery thrombosis.[78]

3. Everolimus (Zortress; Afinitor)[70,80]

    a. Everolimus—Mechanism of action

      i. Modulates the immune response by inhibiting the activity of a regulatory protein critical to the coordination of events required for cells to move from G_1 to the S phase of the cell cycle.

      ii. Everolimus has e potent antiviral and antineoplastic properties.

    b. Everolimus—Dosing and administration

      i. 0.75 mg orally twice daily when adding to CNI

      ii. Adjusted to achieve a trough target of 3 to 8 ng/mL

    c. Everolimus—Therapeutic drug monitoring

      i. Routine monitoring of everolimus trough level is recommended.

      ii. The upper limit to the therapeutic range is recommended at 8 ng/mL.

      iii. Optimally, dose adjustments of everolimus should be based on trough levels obtained more than 4 to 5 days after previous dosing change.

    d. Everolimus—Drug interactions.

      i. Metabolized by the CYP3A enzyme system, its drug interaction profile is very similar to that of cyclosporine and tacrolimus.

    e. Everolimus—Adverse effects[70,79,80]

      i. The adverse effects of everolimus and sirolimus are very similar.

      ii. The most common side effects are as follows:

- Diarrhea
- Acne
- Mouth sores
- Edema
- Hypertension
- Hypercholesterolemia
- Hypertriglyceridemia
- Hyperlipidemia
- Thrombocytopenia
- Anemia
- Rash

  iii. As noted above, both sirolimus and everolimus have been associated with
    - Pneumonitis[72,81]
    - Proteinuria with risk for worsening renal function[82]
    - Delayed wound healing and wound complications and delayed renal allograft recovery[79,80]

F. Costimulation inhibitor: Belatacept (Nulojix)[83–87]

  1. Role in solid organ transplantation
    a. Immunosuppression in patients who are poor candidates for CNI-based immunosuppression or who are subsequently intolerant of CNI-based immunosuppression after renal transplantation.
    b. Risk-benefit profile does not favor belatacept after liver transplantation due to the risk of posttransplant lymphoproliferative disease (PTLD) and rejection.
    c. Limited data exist at present with belatacept in nonrenal/liver allografts.
    d. First used clinically in renal transplantation in 2012.
    e. Intended to replace the CNI in a triple drug immunosuppression and use with MMF and corticosteroids.
    f. Theoretical benefit over CNI with less calcineurin nephropathy to provide improved long-term renal allograft function over CNI-based immunosuppression.
    g. Significantly improved cardiovascular risk profile has been demonstrated with belatacept versus CNI-based immunosuppression.

  2. Belatacept—Mechanism of action[87]
    a. Blocks the costimulatory signal, the binding of CD86 to CD28 on the surface of T cells, which is required for most T-cell activation.

  3. Belatacept—Dosing and administration
    a. *De novo*: 10 mg/kg IV on days 1 and 5, and weeks 2, 4, 8, and 12, then 5 mg/kg IV monthly thereafter.
    b. CNI switch: Slowly taper CNI over 2 to 4 weeks and begin belatacept 5 mg/kg IV on days 1 and 5, and weeks 2, 4, and monthly thereafter
       i. May be administered in an infusion center that is able to administer belatacept or by home infusion.
    c. Note: The transplant recipient must be seropositive for Epstein-Barr virus IgG to decrease the risk of developing PTLD[84,86]

  4. Belatacept—Adverse effects[87]
    a. GI : nausea, diarrhea.
    b. Infusion-related reactions, no prophylaxis medicines are necessary.
    c. Peripheral edema.
    d. Infections, particularly fungal infections.
    e. PTLD.

  5. Belatacept—Therapeutic drug monitoring
    a. No monitoring of levels are necessary.

  6. Belatacept—Clinical trials[83–86]
    a. The BENEFIT and BENEFIT-EXT trial programs compared cyclosporine-based immunosuppression to belatacept after basiliximab induction in addition to MMF and corticosteroids in renal transplant recipients of standard criteria and extended criteria donors. Generally, cellular rejection occurred more commonly in the belatacept arms versus cyclosporine. However, renal allograft function was generally better preserved in the belatacept arms versus cyclosporine. Cardiovascular risk was also substantially lower in the belatacept arms versus cyclosporine.

IV. ADJUVANT PHARMACOTHERAPY IN SOLID ORGAN TRANSPLANT RECIPIENTS

A. Antimicrobials

1. Infections continue to represent an important cause of morbidity and mortality after solid organ transplantation. This population is at risk for
   a. Postoperative and surgical site infections
   b. Nosocomial or hospital-associated infections.
   c. Community-acquired infections
   d. Opportunistic infections
      i. Opportunistic fungal and viral infections are another major concern in the first months after transplantation. Selected organs, such as the transplanted lung, are at substantially higher risk for these infections relative to the other organs.
   e. Reactivation of latent infections as a consequence of immunosuppressive therapy

2. Predicting infectious complications[88] is often a function of the amount of time that has lapsed since the transplant surgery (Figure 4-2).
   a. Posttransplant infectious complications are generally classified as occurring in the following timeframes:
      i. Early (first month).
      ii. Mid (months 2 to 6)
      iii. Late (>6 months) posttransplant period
   b. This classification scheme serves to guide diagnostic and therapeutic strategies for managing infectious complications in this population

3. Antibacterial therapy
   a. Perioperative antibiotics are required to prevent surgical site infections to cover the most common organisms in the hospital environment and those relevant to the specific organ transplanted.[88,89]

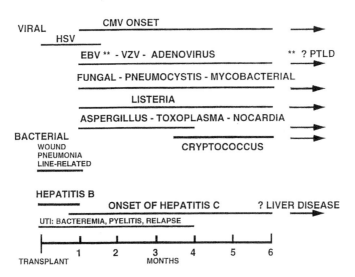

FIGURE 4-2 Timetable for infectious complications after transplantation. *Arrows* indicate infections or other manifestations that may present more than 6 months to years after transplantation. **?, indicates possible relationship of EBV to PTLD; CMV, cytomegalovirus; EBV, Epstein-Barr virus; HSV, herpes simplex virus; PTLD, posttransplantation lymphoproliferative disease; UTI, urinary tract infection; VZV, varicella-zoster virus; ? indicates possible relationship. (Modified from Rubin RH. Infection in the organ transplant patient. In: Rubin RH, Young LS, eds. *Clinical Approach to Infection in the Compromised Host.* New York: Plenum; 1994:629–669, with permission.)

b. Most transplant programs routinely administer antibiotic prophylaxis with trimethoprim/sulfamethoxazole (Bactrim, Septra) to prevent *Pneumocystis jiroveci* pneumonitis
  i. Trimethoprim/sulfamethoxazole is also effective for preventing infections with *Toxoplasma gondii*, selected *Nocardia spp.*, and *Listeria monocytogenes.*[89]
c. Detailed pharmacologic information regarding selected antibiotics that are more commonly used in transplant patients is provided in Table 4-3.[88-91]

4. Antiviral therapy
  a. Viral infections with CMV are a major cause of morbidity and mortality in solid organ transplant recipients.[90,91]
  b. Prevention and mitigation strategies for CMV infections are specific to the transplanted organ, the transplant program, and the serostatus of the donor and recipient pair.
  c. Strategies[91]:
    i. Universal prophylaxis: Patients who are either donor CMV IgG seropositive and/or recipient CMV IgG seropositive receive antiviral prophylaxis for a period of time.
    ii. Preemptive therapy: Patients undergo intensive serological monitoring until they develop an infection, at which point the infection is treated.
    iii. Mixed approach: Shorter duration prophylaxis followed by a period of preemptive therapy.
  d. In high-risk patients (the CMV mismatch: Seronegative recipient of a seropositive donor organ):
    i. Prophylactic use of IV ganciclovir (Cytovene) or oral valganciclovir (Valcyte) is common practice to prevent CMV infections.[89-91]
  e. CMV seropositive recipients
    i. Employ either a universal prophylaxis for a reduced duration relative to the high-risk patient or a preemptive therapy approach with IV ganciclovir or oral valganciclovir, as necessary.[91]
  f. If both the patient and donor are CMV negative, no CMV prophylaxis is required however most programs use Acyclovir for HSV prevention.[89-91]
  g. Antiviral therapies which are commonly employed in the prophylaxis and treatment of viral complications in immunosuppressed transplant patients are summarized in Table 4-4.[89-91]

5. Antifungal therapy
  a. Localized or systemic fungal infections are treated with more potent antifungal agents. See Table 4-5[89-91] for a review of the pharmacology of these agents.
  b. *Aspergillus* and *Candida* species are common fungal infections after transplantation.[88]
    i. Prophylaxis for oropharyngeal candidiasis with nystatin oral solution or clotrimazole (Mycelex) troches for 3 to 12 months after surgery in most transplant centers unless a systemic azole is used.[88,91]
    ii. Prevention of oral candidiasis with nystatin or clotrimazole should also be considered during periods of enhanced immunosuppression.[91]
  c. Systemic infections may be treated with fluconazole (Diflucan), voriconazole (Vfend), or posaconazole (Noxafil).[88,91]
  d. Mechanism of action: These antifungal agents work by blocking fungal cell wall growth resulting in death of the fungus.

TABLE 4-3 Antibacterial Agents

Drug	Indication	Mechanism of Action	Dosage	Common Side Effects	Common Drug Interactions
Vancomycin HCl	Prophylaxis of surgical site infections in patients unable to take penicillin or cephalosporin or in settings with a high prevalence of MRSA; severe or life-threatening infections	Bactericidal against gram (+) bacteria through the inhibition of cell wall synthesis; also selectively inhibits RNA synthesis and alters the permeability of the cell membrane in susceptible bacteria	Prophylaxis: 1 g IV on-call to the operating room Treatment: 15 mg/kg IV Q12 h* for systemic infections; 125 mg po Q12 × 10–14 d for *Clostridium difficile* colitis *renal dose adjustment required	Infusion reactions histamine-mediated (nausea, chills, fever, wheezing, dyspnea, pruritus, urticaria, and rash), nephrotoxicity, neutropenia, and thrombocytopenia Advise slow infusion to reduce risk for infusion reaction	May ↓ efficacy of mycophenolate mofetil due to a ↓ in enterohepatic recirculation Potential ↑ risk of nephrotoxicity when combined with other nephrotoxic drugs such as CNIs
Metronidazole	Second-line therapy to oral vancomycin for *Clostridium difficile* infections	Amebicidal, trichomonacidal, and bactericidal through the inhibition of DNA replication; active against both anaerobic gram (−) bacilli and anaerobic gram (+) cocci	500 mg po TID for 14 d for *Clostridium difficile*	Nausea, diarrhea, vomiting, metabolic taste disturbance, dyspepsia, dysuria, and darkening of urine (no clinical significance), transient eosinophilia or leukopenia	May ↓ efficacy of mycophenolate mofetil due to a ↓ in enterohepatic recirculation May ↑ tacrolimus and cyclosporine levels (weak CYP 3A4 inhibitor)
Trimethoprim (TMP)/ sulfamethoxazole (SMX) [Cotrimoxazole]	Prevention and treatment of: *Pneumocystis jiroveci* pneumonitis (PJP), *Toxoplasma gondii*, selected *Nocardia spp.,* and *Listeria monocytogenes*	Synergistic, bactericidal combination of antibacterial agents, which act sequentially in two successive steps to inhibit the biosynthesis of nucleic acids	Prophylaxis: 80 mg TMP/ 400 mg SMX or 160 mg TMP/800 mg SMX once daily or three times/week daily or three times/week 12 mo posttransplant; some lifelong, also reinstituted during periods of augmented immunosuppression (treatment of rejection)	Hyperkalemia, anorexia, headache, GI disturbances, neutropenia, leukopenia, thrombocytopenia (bone marrow suppression), allergic rash, and photosensitivity	May ↓ efficacy of mycophenolate mofetil due to a ↓ in enterohepatic recirculation. May ↑ voriconazole levels since SMX is a CYP P-450 2C9 inhibitor *Sulfa-allergic patient alternatives (PJP coverage only): dapsone 100 mg po daily; atovaquone 1,500 mg po daily with food, pentamidine 300 mg inhalation monthly

* denotes special conditions.

Burguete S, Sergio R, Maselli DJ, et al. Lung transplant infection. *Respirology.* 2013;18(1):27–38; Costanzo MR, Dipchand A, Starling R, et al. The International Society of Heart and Lung Transplantation Guidelines for the care of heart transplant recipients. *J Heart Lung Transplant.* 2010;29(8):914–956; Fallatah SM, Marquez MA, Bazerbachi F, et al. Cytomegalovirus infection post-pancreas-kidney transplantation—results of antiviral prophylaxis in high-risk patients. *Clin Transplant.* 2013;27(4):503–509; Kotton C. CMV: prevention, diagnosis and therapy. *Am J Transplant.* 2013;S3:24–40

TABLE 4-4 Antiviral Agents

Drug	Indication	Mechanism of Action	Dosage	Common Side Effects	Common Drug Interactions
Acyclovir	Treatment and suppression of the following infections: herpes zoster (shingles), varicella (chickenpox), and herpes simplex	Intracellular conversion to active form—acyclovir triphosphate—which selectively inhibits DNA synthesis and viral replication through competition with deoxy guanosine triphosphate for DNA polymerase and integration into viral DNA. Active in vitro against: herpes simplex virus types 1 and 2 (HSV-1 and HSV-2), varicella-zoster virus (VZV), Epstein-Barr virus (EBV)	*Varies by indication:* Herpes zoster: 800 mg orally 5×/day × 7–10 d *(initiate therapy within 48 h of symptom onset). Varicella: 800 mg orally 4–5×/d × 5–7 d HSV infections: 200 mg orally 5×/d × 10 d or 400 mg orally TID × 7–10 d; *Chronic suppressive therapy* 400 mg orally BID × up to 12 mo IV dosing: 5–20 mg/kg IV every 8 h × 5–10 d *renal dose adjustment required	↑ liver enzymes, headaches, gastrointestinal symptoms (nausea, vomiting, diarrhea, abdominal pain), dizziness, paresthesia	An ↑ in plasma AUC of acyclovir and the inactive metabolite of mycophenolate mofetil occur when coadministered—no dosage adjustment is necessary because of the wide therapeutic index of acyclovir
Valacyclovir	infections: herpes labialis (cold sores); varicella, herpes zoster (shingles); genital herpes	The L-valyl ester prodrug of acyclovir; rapidly and extensively converted to acyclovir. Oral bioavailability is significantly greater than acyclovir.	*Varies by indication:* Herpes labialis: 2,000 mg orally q12 h × 2 doses *(initiate therapy at earliest symptom). Herpes zoster: 1,000 mg orally TID × 7 d *(initiate therapy within 48 h of symptom onset) Genital herpes: 1,000 mg orally BID × 7–10 d for first episode; 500 mg BID × 3–5 d if recurrent, chronic suppression 500 mg BID *renal dose adjustment required	Nephrotoxicity, thrombocytopenia, neurotoxicity (delirium, psychosis, encephalopathy), nausea, headache, dizziness, depression. ↑ AST, AST ↓platelets	↑ Valacyclovir levels if taken with cyclosporine. ↑both levels if taken with MMF, tacrolimus, sirolimus. ↑Nephrotoxocity when taken together (monitor Cr)

(continued)

TABLE 4-4 **Antiviral Agents** (*Continued*)

Drug	Indication	Mechanism of Action	Dosage	Common Side Effects	Common Drug Interactions
Ganciclovir	The prevention and treatment of CMV infection and EBV infection	Intracellular conversion to active form—ganciclovir triphosphate—which inhibits DNA synthesis and viral replication through competition with deoxy guanosine triphosphate for DNA polymerase and integration into viral DNA	*Varies by indication:* CMV disease: Induction: 5 mg/kg 12 h × 14–21 d, given IV infusion over 1 h. Maintenance: 5 mg/kg given as an IV infusion over 1 h once/day × 7 d/wk CMV retinitis: Induction: 5 mg/kg 12 h × 14–21 d, given as an IV infusion over 1 h. Maintenance: 5 mg/kg given as an IV infusion over 1 h once/day × 7 d/wk *renal dose adjustment required	Nephrotoxicity, ↑ liver enzymes, neurotoxicity (confusion agitation, seizures, peripheral neuropathy), hematologic toxicity (neutropenia, anemia, leukopenia thrombocytopenia,) gastrointestinal symptoms (anorexia, N/V, diarrhea, abdominal pain), fever, chills, confusion, pruritus, phlebitis.	↑ risk of hematologic toxicity when administered with or other bone marrow suppressive agents nephrotoxic drugs. ↑ risk of generalized seizures when coadministered with imipenem-cilastatin
Valganciclovir	Prevention and treatment of cytomegalovirus (CMV) and EBV infections	The ʟ-valyl ester prodrug of ganciclovir; rapidly and extensively converted to ganciclovir. Oral bioavailability is significantly greater than ganciclovir	*Varies by indication:* CMV disease and CMV retinitis: Induction: 900 mg po BID × 21 d Maintenance: 900 mg po once daily CMV prevention: 900 mg po once daily *administered with food *renal dose adjustment required	Leukopenia (↓WBCs) Diarrhea, nausea, headache, ↑Cr *Black box warning: thrombocytopenia, granulocytopenia, anemia	Monitor creatinine if taken with Cyclosporine, Tacrolimus, MMF, Sirolimus (may ↑, risk for nephrotoxicity)

* denotes special conditions.
BID, twice daily; TID, three times daily; AUC, area under the curve; h, hours; MMF, mycophenolate mofetil; Cr, creatinine; CMV, cytomegalovirus; IV intravenous; N/V, nausea and vomiting; po, per mouth; wk, week.
From Costanzo MR, Dipchand A, Starling R, et al. The International Society of Heart and Lung Transplantation Guidelines for the care of heart transplant recipients. *J Heart Lung Transplant.* 2010;29(8):914–956; Fallatah SM, Marquez MA, Bazerbachi F, et al. Cytomegalovirus infection post-pancreas-kidney transplantation—results of antiviral prophylaxis in high-risk patients. *Clin Transplant.* 2013;27(4):503–509; Kotton C. CMV: prevention, diagnosis and therapy. *Am J Transplant.* 2013;S3:24–40.

TABLE 4-5 **Antifungal Agents**

Drug	Indication	Mechanism of Action	Dosage	Common Side Effects	Common Drug Interactions
Fluconazole	Candidiasis; cryptococcal meningitis	Highly selective inhibitor of fungal cytochrome P-450 sterol C-14-α-demethylation in the cell membrane of fungi; an essential step in ergosterol biosynthesis	100–400 mg po or IV daily *renal dose adjustment required	Hepatotoxicity (↑ liver enzymes) GI disturbances (nausea, vomiting, diarrhea, abdominal pain, dyspepsia), rash, and headache	↑ toxicity of CYP P-450 3A4 metabolized drugs: cyclosporine, tacrolimus, sirolimus, everolimus, statins, erythromycin, Phenytoin, warfarin. Rifampin ↓ effect of fluconazole by ↑ hepatic metabolism
Itraconazole	Invasive/ noninvasive aspergillosis; candidiasis; histoplasmosis; sporotrichosis; Para cocci-dioidomycosis; chromomycosis; blastomycosis; dermatomycosis; onychomycosis	Highly selective inhibitor of fungal cytochrome P-450 sterol C-14-α-demethylation in the cell membrane of fungi; an essential step in ergosterol biosynthesis	200 mg IV or PO BID -Systemic mycoses required 3 to 6 mo of treatment	Hepatotoxicity (↑ liver enzymes) GI disturbances (nausea, vomiting, diarrhea, abdominal pain, dyspepsia), rash, headache, hypertension, and hypertriglyceridemia	↑ toxicity of CYP P-450 3A4 metabolized drugs: cyclosporine, tacrolimus, sirolimus, everolimus, statins, erythromycin, phenytoin, warfarin. Efficacy of itraconazole ↓ by carbamazepine, isoniazid, phenobarbital, phenytoin, and rifampin (inducers of hepatic enzyme metabolism) Oral drug absorption ↓ by antacids, H$_2$-antagonists, proton pump inhibitors, and sulcrate
Voriconazole	Invasive aspergillosis	Highly selective inhibitor of fungal cytochrome P-450 sterol C-14-α-demethylation in the cell membrane of fungi; an essential step in ergosterol biosynthesis	Intravenous: 6 mg/kg × 2 doses 12 h apart for loading dose (LD) followed by maintenance dose (MD) of 4 mg/kg Q12h. Oral: 400 mg Q12 h × 2 doses (LD) followed by MD of 200 mg BID	Hepatotoxicity (↑ liver enzymes) visual disturbances, fever, rash, nausea, vomiting, diarrhea, headache, and abdominal pain	Voriconazole inhibits CYP P-450 isoenzymes (2C19, 2C9, 3A4) therefore, potential to ↑ plasma concentrations of drugs metabolized by these isoenzymes and ↑ risk of toxicity. Significant ↑ in cyclosporine and tacrolimus levels; sirolimus in contraindicated with voriconazole Efficacy ↓ with enzyme inducers.

(continued)

TABLE 4-5 Antifungal Agents (Continued)

Drug	Indication	Mechanism of Action	Dosage	Common Side Effects	Common Drug Interactions
Clotrimazole	Treatment or prophylaxis of oropharyngeal candidiasis	Clotrimazole and nystatin appear to inhibit the enzymatic conversion of 2, 4-methyl-enedihydrol-anosterol to demethylsterol, the precursor to ergosterol, which is an essential building block of the cytoplasmic membrane of the fungi.	Treatment: 10 mg 4–5×/day dissolved orally × 14 d Prophylaxis: 10 mg TID dissolved orally × 3–6 mo *patients should be instructed not to chew or swallow troches whole.	Hepatotoxicity (↑ liver enzymes), nausea vomiting, abdominal cramps	None.
Nystatin Oral Suspension	Treatment or prophylaxis of oropharyngeal candidiasis		Treatment: 5 mL (500,000 units) QID swish and swallow × 14 days or at least 48 h after perioral symptoms have resolved Prophylaxis: 5 mL (500,000 units) TID to QID swish & swallow × 3–6 mo	Nausea, vomiting, diarrhea abdominal pain	None.
Caspofungin	Candidiasis and salvage for invasive aspergillosis in addition to azole	Inhibits the synthesis of B (1, 3)—D-glucan which is an integral component of the fungal cell wall	70 mg IV or day 1 (LD); then 50 mg IV daily (MD) *dose adjustment required for patients with hepatic impairment—35 mg IV daily (MD) for Child–Pugh Class B	Fever, headaches, hepatotoxicity (↑liver enzymes), infusion reactions, pruritus, nausea, vomiting, and skin rash	May ↓ tacrolimus and sirolimus levels—monitor carefully. Cyclosporine may ↑ caspofungin levels and ↑ liver enzymes (ALT. AST). Combination with carbamazepine, phenytoin, rifampin, and dexamethasone may ↓ caspofungin levels and efficacy (↑ clearance).

* denotes special conditions.

From Costanzo MR, Dipchand A, Starling R, et al. The International Society of Heart and Lung Transplantation Guidelines for the care of heart transplant recipients. *J Heart Lung Transplant.* 2010;29(8):914–956; Fallatah SM, Marquez MA, Bazerbachi F, et al. Cytomegalovirus infection post-pancreas-kidney transplantation—results of antiviral prophylaxis in high-risk patients. *Clin Transplant.* 2013;27(4):503–509; Kotton C. CMV: prevention, diagnosis and therapy. *Am J Transplant.* 2013;53:24–40.

B. Analgesics[92-95]

1. Acute pain management in the postoperative period is managed with routine opioid agents (narcotics), such as morphine, oxycodone, and hydrocodone.
   a. Postsurgical principles of good pain management apply to this population.
      i. Comprehensive review of pain management is beyond the scope of this chapter.
      ii. The use of some nonnarcotic analgesics for intermittent pain management is generally safe.
      iii. Epidural anesthesia has been proven effective after lung transplantation.[94]
2. Nonsteroidal anti-inflammatory drugs (including COX-2 inhibitors) should generally be avoided because of the increased risk of toxicities, especially renal dysfunction.[96]
3. The nonprescription analgesic of choice for transplant patients is acetaminophen, based upon its proven safety profile.
   a. It is also the antipyretic of choice for this group.
   b. This agent is not without toxicities, most notably liver dysfunction with excessive acute or chronic consumption.
   c. Careful patient monitoring is recommended.

C. Medications to manage DM[97-99]

1. DM is a well-known complication of transplantation.
   a. Decreases patients' quality of life.
   b. Worsens long-term outcomes.[97,98]
2. DM after transplantation occurs in up to 50% of solid organ transplant recipients within the first 3 months.[98,99]
   a. High-dose corticosteroid use in many immunosuppressive protocols is implicated as a major cause of DM.
   b. CNIs also contribute to the development of DM.[98]
3. Management of DM is essentially the same as in the nontransplant population and includes the following:
   a. Dietary and lifestyle modifications
   b. Pharmacotherapy
4. Table 4-6[98,99] summarizes the pharmacology of the major categories of insulin and oral-hypoglycemic medications used in the management of DM

D. Medications to manage GI symptoms

1. GI issues such as peptic ulcers and gastroesophageal reflux disease (GERD) symptoms are very common in the transplant population, especially in the early postoperative period.
   a. The increased rates of peptic ulceration have been attributed to the use of steroids for immunosuppression.[69]
   b. Other medications used in prophylaxis or treatment of transplant patients are associated with significant GI toxicities.
2. Prophylactic therapy is commonly prescribed to patients posttransplantation.
3. Table 4-7 summarizes the pharmacology of the common antiulcer medication classes.
4. Use proton pump inhibitors with caution as studies have shown that when combined with MMF, mycophenolic acid levels are lower and may lead to rejection if medications are not adjusted.[100,101]

TABLE 4-6 Antihyperglycemic Agents

Drug	Indication	Mechanism of Action	Dosage	Common Side Effects	Common Drug Interactions
Insulin various formulations): Rapid Acting: Humalog (insulin lispro); Novolog (insulin aspart) Short Acting: Humulin R; Novolin R Intermediate Acting: NPH; Humulin N; Lantus (insulin glargine); Levemir (insulin detemir)	For the treatment of hyperglycemia in insulin-requiring or insulin-dependent diabetic patients.	The primary activity of insulin is the regulation of glucose metabolism. In addition, all insulins have several anabolic and anticatabolic actions on many tissues in the body. In muscle and other tissues (except the brain), insulin causes rapid transport of glucose and amino acids intracellularly, promotes anabolism, and inhibits protein catabolism. In the liver, insulin promotes the uptake and storage of glucose in the form of glycogen, inhibits gluconeogenesis and promotes the conversion of excess glucose into fat. Insulin preparations differ in onset, peak and duration of action.	The dosage of insulin is individually determined in accordance with the requirements of the patient.	Hypoglycemia; prolonged administration of insulin subcutaneously can result in lipoatrophy (depression in the skin) or lipohypertrophy (enlargement or thickening of tissue) in rare cases.	Insulin requirements may be increased by medications with hyperglycemic activity such as corticosteroids, isoniazid, estrogens, oral contraceptives, and thyroid replacement therapy.
Sulfonylureas Glimepirimide (preferred)	Control of hyperglycemia in type 2 diabetics	Stimulates an ↑ in insulin release from functional β-cells in the pancreas. Binds to an ATP-dependent K⁺ channel in the β-cell plasma membrane which causes a depolarization of the membrane and opening of the voltage-dependent Ca⁺ channels—it is the ↑ in intracellular Ca⁺ that produces the insulin secretion.	Glimepirimide 1–8 mg orally daily; taken with first main meal	Hypoglycemia, dizziness, asthenia, headache, nausea	Hypoglycemia may be potentiated when a sulfonylurea is used concurrently with agents that also decrease blood glucose.
Insulin secretagogues Repaglinide (preferred)	Control of hyperglycemia in type 2 diabetics	Chemically unrelated to oral sulphonylureas, but similar mechanism of action (see above). Insulin release with these agents is glucose dependent and diminishes at low blood glucose concentrations.	Repaglinide 0.5–4 mg orally TID with meals	Hypoglycemia, nausea, vomiting, diarrhea, constipation, dyspepsia, headache, arthralgia, back pain, chest pain.	

| *Thiazolidine-diones* Pioglitazone | Control of hyperglycemia in type 2 diabetics | Potent and highly selective agonist for peroxisome proliferator-activated receptor-gamma (PPARγ) which are found in tissues important for insulin action such as adipose tissue, skeletal muscle, and liver. Activation of PPARγ nuclear receptors modulates the transcription of numerous insulin responsive genes involved in the control of glucose and lipid metabolism, and in the maturation of pre-adipocytes. These agents ↓ insulin resistance in the periphery and liver, resulting in ↑ insulin-dependent glucose disposal and ↓ hepatic glucose output respectively. | Pioglitazone 15–45 mg orally once daily | Hypoglycemia, headache, sinusitis, pharyngitis, myalgias, fluid retention, edema, weight gain, abnormal liver function tests. Contraindicated in patients with known congestive heart failure (CHF), as well as those with ↑ ALT >2.5 times the upper limit of normal. | As above, for hypoglycemic and hyperglycemic drugs. The CYP P-450 isoform 3A4 is partially responsible for the metabolism of these agents. Specific formal pharmacokinetic interaction studies have not been conducted with the thiazolidinediones and other drugs metabolized by this enzyme; therefore, monitor carefully when used together. |

Notes: Biguanides such as metformin should be avoided after transplantation. Newer oral agents such as DPP-4 inhibitors do not carry enough data to be recommended routinely after transplantation. From Kesiraju S, Paritala P, Rao Ch UM, et al. New onset of diabetes after transplantation—an overview of epidemiology, mechanism of development and diagnosis. *Transpl Immunol.* 2014;30(1): 52–58; Stevens KK, Patel RK, Jardine AG. How to identify and manage diabetes melitus after renal transplantation. *J Ren Care,* 2012;38(suppl 1):125–137.

TABLE 4-7 **Antiulcer Agents**

Drug	Indication	Mechanism of Action	Dosage	Common Side Effects	Common Drug Interactions
H$_2$-antagonists Famotidine Ranitidine (avoid cimetidine)	Treatment of ulcers, erosions and their gastrointestinal symptoms and prevention of their recurrence; the prophylaxis of gastrointestinal hemorrhage from stress ulceration in seriously ill patients; the prophylaxis of recurrent hemorrhage from bleeding ulcer; prophylaxis and maintenance treatment of duodenal or benign gastric ulcer in patients with a history of recurrent ulceration	Antagonists of histamine at gastric H$_2$-receptor sites—results in the inhibition of both basal gastric secretion and gastric acid secretion induced by histamine, pentagastrin and other secretagogues.	Famotidine* 20–40 mg BID or 40 mg QHS orally; 20 mg q12 h IV Ranitidine 150 mg BID or 300 mg QHS orally; 50 mg q6–8 h IV *renal dose adjustment required for famotidine only	Headache, fatigue, malaise; dizziness; somnolence; insomnia, constipation, diarrhea, nausea, vomiting, abdominal discomfort/pain, dry mouth, dry skin, rash.	May ↓ the bioavailability of itraconazole and ketoconazole by a pH-dependent ↓ on absorption or a change in volume of distribution.
Proton pump inhibitors Esomeprazole Lansoprazole Omeprazole Pantoprazole Others	Treatment of conditions where a reduction of gastric acid secretion is required, such as: duodenal ulcer, gastric ulcer; reflux esophagitis; symptomatic gastroesophageal reflux disease (GERD), Zollinger-Ellison syndrome (pathological hypersecretory condition); and eradication of *Helicobacter pylori*	Inhibits the gastric enzyme H$^+$,K$^+$-ATPase (the proton pump) which catalyzes the exchange of H$^+$ and K$^+$, which inhibits both basal acid secretion and stimulates acid secretion in a dose-dependent manner.	Esomeprazole 40 mg daily or BID orally, Lansoprazole 30 mg daily orally; 30 mg/day IV infusion over 30 min Omeprazole 20 mg daily or 20 mg BID orally Pantoprazole 40 mg daily orally; 8 mg/h IV x 72 h for upper GI bleed *renal dose adjustment required	Diarrhea, headache, flatulence, abdominal pain, constipation, nausea, vomiting, dry mouth and dizziness/vertigo.	Extensive liver metabolism; CYP P-450: 2C19inhibitor and 3A4 substrate; therefore, other drugs metabolized through these cytochrome P-450 isoenzymes should be carefully monitored when co-administered.

* denotes special conditions.

E. Medications to manage cardiovascular complications
   1. Hypertension
      a. The most common medical problem in the posttransplant population.[102,103]
         i. Hypertension has the propensity to cause arteriolar vasoconstriction.
         ii. CNIs are the major cause of this problem.
      b. Postulated mechanisms
         i. Decreased prostacyclin and nitric oxide production
         ii. Increased sodium water retention associated with increased sodium retention in the proximal tubule
      c. Medications of choice for CNI-associated hypertension include the following:
         i. Calcium channel blockers (CCB) such as
            * Amlodipine (Norvasc) and diltiazem (Cardizem)
            * Note: Use with caution when combining CNI and CCB as drug-drug interactions may cause toxicities, such as
               ○ Amlodipine levels increase (risk for hypotension)
               ○ Cyclosporine, tacrolimus, and sirolimus levels increase, assess drug levels for toxicity
         ii. Angiotensin-converting enzyme (ACE) inhibitors
            * Caution when used in combination with CNIs: Risk for hyperkalemia and renal insufficiency
         iii. Angiotensin II AT_1 receptor blockers (ARB)
            * Caution when used in combination with CNIs: Risk for hyperkalemia and renal insufficiency
         iv. These and other antihypertensive mediation classes are reviewed in more detail in Table 4-8.[64,66,67]
      d. Many hypertensive transplant patients will require multiple drugs to achieve control of their blood pressure.
   2. Dyslipidemia[104–107]
      a. Immunosuppressive agents known to increase cholesterol and triglyceride levels include the following:
         i. CNI
         ii. Corticosteroids
         iii. Proliferation signal inhibitors
      b. Management of dyslipidemia is common in transplant patients, with the 3-hydroxy-3-methylglutaryl coenzyme A (HMG-CoA) reductase inhibitors (statins) serving as the primary pharmacotherapeutic approach.[104–107]
      c. Importantly, both tacrolimus and cyclosporine inhibit the organic Anion–transporting polypeptide 1, which is responsible for statin metabolism; thus, statin exposure is increased substantially in the presence of CNI. This typically leads to enhanced myalgia and increased risk for rhabdomyolysis, particularly with lyophilic statins such as simvastatin (Zocor) and atorvastatin (Lipitor). Pravastatin (Pravachol) and rosuvastatin (Crestor) tend to be preferred for patients managed with CNI-based immunosuppression.
      d. The pharmacologic details of this class of medications are also reviewed in Table 4-8.[64,66,67]

TABLE 4-8 Cardiovascular Medications

Drug	Indication	Mechanism of Action	Dosage	Common Side-Effects	Common Drug Interactions
β-Adrenoreceptor Blockers					
Cardio-selective agents (β₁-selective) Atenolol Metoprolol Bisoprolol	Used in treatment of HTN angina pectoris and to reduce mortality in patients with MI selected agents also used in treatment of LV systolic dysfunction (Carvedilol) and cardiac arrhythmias (including: SVT,VT).	Competitive ability to selectively antagonize catecholamine-induced tachycardia at β₁-adrenoreceptors sites in the heart, thus ↓ heart rate, cardiac contractility and CO.	Atenolol 50–200 mg/d po Metoprolol 50–400 mg/d po given daily or BID Bisoprolol 10–20 mg/d	Exertional tiredness, GI disorders (diarrhea, constipation, flatulence, N/V), disturbance of sleep patterns, syncope, vertigo, light-headedness, postural hypotension; 2nd and 3rd degree AV block; may mask hypoglycemia in insulin-dependent diabetics c/i in patients with: unprotected SB and 2nd or 3rd degree AV block	Negative inotropy may occur when metoprolol is given together with calcium antagonists. Verapamil and diltiazem ↓ metoprolol clearance. β-blockers may enhance the negative inotropy of antiarrhythmic agents such as amiodarone.
Calcium Channel Blockers (CCB)					
Non-dihydropyridine type Diltiazem Verapamil	HTN; chronic stable angina; coronary artery disease due to vasospasm; atrial fibrillation/flutter	Selectively inhibits the influx of calcium ions at the voltage-gated (or slow) calcium channels of the plasma membrane into cardiac muscle and vascular smooth muscle. This results in a ↓ of free calcium ions in the muscle tissue, leading to a depression of mechanical contraction of myocardial and smooth muscle and depression of both impulse formation (automaticity) and conduction velocity in the CV system. The non-dihydropyridines have an ↑ effect on AV nodal conduction and weaker vasodilatory effects.	Diltiazem 120–360 mg/d po given QD to QID; 0.25–0.35 mg/kg IV bolus over 2 min; then 5–15 mg/h infusion. Verapamil 188–480 mg/d po given once daily to QID	N/V, swelling/ edema, arrhythmia (AV block, bradycardia, tachycardia and sinus arrest), headache, dizziness, lightheadedness, rash, anorexia, constipation, diarrhea, dyspepsia,	May ↑ cyclosporine, tacrolimus and sirolimus levels—CYP 3A4 inhibitors. When combined with a β-blockers, amiodarone, or other anti-arrhythmic agents ↑ risk of hypotension, bradycardia and AV block. Toxicity ↑ with 3A4 isoenzyme Inhibitors (azole antifungals, erythromycin grapefruit juice) and efficacy ↓ with 3A4 isoenzyme inducers (phenobarbital. Phenytoin, rifampin).

Dihydropyridine type Amlodipine Nifedipine XL	HTN; chronic stable angina.	Dihydropyridines are strong vasodilators, acting via relaxation of vascular smooth muscle cells, with little direct effect on myocardial contractility or SA/AV nodal conduction.	Amlodipine 5–10 mg po QD, Nifedipine 30 mg daily—120 mg BID	Pedal edema, flushing, palpitations, headache, dizziness, lightheadedness, N/V, diarrhea, constipation, and gingival hyperplasia.	These agents under-go biotransformation by the CYP 3A4 isoenzyme. Co-administration of these drugs with others that follow the same route of biotransformation may result in altered bioavailability of one or the other. Toxicity ↑ with 3A4 isoenzyme inhibitors (azole antifungals, erythromycin grapefruit juice) and efficacy ↓ with 3A4 isoenzyme inducers (phenobarbital, phenytoin, rifampin).
Angiotensin Converting Enzyme Inhibitors (ACE-inhibitors)					
Enalapril Lisinopril Quinapril Ramipril	HTN (1st line); CHF and LV dysfunction: post-MI; prevention of CV events; diabetic nephropathy.	ACE catalyzes the conversion of angiotensin I to angiotensin II. ACE-inhibitors suppress the production of angiotensin II, the most vasoactive product of the RAS. ACE-inhibition leads to ↓ systemic arteriolar resistance and mean diastolic and SBP In patients with CHF, inhibition of ACE results in ↓ afterload and heart rate as well as ↑ CO, SV and stroke work.	Enalapril 5–40 mg/d po given QD or BID Lisinopril 10–40 mg QD Quinapril 10–40 mg once daily Ramipril 2.5–20 mg QD	Impaired renal function (↑ serum Cr), hypotension, hyper-kalemia, dizziness, maculopapular rash, N/V, angioedema. Persistent, dry cough attributed to the accumulation of kinins in the respiratory tract due to inhibition of Kinase II.	When combined with agents such as potassium-sparing diuretics, potassium supplements or potassium-containing salt substitutes, severe hyperkalemia may occur. Antihypertensive effect of ACE-inhibitors is augmented by antihypertensive agents that cause renin release, such as thiazide diuretics. Lithium toxicity, with co-administration due to ↓ renal elimination of lithium due to ↓ aldosterone secretion or ↓ renal function.

(continued)

TABLE 4-8 Cardiovascular Medications (Continued)

Drug	Indication	Mechanism of Action	Dosage	Common Side-Effects	Common Drug Interactions
Angiotensin II AT₁ Receptor Blockers (ARB)					
Candesartan Losartan Telmisartan Valsartan	HTN; congestive heart failure, LVdysfunction and post-MI (in ACE-inhibitor intolerant patients); diabetic nephropathy.	Antagonizes angiotensin II by blocking the angiotensin type 1 (AT₁) receptor. Angiotensin II AT₁ receptor blockers act selectively on AT₁, the receptor subtype that mediates the known CV actions of angiotensin II, the primary vaso-active hormone of the RAS.	Candesartan 8–32 mg/d po given QD or BID Losartan 25–100 mg/d po given QD or BID Telmisartan 20–80 mg/d po QD or BID Valsartan 80–320 mg/d po given QD	Similar to ACE-inhibitors. No drug-induced cough.	Similar to ACE-inhibitors.
3-Hydroxy-3methylglutaryl Coenzyme A (HMG-CoA) Reductase Inhibitors (Statins)					
Atorvastatin Pravastatin Rosuvastatin Simvastatin	Management of dyslipidemias; CV event risk reduction	Blocks hepatic synthesis of cholesterol by inhibiting HMG CoA reductase-mediated conversion of HMG CoA to mevalonic acid, an early precursor of cholesterol. This leads to a compensatory ↑ in the number of LDL receptors, principally in the liver, that play a role in clearance of LDL from plasma and reduction of VLDL assembly and secretion, leading to a ↓ in LDL production.	Atorvastatin 10–80 mg po QD Pravastatin 10–80 mg po QD Rosuvastatin 5–40 mg po QD, Simvastatin 10–40 mg po QD *(10 mg/d max. dose recommended in U.S. product monograph for patients on CNI)	GI problems (abdominal pain/cramps, constipation, diarrhea, flatulence, N/V, heartburn), headache, dizziness, rash, pruritus, arthralgias, myalgias, ↑ creatinine kinase (CK), ↑ liver transaminases.	CYP3A4 inhibitors and substrates (amiodarone, clarithromycin, cyclosporine, diltiazem. erythromycin, grapefruit juice, itraconazole, ketoconazole) lead to ↑ plasma concentrations of atorvastatin and simvastatin due to ↓ metabolism potentially resulting in ↑ myopathy. Rifampin ↓ plasma levels of statins secondary to induction of CYP2C9 and CYP3A4. Additive pharmacodynamic interaction with drugs that possess inherent myotoxic potential such as fibric acid derivatives and niacin.

* denotes special conditions.

HTN, hypertension; MI, myocardial infarction;. LV, left ventricular; SVT, supraventricular tachycardia;. VT, ventricular tachycardia; cardiac output; Po, per mouth, QD, once daily, CV, cardiovascular, SBP, Systolic blood pressure; GI-gastrointestinal; N/V, nausea and vomiting; c/i, contraindicated; SB, sinus bradycardia; AV, atrioventricular; BID, twice daily; QID, four times a day; CV, cardiovascular; SA, sinoatrial; ACE, angiotensin converting enzyme, RAS-renin angiotensin system; CHF, congestive heart failure; Cr, creatinine; SV-stroke volume; LDL, low density lipoprotein; VLDL, very low density lipoprotein; CNI, calcineurin inhibitor.

Thierry A, Mourad G, Buchler M, et al. Three-year outcomes in kidney transplant patients randomized to steroid-free immunosuppression or steroid withdrawal, with enteric-coated mycophenolate sodium and cyclosporine: the infinity study. *J Transplant.* 2014;14:171896. doi:10.1155/2014/171898; Kobashigawa J, Ross H, Bara C, et al. Everolimus is associated with a reduced incidence of cytomegalovirus infection following de novo cardiac transplantation. *Transpl Infect Dis.* 2013;15(2):150–162; Rayos® (Prednisone). [Package Insert]. Deerfield, IL. Horizon Pharma USA. Available at http://www.rayosrx. com/PI/RAYOS-Prescribing-Information.pdf. Accessed October 17, 2015.

V. SUMMARY

A. Immunosuppression has evolved over the past few decades, from single agent to multiple agents.

B. More options are now available to
   1. Individualize therapies
   2. Achieve the fine balance between infection and rejection
   3. Prevent short- and long-term complications and toxicities of immunosuppression

C. Medical complications are common in transplant patients.
   1. Understanding the mechanism of these complications helps guide the appropriate selection of medications, which are likely to be most effective.
   2. Clinicians must understand the complexities of posttransplant care including:
      a. Additive medication toxicities
      b. Drug-drug interactions between the immunosuppressive agents
      c. Adjuvant medications prescribed to manage medical complications
      d. Potential opportunistic infections
      e. Predictable metabolic, GI, and cardiovascular complications associated with immunosuppressive therapy
      f. Appropriate prophylactic and treatment pharmacotherapeutic strategies for each transplant organ program

REFERENCES

1. Snyder LD, Gray AL, Reynolds JM, et al. Antibody desensitization therapy in highly sensitized lung transplant candidates. *Am J Transplant.* 2014;14:849–856.
2. Tinckam KJ, Keshavjee SC, Barth CC, et al. Survival in sensitized lung transplant recipients with perioperative desensitization. *Am J Transplant.* 2015;15:417–426.
3. Hanaway MJ. Alemtuzumab in kidney-transplant recipients. *N Engl J Med.* 2011;365(7):671–672.
4. Hanaway MJ, Woodle ES, Mulgaonkar S. Alemtuzumab induction in renal transplantation. *N Engl J Med.* 2011;364:1909–1919.
5. Markmann J, Fishman J. Alemtuzumab in kidney-transplant recipients. *N Engl J Med.* 2011;364(20):1968–1969.
6. Cannon R, Borck G, Marvin M, et al. Analysis of BK viral infection after alemtuzumab induction for renal transplant. Alemtuzumab. *Transpl Infect Dis.* 2012;14(4):374–379.
7. Vadnerkar A, Nguyen M, Toyoda Y, et al. Infectious complications among elderly lung transplant recipients receiving alemtuzumab. *J Heart Lung Transplant.* 2009;28(2):S288–S289.
8. Aggarwal A, Pyle J, Hamilton J, et al. Low-dose rituximab therapy for antibody-mediated rejection in a highly sensitized heart-transplant recipient. *Tex Heart Inst J.* 2012;39(6):901–905.
9. Yelken B, Arpali E, Gorcin S, et al. Eculizumab for treatment of refractory antibody-mediated rejection in kidney transplant patients: a single center experience. *Transplant Proc.* 2015;47(6):1754–1759.
10. Barnett A, Asgari E, Chowdhury P, et al. The use of eculizumab in renal transplantation. *Clin Transplant.* 2013;27(3):E216–E229.
11. Kwiatkowski M, Welch P, McComb J, et al. Evaluating the use of bortezomib and eculizumab in desensitization of transplant patients. *J Pharma Technol.* 2014;30(1):31–38.
12. Patel J, Everly M, Kittleson M, et al. Use of bortezomin as adjunctive therapy for desensitization in combined heart and kidney transplant—a case report. *Clin Transplant.* 2009;347.
13. Kim M, Martin ST, Townsend RK, et al. Antibody-mediated rejection in kidney transplantation: a review of pathophysiology, diagnosis and treatment options. *Pharmacotherapy.* 2014;34(7):733–744.
14. Hendrikx TK, Klepper M, Ijzermans J, et al. Clinical rejection and persistent immune regulation in kidney transplant patients. *Transpl Immunol.* 2009;21(3):129–135.
15. Colaneri J. An overview of transplant immunosuppression: history, principles, and current practices in kidney transplantation. *Nephrol Nurs J.* 2014;41(6):549–561.
16. Jordan SC, Totoda M, Kahwaii J, et al. Clinical aspects of intravenous immunoglobulin use in solid organ transplant recipients. *Am J Transplant.* 2011;11(2):196–202.

17. Kaczorowski DJ, Datta J, Kamoun M, et al. Profound hyperacute cardiac allograft rejection rescue with biventricular mechanical circulatory support and plasmapheresis, intravenous immunoglobulin, and rituximab therapy. *J Cardiothorac Surg.* 2013;8:48.

18. Ahmed T, Senzel L. The role of therapeutic apheresis in the treatment of acute antibody-mediated kidney rejection. *J Clin Apher.* 2012;27:173–177.

19. Hechem R. Antibody-mediated lung transplant rejection. *Curr Respir Care Rep.* 2012;1(3):157–161.

20. Chih S, Tinckam KJ, Ross HJ. A survey of current practice for antibody-mediated rejection in heart transplantation. *Am J Transplant.* 2013;13(4):1069–1074.

21. Wagner S, Brennan D. Induction therapy in renal transplant recipients. How convincing in the current evidence? *Drugs.* 2012;72(5):671–683.

22. Ansari D, Lund LH, Stehlik J, et al. Induction with anti-thymocyte globulin in heart transplantation is associated with better long-term survival compared with basiliximab. *J Heart Lung Transplant.* 2015;34(10):1283–1291.

23. Cantarovich D, Rostaing L, Kamar N, et al. Early corticosteroid avoidance in kidney transplant recipients receiving atg-f induction: 5 year actual results of a prospective and randomized study. *Am J Transplant.* 2014;14(11):2556–2564.

24. Patel J, Kobashigawa J. Minimization of immunosuppression. *Transpl Immunol.* 2008;20(1):48–54.

25. Lee R, Gabardi S. Current trends in immunosuppressive therapies for renal transplant recipients. *Am J Health Syst Pharm.* 2012;69(22):1961–1975.

26. Ponticelli C. Present and future of immunosuppressive therapy in kidney transplantation. *Transplant Proc.* 2011;43(6):2439–2440.

27. Moini M, Schilsky ML, Tichy EM. Review on immunosuppression in liver transplantation. *World J Hepatol.* 2015;7(10):355–1368.

28. Knechtle S. Guidance for liver transplant immunosuppression. *Am J Transplant.* 2011;11(5):886–887.

29. Afshar K. Future direction of immunosuppression in lung transplantation. *Curr Opin Organ Transplant.* 2014;19(6):583–590.

30. Bhorade SM, Stern E. Immunosuppression for lung transplantation. *Proc Am Thorac Soc.* 2009;6(1):47–53.

31. Kahan BD. Forty years of publication of transplantation proceedings—the second decade: the cyclosporine revolution. *Transplant Proc.* 2009;41(5):1423–1437.

32. Moten MA, Doligalski CT. Postoperative transplant immunosuppression in the critical care unit. *AACN Adv Crit Care.* 2013;24(4):345–350.

33. Soderlund C, Radegran G. Immunosuppressive therapies after heart transplantation—the balance between under- and over-immunosuppression. *Transplant Rev.* 2015;29(3):181–189.

34. Witt CA, Puri V, Geiman AE, et al. Lung transplant immunosuppression—time for a new approach? *Expert Rev Clin Immunol.* 2014;10(11):1419–1421.

35. Floreth T, Bhorade SM. Current trends in immunosuppression for lung transplantation. *Semin Respir Crit Care Med.* 2010;31(2):172–178.

36. Treede H, Glanville AR, Klepetko W, et al. Tacrolimus and cyclosporine have differential effects on the risk of development of bronchiolitis obliterans syndrome: results of a prospective, randomized international trial in lung transplantation. *J Heart Lung Transplant.* 2012;31:797–804.

37. Neoral® [Package Insert]. East Hanover, NJ: Novartis Pharmaceutical Corp.; March 2015. Available at https://www.pharma.us.novartis.com/product/pi/pdf/neoral.pdf. Accessed October 17, 2015.

38. Issa N, Kukla A, Ibrahim HN. Calcineurin inhibitor toxicity: a review and perspective of the evidence. *Am J Nephrol.* 2013;37(6):602–612.

39. Castrogudin JF, Molina E, Vara E. Calcineurin inhibitors in liver transplantation: to be or not to be. *Transplant Proc.* 2011;43(6):2220–2223.

40. Prograf® [Package Insert]. Deerfield, IL: Astellas Pharma U.S., Inc.; May 2015. Available at https://www.astellas.us/docs/prograf.pdf. Accessed October 17, 2015.

41. Patel JK, Kobashigawa JA. Tacrolimus in heart transplant recipients: an overview. *BioDrugs.* 2007;21(3):139–143.

42. Kobashigawa JA, Miller LW, Russell SD, et al. Tacrolimus with mycophenolate mofetil (MMF) or sirolimus vs. cyclosporine with MMF in cardiac transplant patients: 1-year report. *Am J Transplant.* 2006;6(6):1377–1386.

43. Eisen HJ, Kobashigawa JA, Starling RC, et al. Everolimus versus mycophenolate mofetil in heart transplantation: a randomized, multicenter trial. *Am J Transplant.* 2013;3(5):1203–1216.

44. Baraldo M, Gregoraci G, Livi U. Steroid-free and steroid withdrawal protocols in heart transplantation: the review of literature. *Transpl Int.* 2014;27(6):515–529.

45. Budde K, Rath T, Sommerer C, et al. Renal efficacy and safety outcomes following late conversion of kidney transplant patients from calcineurin inhibitor therapy to everolimus: the randomized APOLLO study. *Clin Nephrol.* 2015;83(1):11–21.

46. Kaplan B, Qazi Y, Wellen JR. Strategies for the management of adverse events associated with mTOR inhibitors. *Transplant Rev.* 2014;28(3):126–133.

47. Asrani AK, Leise MD, West CP, et al. Use of sirolimus in liver transplant recipients with renal insufficiency: systematic review and meta-analysis. *Hepatology.* 2010;52(4):1360–1370.

48. Cicora F, Massari P, Acosta F, et al. Use of everolimus in renal transplant recipients: data from a national registry. *Transplant Proc.* 2014;46(9):2991–2995.

49. Diekmann F. Immunosuppressive minimization with mTOR inhibitors and belatacept. *Transpl Int.* 2015;28(8):921–927.

50. Carvalha C, Coentrão L, Bustorff M, et al. Conversion from sirolimus to everolimus in kidney transplant recipients receiving a calcineurin-free regimen. *Clin Transplant.* 2011;25(4):E401–E405.

51. Guethoff S, Stroeh K, Grinninger C, et al. De novo sirolimus with low-dose tacrolimus versus full dose tacrolimus with mycophenolate mofetil after heart transplantation—8 year results. *J Heart Lung Transplant.* 2015; 34(5):634–642.

52. Imuran® [Package Insert]. San Diego, CA: Prometheus Laboratories Inc.; December 2011. Available at: http://www.accessdata.fda.gov/drugsatfda_docs/label/2014/016324s037,017391s016lbl.pdf. Accessed October 17, 2015.

53. Cellcept® [Package Insert]. San Francisco, CA: Roche Pharmaceutical, Genentech Inc.; 2015. Available at http://www.gene.com/download/pdf/cellcept_prescribing.pdf. Accessed October 17, 2015.

54. Myfortic® [Package Insert]. East Hanover, NJ: Novartis Pharmaceutical Corp.; September 2015. Available at https://www.pharma.us.novartis.com/product/pi/pdf/myfortic.pdf. Accessed October 17, 2015.

55. Cristelli MP, Tedesco-Silva H, Medina-Pestana JO, et al. Safety profile comparing azathioprine and mycophenolate in kidney transplant recipients receiving tacrolimus and corticosteroids. *Transpl Infect Dis.* 2013;15:369–378.

56. Kim M, Rostas S, Gabardi S. Mycophenolate fetal toxicity and risk evaluation and mitigation strategies. *Am J Transplant.* 2013;13(6):1383–1389.

57. Narayan M, Pankewycz O, Shihab F, et al. Long-term outcomes in African American kidney transplant recipients undergoing contemporary immunosuppression: a four-yr analysis of the Mycophenolic acid Observational REnal Transplant (MORE) study. *Clin Transplant.* 2014;28:184–191.

58. Sarvary E, Nemes B, Varga M, et al. Significance of mycophenolate monitoring in liver transplant recipients: toward the cut-off level. *Transplant Proc.* 2012;44(7):2157–2161.

59. Zuk D, Pearson GJ. Monitoring of mycophenolate mofetil in orthotopic heart transplant recipients—a systematic review. *Transplant Rev.* 2009;23(3):171–177.

60. Bolin P, Guhh R, Kandaswamy R, et al. Mycophenolic acid in kidney transplant patients with diabetes mellitus: does the formulation matter? *Transplant Rev.* 2011;25(3):117–123.

61. Toledo A, Hendrix L, Buchholz V, et al. Improvement of gastrointestinal symptoms after conversion from mycophenolic mofetil to enteric-coated mycophenolate sodium in liver transplant patients. *Clin Transplant.* 2012;26(1):156–163.

62. Steiner R, Awdishu L. Steroids in kidney transplant patients. *Semin Immunopathol.* 2011;33(2):157–167.

63. Vincenti F, Schena FP, Paraskevas S, et al. A randomized multicenter study of steroid avoidance, early steroid withdrawal or standard steroid therapy in kidney transplant recipients. *Am J Transplant.* 2008;8(2):307–316.

64. Thierry A, Mourad G, Buchler M, et al. Three-year outcomes in kidney transplant patients randomized to steroid-free immunosuppression or steroid withdrawal, with enteric-coated mycophenolate sodium and cyclosporine: the infinity study. *J Transplant.* 2014;14:171896. doi:10.1155/2014/171898.

65. Montero N, Webster A, Royela A, et al. Steroid avoidance or withdrawal for pancreas and pancreas with kidney transplant recipients. *Cochrane Database Syst Rev.* 2014;9(9):CD007669–CD007648.

66. Kobashigawa J, Ross H, Bara C, et al. Everolimus is associated with a reduced incidence of cytomegalovirus infection following de novo cardiac transplantation. *Transpl Infect Dis.* 2013;15(2):150–162.

67. Rayos® (Prednisone). [Package Insert]. Deerfield, IL. Horizon Pharma USA. Available at http://www.rayosrx.com/PI/RAYOS-Prescribing-Information.pdf. Accessed October 17, 2015.

68. Meadows H, Taber D, Pilch N, et al. The impact of early corticosteroid withdrawal on graft survival in liver transplant recipients. *Transplant Proc.* 2012;44(5):1323–1328.

69. Chou H, Chi N, Lin M, et al. Steroid pulse therapy combined with plasmapheresis for clinically compromised patients after heart transplantation. *Transplant Proc.* 2012;44(4):900–902.

70. Zuckermann A, Wang S, Epailly E, et al. Everolimus immunosuppression in de novo heart transplant recipients: what does the evidence tell us now? *Transplant Rev.* 2013;27(3):76–84.

71. Meier-Kriesche HU, Schold JD, Srinivas TR, et al. Sirolimus in combination with tacrolimus is associated with worse renal allograft survival compared to mycophenolate mofetil combined with tacrolimus. *Am J Transplant.* 2005;5(9):2273–2280.

72. Champion L, Stern M, Israel-Biet D, et al. Brief communication: sirolimus-associated pneumonitis: 24 cases in renal transplant recipient. *Ann Intern Med.* 2006;144:505–509.

73. Topilsky Y, Hasin T, Raichlin E, et al. Sirolimus as primary immunosuppression attenuates allograft vasculopathy with improved late survival and decreased cardiac events after cardiac transplantation. *Circulation.* 2012;125:708–720.

74. Ciancio G, Burke GW, Gaynor JJ, et al. A randomized long-term trial of tacrolimus/sirolimus versus tacrolimus/mycophenolate versus cyclosporine/sirolimus in renal transplantation: three-year analysis. *Transplantation.* 2006;81:845–852.

75. Larson TS, Dean PG, Stegall MD, et al. Complete avoidance of calcineurin inhibitors in renal transplantation: a randomized trial comparing sirolimus and tacrolimus. *Am J Transplant.* 2006;6(3):514–522.

76. Demopoulos L, Polinsky M, Steele G, et al. Reduced risk of cytomegalovirus infection in solid organ transplant recipients treated with sirolimus: a pooled analysis of clinical trials. *Transplant Proc.* 2008;40(5):1407–1410.

77. Gleissner CA, Doesch A, Ehlermann P, et al. Cyclosporine withdrawal improves renal function in heart transplant patients on reduced-dose cyclosporine therapy. *Am J Transplant.* 2006;6:2750–2758.

78. Rapamune®[Package Insert]. Philadelphia, PA: Pfizer, Wyeth Pharma USA; July 2011. Available at http://labeling.pfizer.com/showlabeling.aspx?id=139. Accessed October 17, 2015.

79. Dean PG, Lund WJ, Larson TS, et al. Wound-healing complications after kidney transplantation: a prospective, randomized comparison of sirolimus and tacrolimus. *Transplantation,* 2004;77(10):1555–1561.

80. Zortress® [Package Insert]. East Hanover, NJ: Novartis Pharmaceuticals; January 2015. Available at https://www.pharma.us.novartis.com/product/pi/pdf/zortress.pdf. Accessed October 17, 2015.

81. White DA, Camus P, Endo M, et al. Noninfectious pneumonitis after everolimus therapy for advanced renal cell carcinoma. *Am J Respir Crit Care Med.* 2010;182(3):396–403.

82. Chapman JR, Rangan GK. Why do patients develop proteinuria with Sirolimus? Do we have the answer? *Am J Kidney Dis.* 2010;55(2):213–216.

83. Pestana JO, Grinyo JM, Vanrenterghem Y, et al. Three-year outcomes from BENEFIT-EXT: a phase II study of belatacept versus cyclosporine in recipients of extended criteria donor kidneys. *Am J Transplant.* 2012;12(3):630–639.

84. Vincenti F, Larsen CP, Alberu J, et al. Three-year outcomes from BENEFIT, a randomized active-controlled, parallel-group study in adult kidney transplant recipients. *Am J Transplant.* 2012;12(1):210–217.

85. Vanreterghem Y, Bresnahan B, Campistol J, et al. Belatacept-based regimens are associated with improved cardiovascular and metabolic risk factors compared with cyclosporine in kidney transplant recipients (BENEFIT and BENEFIT-EXT studies). *Transplantation.* 2011;91:976–983.

86. Vincenti F, Charpentier B, Vanreterghem Y, et al. A phase III study of belatacept-based immunosuppression regimens versus cyclosporine in renal transplant recipients (BENEFIT study). *Am J Transplant.* 2010;10:535–546.

87. Nulojix ® [Package Insert]. Princeton, NJ. Bristol Meyers Squib; September 2014. Available at http://packageinserts.bms.com/pi/pi_nulojix.pdf. Accessed October 17, 2015.

88. Burguete S, Sergio R, Maselli DJ, et al. Lung transplant infection. *Respirology.* 2013;18(1):27–38.

89. Costanzo MR, Dipchand A, Starling R, et al. The International Society of Heart and Lung Transplantation Guidelines for the care of heart transplant recipients. *J Heart Lung Transplant.* 2010;29(8):914–956.

90. Fallatah SM, Marquez MA, Bazerbachi F, et al. Cytomegalovirus infection post-pancreas-kidney transplantation—results of antiviral prophylaxis in high-risk patients. *Clin Transplant.* 2013;27(4):503–509.

91. Kotton C. CMV: prevention, diagnosis and therapy. *Am J Transplant.* 2013;S3:24–40.

92. Huprikar S. Revisiting antifungal prophylaxis in high-risk liver transplant recipients. *Am J Transplant.* 2014;14(12):2683–2684.

93. Villamor R, Lee A, Sommer S, et al. Pain after lung transplant: high-frequency chest oscillation vs chest physiotherapy. *Am J Crit Care.* 2013;22(2):115–124.

94. Richard C, Girard D, Girard F, et al. Acute postoperative pain in lung transplant recipients. *Ann Thorac Surg.* 2004;77(6):1951–1955.

95. Madan A, Barth K, Reuben A, et al. Chronic pain among liver transplant candidates. *Prog Transplant.* 2012;22(4):379–384.

96. Gabardi S, Luu L. Nonprescription analgesics and their use in solid-organ transplantation: a review. *Prog Transplant.* 2004;14:182–190.

97. Palepu S, Prasad GV. New-onset diabetes mellitus after kidney transplantation: current status and future directions. *World J Diabetes.* 2015;6(3):445–455.

98. Kesiraju S, Paritala P, Rao Ch UM, et al. New onset of diabetes after transplantation—an overview of epidemiology, mechanism of development and diagnosis. *Transpl Immunol.* 2014;30(1):52–58.

99. Stevens KK, Patel RK, Jardine AG. How to identify and manage diabetes mellitus after renal transplantation. *J Ren Care.* 2012;38(suppl 1):125–137.

100. Kofler S, Deutsch M, Bigdeli A, et al. Proton pump inhibitor co-mediation reduces mycophenolate acid drug exposure in heart transplant recipients. *J Heart Lung Transplant.* 2009;28(6):605–611.

101. Knorr J, Sjeine M, Braitman L, et al. Concomitant proton pump inhibitors with mycophenolate mofetil and risk of rejection in kidney transplant recipients. *Transplantation.* 2014;97(5):518–524.

102. Kittleson MM, Kobashigawa JA. Long-term care of the heart transplant recipient. *Curr Opin Organ Transplant.* 2014;19(5):515–524.

103. Adamczak M, Gazda M, Gojowy D, et al. Hypertension in patients after liver transplantation. *J Hypertens.* 2015;33(suppl 1):e32.

104. Eckel RH, Cornier MA. Update on the NCEP ATP-III emerging cardiometabolic risk factors. *BMC Med.* 2014;12:115–124.

105. Charlton M. Obesity, hyperlipidemia and metabolic syndrome. *Liver Transpl.* 2009;15(suppl 2):S83–S89.

106. Kobashigawa JA, Moriguchi JD, Laks H, et al. Ten-year follow-up of a randomized trial of pravastatin in heart transplant patients. *J Heart Lung Transplant.* 2005;24(11):1736–1740.

107. Chawla C, Greene T, Beck G, et al. Hyperlipidemia and long term outcomes in nondiabetic chronic kidney disease. *Clin J Am Soc Nephrol.* 2010;5(9):1582–1587.

SELF-ASSESSMENT QUESTIONS

1. Which of the following agents is used to prevent cellular rejection within the first 6 months after transplantation and is given once at the time of transplantation?
   a. Sirolimus
   b. Alemtuzumab
   c. Basiliximab
   d. Tacrolimus

2. Which of the following combinations of medicines represent the classic and most often used triple-drug maintenance immunosuppression regimen?
   a. Cyclosporine, azathioprine, methylprednisolone
   b. Tacrolimus, azathioprine, prednisone
   c. Tacrolimus, mycophenolate mofetil, prednisone
   d. Cyclosporine, everolimus, methylprednisolone

3. Which of the following are acceptable agents to replace calcineurin inhibitors after transplantation?
   1. Sirolimus
   2. Belatacept
   3. Methotrexate
   a. 1 only
   b. 1 and 2
   c. 2 and 3
   d. 1, 2, and 3

4. Which of the following maintenance immunosuppressive agents requires the transplant recipient to be EBV IgG seropositive to minimize the risk of posttransplant lymphoproliferative disorder?
   a. Belatacept
   b. Sirolimus
   c. Tacrolimus
   d. Azathioprine

5. Which of the following immunosuppressive agents should *only* be used as induction immunosuppression?
   a. Antithymocyte globulin
   b. Alemtuzumab
   c. Belatacept
   d. Basiliximab

6. Which of the following maintenance immunosuppressive agents is associated with renal dysfunction due to worsening proteinuria?
   a. Mycophenolate sodium
   b. Azathioprine
   c. Sirolimus
   d. Cyclosporine

7. Which corticosteroid strategy is associated with the greatest risk/benefit profile after renal transplantation performed with rabbit antithymocyte globulin?
   a. Early avoidance
   b. Slow taper
   c. Late minimization
   d. Chronic maintenance

8. Hypertension is common after transplantation and is likely associated with which of the following immunosuppressive classes of medicines?
   a. Proliferation signal inhibitors
   b. Costimulatory inhibitors
   c. Induction immunosuppression
   d. Calcineurin inhibitors

9. Which of the following immunosuppressive agents is not recommended for use immediately after heart or lung transplantation due to impaired wound healing?
   a. Tacrolimus
   b. Cyclosporine
   c. Sirolimus
   d. Azathioprine

10. Voriconazole has significant drug-drug interactions. Which of the following immunosuppressive medicines requires dose adjustment for this drug interaction?
   1. Tacrolimus
   2. Everolimus
   3. Cyclosporine
   a. 1 only
   b. 1 and 2
   c. 2 and 3
   d. 1, 2, and 3

Correct Answers:
1.b   2.c   3.b   4.a   5.c   6.c   7.a   8.d   9.c   10.d

CHAPTER 5

Transplant Complications: Infectious Diseases

Debra Dumas-Hicks, RN, BS, CCTC, CCTN

Fawn Fitzmorris, RN, CCTC

Cynthia Cassidy, RN, BSN, CCTC

Karýn Ryan Canales, RN, BSN, CCTC

I. INTRODUCTION

A. Solid organ transplantation (SOT) has been established as an accepted therapy for end-stage disease of the kidneys, liver, heart, and lungs for nearly 30 years. When infection occurs after SOT, early and specific diagnosis and rapid and aggressive treatment are essential to good clinical outcomes.[1]

1. Recognition of infection is challenging in transplant recipients as presentation is often complicated by noninfectious causes of fever, such as drug interactions or graft rejection.

2. As a result of the growing population of immunosuppressed patients with prolonged survival, an increased incidence and spectrum of opportunistic infections has been observed.

3. Guidelines for the diagnosis and treatment of infection in transplant recipients have been developed.[2]

4. While there is general agreement on the major infections for which routine screening is performed, centers vary in the extent of infectious disease investigation and the actions taken as a result of those investigations.[3]

II. INFECTIOUS DISEASE EVALUATION OF THE PRETRANSPLANT CANDIDATE

A. Key Points

1. The successful outcome of SOT requires the careful selection of transplant recipients through a process of medical evaluation and screening.

2. The identification of active and latent infection, along with the optimization of treatment, is an important role of the transplant specialist.

3. Early identification of risk factors that predispose transplant candidates to infection and prompt referral to an experienced infectious diseases (ID) specialist when indicated can prevent posttransplant infections and improve patient outcomes.

B. Goals of Pretransplant Screening
   1. Identify conditions that may indicate a contraindication to transplantation.
   2. Treat active infection in the pretransplant phase, as clinically indicated.
   3. Recognize the risk of posttransplant infection and develop strategies for prophylaxis.
   4. Implement preventative measures, including updating immunizations.

C. History Review
   1. Childhood infections such as measles, mumps, chickenpox, mononucleosis
   2. Underlying illness causing organ failure including, but not limited to, cystic fibrosis (respiratory failure), hepatitis C virus (HCV cirrhosis/liver failure)
   3. Adulthood infections that can include the following:
      a. Hepatitis B virus (HBV) and hepatitis C virus (HCV)
      b. Human immunodeficiency virus (HIV)
      c. Tuberculosis (TB)
      d. Sexually transmitted diseases
      e. Endemic mycoses (histoplasmosis, blastomycosis, coccidioidomycosis)
      f. Recurrent infections (e.g., urinary tract, pneumonia, staphylococcal skin soft tissue infection, line-related infections)
   4. Concurrent/nosocomial infections such as
      a. Urinary tract infection
      b. Pneumonia
      c. Peritonitis
      d. Wound infection
      e. Occult abscess
      f. Catheter/ventricular assist device–related infection
   5. Immunizations
   6. Travel history
   7. Social risk factors such as
      a. Alcohol/drug abuse
      b. Incarceration
      c. High-risk sexual behavior
         i. Lack of contraceptive barrier use
         ii. Multiple sex partners
      d. Tattoos
      e. Body piercings
      f. Socioeconomic challenges
         i. Limited health care access
         ii. Poverty
         iii. Language barriers
         iv. Low health literacy
   8. Environmental exposure such as industrial chemicals, cigarette smoke
   9. Nutritional practices such as the following:
      a. Unsafe source of drinking water
      b. Consumption of raw/undercooked meat, unpasteurized dairy products, seafood
   10. Allergies to antimicrobial agents
   11. See Table 5-1 for Pretransplant Diagnostic Tests and Team Evaluations

TABLE 5-1 Infectious Disease Evaluation

Physical examination	Nutritional status: cachexia, obesity, integumentary (skin lesions)
	Eyes, ears, nose, throat
	Respiratory (rales, rhonchi, breath sounds)
	Cardiac (rub, murmur, endocarditis)
	Gastrointestinal (diarrhea, bleeding, ulcers)
	Genitourinary (prostate examination, Papanicolaou test)
Blood work	Complete blood cell count with differential leukocyte count
	Complete metabolic panel
	Cytomegalovirus IgG and IgM antibodies
	Toxoplasma gondii IgG and IgM antibodies
	Herpes simplex virus I and II IgG and IgM antibodies
	Varicella zoster titers
	Epstein-Barr virus IgG and IgM antibodies
	Serologic screening for syphilis (rapid plasma reagin test)
	Human immunodeficiency virus (HIV) 1 and 2
	Hepatitis A, B, and C
	Lyme titers (if indicated)
	Glycosylated hemoglobin (if indicated)
Other	Chest radiograph
	Computed tomography scan (if indicated)
	CT scan of paranasal sinuses (particularly for patients with cystic fibrosis or a history of recurrent sinus infections)
	Abdominal ultrasound
	Tuberculin skin test
	Quantiferon gold lab
	Urinalysis and urine culture
	Stool culture (if indicated)
	Stool for ova and parasites (if indicated)
	Dental screening
Organ-specific	Heart transplantation: *Toxoplasma gondii* IgG and IgM antibodies
	Lung transplantation: Sputum cultures to detect colonization of respiratory tract by *Aspergillus* species, *Burkholderia cepacia*

From Fischer SA, Lu K. Screening of donor and recipient in solid organ transplantation. *Am J Transplant.* 2013;13(suppl 4):9–21; Danziger-Isakov L, Kumar D. Vaccination in solid organ transplantation. *Am J Transplant.* 2013;13(suppl 4):311–317; Ison MG, Grossi P. Donor-derived infections in solid organ transplantation. *Am J Transplant.* 2013;13(suppl 4):22–30; Ison MG, Nalesnik MA. An update on donor-derived disease transmission in organ transplantation. *Am J Transplant.* 2011;11:1123–1130; Greenwald MA, Kuehnert MJ, Fishman JA. Infectious disease transmission during organ and tissue transplantation. *Emerg Infect Dis.* 2012;18(8):e1.

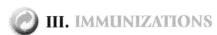 **III. IMMUNIZATIONS**

    A.   Key Points[4]

         1.   Transplant candidates and recipients are at increased risk of infectious complications due to end-organ failure and immunosuppression.

         2.   Every effort should be made to immunize patients in the early phase of disease because the response to many vaccines is diminished in organ failure.

         3.   Transplant recipients may have a suboptimal response to vaccinations due to their immunosuppressed status; therefore, it is critical to update immunizations prior to transplantation.

4. The ideal time to give vaccines following transplantation is unknown; however, most centers restart vaccinations approximately 3 to 6 months posttransplant.

B. Recommended Pretransplant Immunizations[4]
   1. Adult Candidates
      a. Influenza (administered yearly posttransplantation: *inactive* vaccine only)
      b. Hepatitis B:
         i. Assess before and monitor after transplant
         ii. Administer booster if titers fall below 10 IU/L5
      c. Hepatitis A (liver transplant candidates or patients at high risk for exposure)
      d. Tetanus
      e. Pertussis (Tdap) if no tetanus booster in last 10 years
      f. Inactive polio
      g. Pneumococcal
      h. Meningococcal, especially for
         i. Military personnel
         ii. Travelers to high-risk areas
         iii. Postsplenectomy patients
         iv. College freshmen living on campus
      i. Rabies (exposure or potential exposures due to vocations only)
      j. Human papillomavirus (HPV): males and females ages 9 to 26 years
      k. Measles, mumps, rubella (MMR): if seronegative (see Pediatric Candidates section)
      l. Varicella—if seronegative
      m. Note: Live vaccine: must avoid transplantation 4 weeks following administration
      n. Bacille Calmette-Guérin (BCG)—unavoidable exposure to TB
   2. Pediatric Candidates: same as adult candidates with the following exceptions:
      a. Hepatitis A: all pediatric candidates.
      b. *N. meningitidis* (MCV4): all candidates 11 to 18 years of age and as young as 9 months with special circumstances (see Adult Candidates section).
      c. Varicella: vaccine should be administered after 12 months of age with second dose approximately 3 months later.
      d. Measles, mumps, rubella (MMR) may be administered as early as 6 months of age and repeated after 4 weeks following the first injection.
      e. Wait at least 4 weeks between administration of live vaccines and transplant procedure for *all* adult and pediatric candidates.

IV. DONOR-TRANSMITTED INFECTIONS

A. Key Points[5]
   1. Donor-transmitted infection is frequently associated with significant recipient morbidity and mortality.[6]
   2. Despite advances in surgical technique, immunosuppression, and infection prevention, unexpected transmission of infections from donor to recipient is an infrequent complication of transplantation.[7]

B. Donor Risk Assessment
   1. Donor chart review

2. Discussion with available family, friends, and/or acquaintances for knowledge of
    a. Prior infections
    b. Immunizations
    c. Unusual exposures to infection
    d. Psychosocial history
        i. Alcohol/drug abuse
        ii. Incarceration
        iii. High-risk sexual behavior/multiple sex partners
        iv. Tattoos
        v. Body piercing
    e. Socioeconomic status/challenges
        i. Living conditions
        ii. Health care access
        iii. Medical adherence
        iv. Poverty
        v. Language barriers

C. Physical Examination
    1. Performed by organ procurement team and procuring surgeon
    2. Evidence of active infections including abscesses, ulcers, genital/anal trauma, lymphadenopathy
    3. Evidence of recent drug use such as track marks
    4. Evidence of underlying disease (cirrhosis, skin lesions, or other malignancies)
    5. Other abnormalities such as free spillage of intestinal contents or obvious pus or sign of infection involving specific donor organs and/or vessels

D. Laboratory Studies
    1. Donor testing includes the following:
        a. Complete blood cell count (CBC)
        b. Microbial cultures (e.g., blood, urine)
        c. Serologic assay (e.g., antibodies against HIV, hepatitis B virus [HBV]), and hepatitis C virus [HCV]) and, in certain cases, nucleic acid testing (NAT) (including assays for HIV, HCV, or HBV).[7]
    2. Ideally, serologic testing should be performed before and after blood product administration.
    3. If serologic testing is done after the donor is transfused, the number of blood product units should be recorded.

E. High-Risk Donors
    1. Public Health Service (PHS) guidelines developed in 1994 provide guidance to minimize the risk of HIV transmission and to monitor recipients following the transplantation of "high-risk" organs.[8]
    2. The intent of the PHS guideline is to improve organ transplant recipient outcomes by reducing the risk of unexpected HIV, HBV, and HCV transmission, while preserving the availability of high-quality organs using an evidence-based approach to formulate the recommendations.[8]
    3. Transplant programs must obtain specific informed consent from the intended recipient according to the guidelines specified in the Organ Procurement and Transplant Network (OPTN) Policy 15.3 (Figure 5-1).[8,9]
    4. Behavior/History Criteria established by the PHS as "high risk" for transmitting HIV or other infectious diseases despite negative preliminary testing:
        a. People who have had sex with a person known or suspected to have HIV, HBV, or HCV infections in the preceding 12 months

Transplant programs must obtain specific informed consent before transplant of an organ when, in the transplant program's medical judgment, any of the following occurs:

- The deceased donor has a known medical condition that may be transmissible to the recipient, with the exception of HIV, which must be handled according to Policy 2.7: *HIV Screening of Potential Deceased Donors or exclusion criteria in* Table 14:2: *Requirements for Living Donor Kidney Medical Evaluations.*
- The deceased donor meets the guidelines for an increased risk of transmitting HIV, hepatitis B, and hepatitis C as specified in the *U.S. Public Health Services (PHS) Guideline.*
- When a hemodiluted specimen is used for deceased donor HIV, hepatitis B, or hepatitis C screening, according to Policy 2.5: *Hemodilution Assessment.*

Transplant programs must also inform potential candidates of the general risks of potential transmission of malignancies and disease from organ donors, including all of the following information:

- Deceased donors are evaluated and screened as outlined in Policy 2.3: Evaluating and Screening Potential Deceased Donors.
- Living donors are only required to undergo screening for the diseases listed in Policy 14.4: Medical Evaluation Requirements for Living Donor.
- That there is no comprehensive way to screen potential deceased and living donors for all transmissible diseases.
- That transmissible diseases and malignancies may be identified after transplant.

The transplant program must do **both** of the following:

- Explain these risks and obtain informed consent from the potential candidate or candidate's agent before transplant.
- Document consent in the potential candidate's medical record.

15.3.A: Deceased Donors with Additional Risk Identified Pretransplant

If additional deceased donor disease or malignancy transmission risk is identified pretransplant, the transplant program must do **all** of the following:

- Explain the risks and obtain informed consent from the potential transplant recipient or the potential recipient's agent before transplant.
- Document this consent in the potential recipient's medical record.
- Follow any recipient of the deceased donor organs for the development of potential donor-derived disease after transplantation.

15.3.B: Donors at Increased Risk for Transmission of Blood-borne Pathogens

If a deceased donor is found to have an increased risk for transmitting blood-borne pathogens, the transplant program must offer recipients of the donor organs **all** of the following in addition to routine posttransplant care:

- Additional posttransplant testing for HIV, hepatitis C, and hepatitis B as appropriate based on the recipient's pretransplant status
- Treatment of or prophylaxis for the transmissible disease, when available

FIGURE 5-1   Organ Procurement and Transplantation Network Policy 15.3: informed consent of transmissible disease risk (available at: www.optn.transplant.hrsa.gov/ContentDocuments/OPTN_Policies.pdf).

b. Male with male (MSM) sex in the preceding 12 months
c. Women who have had sex with a man with a history of MSM behavior in the preceding 12 months.
d. People who have had sex in exchange for money or drugs in the preceding 12 months.
e. People who have had sex with a person who had sex in exchange for money or drugs in the preceding 12 months.
f. People who have had sex with a person who has injected drugs by IV, IM, or SQ route for nonmedical reasons in the preceding 12 months.

g. A child who is <18 months of age and born to a mother known to be infected with or at increased risk for HIV, HBV, or HCV infection.

h. A child who has been breast-fed within the preceding 12 months and the mother is known to be infected with or at increased risk for HIV infection.

i. People who have injected drugs by IV, IM, or SQ route for nonmedical reasons in the preceding 12 months.

j. People who have been in lockup, jail, prison, or a juvenile correction facility for more than 72 hours in the preceding 12 months.

k. People who have been newly diagnosed with or have been treated for syphilis, gonorrhea, *Chlamydia*, or genital ulcers for the preceding 12 months.

l. People who have been on hemodialysis in the preceding 13 months should be identified as high risk for HCV infection only.

 V. POSTTRANSPLANT INFECTION[10]

A. Key Points

1. Early, specific diagnosis and rapid, aggressive treatment are essential in obtaining favorable outcomes when infection occurs posttransplantation.

2. Etiologies of infections are diverse and include common viral and bacterial diseases and uncommon opportunistic infections that are clinically significant only in immunocompromised hosts.

3. Immunosuppression impairs inflammatory responses normally associated with microbial invasion.

B. Exposure to Infection

1. Epidemiologic exposure

2. Latent pathogens can reactivate in the setting of immunosuppression

a. Cytomegalovirus (CMV), herpes simplex virus (HSV), varicella-zoster virus (VZV, shingles), HBV, HCV, papillomavirus, and BK polyomavirus frequently reactivate after transplantation.

b. Geographically restricted systemic mycoses (histoplasmosis, coccidioidomycosis, diseases caused by the parasite *Trypanosoma cruzi*) may have occurred many years pretransplantation.

c. Significance of exposure varies based upon specific immune deficit(s).

d. Bacterial (*Staphylococcus* spp., *Streptococcus* spp.) and fungal (*Candida* spp., *Aspergillus* spp.) pathogens are more significant in the setting of neutropenia.[11]

e. Viral (CMV) and intracellular (TB) infections are more common with T-cell immune deficits.

f. *Strongyloides stercoralis* may reactivate many years after exposure.

3. Community-acquired pathogens

a. Respiratory viruses such as influenza, respiratory syncytial virus (RSV), and adenovirus

b. Bacterial pathogens such as *Streptococcus pneumoniae*, *Legionella*, and *Salmonella*

4. Food-borne illnesses caused by organisms such as *Escherichia coli*, *Cryptosporidium*, *Salmonella*, *Toxoplasma gondii* (usually related to contact with cat feces), *Vibrio vulnificus*, and *Campylobacter*

5. Nosocomial infections

a. Prolonged hospitalization and mechanical ventilation increase vulnerability to hospital-acquired infections in the early postoperative period.

    b. Gram-negative bacilli (*Pseudomonas aeruginosa, Legionella*)

    c. Antimicrobial-resistant gram-positive organisms (vancomycin-resistant enterococci [VRE], methicillin-resistant *Staphylococcus aureus* [MRSA])

    d. Fungi (*Aspergillus* spp. and nonalbicans or azole-resistant *Candida* species)

    e. *Clostridium difficile* colitis[12]

    f. See Table 5-2 for major pathogens that cause infectious disease in SOT recipients

C. Periods of Increased Risk

    1. Early postoperative period when immunosuppression doses are highest

    2. Increase in immunosuppressant therapy to treat acute rejection

D. Posttransplant Infection Timetable[10,13]

    1. The posttransplant course can be divided into three time periods related to the risk of infection by specific pathogens (see Figure 5-2):

        a. Early posttransplant period (days 0 to 30)

           i. Infection from either donor or recipient

           ii. Infectious complications from surgery and/or hospitalization

        b. Intermediate period (months 1 to 6)

           i. Highest risk for developing opportunistic infections

           ii. Reflective of local epidemiology, immunosuppression, and antimicrobial prophylaxis

TABLE 5-2 Major Pathogens that Cause Infection in Transplant Recipients

Bacterial	Viral	Fungal	Parasitic
Enteric gram-negative bacteria	Cytomegalovirus	*Candida* species	*Toxoplasma gondii*
Pseudomonas aeruginosa	Epstein-Barr virus	*Aspergillus* species	*Cryptosporidium*
Legionella species	Herpes simplex virus	*Cryptococcus neoformans*	*Strongyloides stercoralis*
Nocardia asteroides	Varicella zoster virus	*Pneumocystis carinii*	
Listeria monocytogenes	Hepatitis B virus	*Coccidioides immitis*	
Salmonella species	Hepatitis C virus	*Histoplasma capsulatum*	
Mycobacterium tuberculosis	Human herpesvirus 6	*Blastomyces dermatitidis*	
Nontuberculous mycobacteria	Papillomavirus		
	Adenoviruses		
	Respiratory syncytial virus		
	Influenza virus		
	Enterovirus		
	Papovavirus		

From Green M. Introduction: infections in solid organ transplantation. *Am J Transplant*. 2013;13(suppl 4):3–8; Jani AA. Infections after solid organ transplantation. *Medscape*. 2014. Available at http://emedicine.medscape.com/article.430550-overview. Accessed August 26, 2015; Fishman J. Infection in the solid organ transplant. In: Marr K, ed. *Up to Date*. Waltham, MA: Wolters Kluwer; 2015. Available at http://www.uptodate.com/contents/infection-in-the-solid-organ-transplant-recipient#H5. Accessed August 1, 2015.

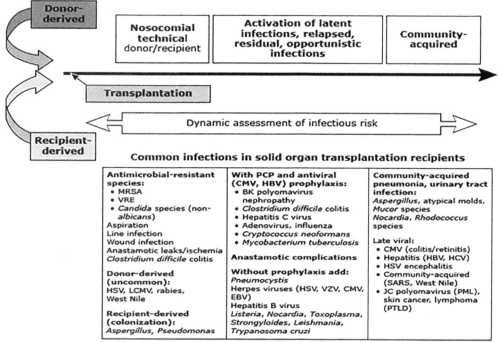

FIGURE 5-2   Infections in solid organ transplant recipients. CMV, cytomegalovirus; EBV, Epstein-Barr virus; HSV, herpes simplex virus; MRSA, methicillin-resistant *Staphylococcus aureus*; PML, progressive multifocal leukoencephalopathy; PTLD, posttransplant lymphoproliferative disorder; SARS, severe acute respiratory syndrome; VRE, vancomycin-resistant *Enterococcus*; VZV, varicella-zoster virus. (From Fishman JA; the AST Infectious Diseases Community of Practice. Introduction: infection in solid organ transplant recipients. *Am J Transplant*. 2009;9(suppl 4):S3. Copyright © 2009 American Society of Transplantation and the American Society of Transplant Surgeons. Reproduced with permission of John Wiley & Sons, Inc. Graphic 58770 Version 5.0.)

    c. Late posttransplant period (>6 months)
       i. Stable and reduced levels of immunosuppression for most patients.
      ii. Subject to community-acquired pneumonias and late viral infections.
     iii. Patients with suboptimal graft function require higher than normal levels of immunosuppression and are at highest risk for opportunistic infections (i.e., pneumocystis pneumonia [PCP], cryptococcosis, nocardiosis) and severe illness.
  2. Significance of timetable
    a. Common patterns of opportunistic infection are observed following solid organ transplantation based on epidemiologic exposures and the "net state of immunosuppression."
    b. The time line is altered based on the immunosuppressive regimen and prophylactic medications. The dynamic assessment of infectious risk represents assays that will measure an individual's risk for infection due to specific pathogens or in general.
    c. See Table 5-3 for posttransplant intervals for infection.[10,14,15]
  3. Guide to develop antimicrobial strategies[10,14,15]
    a. Develop differential diagnosis for the SOT recipient with clinical manifestations of infection.
    b. Detect presence of excessive environmental risks (individual, community, nosocomial).

TABLE 5-3 Posttransplant Intervals of Infection

Time Period	Type of Infection	Example
First month	Continuation of recipient's pretransplant infection	*Pseudomonas aeruginosa* infections in lung transplant candidates with cystic fibrosis
	Infections related to the surgical procedure, other iatrogenic procedures, and indwelling lines and catheters	Anastomotic leaks, obstructions lymphoceles Infection related to invasive lines, catheters[1]
	Transmission of infection by the donor allograft	*Staphylococcus, Streptococcus, Pseudomonas* spp., *Salmonella* spp., *Aspergillus* spp., *Candida* spp. CMV, EBV, HHV-6, HSV, VZV, HTLV-1 and HTLV-2, HIV, HBV, HCV, LCMV, mycobacteria, West Nile virus, rabies, Chagas' disease, *Leishmania*, toxoplasmosis, respiratory viruses
	Early reactivation of latent viruses	Reactivation of herpes viruses
Months 2–6	Infections caused by opportunistic organisms or immunomodulating viruses	Reactivation of latent viral infections: CMV, EBV, HSV, VZV, HBV, HCV, BK polyomavirus

CMV, cytomegalovirus; EBV, Epstein-Barr virus; HHV-6, human herpesvirus 6; HSV, herpes simplex virus; VZV, varicella zoster virus; HTLV, human T-cell lymphotropic virus; HIV, human immunodeficiency virus; HBV, hepatitis B virus; HCV, hepatitis C virus; LCMV, lymphocytic choriomeningitis virus.
From Jani AA. Infections after solid organ transplantation. *Medscape.* 2014. Available at http://emedicine.medscape.com/article.430550-overview. Accessed August 26, 2015; Morris MI, Fischer SA, Ison MG. Infections transmitted by transplantation. *Infect Dis Clin North Am.* 2010;24(2):497–514; Chong PP, Razonable RR. Diagnostic and management strategies for donor-derived infections. *Infect Dis Clin North Am.* 2013;27(2):253–270.

E. Other Factors Associated with Posttransplant Risks
1. Donor-derived infections[6,7,14]
    a. Latent or unappreciated active infection in donor at time of transplant (CMV or Epstein-Barr virus [EBV] infection; toxoplasmosis)
    b. Bloodstream infections (*Staphylococcus, Pneumococcus, E. coli, Candida*); adequate therapy should be confirmed prior to organ acceptance
2. Net state of immunosuppression: determined by interaction of several factors[10]
    a. Immunosuppressive therapies
        i.   Type/dose of medications, plasmapheresis, IgG
    b. Comorbidities such as
        i.   Diabetes
        ii. Malnutrition
    c. Graft abnormalities
    d. Concurrent neutropenia or lymphopenia
    e. Invasive devices—vascular access devices, urinary catheters, drains
    f. Concomitant infection with immunomodulating viruses
        i.   CMV
        ii. EBV
        iii. HHV-6
        iv. HBV
        v.   HCV
    g. See Table 5-4 regarding factors that affect the diagnosis of posttransplant infection.[1,10,15]

TABLE 5-4 Factors to Consider in Diagnosis of Posttransplant Infection

Factor	Example
Pretransplant host factors	Age, nutritional status, comorbidities (e.g., diabetes mellitus), medications (e.g., steroid use), infection history (particularly infections that further suppress the immune system, such as CMV, EBV, HBV, HCV)
Preoperative factors	Invasive devices (e.g., intra-aortic balloon pump, assist devices, mechanical ventilation, hemodialysis)
Type of organ transplanted	Risk of infection greater for lung transplant recipients
Perioperative factors	Ischemic time, blood loss, transfusions
Donor factors	Donor CMV seropositive, recipient CMV seronegative
Immunosuppression regimen	Maintenance therapy (medications, doses, frequency), use of antilymphocyte therapy, net state of immunosuppression
Rejection history	Severity, treatment, and response to treatment
Current antimicrobial regimen (if any)	Use of prophylactic antiviral, antifungal, and antibiotic therapy
Posttransplant exposure to nosocomial, community, or geographic sources of infection	Any recent hospitalizations, community outbreaks of infection, exposure to endemic bacteria, virus, and fungi
Onset of symptoms	Bacterial infections usually manifest over a 24–48 h time period, but they can evolve over several (3–5) days

From Green M. Introduction: Infections in solid organ transplantation. *Am J Transplant.* 2013;13(suppl 4):3–8; Jani AA. Infections after solid organ transplantation. *Medscape.* 2014. Available at http://emedicine.medscape.com/article.430550-overview. Accessed August 26, 2015; Chong PP, Razonable RR. Diagnostic and management strategies for donor-derived infections. *Infect Dis Clin North Am.* 2013;27(2):253–270.

 VI. CLINICAL MANIFESTATIONS OF INFECTION

A. Key Points

1. Significant clinical manifestations of infection include the following[10]:

a. Usual signs of infection (e.g., fever, chills, generalized malaise) may be replaced by nonspecific symptoms (altered mental status, elevated liver function tests) due to immunosuppression

b. Fever without localizing findings or fever with headache

c. Central nervous system (CNS) changes, including changes in level of consciousness

d. Unexplained skin lesions

2. Important characteristics of CNS infections include the following[5,7,10]:

a. The signs of meningeal irritation may be masked by immunosuppression.

i. Changes in level of consciousness may be subtle.

ii. The most reliable indication of a CNS infection is the simultaneous presence of unexplained fever and headache.

• Patients presenting with these manifestations should have an immediate and complete neurologic workup (CT scan or magnetic resonance imaging [MRI] of brain; lumbar puncture [unless otherwise contraindicated]).

VII. CLASSES OF INFECTIONS

   A.   Key Points

      1. The four classes of infection most prevalent after transplant include the following:

         a. Bacterial

         b. Viral

         c. Fungal

         d. Parasitic

      2. Major infection causing pathogens

         a. The major pathogens that cause infections in transplant recipients are listed in Table 5-2.[1,10]

 VIII. PREVENTION AND SAFE LIVING AFTER TRANSPLANTATION[15,16]

   A.   Key Points

      1. Leading a healthy and normal life is possible after transplantation.

      2. The risk of exposure to infectious agents will always be present. Therefore, transplant recipients should be counseled on the modes of transmission and means to reduce the risk of infection.

         a. Direct contact

            i. Frequent and thorough hand washing is imperative and should take place

- Before cooking and eating
- Before and after touching wounds, even when using gloves
- Before touching mucous membranes
- After blowing nose or touching other secretions
- After touching or cleaning up after pets or other animals
- After gardening, touching soil or plants
- After using the rest room or touching any items having contact with human or animal feces (toilets, bedpans, litter boxes)

         b. Percutaneous exposures

            i. Avoid intravenous and intradermal illicit drug use.

           ii. Tattoos and body piercings represent break in skin; all nonsterile practices should be avoided.

         c. Pet safety and animal contact

            i. Wash hands carefully after handling pets.

           ii. Avoid cleaning bird cages and feeders, litter boxes, and handling animal feces.

           iii. Avoid stray animals.

           iv. Avoid animal bites, scratches, and contact with animals having diarrhea.

           v. Avoid contact with nonhuman primates (monkeys).

           vi. Wait approximately 6 to 12 months after transplantation before acquiring a new pet.

         d. Safe sexual practices

            i. Use latex condoms during periods of increased immunosuppression and/or outside of long-term monogamous relationships.

           ii. Avoid exposure to feces during sexual contact.

         e. Inhalation

            i. Avoid close contact with persons with respiratory illnesses.

           ii. Avoid crowded areas (elevators, subways, shopping malls) during periods of increased immunosuppression and epidemic illness circulation.

        iii. Avoid tobacco and marijuana smoke, which is associated with fungal spores.

        iv. TB exposure
- Avoid individuals with known active disease.
- Avoid persons with increased risk (i.e., those working in prisons, jails, homeless shelters).

        v. Construction sites, excavations, and some home remodeling projects may have high concentration of dust with increased risk of mold exposure (*Histoplasma, Aspergillus*)

    f. Ingestion

        i. Water safety
- Cryptosporidiosis may occur from drinking contaminated drinking water during recreational activities.
- Using filters and/or drinking bottled water may reduce risk.
- Abrasions acquired during swimming or bathing in contaminated water may pose risk to exposure to organisms such as *Vibrio* species, *Mycobacterium marinum*, or *Aeromonas*.

        ii. Food safety (items to avoid)
- Unpasteurized milk, fruit, or vegetable juice (*E. coli, Salmonella, Cryptosporidium*)
- Cheeses made with unpasteurized milk such as brie, feta (*Listeria*)
- Raw or undercooked eggs (*Salmonella*)
- Raw or undercooked meat, poultry, or fish (bacterial and parasitic infections such as tapeworms and *Toxoplasma gondii*)
- Raw or undercooked seafood (*Vibrio* species, viruses that cause gastroenteritis or hepatitis, *Cryptosporidium*)
- Cross-contamination of raw and cooked foods

IX. VIRAL INFECTIONS

  A. Overview[13,17]

    1. Epidemiology

      a. Community exposure: influenza, adenovirus, parainfluenza, varicella

      b. Allograft transmission: CMV, EBV, viral hepatitis, HSV

      c. Reactivation of distant viruses: herpes simplex virus, BK virus, herpes zoster as shingles

    2. Clinical

      a. Direct effects: fever, neutropenia, and invasive disease (e.g., pneumonia, hepatitis, meningitis)

      b. Indirect effects:

        i. Alteration in the net state of immunosuppression and increased susceptibility to opportunistic infections

        ii. Potential allograft injury

        iii. Potential oncogenesis

  B. Herpes viruses

    1. Eight members of the herpes viruses family that can cause disease after SOT:

      a. Herpes simplex virus 1 and 2

      b. Varicella-zoster virus (VZV)

      c. Epstein-Barr virus or HHV-4

      d. Cytomegalovirus or HHV-5

e. HHV-6, HHV-7: roseola infantum[18]

    i. Primary infection first 5 years of life and then latent.

    ii. In SOT, cases due to reactivation/reinfection and transient with few clinical symptoms. No antiviral therapy needed.

f. HHV-8

    i. After SOT, endemic in certain regions (i.e., Saudi Arabia; South Africa) causing Kaposi's sarcoma (KS), Castleman's disease, and primary effusion lymphoma.

    ii. Treatment consists of reduction/withdrawal of immunosuppression, chemotherapy, and possible conversion to mammalian target of rapamycin (mTOR) inhibitors.

2. Can be transmitted directly but usually characterized by viral latency.

3. Replication of latent herpes viruses can be triggered by net immunosuppression in the SOT recipient.[17]

4. Herpes virus "infection" versus "disease"

a. The term "infection" refers to the presence of viral replication as indicated by cultures or serological testing (i.e., polymerase chain reaction [PCR] from cerebrospinal fluid, visceral tissue samples, and/or direct fluorescence antibody from vesicular lesions).

b. The term "disease" indicates that the patient has specific symptoms that are caused by a herpes virus. Viremia and/or tissue invasion are present. Tissue invasion can manifest as esophagitis, hepatitis, tracheobronchitis, and, often, disseminated disease.

C. Herpes simplex virus (HSV)[13,17]

1. Overview

a. Approximately 80% of adult transplant recipients are HSV seropositive.

b. Incidence highest in kidney transplant recipients.

c. Most common strains associated with mucocutaneous ulcerative infections: HSV-1 and HSV-2.

d. HSV-1 is more common with oral lesions, which may extend beyond the lip into the oral cavity and esophagus.

    i. Herpes labialis is the most common clinical manifestation of HSV-1.

    ii. Lesions may bleed, interfere with nutritional intake, and require local analgesia to control pain.

e. HSV-2 involves the perianal and genital areas.

f. After a primary HSV infection, the virus remains latent in the sensory nerve ganglia.

g. Reactivation infection occurs in up to 40% of recipients, typically during the first posttransplant month.

2. See Table 5-5 for the clinical manifestations, prevention/prophylaxis, diagnosis, and treatment of HSV.

D. Varicella zoster virus (VZV)—Human herpesvirus 3 (HHV-3)[13]

1. Overview

a. VZV is a highly infectious alphaherpesvirus that is acquired through skin-to-skin contact or airborne respiratory droplets.

b. VZV causes chickenpox as a primary infection and then becomes latent in nerve root ganglia until possible reactivation later in life as shingles.

c. Most SOT recipients have developed VZV antibodies so that reactivation of the virus accounts for 90% of adult recipients.

(text continues on page 158)

TABLE 5-5 Major Organisms Causing Posttransplant Infection: Clinical Manifestations, Prevention/Prophylaxis, Diagnostic Tests, and Treatment Options

Organism	May Cause	Clinical Manifestations	Prophylaxis/Preemptive Therapy	Diagnostic Tests	Treatment Options
CMV[10,17,19-21]	CMV syndrome Tissue-invasive disease: Gastroenteritis Myocarditis Pneumonitis Retinitis (rare) Encephalitis (rare) Pancreatitis (rare)	CMV syndrome: Fever Fatigue Malaise Leukopenia Thrombocytopenia Elevated LFTs Gastroenteritis: Anorexia, dysphagia Abdominal cramping Nausea, vomiting, diarrhea Ulceration, bleeding Pneumonitis: Fever Dyspnea	CMV-negative, filtered, or leukocyte-poor blood products Prophylaxis: valganciclovir is first choice Oral ganciclovir IV ganciclovir Valacyclovir used for minimal risk recipients or if cost an issue Done for 3–12 mo posttransplant Preemptive: Weekly quantitative CMV-PCR assays for at least 3 mo posttransplant If positive, may treat Duration of prophylaxis: range: 3–12 mo posttransplant	Serologic: helpful pretransplant but not diagnostic for infection Complement fixing assay Immunofluorescence ELISA Latex agglutination systems Virologic: Antigenemia assay Quantitative PCR Tissue culture Biopsy Antigenemia: CMV pp65 detected in leukocytes CMV DNA detected in plasma, whole blood, isolated peripheral blood leukocytes, or buffy coat specimens RNAemia: CMV RNA detected in plasma, whole blood, isolated peripheral blood leukocytes	IV ganciclovir Oral ganciclovir CMV hyperimmune globulin for tissue-invasive disease Immunoglobulin For ganciclovir-resistant organisms: Foscarnet Ganciclovir + foscarnet Foscarnet+ Cidofovir Intravenous immune globulin (IVIG)

(continued)

TABLE 5-5 Major Organisms Causing Posttransplant Infection: Clinical Manifestations, Prevention/Prophylaxis, Diagnostic Tests, and Treatment Options (Continued)

Organism	May Cause	Clinical Manifestations	Prophylaxis/Preemptive Therapy	Diagnostic Tests	Treatment Options
Epstein-Barr virus[10,17]	Mononucleosis PTLD: nodal or extranodal disease of CNS, GI tract, lungs, or bone marrow	Mononucleosis: Lymph node hyperplasia Splenomegaly Atypical mononuclear leukocytes Abnormal LFTs Fever Sore throat PTLD: Mononucleosis-like syndrome Weight loss Fever of unknown origin Abdominal pain Anorexia Jaundice Bowel perforation GI bleeding Renal and hepatic dysfunction Pneumothorax Pulmonary infiltrates CNS findings (seizures, altered LOC) Allograft involvement	Preemptive therapy for patients at high risk (e.g., IV ganciclovir during antilymphocyte antibody therapy)	Mononucleosis: CBC EBV antibody LFTs . Heterophil agglutination antibody test PTLD: CT scan: Note: absence of adenopathy does not rule out PTLD; disease can be entirely extranodal Tissue biopsy	Mononucleosis: Acyclovir PTLD: benign polyclonal polymorphic B-cell hyperplasia: May consider acyclovir Ganciclovir Decreased immunosuppression (possibly) PTLD: early malignant polyclonal polymorphic B-cell lymphoma: Acyclovir Ganciclovir Interferon-α Gamma globulin Anti–B-cell antibodies (anti-CD20) Decreased immunosuppression (possibly) PTLD: monoclonal polymorphic B-cell lymphoma: Chemotherapy Radiation Resection Decreased immunosuppression

Pathogen	Clinical features	Manifestations	Prevention	Diagnosis	Treatment
Herpes simplex virus 1[17] Herpes simplex virus 2[17]	Herpes labialis Herpetic esophagitis Anogenital lesions Visceral infection is rare	HSV-1: Crusted ulcerations HSV-2: Coalescing ulcerations without clear-cut vesicles	Acyclovir (low-dose) Ganciclovir (has low oral bioavailability) Valacyclovir Famciclovir Duration of prophylaxis: typically 30–90 d	Viral culture Direct immunofluorescence studies Tzanck smear PCR	Acyclovir Ganciclovir Valacyclovir Famciclovir Foscarnet for resistant strains
Varicella zoster[15,17,22]	Localized dermatomal zoster Disseminated infection Bone marrow suppression Encephalitis	Localized dermatomal zoster that involves two or three adjoining dermatomes without visceral involvement (viral reactivation) Primary, disseminated infection: associated with hemorrhagic pneumonia, skin lesions, encephalitis, pancreatitis, hepatitis, and disseminated intravascular coagulation	Seronegative recipients with significant exposure (same room contact with diagnosed case of chickenpox or direct contact with skin lesion of shingles) Varicella zoster hyperimmune globulin within 72 h of significant exposure IV acyclovir within 24 h of eruption of skin rash	Characteristic unilateral vesicular lesions VZV antibody titer Tzanck smear Direct immunofluorescence studies PCR Serologic testing PCR assay	Localized infection: Acyclovir (oral) Famciclovir (oral) Valacyclovir (oral) Disseminated infection: Acyclovir (IV; high-dose) VZV immune globulin for VZV-seronegative recipients within 72 h of exposure to VZV Ganciclovir Foscarnet
HHV-6[18]	Interstitial pneumonitis	Two noncontiguous dermatomal involvement Fever Malaise Rash Bone marrow dysfunction	None at present		
Hepatitis viruses[17,23,24]	Acute or chronic hepatitis Cirrhosis	Recurrent HBV infection: + HbsAg (typically 2–6 mo posttransplant) Hepatocellular symptoms that can range from mild hepatitis to fulminant liver failure HCV: chronic hepatitis	HBV vaccine for nonimmune transplant candidates Perioperative anti-HBV immune globulin for liver transplant candidates with HBV infection	HBV: Serologic testing HCV: Detection of HCV-RNA by reverse transcriptase PCR Liver biopsy	HBV: Immune globulin

(continued)

TABLE 5-5 Major Organisms Causing Posttransplant Infection: Clinical Manifestations, Prevention/Prophylaxis, Diagnostic Tests, and Treatment Options (Continued)

Organism	May Cause	Clinical Manifestations	Prophylaxis/Preemptive Therapy	Diagnostic Tests	Treatment Options
Polyomavirus: BK virus[15,25,26]	Tubulointerstitial nephritis Ureteral stenosis Obstructive nephropathy Progressive graft dysfunction Graft loss	Fever Persistent hematuria Elevated serum creatinine level		Plasma and urine assays: detection of virus DNA by PCR Urine cytology: detection of characteristic "decoy" cells Immunohistochemistry Tissue biopsy (gold standard) May be difficult to differentiate virus infection from rejection; definitive diagnosis requires visualization of polyomavirus inclusion bodies in biopsy specimen	Decrease immunosuppression agents under investigation Cidofovir Leflunomide Quinolone antibiotics IVIG Supportive care

Polyomavirus: JC virus[15,25,26]	Multifocal demyelination in brain
	Progressive demyelinating
	PML progressive multifocal leukoencephalopathy
	Progressive neurologic deficits
		May involve cerebral cortex, brain stem, or cerebellum
		Cortical syndromes:
		  Visual deficits (hemianopsia)
		  Hemiparesis
		  Frontal lobe dementia
		Brain stem lesions:
		  Contralateral hemiparesis or hemisensory deficits
		Unilateral lesions:
		  Clumsiness
		  Limb incoordination
				MRI of head
				CT scan
				EEG
				PCR analysis of spinal blood and spinal fluid
				Biopsy of brain with in situ hybridization for JC virus
					Cessation of immunosuppression
					Corticosteroid therapy
					Nucleoside analogs: interfere with DNA synthesis:
					  Cytosine arabinoside
					  Adenosine arabinoside
					  Iododeoxyuridine
					  Zidovudine
					Interferons: stimulate natural killer cells
					Nucleoside analogs: interfere with DNA synthesis:
					  Cytosine arabinoside
					  Adenosine arabinoside

Organism	Disease/Syndrome	Clinical manifestations	Prevention/Control	Diagnosis	Treatment
Polyomavirus: JC virus[5,25,26] (Continued)		Midline lesions: Imbalance, falls; Disequilibrium; Gait disturbance; Cerebellar lesions: Blurred vision; Dysarthria; Classic triad: dementia, hemiparesis, hemianopsia			Iododeoxyuridine; Zidovudine
Respiratory syncytial virus[27,28]	Upper respiratory infection; Lower respiratory tract disease; Organ rejection; Bronchiolitis obliterans	Rhinorrhea; Sinus congestion; Otalgia; Nausea; abdominal pain; Cough; Dyspnea; Fever >100.4°F (38°C); Wheezing, rales, rhonchi; Infiltrates on chest radiograph; Sinusitis on sinus radiograph	Aggressive infection control measures; Aerosolized ribavirin; IVIG	Antigen detection by immunofluorescence assay; Antigen detection by immunoassay; RNA detection by reverse transcription PCR; Serology: Demonstration of RSV-IgM antibody (acute infection); Significant ↑ in RSV-IgG antibody between acute- and convalescent-stage sera; Culture: less sensitive and specific in adult vs. pediatric population	Aerosolized ribavirin; IVIG; RSV pneumonitis: Aerosolized ribavirin; Palivizumab (RSV monoclonal antibody) plus aerosolized ribavirin
Influenza virus[27,28]	Influenza syndrome; Secondary bacterial complications	Fever; Chills; Rigors; Cough (typically nonproductive); Sore throat; Fatigue; Headache; Myalgia	Aggressive infection control measures; Annual vaccination of patients and household contacts (unless otherwise contraindicated); Annual vaccination of health care workers	History and clinical examination; Detection of virus-infected cells (via nasopharyngeal washing or respiratory secretions) with specific fluorescent-labeled antibody probes	Influenza A: early administration of: Amantadine; Rimantadine; Influenza B: Oseltamivir; Zanamivir; If started within 36–48 h of symptom onset

(continued)

TABLE 5-5 Major Organisms Causing Posttransplant Infection: Clinical Manifestations, Prevention/Prophylaxis, Diagnostic Tests, and Treatment Options (Continued)

Organism	May Cause	Clinical Manifestations	Prophylaxis/Preemptive Therapy	Diagnostic Tests	Treatment Options
Parainfluenza virus[27,28]	Can cause mild upper respiratory disease May progress to pneumonia	May mimic influenza	No definitive recommendations	Viral isolation Viral shell assays Rapid antigen detection	Ribavirin has been used for lower respiratory tract disease
Coronavirus[10,22]	Asymptomatic or mild respiratory illness that may progress to fatal respiratory failure (SARS)	Fever >100.4°F (38°C) Chills Headache Myalgia Cough Shortness of breath Dyspnea Hypoxia Lymphopenia Thrombocytopenia Mild ↑ in transaminases	No definitive recommendations	Chest radiograph (evidence of pneumonia or adult respiratory distress syndrome) Detection of viral RNA by real-time reverse transcription-PCR Detection of acute and convalescent antibodies to SARS by enzyme immunoassay	Supportive care Empiric antimicrobial agents Intravenous administration of ribavirin Corticosteroids Investigational
Parvovirus B19[10,15]	Severe, refractory anemia Pancytopenia Thrombotic microangiopathy Fibrosing cholestatic hepatitis Graft dysfunction	Chronic anemia ↓ platelets ↓ white blood cell count Fever Malaise Pancytopenia	No definitive recommendations	Detection of parvovirus B19 DNA in serum by PCR assay	High-dose IVIG ↓ in immunosuppression Discontinuing tacrolimus (if possible)

Human papillomavirus[10,15]	Cutaneous warts
	Anogenital warts
	Carcinoma of cervix and bladder
	Squamous cell carcinoma
	Anogenital carcinoma
		Warts
		  Cutaneous
		  Urogenital
		  Anal
		Squamous cell carcinoma that arises in beds of flat warts
			Avoidance of excessive sun exposure and ultraviolet light
			Sun precautions
			Sunscreen with high sun protection factor (≥15)
				Tissue biopsy	Topical keratolytic agents
					Caustic agents
					Topical retinoids
					Oral retinoids
					Podophyllin, 5-fluorouracil
					Bleomycin
					Ablation
					Carcinoma (skin, cervix, urinary tract):
					  Resection
					  Reduction or withdrawal of immunosuppression
					  Radiation chemotherapy

Listeria monocytogene[10,22]	Bacteremia
	Meningitis
	Meningoencephalitis
	Myocarditis
	Cerebritis without meningitis
	Less common manifestations:
	  Pneumonia
	  Arthritis
	  Endophthalmitis
	  Endocarditis
	  Peritonitis
	  Myocarditis
	  Hepatitis
		Fever (1–5 d)
		Headache
		Decreased LOC
		Focal neurological deficits
		Meningismus
		Nuchal rigidity
		Spinal fluid: neutrophils, lymphocytes; glucose may be normal
		Abdominal cramps, diarrhea
		Seizures
			TMP-SMZ
			Dietary precautions regarding milk, cheeses, undercooked meats, and uncooked vegetables
				Blood, sputum cultures
				CT scan
				MRI
				CSF cell count, Gram stain, culture, and protein and sugar determination
				Note: organism may be confused with diphtheroids in Gram stain smears of pus or sputum
				Diagnosis confirmed by isolation of Listeria monocytogenes from culture of blood, CSF, or other sterile source
					Treatment of choice: ampicillin + aminoglycoside
					Meningeal doses of penicillin or ampicillin
					Gentamicin
					TMP-SMZ for penicillin-allergic patients

(continued)

TABLE 5-5 Major Organisms Causing Posttransplant Infection: Clinical Manifestations, Prevention/Prophylaxis, Diagnostic Tests, and Treatment Options (Continued)

Organism	May Cause	Clinical Manifestations	Prophylaxis/Preemptive Therapy	Diagnostic Tests	Treatment Options
Nocardia[10,29]	Pulmonary and extrapulmonary infection (CNS, skin, and bone)	Subacute onset is typical Subacute symptoms: Fever Cough Chest pain Pulmonary nodules, abscesses, cavitating lesions, infiltrates, effusions	TMP-SMZ Typical pneumocystis pneumonia prophylaxis with TMP-SMZ offers some protection	Cultures: sputum, BAL fluid Gram stain Modified acid-fast stain Diagnosis confirmed by the presence of Nocardia species in culture	Sulfonamides preferred Sulfisoxazole TMP-SMZ Amikacin Imipenem Third-generation cephalosporins Minocycline Linezolid Isolated pulmonary infection: 3–6 mo of therapy Disseminated disease: 12 mo of therapy
Legionella[22]	Pneumonia	Fever, chills Focal pulmonary infiltrate Headache Confusion Minimally productive cough Diarrhea Chest pain Malaise Dyspnea	Routine culture of hospital water supply Water treatment to control nosocomial infection	Cultures: sputum, BAL fluid Direct fluorescent antibody stain of respiratory secretions Urinary antigen detection: can only detect serogroup 1 of Legionella pneumophila species Fine needle aspiration of lung Open lung biopsy Chest radiograph: dense infiltrates (unilateral or bilateral) that may → cavitation Diagnosis confirmed by: Legionella antigen in urine Direct fluorescent antibody stain (respiratory secretions or tissue biopsy) Culture of lower respiratory tract secretions	Quinolones (particularly levofloxacin or ciprofloxacin) Rifampin (may interact with other drugs via the hepatic cytochrome p450 system) Macrolides (azithromycin, erythromycin) interact with immunosuppressive medications and should generally be avoided) TMP-SMZ (but the side effects include bone marrow suppression, hepatitis, rash)

Mycobacteria[22,30]	Pulmonary infection Extrapulmonary infection (intestinal, skeletal, bone, genitourinary, cutaneous, CNS) Disseminated disease[3]	Pulmonary: Nonproductive cough Mucopurulent secretions Hemoptysis Dyspnea Chest pain Fever Excessive sweating Weight loss Organ-specific manifestations	Test and treat before transplantation Isoniazid (controversial)	Tuberculin test: positive in 25%–33% of recipients infected with this disease Chest radiograph Bronchoscopy with BAL Transbronchial biopsy Pleural needle biopsy Tuberculin test: often negative Smears for acid-fast bacilli and mycobacterial culture Organ-specific histology Isolates require antimicrobial susceptibility testing	Isoniazid (hepatotoxic) Rifampin (hepatotoxic) Pyrazinamide Ethambutol (may → optic neuritis) Streptomycin (ototoxic; nephrotoxic) Increases catabolism of steroids and cyclosporine and tacrolimus; monitor levels of cyclosporine and tacrolimus; monitor patient for rejection Monitor renal and hepatic function Recipients with active disease: 9–12 mo of therapy with two agents to which pathogen is susceptible
Aspergillus[31,32]	Pulmonary and extrapulmonary infection Disseminates to: Brain Liver Spleen Kidneys Heart Blood vessels Bones Joints GI tract	Depend on site(s) involved Pulmonary involvement: Nonproductive cough Pleuritic chest pain Pulmonary infiltrates or nodules Dyspnea Low-grade fever Invasive/disseminated infection: Refractory fever Sinusitis Epistaxis; nasal pain Periorbital pain or swelling	No definitive recommendations Heart, lung, heart-lung recipients: aerosolized amphotericin B Lung recipients: oral itraconazole for patients with airway colonization Epidemiologic: minimize contact with fungal spores; shield patient from nosocomial environmental hazards: high-efficiency particulate air filters; high-performance masks Preemptive: amphotericin B if respiratory tract is colonized	Chest radiography Note: may be normal BAL Transbronchial biopsy Open lung biopsy CT scan (e.g., lung, sinuses) Tissue biopsy CT or MRI for brain abscesses Sputum cultures Repeated positive cultures suggest invasive disease Positive sputum cultures plus cavitary lung disease suggest invasive disease	Amphotericin B Itraconazole (oral or IV) Voriconazole: recently shown to have greater efficacy than amphotericin B for invasive disease Use of voriconazole with sirolimus is contraindicated Caspofungin: approved for refractory aspergillosis Absorption may be erratic, especially in patients with low gastric acidity; monitor plasma concentration of drug

(continued)

TABLE 5-5 Major Organisms Causing Posttransplant Infection: Clinical Manifestations, Prevention/Prophylaxis, Diagnostic Tests, and Treatment Options (Continued)

Organism	May Cause	Clinical Manifestations	Prophylaxis/Preemptive Therapy	Diagnostic Tests	Treatment Options
Aspergillus[31,32] (Continued)		Cutaneous embolic lesions Progressive erythema or induration along tunneled venous catheter Focal neurologic findings Hemoptysis: sign of invasive disease			May → nephrotoxicity in patients on calcineurin inhibitors; monitor renal function (lipid formulations are less likely to be nephrotoxic; may be preferable for chronic treatment) Associated with higher relapse rates than amphotericin B

Candida[10,33,34]	Mucocutaneous candidiasis
	
	Oropharyngeal thrush
	
	Candidal esophagitis
	
	Vaginitis
	
	Intertrigo
	
	Paronychia
	
	Onychomycosis
	
	Sternal wound infection; mediastinitis
	
	Intra-abdominal abscesses
	
	UTI
	
	Endocarditis
	
	Disseminated infection
		Thrush:
		  White patches or ulcers in mouth
		
		Vaginitis:
		  White or yellow vaginal discharge
		  Pruritus
		
		Intertrigo:
		  Erythematous, popular skin rash
		
		Paronychia:
		  Redness, swelling, suppuration around nail edge
		
		Onychomycosis:
		  Thickened, discolored nails
		
		Intravascular catheter infections
		
		Fever, sepsis
			Clotrimazole troches
			
			Oral Nystatin
			
			Liver transplant recipients:
			  Preoperative oral bowel decontamination with nystatin to ↓ gut colonization
			
			Kidney and pancreas-kidney transplant recipients:
			  Preemptive therapy for asymptomatic candiduria
			
			Pancreas transplant recipients:
			  Anecdotal reports of fluconazole prophylaxis for high-risk patients:
			    Enteric drainage
			    Pretransplant peritoneal dialysis
				Direct fluorescent antibody stain of respiratory secretions
				
				Localized infection:
				  Cultures with Gram stain
				
				Disseminated candidiasis:
				  Blood cultures
				  CT scan
				  Biopsy of skin lesions
				  Tissue biopsy
				
				Diagnosis confirmed by isolating Candida species from culture specimens
					Amphotericin B and lipid-based preparations
					
					Lipid-based preparations: less nephrotoxic
					
					Clotrimazole
					
					Mycostatin
					
					Fluconazole for esophagitis and refractory candidiasis
					
					Candidemia in unstable or critically ill patients:
					  Amphotericin B followed by fluconazole if organism is sensitive to fluconazole
					
					Candidemia in stable patients:
					  Fluconazole, if organism is sensitive to fluconazole
					
					Candida albicans:
					  Fluconazole
					  Itraconazole
					
					Candida krusei:
					  Typically resistant to fluconazole

Organism	Epidemiology/Risk factors	Clinical features	Prophylaxis	Diagnosis	Treatment/Comments
Candida[10,33,34] (*Continued*)			Pancreas after kidney transplant; Reperfusion pancreatitis; Retransplantation		Requires maximal doses of amphotericin B. Newer agents: for *Candida* species — Caspofungin, Voriconazole. Monitor renal function and cyclosporine levels; adjust dose accordingly. Effective for most *Candida* species except *Candida krusei* and *Candida glabrata*. When used with cyclosporine, may ↑ risk of hepatotoxicity; monitor liver function. When used with tacrolimus, may → ↓ tacrolimus levels; monitor tacrolimus levels
Cryptococcus neoformans[31,35]	Predilection for CNS; Meningitis; Brain abscesses; Secondary seeding of skin, CNS, eye, urinary tract, and skeletal system; Pulmonary infection	Pulmonary infection: cough; Lung nodules; CNS involvement:; Progressive headache; Memory or attention deficits; Emotional disturbance; Disorders of balance; Cranial nerve dysfunction; Fever; Meningismus; Confusion; Dysphagia; Muscle weakness, tremor	Primary prophylaxis: not recommended	Lumbar puncture; CT scan; MRI; Blood culture; CSF analysis: cell count; protein and sugar; Gram stain; acid-fast and fungal stains and cultures (fungal, bacterial, and mycobacterial); Cryptococcal antigen test on blood, CSF, and pleural fluid; CSF in meningitis: Lymphocytic pleocytosis, ↑ protein, ↓ sugar, ↑ opening pressure	Amphotericin B; Amphotericin B with 5-flucytosine; Fluconazole with 5-flucytosine; Fluconazole; Course of treatment: minimum of 8–10 wk; Requires monitoring of renal function and cyclosporine levels; Requires monitoring of 5-flucytosine levels to minimize hepatic and bone marrow toxicity

(continued)

TABLE 5-5 Major Organisms Causing Posttransplant Infection: Clinical Manifestations, Prevention/Prophylaxis, Diagnostic Tests, and Treatment Options (*Continued*)

Organism	May Cause	Clinical Manifestations	Prophylaxis/Preemptive Therapy	Diagnostic Tests	Treatment Options
Cryptococcus neoformans[31,35] (*Continued*)		Urinary incontinence Focal neurologic signs Seizures Subacute presentation: Low-grade fever Headache Altered mental status Cutaneous involvement: Ulcers Papules or pustules Subcutaneous swelling or tumors Ecchymoses Granulomata Abscesses Vesicles Palpable purpura or papules Necrotizing vasculitis Cellulitis		Definitive diagnosis: detection of antigen in serum and CSF	
Pneumocystis carinii[36,37]	Pneumonitis	Presentation typically subacute Fever Nonproductive cough Dyspnea Hypoxemia Tachypnea Diffuse pulmonary infiltrates	TMP-SMZ (low dose for 6 mo) Dapsone Aerosolized pentamidine Atovaquone In patients with G6PD deficiency, evaluate risk of dose-dependent hemolytic anemia	Transbronchial lung biopsy Needle biopsy of lung Bronchoalveolar lavage Chest radiograph (may be negative) Confirmatory diagnosis: direct staining of specimens: sputum, BAL lavage or lung tissue	TMP-SMZ (high-dose) for 21 d Pentamidine Dapsone-trimethoprim Clindamycin-primaquine (if not G6PD deficient) Dose may have to be adjusted for renal dysfunction

Histoplasma capsulatum[38]	Disseminated infection (most common presentation)	Subacute respiratory illness with either focal or disseminated interstitial or miliary infiltrates Fever (not always present) Night sweats Chills Cough Headache Arthritis, myalgias CNS manifestations Hepatosplenomegaly Cutaneous, intestinal, oral mucosal lesions	No firm recommendations; some centers use itraconazole for seropositive recipients	Methenamine-silver stain Peripheral blood stains Cultures: blood, respiratory secretions, tissue Serology Antigen detection (urine, serum, CSF, BAL fluid) Chest radiography (may be normal)	Amphotericin B Itraconazole for maintenance therapy Requires monitoring of renal function and cyclosporine levels Absorption may be erratic, especially in patients with low gastric acidity; monitor plasma concentration of drug
Toxoplasma gondii[39]	Myocarditis Pericarditis Pneumonitis Encephalitis Hepatitis Retinochoroiditis	Mononucleosis-like syndrome of fever, malaise, and lymphadenopathy Myocardial dysfunction that mimics rejection Pulmonary: fever, dyspnea, cough, hemoptysis CNS involvement: multiple focal neurologic deficits, altered mental status; fever with headache	Particularly for seronegative recipient/ seropositive donor: Pyrimethamine (for sulfa allergy) Pyrimethamine + sulfonamide Pyrimethamine + folinic acid Co-trimoxazole Atovaquone TMP-SMZ Avoid changing cat litter boxes Avoid raw or undercooked meat	Endomyocardial biopsy Antibody titers Lung lavage and/or biopsy CT scan of head Chest radiograph Tissue and/or blood culture Serologic assays Definitive diagnosis: histological detection of trophozoites + inflammation	Pyrimethamine with folinic acid and sulfadiazine Sulfa allergy: dapsone used instead of sulfadiazine Clindamycin and pyrimethamine with folinic acid Folinic acid given to prevent myelotoxicity Continue therapy for 2–3 wk after acute infection has resolved

(continued)

TABLE 5-5 Major Organisms Causing Posttransplant Infection: Clinical Manifestations, Prevention/Prophylaxis, Diagnostic Tests, and Treatment Options (Continued)

Organism	May Cause	Clinical Manifestations	Prophylaxis/Preemptive Therapy	Diagnostic Tests	Treatment Options
Cryptosporidium[40]	Gastroenteritis Gallbladder infection	Profuse, watery diarrhea Abdominal pain Nausea and vomiting Fever Myalgias	Boil water for 5 min or use distilled or filtered water Avoid ice cubes in restaurants Avoid soda fountain drinks	Stool testing Antibody detection assays Small or large bowel biopsy	Replace fluid and electrolytes Maintain nutritional status Spiramycin effective for some patients; adverse effects reported (increased stool output and volume loss)

Strongyloides stercoralis[41]	Ulcerating hemorrhagic enterocolitis
	Hemorrhagic pneumonia
	Disseminated disease:
	  Pulmonary
	  CNS (gram-negative meningitis)
		GI:
		  Abdominal pain and distention
		  Diarrhea
		  Nausea and vomiting
		  Adynamic ileus
		  Small bowel obstruction
		  Hemorrhage
		Pulmonary:
		  Tachypnea
		  Dyspnea
		  Bronchospasm
		  Cough
		  Hemoptysis CNS:
		  Headache
		  Fever
		  Eosinophilic meningitis
		  Mental status changes
		  Coma
		  Focal neurologic deficits
			Consider preemptive ivermectin for transplant candidates who have traveled to or lived in endemic areas
			Screen at-risk candidates for infection
			Treat established infection before transplantation
				Stool specimen for rhabditiform larvae (may be negative)
				Papanicolaou stain of duodenal aspirates, urine, ascitic fluid, sputum, and stool
				Jejunal biopsy
				Serologic testing
				Chest radiograph (frequently inconclusive)
				Definitive diagnosis: presence of larvae in stool
					Albendazole
					Ivermectin
					Thiabendazole
					Taper immunosuppressive agents
					Systemic antibacterial therapy for bacteremia or meningitis
					Periodic retreatments may be necessary
					Hyperinfection: 7–10 d of antimicrobial therapy

Strongyloides stercoralis[1] (Continued)	Gram-negative meningitis	
	Skin manifestations:	
		Migratory, raised, linear rash that may move at a rate of 10 cm/hr
		Crops of urticarial eruptions; immediate hypersensitive reactions to migrating worms, especially on the waist and buttocks)

BAL, bronchoalveolar lavage; CT, computed tomography; CMV, cytomegalovirus; CSF, cerebrospinal fluid; CBC, complete blood count; CNS, central nervous system; EBV, Epstein-Barr virus; ELISA, enzyme-linked immunosorbent assay; EEG, electroencephalogram; G6PD, glucose-6-phosphate dehydrogenase; GI, gastrointestinal; LFT, liver function tests; HBV, hepatitis B virus; HbsAg, hepatitis B surface antigen; HCV, hepatitis C virus; HCV-RNA, hepatitis C virus ribonucleic acid; HHV, human herpesvirus 6; HSV, herpes simplex virus; IV, intravenous; IVIG, intravenous immunoglobulin; LOC, level of consciousness; MRI, magnetic resonance imaging; PCR, polymerase chain reaction; PTLD, posttransplant lymphoproliferative disease; SARS, severe acute respiratory syndrome; TMP-SMZ, trimethoprim-sulfamethoxazole; VZV, varicella zoster virus; UTI, urinary tract infection.

        i.   SOT recipients that are seronegative (2% to 3%) are at high risk for developing severe VZV.

        ii. Typically occurs between 3 months and 3 years posttransplant with a median time of 14 months.

        iii. Infection is defined by cutaneous involvement of greater than two noncontiguous dermatomes and/or visceral involvement.

    d. Herpes zoster in a transplant recipient requires urgent medical evaluation to determine extent of disease. If disseminated infection occurs, hospitalization is indicated for administration of intravenous antiviral therapy.

    e. VZV-seronegative recipients are advised to report any exposure to VZV so that zoster immune globulin may be promptly administered.

    f. Cutaneous manifestations may be muted, especially if immune globulin is given; patient should be observed for primarily visceral manifestations.

    g. Dermatomal pain without typical skin eruptions has been observed.

  2. See Table 5-5 for the clinical manifestations, prevention/prophylaxis, diagnosis, and treatment of VZV.

E. Epstein-Barr virus (EBV)[17,18,42]

  1. Overview

    a. Human herpesvirus 4 (HHV-4).

    b. Because approximately 90% of adults are EBV seropositive, the majority of EBV infections in transplant recipients are reactivation infections.

        i.   EBV latency occurs because the virus establishes a persistent infection in B cells.

        ii. In immunocompetent individuals, this persistent infection is optimally controlled by EBV-specific cytotoxic T lymphocytes.

        iii. In immunocompromised individuals, the cytotoxic T-lymphocyte response is impaired, thus increasing the potential for EBV-driven B-cell proliferation.

    c. EBV-seronegative recipients can acquire primary EBV infection from

        i.   The community

        ii. The allograft itself

        iii. Blood transfusions

  2. Incidence

    a. EBV replication occurs in approximately 20% to 30% of all solid organ transplant recipients and in 80% of recipients who receive antilymphocyte antibody therapy.

    b. Reactivation infections occur in approximately 30% to 40% of EBV-seropositive recipients.

    c. Primary infections occur in approximately 70% to 80% of EBV-seronegative recipients.

        i.   EBV infection typically occurs during the first 6 months posttransplant.

        ii. Effects of EBV infection: the sequelae of EBV infection range from a mononucleosis-like syndrome to posttransplant lymphoproliferative disease (PTLD).

  3. Risk factors for PTLD

    a. Most important risk factor is the transplantation of an EBV-seropositive donor organ into an EBV-seronegative recipient

    b. High EBV viral load

    c. Primary EBV infection

    d. CMV mismatch (donor CMV seropositive; recipient CMV seronegative)

    e. CMV disease

    f. Potent immunosuppression

TABLE 5-6 Incidence of EBV by Type of Allograft

Type of Allograft	Incidence
Multiorgan	13%–33%
Small intestine	32%
Kidney-pancreas	3%–12%
Lung	3%–12%
Heart	3%–12%
Liver	3%–12%
Kidney	1%–2%

From Allen UD, Preiksitis JK; AST Infectious Disease Community of Practice. Epstein-Barr and post transplant lymphoproliferative disease in solid organ transplant recipients. *Am J Transplant.* 2013;(13):107–120. Ref.[43]

  g. Type of allograft (see Table 5-6 for the incidence of EBV infection by allograft type)
  h. Age: young (infants and young children) and older age recipients

F. Cytomegalovirus[19–21]
  1. Overview
    a. Member of the herpesviridae family; human herpesvirus.[5]
    b. Sixty percent of US population exposed to CMV; prevalence of 90% in high-risk groups.
    c. Most common viral pathogen after SOT.
    d. Over the course of the first year posttransplant, over 50% of transplant recipients demonstrate evidence of CMV viral replication.
    e. See Table 5-7 for the risk of CMV by type of allograft.
  2. Risk factors for CMV disease[15,19]
    a. Most important risk factor is CMV mismatch status:
      i. Donor CMV positive (D+); recipient CMV negative (R–): high risk
      ii. Donor CMV positive (D+); recipient CMV positive (R+): intermediate risk
      iii. Donor CMV negative (D–); recipient CMV positive (R+): intermediate risk
      iv. Donor CMV negative (D–); recipient CMV negative (R–): low risk
    b. Potent immunosuppressive drug regimens[15]
    c. Net state of immunosuppression
    d. High CMV viral load
    e. Multiple episodes of CMV disease

TABLE 5-7 Level of Risk of CMV by Type of Allograft

Level of Risk	Type of Allograft
High	Lung
	Small bowel
Intermediate	Liver
	Pancreas
	Heart
Low	Kidney

From Kotton D, Kumar D, Caliendo A, et al. International consensus guidelines on the management of cytomegalovirus in solid organ transplantation. *Transplantation.* 2010;89:779–795; Vella J, Bennett W, Brennan D. Cytomegalovirus in renal transplant recipients. In: Murphy B, ed. *Up to Date.* Waltham, MA: Wolters Kluwer; 2015. Available at http://www.uptodate.com/contents/cytomegalovirus-infection-in-renal-transplant-recipients. Accessed September 7, 2015.

    f. Prolonged CMV prophylaxis with oral ganciclovir[21]

    g. Suboptimal antiviral drug concentration

    h. Type of solid organ transplant procedure: in descending order (highest to lowest risk):

        i. Kidney/pancreas

        ii. Lung

        iii. Heart and kidney

        iv. Liver

3. Time line

    a. Most commonly seen 2 to 6 months after SOT without prophylaxis.

    b. Use of oral antiviral prophylaxis (valgancyclovir [Valcyte]) has delayed onset of CMV disease until completion of drug prophylaxis.

4. Detection[15,19-21]

    a. Serology testing used in pretransplant setting to determine transplant candidate's risk of developing CMV after SOT.

        i. CMV immunoglobulin (IgG) confirms previous exposure to CMV.

        ii. Comparison of the donor and recipient CMV IgG status will determine risk category and management (CMV preemptive vs. prophylactic therapy) after transplant.

        iii. See Table 5-8 for CMV risk by CMV serology.

    b. Qualitative and quantitative CMV PCR blood assays are the most rapid and sensitive detection methods utilized currently.

        i. Viral load results are currently reported as international units/mL.

        ii. Note: It is important to use the same test and specimen type (whole blood or plasma) when monitoring patients over time in order to accurately assess changes in viral load.

    c. CMV is slow growing in conventional cultures; these are not often used often due to modest sensitivity and slow turnaround for results.

    d. Histologic examinations of tissue specimens are useful for the identification of CMV tissue invasive disease.

5. CMV prevention: prophylaxis versus preemptive therapy[19]

    a. Prophylaxis: administration of antiviral agent to high- and moderate-risk recipients

        i. Oral valganciclovir (Valcyte) for 3 to 6 months after SOT for kidney, liver, pancreas, and heart transplant recipients; 1 year for lung transplant recipients.

        ii. Major drawbacks to antiviral drug therapy

           • Myelosuppression (mainly leukopenia)

           • Drug cost

TABLE 5-8 Risk of Cytomegalovirus (CMV) by CMV Serology

Risk Level	Serology
High	Donor +, Recipient −
Moderate	Donor +, Recipient +
	Donor −, Recipient +
Low	Donor −, Recipient −

From Ramanan P, Razonable R. Cytomegalovirus infections in solid organ transplantation: a review. *J Infect Chemother.* 2013;45(3):260–271.; Kotton D, Kumar D, Caliendo A, et al. International consensus guidelines on the management of cytomegalovirus in solid organ transplantation. *Transplantation.* 2010;89:779–795.

- Late-onset CMV occurs more commonly among CMV D+/R−
- Potential drug resistance
  b. Preemptive therapy: administration of antiviral agent to a select group of recipients at high risk for developing CMV
    i. Determined with weekly quantitative CMV PCR assays for the first 3 months after SOT.[19]
    ii. Treatment for CMV given if CMV PCR results are positive.
    iii. Drawbacks to preemptive therapy are the cost and logistics of weekly laboratory tests.
6. Effects of CMV[21]
  a. Direct effects: CMV infection and CMV disease[21]
    i. CMV infection is considered present if CMV is detected through molecular techniques, viral cultures, and/or changes in serology.
    ii. CMV disease is accompanied by clinical signs and symptoms.
      - CMV syndrome, which manifests as fever and/or malaise, leukopenia, or thrombocytopenia
      - Tissue-invasive CMV disease (see Table 5-9)
  b. Indirect effects:
    i. Opportunistic infections
    ii. Allograft injury
    iii. Rejection
7. Bidirectional relationship between CMV and rejection
  a. CMV can trigger rejection.
  b. Inflammation associated with rejection (and rejection therapy) can increase CMV viral replication.

TABLE 5-9 Types of CMV Disease

Type	Definition: Combination of
Pneumonia	Signs and/or symptoms of pulmonary disease and detection of CMV in fluid obtained from bronchoalveolar lavage or from tissue samples
Gastrointestinal disease	Clinical symptoms (upper or lower gastrointestinal tract) and endoscopy-detected macroscopic mucosal lesions and detection of CMV infection in tissue obtained from gastrointestinal tract biopsy
Hepatitis	↑ bilirubin and/or liver enzymes and absence of any other documented etiology of hepatitis and detection of CMV infection in tissue obtained from liver biopsy
Central nervous system	Central nervous system symptoms and detection of CMV in cerebrospinal fluid or in tissue obtained from brain biopsy
Nephritis	In patient with renal dysfunction: detection of CMV infection and histological identification of CMV in tissue obtained from kidney biopsy
Cystitis	In patient with cystitis: detection of CMV infection and histological identification of CMV in tissue obtained from bladder biopsy
Myocarditis	In patient with myocarditis: detection of CMV infection and histological identification of CMV in tissue obtained from heart biopsy
Pancreatitis	In patient with pancreatitis: detection of CMV infection and histological identification of CMV in tissue obtained from biopsy of pancreas tissue

From Kotton D, Kumar D, Caliendo A, et al. International consensus guidelines on the management of cytomegalovirus in solid organ transplantation. *Transplantation.* 2010;89:779–795; Vella J, Bennett W, Brennan D. Cytomegalovirus in renal transplant recipients. In: Murphy B, ed. *Up to Date.* Waltham, MA: Wolters Kluwer; 2015. Available at http://www.uptodate.com/contents/cytomegalovirus-infection-in-renal-transplant-recipients. Accessed September 7, 2015.

8. Organ-specific effects on allograft:
   a. Liver: vanishing bile duct syndrome
   b. Heart: coronary artery vasculopathy
   c. Lung: bronchiolitis obliterans
   d. Kidney: glomerulopathy
9. Epidemiological patterns[15]
   a. Primary infection: CMV-seronegative recipient receives cells that are latently infected with CMV from a CMV-seropositive donor; viral replication ensues.
      i. Compared with reactivation infection and superinfection (below), primary CMV infections have the following:
         • Higher rates of CMV infection, symptomatic disease, and recurrence
         • Higher mortality rates
         • Earlier onset posttransplant
         • Increased risk of disseminated disease
   b. Reactivation infection: Recipient is CMV seropositive and endogenous latent virus reactivates.
      i. An inflammatory process or stress can promote reactivation (e.g., rejection, antilymphocyte therapy, sepsis).
   c. Superinfection: CMV-seropositive recipient receives an allograft from a CMV-seropositive donor, and the strain of CMV virus that reactivates is from the donor.
10. Ganciclovir-resistant CMV[15,21]
   a. Often a late-onset complication of SOT:
      i. Median onset, lung transplantation: 4.4 months
      ii. Median onset, nonlung transplantation: 10 months
   b. Indications that CMV strain may be resistant:
      i. Patient shows no significant improvement or resolution of symptoms after a 14-day course of full-dose IV ganciclovir.
      ii. There is no decrease in viral load after a 14-day course of full-dose IV ganciclovir.
11. See Table 5-5 for the clinical manifestations, prevention/prophylaxis, diagnosis, and treatment of CMV.

G. Human herpesvirus 6 (HHV-6)[18]
   1. Usually reactivation of endogenous latent virus.
   2. Onset typically occurs between 2 and 4 weeks posttransplantation.
   3. CMV coinfection is common.
   4. See Table 5-5 for the clinical manifestations, prevention/prophylaxis, diagnosis, and treatment of HHV-6.

H. HHV-8[18]
   1. After SOT, endemic in certain regions (i.e., Saudi Arabia; South Africa)
   2. May contribute to development of Kaposi's sarcoma, Castleman's disease, primary effusion lymphoma, cutaneous lesions, and some visceral (gastrointestinal and/or lung) lesions.
   3. Treatment consists of reduction/withdrawal of immunosuppression, chemotherapy, and possible conversion to mTOR inhibitors.

I. Hepatitis viruses[23,24]
   1. Overview

    a. Posttransplant liver disease may be due to drug-induced hepatotoxicity or virus-induced disease.

    b. Hepatotoxic drugs

       i. Immunosuppressants

       ii. Antimicrobial agents: particularly those used to treat tuberculosis (e.g., isoniazid, pyrazinamide, rifampin [Rifadin])

       iii. Statins/HMG-CoA reductase inhibitors

       iv. Antihypertensive agents

       v. Diuretics

       vi. Acetaminophen

       vii. Herbs (alternative medicines)

    c. Virus-induced disease: hepatitis virus A (HAV), hepatitis B virus (HBV), hepatitis C virus (HCV), and hepatitis E virus (HEV)

       i. HBV and HCV are more common causes of morbidity and mortality after SOT, but along with HAV, HEV has emerged in developing countries.[24]

       ii. Risk of recurrence of either hepatitis B or C >80%.

       iii. Viral hepatitis may be transmitted via the allograft.[5]

2. Hepatitis B virus (HBV)

    a. In SOT, HBV can cause hepatitis, cirrhosis, and hepatocellular carcinoma.

    b. Approximately 50% of recipients with HBV infection will have end-stage liver disease and/or hepatocellular carcinoma at 10 years posttransplant.[23]

    c. Mode of transmission

       i. Allograft

       ii. Sexual transmission

       iii. Parenteral

       iv. Reactivation of latent virus

    d. Diagnosis

       i. Screening tests for antibodies:

          • HBsAb: hepatitis B surface antibody

          • HBcAb: hepatitis B core antibody

          • HBeAb: hepatitis B e-antibody

       ii. Screening tests for antigens:

          • HBsAg: hepatitis B surface antigen

       iii. Nucleic acid tests to detect HBV-DNA in the blood:

          • PCR

          • Hybridization assays

    e. Treatment[15,23]

       i. Lamivudine (Epivir); adefovir (Hepsera)

       ii. Tenofovir (Viread) or entecavir (Baraclude); more effective in nonrenal SOT recipients)

       iii. Hepatitis immune globulin (HBIG)

    f. Prophylaxis

       i. HBV serology screening pretransplant

       ii. HBV vaccine series (preferably pretransplant; better efficacy)

          • Dialysis patients and prospective kidney transplant patients should be given vaccine early in renal failure with 3- to 5-year booster vaccinations to improve immunogenicity.

          • Mandatory as part of evaluation for SOT.

3. Hepatitis C virus (HCV)
  a. End-stage liver disease secondary to HCV is currently a leading indication for liver transplantation.
    i. HCV reinfection of new liver allograft is universal with 10%, and 20% of recipients with HCV infection will have end-stage liver disease and/or hepatocellular carcinoma at 10 years posttransplant.
    ii. Main causes for HCV progression after SOT:
      • Intense immunosuppression, particularly T-cell–depleting therapies
      • Advanced donor and recipient age
      • Prolonged warm and cold ischemic times
      • Coinfections with CMV and HIV
      • Genotype 1b; HLA mismatch
  b. Diagnosis:
    i. Screening tests for antibody to HCV enzyme immunoassay (EIA) and HCV chemiluminescence immunoassay (CIA)
    ii. HCV PCR (qualitative; quantitative)
  c. Treatment[24]:
    i. In the past, combination therapy with interferon and ribavirin was the most effective therapeutic regimen for posttransplant HCV infection, but this combination is problematic because
      • It is effective in <50% of patients who are infected with the most common HCV genotype found in the United States.
      • Many recipients find this regimen intolerable.
    ii. Current treatment for hepatitis C is rapidly evolving with the introduction of protease inhibitors. The treatment guidelines are determined by the genotype, whether the patient is treatment naive, and whether the patient has failed prior interferon or ribavirin treatment.
      • Simeprevir (Olysio)-sofosbuvir (Sovaldi)
      • Ombitasvir-paritaprevi-ritonavir-dasabuvir (Viekira Pak)
      • Ledipasvir-dofosbuvir (Harvoni)
      • Daclatasvir (Daklinza)
    iii. Most hepatitis C patients are treated prior to transplantation; this may eliminate the need for transplantation as the disease has not progressed to cirrhosis and fibrosis.
  d. Prevention
    i. No vaccine available for HCV
    ii. Infection control
4. Hepatitis E virus (HEV)[15,23,24]
  a. Newly discovered cause of acute/chronic hepatitis.
  b. Modes of transmission:
    i. In developing countries, preference for fecal-oral mode of transmission.
    ii. With industrialized countries, it has been reported with zoonotic mode of transmission.
  c. Prevention includes good hygiene and adequate cooking of meat.
  d. Vaccine is in development.
5. See Table 5-5 for the clinical manifestations, prevention/prophylaxis, diagnosis, and treatment of hepatitis infections.

J. Polyomaviruses[15,25,26]

1. Overview
   a. Polyomavirus hominis 1 (BK virus) and John Cunningham virus (JC virus)
      i.   These names reflect the first patients who exhibited these viruses
      ii. Only two members of polyomavirus family known to naturally infect humans.
   b. Approximately 80% of the general adult population is seropositive for the BK and JC viruses.
   c. Transmission: respiratory route.
   d. BK and JC viruses have latency properties and often reactivate in the immunosuppressed recipient.
      i.   Viruses tend to persist in the kidneys, ureters, brain, and spleen.
2. BK virus
   a. Transplant recipients may have primary and reactivation infections.
   b. BK virus reactivation in kidney transplant recipients is common (prevalence: 45% to 50%), but reactivation progresses to nephropathy only occasionally (prevalence: 1% to 10%).
   c. Reactivation after kidney transplantation may cause significant morbidity:
      i.   Tubulointerstitial nephritis
      ii. Ureteral stenosis that leads to obstructive nephropathy
      iii. Progressive graft dysfunction
      iv. Graft loss: ranges from 10% to 80% in kidney transplant recipients with polyomavirus-associated nephropathy (PyVAN)
   d. Risk factors
      i.   Donor (organ) determinants:
        * HLA mismatches
        * Deceased donation
        * High BKV-specific antibody titers
        * Female gender
      ii. Recipient determinants:
        * Older age
        * Male gender
        * Low or absent BKV-specific antibody titers
      iii. Modulating factors after transplant:
        * Acute and recurrent rejection episodes
        * Ureteric stents
      iv. Intense immunosuppression:
        * Prolonged steroid exposure
        * Higher drug levels
        * Lymphocyte-depleting antibodies
        * Tacrolimus (Prograf)—mycophenolic acid versus other drug combinations
   e. No effective antiviral therapies, so it is imperative that screening for BK virus replication be performed routinely in order to guide reduction of immunosuppression.
   f. See Table 5-5 for the clinical manifestations, prevention/prophylaxis, diagnosis, and treatment of BK virus.
3. JC virus
   a. Causes progressive multifocal leukoencephalopathy (PML)
      i.   Opportunistic JC virus infects and lyses oligodendrocytes; this causes multifocal demyelination in brain and progressive neurological deficits.

        ii. Timing of onset: typically more than 6 months to several years posttransplant.

        iii. Noninflammatory CNS infection; not associated with fever or meningeal signs (nuchal rigidity).

        iv. May occur concurrently in subset of kidney transplant recipients with documented BK virus–induced interstitial nephritis.

    b. Reported in renal, liver, heart, and lung transplant recipients.

    c. See Table 5-5 for the clinical manifestations, prevention/prophylaxis, diagnosis, and treatment of JC virus.

  4. Parvovirus B[15,42]

    a. Typically acquired during school-age period

        i. Results in "slapped cheek" rash that may be accompanied by lacy erythematous exanthem of extremities

        ii. Can cause pure red blood cell aplasia with low hematocrit

    b. See Table 5-5 for the clinical manifestations, prevention/prophylaxis, diagnosis, and treatment of parvovirus B.[42]

  5. Human papillomavirus (HPV)[15,44]

    a. Overview

        i. HPV infects epithelial tissues of skin and mucous membranes.

        ii. Associated with the development of warts or condyloma (cutaneous and anogenital).

        iii. Cause of more than 90% cervical and large proportion of anal, penile, and vaginal cancers.[44]

        iv. Can be associated with development of nonmelanoma skin cancers.

        v. Most HPV is contracted through sexual transmission.

    b. Cutaneous warts

        i. Incidence of warts increases with duration of immunosuppression

        ii. Tend to develop on areas of body exposed to sun

        iii. More common in patients prone to sunburn

        iv. May be refractory to treatment and tend to recur

    c. Squamous cell carcinoma

        i. Rate increases with duration of immunosuppression

        ii. Risk factor: chronic sun exposure

    d. See Table 5-5 for the clinical manifestations, prevention/prophylaxis, diagnosis, and treatment of human papillomavirus.

K. Community-acquired respiratory infections (CARV)[27,28]

  1. Overview

    a. Frequent cause of disease in SOT recipients.[27]

    b. Lower respiratory tract infection with CARV can be associated with significant morbidity and mortality.

    c. Infection control measures such as hand washing and control of air and droplet infection remain the best way to decrease the burden of CARV after SOT.

  2. Epidemiology

    a. Respiratory syncytial virus, influenza, parainfluenza infections typically occur in winter months.

    b. Parainfluenza virus 3 and adenovirus infections occur throughout the year.

    c. Viral respiratory infections can occur at any time after transplantation.

        i. Early posttransplant infection may be associated with nosocomial infection or reactivation of latent virus.

- Transmission of adenovirus from donor organ has been reported.
- Late posttransplant infection: typically community acquired.

    ii. Transplant patients may be the first individuals within a community to become infected with a community-acquired respiratory infection.

3. Mode of transmission
   a. Virus-laden respiratory droplets and aerosols.
   b. Direct contact (person-to-person).
   c. Contact with fomites.
   d. Transmission can occur in community and hospital environment.

4. Clinical presentation (general)
   a. Upper respiratory tract symptoms
   b. Elevated temperature (SOT recipients may not present with fever immediately)
   c. Myalgia, arthralgia
   d. Anorexia
   e. Inflammation of mucosa

5. Range of sequelae: mild, self-limiting upper respiratory infection to:
   a. Viral pneumonia, respiratory failure, and secondary infection with fungal or bacterial pathogens.
   b. CMV may be reactivated secondary to immunomodulation.

6. Respiratory syncytial virus (RSV)
   a. Transmission
      i. Primarily through large droplets and fomites
      ii. Can survive on surfaces (nonporous), skin, and gloves for hours
      iii. Requires close person-to-person contact or contact with contaminated surfaces
   b. See Table 5-5 for the clinical manifestations, prevention/prophylaxis, diagnosis, and treatment of RSV.

7. Influenza viruses (A & B)[27]
   a. Infections with influenza viruses range from mild, self-limiting syndromes to serious secondary infections—typically bacterial.
   b. See Table 5-5 for the clinical manifestations, prevention/prophylaxis, diagnosis, and treatment of influenza virus infections.

8. Parainfluenza viruses (PIV)[27]
   a. Paramyxovirus with four species: PIV 1, 2, 3, 4.
   b. In healthy individuals, viral shedding after PIV infection lasts for approximately 1 week; in transplant recipients, particularly those on long-term steroid therapy, shedding may be prolonged (>4 weeks).[28]
   c. Higher incidences in lung transplant recipients and more severe PIV infections in children have been noted.
   d. See Table 5-5 for the clinical manifestations, prevention/prophylaxis, diagnosis, and treatment of parainfluenza virus infections.

9. Rhinovirus
   a. Most common cause of the common cold in immunocompetent persons and is the most frequently identified respiratory virus in SOT recipients.
   b. Has been associated with lower respiratory tract infections and chronic viral shedding in lung transplant recipients.

10. Coronavirus (HcoV)[28]
    a. Associated with a range of infections from mild upper respiratory infections to severe acute respiratory syndrome (SARS)

11. Other Community-Acquired-Respiratory Infections (CARV)

a. Adenoviruses
   i. Cause a range of respiratory, GI, conjunctival, and disseminated pathology in the SOT recipient
   ii. Type of pathology depends on the offending serotype and the type of transplant
   iii. Most common in the first 3 months after transplant and with higher immunosuppression dosing
b. Human metapneumovirus (HMPV), polyomavirus KI, bocavirus (HboV)[28]
   i. Significance in the SOT population has not been determined. Further study is needed.
   ii. See Table 5-5 for the clinical manifestations, prevention/prophylaxis, diagnosis, and treatment of coronavirus infections.

X. BACTERIAL INFECTIONS[22]

A. Overview
  1. Bacteria are the most common causes of infection in transplant recipients.
    a. Bacterial infections are associated with increased morbidity and mortality in transplant recipients, particularly the rapidly emerging multidrug-resistant bacteria:
      i. Gram negative (e.g., *Pseudomonas aeruginosa*; extended-spectrum B-lactamase [ESBL] producing Enterobacteriaceae)
      ii. Gram positive (e.g., VRE; MRSA)[22]
  2. Bacterial pneumonias are common among all types of solid organ transplant recipients.

B. Bacterial infections in specific transplant populations are listed in Tables 5-5 and 5-10.

C. Listeriosis[22,30]
  1. Caused by *Listeria monocytogenes*.
  2. Typically occurs within first two posttransplant months but can occur years later.
  3. One of the most frequent causes of CNS infection in SOT recipients.
  4. Meningitis secondary to *Listeria monocytogenes* has a high mortality rate (approximately 25%).[22]
  5. Mode of transmission: ingestion of contaminated food.
  6. See Table 5-5 for the clinical manifestations, prevention/prophylaxis, diagnosis, and treatment of listeriosis.

D. Nocardiosis[29,30]
  1. Most common species is *Nocardia asteroides*.
  2. There is an increased incidence of *Nocardia* infection as there are better diagnostics as well as more immunocompromised patients.
  3. Most common site: lung (pneumonitis, pulmonary nodules, pulmonary abscesses).
  4. Extrapulmonary sites: brain (abscesses, meningitis), skin, bone.
  5. Transmission: inhalation into the lungs or inoculation into skin.
  6. Note: All patients should have CNS imaging to rule out possibility of brain abscess because up to 1/3 of cases have CNS involvement.
  7. Prevention and prophylaxis:

TABLE 5-10 Bacterial Infections in Specific Transplant Complications

Allograft	General Considerations	Clinical Manifestations	Diagnosis	Treatment	Prevention

Lung	Pneumonia: common
	
	Overall prevalence: 72%[30]
	
	Bacteria are the cause of the majority of infections in lung transplant recipients[30]
	
	The most frequent infection is bacterial pneumonia
	
	Pneumonia: most common pathogens:
	
	Gram-negative bacteria:
	  Enterobacteriaceae
	  Pseudomonas aeruginosa
	
	Other significant pathogens:
	  Staphylococcus aureus
	  Haemophilus influenzae
	  Streptococcus pneumoniae
	
	Lung susceptible to infections due to:
	  Impaired cough reflex
	  Poor mucociliary clearance
	  Ischemia
	  Abnormal lymph drainage
	  Reperfusion injury
	  Airway inflammation secondary to rejection → bacterial colonization
	
	Single lung transplantation:
		Pneumonia:
		
		Persistent respiratory failure
		
		Failure to wean from ventilator
		
		Fever
		
		Purulent respiratory secretions
		
		Lung consolidations
		
		Mediastinitis:
		
		Fever
		
		Leukocytosis
		
		Systemic toxicity
		
		Sternal wound infection:
		
		Early:
		  Poor wound healing
		  Dehiscence
		
		Late:
		  Sinus tract formation
		  Purulent discharge
		
		NOTE: fever and leukocytosis may not be present
			Pneumonia: respiratory tract cultures
			
			Mediastinitis: CT scan
			
			Sternal wound infection: CT scan, nuclear imaging studies
				Pathogen-specific antimicrobials
				
				Dual antimicrobial regimen for:
				
				  Pseudomonas aeruginosa
				  Burkholderia cepacia
				  Enterobacteriaceae (multidrug resistant)
				
				Mediastinitis:
				  Surgical wound debridement
				  Antimicrobial therapy
				
				Sternal wound infection:
				  Surgical wound debridement
				  Antimicrobial therapy
					Antimicrobial prophylaxis guided by respiratory tract cultures from donor and recipient
					
					Patients colonized with *Burkholderia cepacia* or multiple drug-resistant gram-negative bacteria:
					  Double or triple antibiotic therapy
					
					Inhaled aminoglycosides
					
					Perioperative prophylaxis for sternal wound infections:
					  Antimicrobials for gram-positive bacteria

(continued)

TABLE 5-10 Bacterial Infections in Specific Transplant Complications (Continued)

Allograft	General Considerations	Clinical Manifestations	Diagnosis	Treatment	Prevention
Lung (Continued)	Infection spreads from native lung to allograft Pathogens with high morbidity and mortality in lung transplantation for cystic fibrosis: Burkholderia cepacia Pseudomonas pathogens				
Liver	Most common bacterial infections: Intra-abdominal Surgical wound Other bacterial infections: Wound Cholangitis Abscesses Device related[3] Most common sites of infection: Liver Biliary tract Peritoneal cavity Surgical site Bloodstream Risk factors for intra-abdominal infections: Long surgical time Blood transfusions Reoperation	Wound infections or intra-abdominal abscess: Fever Abdominal pain Dehiscence Purulent drainage Pain Guarding Rebound tenderness Cholangitis: Fever RUQ pain Rebound tenderness Hyperbilirubinemia ↑ transaminases ↑ alkaline	Wound infections: Cultures CT scans Ultrasound MRI Cholangitis: Cholangiogram LFTs	Surgical or CT- or US-guided drainage of abscess Pathogen-specific antimicrobials Complicated infections: Cephalosporins Fluoroquinolone Carbapenems Beta-lactam and beta-lactamase inhibitor combinations Cholangitis: Obstruction: ERCP with dilation No obstruction: IV antibiotics	Good surgical technique Gram-negative infections: oral selective bowel decontamination (↓ gram-negative aerobic bacteria and fungi; spares gram-positive and anaerobic microbes that exert antagonistic effect on gram-negative organisms) Wound infections: perioperative administration of extended-spectrum cephalosporin Antibiotic therapy typically continued for 24–48 h after surgery Antimicrobial prophylaxis before posttransplant cholangiograms, biopsies, or any other procedure that involves manipulation of the biliary tract

Liver (Continued)	Kidney				

Early rejection
 	
CMV infection
 	
Retransplantation
 	
Roux-en-y choledocho-jejunostomy anastomosis (due to reflux of intestinal material and microbial flora into biliary system)
	Eighty percent of infections are bacterial[45]
	
	Urinary tract:
	  Site of most bacterial infections
	  Most common primary site associated with secondary bacteremia
	
	UTIs: common pathogens
	  Enterobacteriaceae
	  Pseudomonas aeruginosa
	  Enterococcus sp.
	
	Risk factors:
	  DM
	  Renal insufficiency
	  Prolonged catheter use
	  ↓ urine flow through urinary epithelium
	  Neurogenic bladder
	  Anatomic abnormalities
	
	Risk factors for recurrent UTIs:
	  Serum creatinine >2 mg/dL
	  Prednisone dose >20 mg/day
		UTI:
		  Acute pyelonephritis
		  Fever
		  Pain: graft site
		  Leukocytosis
		  Active urinary sediment
		  Note: UTIs may be asymptomatic
		
		Lymphoceles:
		  Fever
		  Graft tenderness
		  Unilateral leg edema on side of kidney transplant may be a sign of a lymphocele (infected or not infected)
			Surveillance urine cultures:
			  Clean catch, midstream urine specimen
			  Culture of genitourinary stents[46]
			
			Febrile patients:
			  Blood cultures
			
			Recurrent UTIs:
			  Imaging studies to detect anatomic problems or obstruction[3]
				UTIs:
				  Pathogen-specific antimicrobial
				  Fluoroquinolones
				  Cephalosporins
				  Vancomycin for infections due to coagulase-negative staphylococci or ampicillin-resistant enterococci
				
				Pyelonephritis: typically requires 2 or more weeks of therapy
				
				Wound infections:
				  Surgical debridement
				  Antimicrobial therapy
					Incidence of asymptomatic UTIs is high; therefore surveillance cultures are frequently required
					
					Early catheter removal
					
					UTIs:
					  TMP/SMX
					  Ciprofloxacin
					  TMP/SMX to ↓ incidence of septicemia
					
					For patients with sulfa allergy: fluoroquinolones
					
					Surgical wound infections: perioperative cephalosporin antibiotic[3]

(continued)

TABLE 5-10 Bacterial Infections in Specific Transplant Complications (Continued)

Allograft	General Considerations	Clinical Manifestations	Diagnosis	Treatment	Prevention
Kidney (*Continued*)	Multiple treated rejection episodes Chronic viral infections Etiology of surgical wound infections: gram-positive cocci; gram-negative bacilli Lymphoceles can → abscess formation secondary to repeated percutaneous drainage				
Heart	Types of infection: Main infection: ventilator-associated pneumonia due to gram-negative bacteria (*Pseudomonas aeruginosa, Klebsiella pneumoniae,* other *Enterobacteriaceae*) Sternotomy infection: *Staphylococcus aureus,* coagulase-negative staphylococci Mediastinitis Bacteremia Pneumonia: most common bacterial infection Mediastinitis typically caused by gram-positive bacteria (*Staphylococcus aureus, coagulase-negative staphylococcus aureus*); gram-negative organisms can also cause mediastinitis	Pneumonia: Persistent respiratory failure Failure to wean from ventilator Fever Purulent respiratory secretions Lung consolidations Mediastinitis: Fever Leukocytosis Systemic toxicity Sternal wound infection: Early: Poor wound healing Dehiscence Late: Sinus tract formation Purulent discharge	Pneumonia: Respiratory tract cultures Mediastinitis: CT scan Sternal wound infection: CT scan Nuclear imaging studies	Pneumonia: Pathogen-specific antimicrobial Mediastinitis: Surgical wound debridement Antimicrobial therapy directed toward gram-positive organisms Sternal wound infection: Surgical wound debridement Antimicrobial therapy directed toward gram-positive organisms	Pneumonia: Early weaning from ventilator Aggressive pulmonary hygiene Sternal wound infection: Perioperative antimicrobials Endocarditis: Standard dental prophylaxis

Pancreas	Most common:	Wound infections or intra-abdominal abscess:	Wound infections:	Wound infections:	Early catheter removal
	Wound infections	Fever	CT scan	Surgical or CT- or US-guided drainage of abscess	UTIs:
	Intra-abdominal abscesses	Abdominal pain	Abdominal US		TMP/SMX
		Dehiscence	MRI	Pathogen-specific antimicrobials	Ciprofloxacin
	Most common pathogen associated with wound and intra-abdominal infections: enteric bacteria	Purulent drainage	CBC count	UTIs:	TMP/SMX to ↓ incidence of septicemia
		Pain	LFTs	Pathogen-specific antimicrobial	For patients with sulfa allergy:
	UTIs commonly associated with urinary drainage of exocrine secretions (due to bacterial overgrowth in bladder)	Guarding	Fluid cultures[3]	Fluoroquinolones	Fluoroquinolones
		Rebound tenderness[3]	UTIs:	Cephalosporins	Surgical wound infections:
			Surveillance urine cultures: clean catch, midstream urine specimen		Perioperative cephalosporin antibiotic
	Other infections:		Febrile patients:		
	Cellulitis (abdominal wall)		Blood cultures		
	Peripancreatic abscesses		Recurrent UTIs:		
	Peritonitis		Imaging studies to detect anatomic problems or obstruction		
	Common pathogens:				
	Gram-positive cocci				
	Gram-negative bacteria				
	Anaerobic bacteria				
	Pancreatic duct infection: gram-negative bacteria appear to grow more readily in pancreatic secretions than gram-positive bacteria				

CBC, complete blood cell; CT, computed tomography; DM, diabetes mellitus; ERCP, endoscopic retrograde cholangiopancreatography; LFTs, liver function tests; MRI, magnetic resonance imaging; RUQ, right upper quadrant; SPK, simultaneous pancreas kidney; TMP/SMX, trimethoprim/sulfamethoxazole; US, ultrasound; UTI, urinary tract infection.

a. Trimethoprim/sulfamethoxazole (TMP-SMX; Bactrim) is the primary prevention of nocardiosis.
b. However, there are isolates that are able to break through.
   i.   This is most likely due to every other day dosing.
c. Daily dosing may help keep a sustained blood level.

E. Legionellosis[29,47]

1. Caused by *Legionella pneumophila*.
2. May occur at any time after transplantation
   a. Nosocomial sources: contaminated hospital water supply, ventilators, nebulizers
   b. Community-acquired sources: drinking water, water heaters, room humidifiers, water aerosolization sources, and shower heads
3. Should be considered whenever a transplant recipient presents with pneumonia-like symptoms.
4. Simultaneous infection by other pulmonary pathogens may occur.
5. Urine antigen test for *Legionella* only detects *Legionella pneumophila* serotype 1.
6. Mortality in transplant recipients is high (often over 50%).
7. See Table 5-5 for the clinical manifestations, prevention/prophylaxis, diagnosis, and treatment of legionellosis.

F. Tuberculosis[22,30]

1. Most commonly caused by *Mycobacterium tuberculosis*.
2. Worldwide incidence in transplant recipients:
   a. Developed countries: 1% to 6%
   b. Remainder of the world: up to 15%
3. Mortality in transplant recipients: up to 40%.
4. Transplant recipients are at risk for primary and reactivation infections.
5. While 51% to 64% of transplant patients have pulmonary infections, many have atypical and extrapulmonary manifestations that may prolong diagnosis and delay appropriate treatment.
6. Generally, the chest radiograph can show focal, miliary, or nodular patterns.
7. Treatment is prolonged and requires use of three or four medications with risk of hepatotoxicity.
8. See Table 5-5 for the clinical manifestations, prevention/prophylaxis, diagnosis, and treatment of tuberculosis.

G. *Clostridium difficile*[12,22,48,49]

1. Spore-forming anaerobic gram-positive bacillus.
2. Pathogen produces protein endotoxins (Toxin A and Toxin B) that cause cytokine response of neutrophilic infiltrate and cytokine release in the tissues.
3. Of those patients colonized with toxigenic *Clostridium difficile*, 50% do not develop active disease.
4. *C. difficile* produces a toxin that causes mucosal inflammation, secretion of fluids from the colon, and injury to the colon causing yellow plaque formation (pseudomembrane).
5. Risk factors
   a. Antimicrobial agents (but can occur without prior antibiotic therapy)
      i.   Broad-spectrum antibiotics (e.g., ampicillin, clindamycin, and the cephalosporins) disrupt the normal flora in the bowel; this in turn permits the overgrowth of *C. difficile*.
      ii. Hospitalization.
      iii. Older age (65 or older).

     iv. Albuminemia.

     v. Net state of immunosuppression.

     vi. Inflammatory bowel disease.

     vii. Gastric acid suppression with H_2 blockers and proton pump inhibitors may suppress acid that kills *C. difficile* spores.

6. Potential clinical manifestations may include the following: (onset may be abrupt)

  a. Fever

  b. Abdominal cramps, pain, distension

  c. Diarrhea

  d. Stools may be profuse, watery, and/or bloody

  e. Ileus (diarrhea may be absent)

  f. Toxic megacolon

  g. Perforation of colon

  h. Bandemia/leukocytosis

  i. Computerized tomography (CT) scan with evidence of bowel wall edema and ascites

7. Complications

  a. Fluid and electrolyte imbalances

  b. Inadequate absorption of medications

8. Treatment options

  a. Stop antimicrobial agents or change to a more narrow spectrum age

  b. Metronidazole (Flagyl) 250 to 500 mg by mouth, three to four times per day, 10 to 14 days

     i. Intravenous metronidazole may be required for patients with severe dysmotility or ileus, as oral medication may not cross the colonic mucosa and reach the feces.

     ii. Consider interaction with tacrolimus (Prograf; Astagraf) and sirolimus (Rapamune); check levels often as dose adjustments may be indicated to maintain therapeutic immunosuppression levels.

  c. For patients with severe infection or those who do not respond to metronidazole:

     i. Vancomycin 125 mg by mouth four times per day for 10 to 14 days

     ii. Children: 40 mg/kg in 4 doses

     iii. Intravenous vancomycin should not be given as it does not cross into the gut

  d. For patients with multiple relapses[48–50]:

     i. Prolonged vancomycin tapering

     ii. Intravenous immunoglobulin (potential option)

     iii. Fidaxomicin (Dificid)

       • 200 mg by mouth twice a day

       • Consider interaction with cyclosporine (Neoral; Gengraf); check levels frequently to adjust dosing as indicated to maintain a therapeutic level of cyclosporine.

     iv. Fecal microbiota transplant[50]

9. Prevention[49,50]

  a. Prudent use of antibiotics.

  b. Strict adherence to infection control guidelines.

  c. Proper and thorough environmental cleaning.

  d. Probiotics may be useful for prevention of worsening *C. difficile* infection.

H. Vancomycin-resistant *Enterococcus* (VRE)[45,51]
1. After *Staphylococcus* infections, *Enterococcus* infections are the most common nosocomial infection in the United States.
2. Enterococci are typically found in GI tract and female genitourinary tract.
3. Two most common species:
    a. *Enterococcus faecalis*
    b. *Enterococcus faecium*: resistant to both vancomycin and ampicillin in the United States
4. Suspect VRE in patient with gram-positive cocci in pairs and chains in blood cultures.
5. VRE colonization:
    a. Risk of colonization involves exposure to VRE and host susceptibility.
    b. Important risk factors:
        i. Proximity to patients with VRE colonization, especially patients with diarrhea
        ii. Length of hospital stay
    c. Intestinal colonization has no symptoms, may persist for long periods of time, and is a mechanism for transmission of VRE to other patients.
    d. Colonization rates after SOT: 11% to 63%.
    e. VRE-colonized transplant recipients are at risk of infection.
6. VRE infection[45,51]
    a. Develops in patients with VRE colonization.
    b. Infection rate among solid organ transplant recipients: 1% to 16%.
    c. Recipients of abdominal allografts are particularly susceptible to infection.
    d. Potential portals of entry:
        i. Urinary tract
        ii. Intra-abdominal or pelvic sources
        iii. Wounds
        iv. Intravascular catheters
    e. Risk factors of VRE Infection:
        i. Immunosuppressive therapy
        ii. Lengthy intensive care unit stay
        iii. Prolonged hospitalization
        iv. Severity of illness
        v. Exposure to patients with VRE
        vi. Administration of broad-spectrum antibiotics
        vii. Renal insufficiency
        viii. Hemodialysis
        ix. CMV-seropositive donor; CMV-seronegative recipient
        x. Prolonged surgical time
        xi. Reoperation
        xii. Total parental nutrition
        xiii. Enteral tube feedings
        xiv. Indwelling bladder catheters
    f. Transmission:
        i. Within institution: direct or indirect contact
            * Staff hands.
            * Organism has been isolated from virtually all objects in health care environment (e.g., organism survival: stethoscope diaphragm 30 minutes; on countertop 1 week).
        ii. Between institutions
            * Via health care professionals who work at more than one hospital
            * Transfer of infected patients between institutions

g. Potential treatment options:
   i. Removal of nidus of infection (e.g., by draining abscesses, surgical debridement of wounds)
   ii. Antimicrobial agents
   * For ampicillin-susceptible organisms: ampicillin, aminopenicillin, or ureidopenicillin derivatives
   * For severe infections: combination broad-spectrum therapy with aminoglycosides such as gentamicin, tobramycin (Tobi), amikacin (Amikin)
   * Ordaptomycin: for organisms that are not susceptible to ampicillin or for patients allergic to penicillin and vancomycin
   * Linezolid (Zyvox): oral or intravenous preparation, side effects:
     ○ Bone marrow suppression including anemia and thrombocytopenia (this may preclude long-term therapy with linezolid).
     ○ Serotonin syndrome (fever, hypertension, tachycardia, confusion) when used with some antidepressants.
     ○ Some resistance to linezolid has been noted.
   * Quinupristin/dalfopristin (for *Enterococcus faecium* only): intravenous preparation, requires central catheter to prevent phlebitis, side effects:
     ○ Arthralgias, myalgias.
     ○ Most *Enterococcus faecalis* organisms are intrinsically resistant to this agent.
7. Prevention
   a. Strict adherence to infection control guidelines
      i. Gowns, gloves, hand washing
      ii. Prudent use of antimicrobial agents
   b. Surveillance cultures (rectal or stool) for early identification and isolation of patients colonized with VRE
      i. Tracking of VRE colonization in high-risk units
      ii. Continuation of isolation procedures per protocol (e.g., until three weekly cultures have been negative)
      iii. Proper and thorough environmental cleaning; use dedicated stethoscope, thermometer, and sphygmomanometer
   c. Epidemiological pattern is changing
      i. In the United States: community dissemination is developing.
      ii. In Europe: very resistant enterococci are emerging.

I. Methicillin-resistant *Staphylococcus aureus* (MRSA)[46,52]
   1. MRSA remains a threat to transplant patient. However, incidence is decreasing in the community now.
   2. Colonization occurs mainly in the nasopharynx and on the skin. Those colonized with MRSA or methicillin-susceptible *Staphylococcus aureus* (MSSA) have a high risk of developing a subsequent infection.
   3. Transplant patients have a high risk of colonization with MRSA due to prolonged illness and contact in the health care system.
   4. *S. aureus* infections can occur as the following:
      a. Wound infections
      b. Bacteremia, often associated with central venous catheter infection

    c. Metastatic infections (e.g., arthritis, osteomyelitis, meningitis)

    d. Pneumonia

    e. Endovascular infection (endocarditis, septic thrombophlebitis).

5. Transmission

    a. Colonized or infected patient

    b. Colonized health care worker

    c. Allograft.

6. Reported clinical manifestations

    a. SOT recipients in general

       i. Pneumonia: *Staphylococcus aureus* is the most common gram-positive organism that causes bacterial pneumonia in the first 3 months following SOT

       ii. Wound infections

       iii. Bacteremia

    b. Liver transplant recipients

       i. Wound infection

       ii. Bacteremia

       iii. Pneumonia

    c. Heart, heart-lung, and lung transplant recipients

       i. Mediastinal abscess

       ii. Mediastinitis

       iii. Endocarditis

       iv. Pericarditis

    d. Kidney transplant recipients

       i. Central line infections

7. Treatment options

    a. Vancomycin

    b. Daptomycin

    c. Linezolid (bacteriostatic, limited use due to myelosuppression and adverse effect such as optic neuropathy)

    d. Quinupristin/dalfopristin (infrequently used, not well tolerated)

    e. Others: tigecycline, ceftaroline, dalbavancin

    f. Rifampin added if there is prosthetic device infection

8. Prevention

    a. Surveillance cultures to detect nasal colonization on admission and periodically thereafter.

    b. Intranasal mupirocin to eradicate MRSA in colonized patients.

    c. Strict adherence to and monitoring of infection control measures.

    d. Cohorting for staff and MRSA-positive and MRSA-negative patients.

    e. Use of vascular catheters impregnated with antibiotics.

    f. Proper and thorough environmental cleaning.

    g. Consider decolonization protocol: intranasal 2% mupirocin BID × 5 days coupled with chlorhexidine baths for 7 days.

9. Note: Community-acquired MRSA (CA-MRSA) has also been observed and is rapidly spreading to many communities across the world.

    a. Transmission

       i. Person-to-person

       ii. Person–to inanimate objects–to person

    b. Clinical manifestations

       i. Skin infection: boils

       ii. Soft tissue infection

       iii. Pneumonia

  c. Treatment
   i. Incision and drainage if possible
   ii. Often responds to TMP/SMZ (Bactrim), clindamycin, and doxycycline
 10. Incidence of vancomycin-intermediate *Staphylococcus aureus* (VISA) is increasing worldwide.

J. Multidrug-resistant gram-negative bacteria[52]

1. Extended-spectrum beta-lactamase (ESBL) gram-negative bacilli.
2. The use of broad-spectrum beta-lactam antibiotics has resulted in the development of gram-negative bacilli that produce ESBL.
3. These bacilli are resistant to many antibiotics, including the penicillins, first-generation and newer cephalosporins, cephamycins, carbapenems, and fluoroquinolones.
4. Resistance to these antibiotics has been acquired primarily by the following:
  a. *Klebsiella pneumoniae*
  b. *Escherichia coli*
  c. *Enterobacter*
  d. *Pseudomonas*
  e. *Acinetobacter*
5. Clinical sequelae:
  a. Urinary tract infections (UTI)
  b. Septicemia
  c. Hospital-acquired pneumonia
  d. Intra-abdominal abscesses
  e. Brain abscesses
  f. Device-related infections
6. Risk factors:
  a. Antibiotic therapy (especially with newer cephalosporins)
  b. Surgery
  c. Intensive care unit stay
  d. Prolonged hospitalization
7. Treatment
  a. Removal of source of infection (e.g., colonized intravascular line)
  b. Drainage of abscesses
  c. Antibiotic therapy, taking into consideration site and severity of the infection, liver and renal function, and patient's age
  d. Bacteremia: carbapenems (imipenem, meropenem)
  e. Nonbacteremic UTIs: oral agents (e.g., trimethoprim, nitrofurantoin [Macrobid])
  f. Note: use of aminoglycosides with calcineurin inhibitor can result in nephrotoxicity
  g. Colistin (polymyxin E): highly nephrotoxic
  h. Tigecycline (Tygacil)
8. Prevention
  a. Prudent use of antibiotics
  b. Prompt identification and separation of patients colonized or infected with ESBL bacilli or multidrug-resistant bacteria
  c. Cohorting of nurses and patients
  d. Strict adherence to infection control guidelines
  e. Proper and thorough environmental cleaning

XI. FUNGAL INFECTIONS[31,35]

A. Overview
   1. Fungal infections are a major cause of posttransplant morbidity and mortality.[11,35]
   2. The incidence of fungal infection among transplant recipients is lower than that of bacterial or viral infections; however, the mortality is typically higher.
      a. Reported incidence: 5% (renal transplant recipients) to approximately 50% (liver transplant recipients)
   3. Fungal infections typically occur in first 6 months posttransplant but can occur over the first several years.
   4. Fungal infections may be categorized as follows:
      a. Opportunistic infections (aspergillosis, candidiasis, cryptococcosis, and pneumocystis)
      b. Infections with geographically restricted mycoses (histoplasmosis, coccidioidomycosis, and blastomycosis).
   5. Potential portals of entry[11]:
      a. Respiratory tract (most common)
      b. GI tract
      c. Skin (e.g., via intravascular catheters)
      d. Donor-derived infection.
   6. Risk factors for fungal infections[11]:
      a. High-dose corticosteroid therapy
      b. Broad-spectrum antimicrobial agents
      c. Rejection requiring increased immunosuppression
      d. Allograft dysfunction
      e. Concurrent infection with immunomodulating virus (e.g., CMV).
   7. Fungal colonization: clinical manifestations are frequently nonspecific and often overlap with other infectious and noninfectious processes.[21]
   8. When a fungal infection is diagnosed, it is important to look for *metastatic infection, particularly to skin, skeleton, and CNS.*

B. *Candida* species
   1. Found in human GI tract (oropharynx to anus), gynecological tract, and skin
      a. Pretransplant colonization of GI tract is a risk factor for posttransplant candidal infection.
   2. Most common sources: GI tract and intravascular catheters[11]
   3. Risk factors for invasive disease:
      a. Total parenteral nutrition
      b. Central venous catheters
      c. Acute renal failure
      d. Diabetes mellitus (DM)
      e. Corticosteroid therapy
      f. Neutropenia
      g. Abdominal surgery
      h. Use of broad-spectrum antibiotics
      i. Immunomodulating viral infections (e.g., CMV, HHV-6).
   4. See Table 5-5 for the clinical manifestations, prevention/prophylaxis, diagnosis, and treatment of candidal infections.

C. *Aspergillus* species[31,32,53,54]
   1. Epidemiological characteristics

   a. *Aspergillus* infections occur in 1% to 15% of SOT recipients.
   b. The mortality rate for transplant recipients with invasive aspergillosis ranges from 74% to 92%.
   c. Between 9.3% and 16.9% of all deaths within the first posttransplant year are due to invasive aspergillosis.
2. *Aspergillus fumigatus* is the most common human pathogen.
3. Portal of entry in majority of cases: respiratory tract via environmental exposure[24]
   a. Once the pathogen invades lung tissue, ulceration and necrosis ensue, as well as invasion of the tissues and blood vessels.
   b. If the pathogen invades blood vessels, widespread dissemination can occur.
4. The lung is the most common site of primary infection.[11]
5. Historically, aspergillosis typically occurred during the first 3 months posttransplant; newer data indicate that late-onset infections are becoming more frequent.[3]
6. Chronic obstructive pulmonary disease (COPD) predisposes patients to colonization of the airway with *Aspergillus*.
7. Risk factors for invasive infections[11]:
   a. Neutropenia
   b. Potent immunosuppression (particularly high-dose steroid therapy)
   c. Prolonged operative time
   d. Renal failure
8. See Table 5-5 for the clinical manifestations, prevention/prophylaxis, diagnosis, and treatment of *Aspergillus* infections.

D. *Cryptococcus neoformans*[11,31,40,53,54]
   1. Pathogen is ubiquitous in the environment, especially in soil and bird excrement.
   2. Disease is acquired through inhalation.
   3. Infections can occur throughout the entire posttransplant course.
   4. *Cryptococcus neoformans* is the most common cause of fungal CNS infection.[20,21]
   5. See Table 5-5 for the clinical manifestations, prevention/prophylaxis, diagnosis, and treatment of *Cryptococcus neoformans* infections.

E. *Pneumocystis carinii*[31,33,36,37,54]
   1. Originally classified as a protozoan but now classified as a fungal pathogen.
   2. Infection typically occurs during first 6 months after transplantation in those recipients who do not receive prophylaxis.
   3. A number of diseases may mimic pneumocystis: CMV, influenza, adenovirus infection, miliary TB, disseminated fungal infections, adult respiratory distress syndrome, and RSV.[11]
   4. See Table 5-5 for the clinical manifestations, prevention/prophylaxis, diagnosis, and treatment of *Pneumocystis carinii* infections.

F. Endemic mycoses[34,38]
   1. Overview
      a. Endemic mycoses include *Coccidioides immitis*, *Histoplasma capsulatum*, *Blastomyces dermatitidis*, and *Paracoccidioides brasiliensis*.[11,38]
      b. The endemic mycoses should be considered in symptomatic patients who have traveled to or lived in Central or South America, Southeast Asia, or the midwestern or southwestern areas of the United States.

        i. Endemic areas for *Histoplasma capsulatum* and *Blastomyces dermatitidis* include the Ohio River and Mississippi valleys, respectively.

        ii. Endemic areas for *Coccidioides immitis*: primarily southwestern United States.

    c. Theoretically, infection (primary or reactivation) can occur at any time during the posttransplant period

        i. Blastomycosis: typically develops 1 to 2 years after transplant

        ii. Coccidioidomycosis: typically develops within the first year after transplant

        iii. Histoplasmosis: typically develops within 1 to 2 years posttransplantation.

    d. The pathogenesis of histoplasmosis, coccidioidomycosis, and blastomycosis is similar to that of TB. The following clinical presentations should prompt consideration of endemic disease in differential diagnosis[34]:

        i. Subacute respiratory illness with focal or disseminated infiltrates on chest radiograph

        ii. Nonspecific febrile illness

        iii. Illness in which metastatic aspects predominate, that is, mucocutaneous manifestations in histoplasmosis or blastomycosis, CNS manifestations in coccidioidomycosis[25]

  2. See Table 5-5 for the clinical manifestations, prevention/prophylaxis, diagnosis, and treatment of *Histoplasma capsulatum*.

XII. PARASITIC INFECTIONS[11,55]

  A. Overview

    1. The major protozoal pathogens are *Toxoplasma gondii* and *Cryptosporidium parvum*.

  B. *Toxoplasma gondii*[55]

    1. Toxoplasmosis typically results from reactivation of latent disease.

    2. Toxoplasmosis is more common in heart and heart-lung recipients than in any other transplant groups because the pathogen encysts in the heart muscle.

      a. Incidence increases to more than 50% for *Toxoplasma*-seronegative recipients who receive allografts from *Toxoplasma*-seropositive donors and who do not receive prophylaxis.

      b. The overall incidence of toxoplasmosis in heart transplant recipients ranges from 4% to 12%.

    3. Infection typically occurs during first 2 months following transplantation.

    4. Toxoplasmosis can mimic rejection; endomyocardial biopsy is required for a definitive diagnosis.

    5. See Table 5-5 for the clinical manifestations, prevention/prophylaxis, diagnosis, and treatment of toxoplasmosis.

  C. *Cryptosporidium parvum*[55,56]

    1. Diarrhea caused by this pathogen is frequently fatal in immunocompromised patients; hospitalization may be required to reverse dehydration and wasting. Infection of the proximal small bowel is common; however, organisms can also be harbored in the hepatobiliary tree.

    2. Organisms shed by patients are infectious; universal precautions are mandatory.

3. The disease is transmitted by fecal-oral contamination or water transmission.
4. Transplant recipients whose water supplies may be contaminated with *Cryptosporidium* may be advised to take special precautions such as the following:
    a. Boiling water for 5 minutes prior to drinking or using in food preparation OR using bottled distilled water
    b. Avoiding ice cubes that have been made with tap or well water
    c. Adding a filter to faucet
    d. Avoiding soda fountain drinks that have been reconstituted with tap water
5. See Table 5-5 for the clinical manifestations, prevention/prophylaxis, diagnosis, and treatment of cryptosporidiosis.

D. *Strongyloides stercoralis*[39,41]
1. A helminthic (worm) parasite and intestinal nematode found in 36 states in the United States; endemic in Southeast Asia, the Caribbean, and West Africa.
2. Organism can live (asymptomatically) in the GI tract for decades.
3. Organism causes diarrhea and peripheral eosinophilia (atypical marker for parasitic infection).
    a. Autoinfection: process by which the larvae transform into an infectious form within the intestine.
    b. Larvae invade intestinal mucosa.
    c. Constant reintroduction of infectious forms into the host sustains the infection.
    d. In transplant recipients, autoinfection may precipitate a hyperinfection syndrome (disseminated strongyloidiasis).
    e. Hyperinfection accelerates the organism's lifecycle leading to excessive helminth burden.
        i. Disruption of normal intestinal barrier results in gram-negative bacteremia and shock.
        ii. Mortality rate of hyperinfection: approximately 70%.
4. See Table 5-5 for the clinical manifestations, prevention/prophylaxis, diagnosis, and treatment of strongyloidiasis.

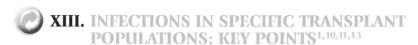

XIII. INFECTIONS IN SPECIFIC TRANSPLANT POPULATIONS: KEY POINTS[1,10,11,13]

A. Lung and heart-lung transplant recipients[1,10]
1. Pneumonia is a common complication: overall prevalence approximately 60%.
    a. Increased susceptibility is associated with the following factors:
        i. Decreased cough reflex
        ii. Impaired mucociliary clearance
        iii. Graft ischemia; reperfusion injury
        iv. Altered lymphatic drainage
        v. Inflammation of airway secondary to rejection
    b. Bacterial pathogens are the most common cause of pulmonary infections.
        i. Most common early pathogens: gram-negative bacteria such as *Enterobacteriaceae* and *Pseudomonas aeruginosa*
    c. Clinical presentation of nosocomial pneumonia:
        i. Respiratory failure that requires mechanical ventilation.
        ii. Consolidation on chest radiograph.

iii. Fever and leukocytosis may be muted or absent.
d. Treatment
   i. Guided by antimicrobial susceptibilities of pathogens.
   ii. Therapy is aggressive and may involve multiple agents.
e. Prevention
   i. Tailored antimicrobial prophylaxis based on respiratory tract cultures of donor and recipient
   ii. Wound infections: perioperative prophylaxis for gram-positive bacteria.
2. CMV is the most lethal infection.
3. The donor lung is only type of allograft that is frequently infected or colonized with bacterial pathogens.
4. The native lung of single lung transplant recipients is also susceptible to infection.
   a. Radiographic changes in the native lung (e.g., those caused by fibrosis) may make diagnosis of infection difficult.
5. Other serious posttransplant infections include the following:
   a. Mediastinitis and sternal wound infections
      i. Wound infections: perioperative prophylaxis for gram-positive bacteria may be given
      ii. May require debridement in addition to antimicrobial agents
   b. Infections that lead to leakage or dehiscence of the bronchial or tracheal anastomoses
      i. Nosocomial bacteria, *Candida* spp., and *Aspergillus* spp. are commonly associated with anastomotic infections.
6. Toxoplasmosis
   a. More common in heart transplant recipients than in any other transplant group because *Toxoplasma gondii* encysts in the heart muscle.
   b. Symptoms of toxoplasmosis may appear from 3 weeks to 6 months posttransplant.
   c. Toxoplasmosis can mimic rejection; therefore, an endomyocardial biopsy is required for definitive diagnosis.

B. Liver transplant recipients[16,17]
1. Early after transplant, intra-abdominal and liver abscesses, peritonitis, wound infections, and cholangitis are common.
2. The abdomen is the most common site of bacterial infection.
   a. The abdomen is the most common source of bacteremia (particularly peritoneal space and biliary tract).
   b. Risk factors for abdominal infections:
      i. Long surgical time
      ii. Biliary leaks, obstruction, stenosis
      iii. Hepatic artery stenosis or thrombosis
      iv. Large number of blood transfusions
      v. Reoperation
      vi. Early rejection
      vii. CMV infection
      viii. Retransplantation.
   c. The type of biliary anastomosis may affect the risk of infection.
      i. Choledochostomy (duct-to-duct): Risk of infection may be less because of maintenance of the native sphincter of Oddi.

      ii. Roux-en-Y choledochojejunostomy anastomoses: Rate of abdominal infections may be higher due to potential for reflux of enteric organisms into the biliary system.

3. The incidence of invasive fungal infections is high.
4. Clinical presentation:
   a. Wound infections and intra-abdominal abscesses
      i. Abdominal pain
      ii. Fever in some, but not all, patients
         * Fever may not develop with some pathogens.
      iii. Wound dehiscence
      iv. Purulent drainage from wound
      v. Pain with palpation
      vi. Guarding, rebound
      vii. Laboratory findings: leukocytosis in some, but not all, patients
   b. Cholangitis
      i. Fever
      ii. Pain in right upper quadrant
      iii. Abdominal tenderness
      iv. Laboratory findings: leukocytosis, elevated bilirubin, transaminases, alkaline phosphatase.
5. Diagnosis requires imaging studies: CT scans, ultrasound, MRI.
6. Treatment[24]
   a. Intra-abdominal and surgical wound infections
      i. Antimicrobial therapy
         * Based on cultures and sensitivities.
         * Empiric therapy for known colonizing pathogens may be initiated until culture and sensitivity results are available.
      ii. Intra-abdominal abscess: drainage
   b. Cholangitis
      i. Intravenous antibiotics in the setting of adequate biliary flow
      ii. In the setting of biliary tree obstruction: endoscopic retrograde cholangiopancreatography (ERCP) with dilatation
7. Prevention
   a. Pre- and posttransplant: selective bowel decontamination
   b. Perioperative antimicrobials to decrease risk of wound infections
   c. Posttransplant: antimicrobial prophylaxis prior to invasive procedures such as liver biopsies
8. Almost all liver transplant recipients who had pretransplant HCV infections remain viremic after transplantation.
   a. Recurrent HCV infection occurs in 30% to 70% of these patients during the first posttransplant year.
9. Without adequate immunoprophylaxis, HBV graft infection recurs in 80% to 100% of hepatitis B surface antigen–positive liver transplant recipients.
   a. With the appropriate use of HBIG and new antiviral agents (e.g., lamivudine [Epivir], adefovir [Hepsera]), this recurrence rate is significantly reduced.

C. Kidney transplant recipients
1. Approximately 80% of infections are caused by bacteria.
   a. Risk factors for bacterial infections:
      i. Decreased urine flow

    ii. Renal insufficiency

    iii. Prolonged catheterization of bladder

    iv. Comorbidities such as DM

2. Common infectious syndromes include the following:
   a. Genitourinary tract infections (particularly UTIs associated with catheters)
   b. Pneumonia
   c. Primary bacteremia (often associated with use of vascular catheters)
   d. Intra-abdominal infections
   e. Surgical site infections (superficial or deep), often associated with fluid collections or devitalized tissues

3. Bloodstream infections
   a. The urinary tract is the most common site of primary infection that is associated with secondary bacteremia.
   b. Poor outcomes are associated with the following causative agents:
      i. Gram-negative bacteria
      ii. Organisms that are multidrug resistant
      iii. *Candida* species

4. Genitourinary tract infections
   a. Incidence of UTIs has decreased due to the routine use of trimethoprim-sulfamethoxazole (TMP-SMX; Bactrim) and early catheter removal.
   b. Risk of genitourinary tract infections is related to surgical complications (e.g., urine leaks, wound hematomas, lymphoceles).
   c. Asymptomatic candiduria can be serious because of the potential for the development of obstructing candidal fungal balls, ascending candidal pyelonephritis, and sepsis, particularly in diabetic recipients with bladder dysfunction.
   d. For patients with suspected UTIs, obtain a clean-catch midstream urine specimen for bacterial and fungal culture (quantitative).
   e. Clinical presentation—UTIs:
      i. Acute pyelonephritis
      ii. High fever
      iii. Pain at site of graft
      iv. Renal allograft dysfunction
      v. Laboratory findings: leukocytosis, urinary sediment
      vi. Note: May be asymptomatic (no urgency, frequency, dysuria); pyuria may be absent

5. Treatment[24]
   a. UTIs:
      i. Antimicrobial therapy is based on the culture and sensitivities.
      ii. Duration of therapy is based on the severity of the infection.
      iii. Pyelonephritis typically requires at least 2 weeks of therapy.
      iv. Recurrent infections require imaging studies to detect any anatomic anomalies or obstruction.
   b. Surgical wound infections:
      i. May require debridement in addition to antimicrobial therapy.
      ii. Empiric coverage may be initiated until results of culture and sensitivities are available.

6. Prevention[10,16]
   a. UTIs and bloodstream infections:

      i. Routine surveillance urine cultures

      ii. Antimicrobial prophylaxis with trimethoprim/sulfamethoxazole (TMP-SMX; Bactrim) or fluoroquinolones in certain situations.

7. Surgical wound infections: perioperative antibiotic such as a cephalosporin.

8. Unilateral leg edema on the side of the kidney transplant may be a sign of a lymphocele, either infected or not infected, near the allograft.

9. Fever

  a. Requires blood cultures.

  b. Differential diagnosis includes the following:

      i. Infection and/or rejection

      ii. Adverse effect of medications

      iii. Noninfectious systemic inflammatory response such as the following:

         • Pancreatitis

         • Cytokine release syndromes associated with the administration of monoclonal or polyclonal antibodies

         • Pulmonary embolism

  c. Fever of unknown origin may be associated with a deep wound infection; diagnosis requires needle aspiration of wound and ultrasound or CT scanning of both pelvic implantation and nephrectomy operative sites.

D. Heart transplant recipients

1. The lung is a common site of infection.

  a. Major bacterial infection: ventilator-associated pneumonia caused by gram-negative bacteria

  b. Clinical presentation[3]

      i. Respiratory failure and inability to wean from ventilator

      ii. Fever in some, but not all, patients

      iii. Purulent respiratory secretions

      iv. Consolidation on chest radiograph

  c. Treatment

      i. Based on results of cultures and sensitivities

  d. Prevention

      i. Early extubation

      ii. Aggressive pulmonary toilet

2. Mediastinitis

  a. Most common during first 2 to 4 weeks posttransplant

  b. Clinical presentation

      i. Initial symptoms may be subtle: mild chest discomfort, slight edema, and/or erythema along sternal incision.

      ii. Some patients may present with fever and bacteremia.

      iii. Laboratory findings: leukocytosis.

  c. Treatment

      i. Surgical debridement

      ii. Antimicrobial therapy

3. Sternal wound infections

  a. Clinical presentation

      i. Early postoperative period

         • Poor wound healing

         • Dehiscence

          ii. Later postoperative period
- Formation of sinus tract
- Purulent drainage

      b. Treatment[3]
        i. Surgical debridement
        ii. Antimicrobial therapy directed at gram-positive pathogens
      c. Prevention: perioperative antimicrobial agents directed at gram-positive pathogens

    4. CMV
      a. Single most common and most important pathogen that affects heart transplant recipients.
      b. The risk of developing symptomatic CMV disease is significantly greater when the virus that is activated is of donor origin rather than recipient origin.
      c. The GI tract is the most common site of CMV infection.
      d. CMV pneumonitis has the highest morbidity and mortality rate of any CMV infection.

    5. Toxoplasmosis
      a. More common in heart transplant recipients than in any other transplant group because *Toxoplasma gondii* encysts in the heart muscle.
      b. Symptoms of toxoplasmosis may appear from 3 weeks to 6 months posttransplant.
      c. Toxoplasmosis can mimic rejection; therefore, an endomyocardial biopsy is required for definitive diagnosis.

E. Pancreas transplant recipients[22]
    1. Recipients are particularly susceptible to candidiasis due to the following:
      a. Underlying DM
      b. Indwelling bladder catheters
      c. Drainage of exocrine secretions into bladder
    2. Bacterial UTIs may also be associated with drainage of exocrine secretions into bladder (promotes bacterial overgrowth).
    3. The most common bacterial infections are wound and intra-abdominal infections.
    4. Treatment: similar to treatment of infections in liver and renal transplant recipients.
    5. Prevention:
      a. Trimethoprim/sulfamethoxazole (TMP-SMX [Bactrim])
      b. Standard perioperative antibiotics

F. Kidney-pancreas transplant recipients[22]
    1. Wound infections and UTIs are more common in kidney-pancreas transplant recipients than in isolated kidney transplant recipients.
    2. Factors associated with increased risk of UTI include the following:
      a. Enzymatic digestion of the glycosaminoglycan layer that normally protects the urothelium
      b. Change in the urinary pH secondary to pancreatic exocrine secretions
      c. Underlying glycosuria
    3. Pancreatic abscess associated with gram-negative organisms or fungi may necessitate surgical draining or removal of the graft.

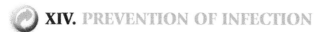 **XIV.** PREVENTION OF INFECTION

  A. Pharmacologic measures

    1. Antimicrobial therapy

      a. Therapeutic: to treat an established infection

      b. Prophylactic: administration of antimicrobials to an entire population of patients to prevent common infections

      c. Preemptive: administration of antimicrobials to a subgroup of patients who are at high risk

    2. Antibiotic prophylaxis against infective endocarditis per American Heart Association guidelines

    3. Periodic posttransplant vaccinations per Centers for Disease Control and Prevention guidelines for immunocompromised individuals[4,57]

      a. Posttransplant vaccination protocols vary among transplant centers; commonly recommended vaccines include the following:

        i. Annual influenza vaccine (for recipients and household contacts unless otherwise contraindicated)

        ii. Pneumococcal vaccine approximately every 5 to 6 years

        iii. Tetanus booster every 10 years; some transplant centers prefer to treat tetanus-related wounds with tetanus immunoglobulin alone

      b. It is important to note that vaccinations in transplant recipients may be less effective due to the following[4]:

        i. Loss of previous immunity due to declining antibody levels and decreased antibody responses to previous vaccine antigens

        ii. Reduced vaccine efficacy: decreased responsiveness to vaccine immunization.

      c. Live attenuated vaccines[24]

        i. Typically *contraindicated* in adults due to the potential for viral replication in the immunocompromised host

- Oral polio vaccine
- MMR vaccine
- Bacilli Calmette-Guérin
- Smallpox vaccine
- TY21a typhoid vaccine
- Yellow fever vaccine—if severely immunocompromised
- Varicella vaccine

        ii. *Household contacts* of transplant recipients can safely receive *inactivated* vaccines based on CDC recommendations, can receive the following live vaccines but MUST follow CDC recommendations regarding contact with SOT recipient.

- MMR
- Rotavirus
- Varicella
- Yellow fever
- Oral typhoid

    4. Nonpharmacologic measures

      a. Health care providers and institutions (Box 5-1)

      b. Patients and family members (Box 5-2)

BOX 5-1   Nonpharmacologic Measures for Health Care Providers and Institutions
Health Care Providers

- Wash hands frequently and thoroughly with antimicrobial soap or alcohol gel products.
- Use aseptic technique per posttransplant protocols (e.g., central line dressing changes).
- Follow reverse isolation procedures per posttransplant protocol.
- Housekeeping per posttransplant hospital protocol
- Use leukocyte-depleted and CMV-negative blood products for CMV-seronegative recipients.
- Use high-efficiency leukocyte blood filters.
- Discontinue indwelling lines and catheters as soon as possible.
- Obtain posttransplant infection surveillance tests per protocols and in a timely manner.
- Avoid cross-contamination by staff members caring for patients with contagious infections.
- Use special masks to transport recipients through high-risk areas of hospital (e.g., construction sites that might contain *Aspergillus* spores).

Institutions

- Monitor showers, toilet facilities, and air-conditioning systems for *Legionella*.
- Use high-efficiency particulate air-filtered air-handling systems if air supply is potentially contaminated, especially from construction.

Chong PP, Razonable RR. Diagnostic and management strategies for donor-derived infections. *Infect Dis Clin North Am.* 2013;27(2):253–270.
Avery RK, Michaels MG. Strategies for safe living after solid organ transplantation. *Am J Transplant.* 2013;13(suppl 4):304–310.

BOX 5-2   Nonpharmacologic Measures for Patients and Family Members

---

- Wash hands frequently and thoroughly with antimicrobial soap.
- Avoid people with obvious signs of illness.
- Avoid raw or partially cooked foods of animal origin.
- Avoid cross-contamination between raw and cooked foods.
- Avoid unpasteurized products.
- Wash raw fruits and vegetables thoroughly before eating.
- Avoid potential animal sources of infection (e.g., cleaning cat litter boxes, bird cages, fish aquaria; petting zoos).
- Avoid close contact with infants and others who have recently received live virus vaccines (oral polio, varicella, or measles-mumps-rubella vaccines).
- Avoid potential sources of fungal infections during first posttransplant year (e.g., live plants, fresh flowers).
- Obtain yearly influenza vaccine (patients and household contacts) unless otherwise contraindicated.
- Use boiled (for at least 1 full minute) water or distilled water if safety of drinking water is questionable.
- Avoid intravenous drug use.
- Follow safer sex guidelines.
- Consult with transplant or infectious disease physician about travel to areas requiring malaria prophylaxis and/or vaccines.

Chong PP, Razonable RR. Diagnostic and management strategies for donor-derived infections. *Infect Dis Clin North Am.* 2013;27(2):253–270.
Avery RK, Michaels MG. Strategies for safe living after solid organ transplantation. *Am J Transplant.* 2013;13(suppl 4):304–310.

XV. SUMMARY: KEY POINTS[20]

A. Because immunosuppressed patients may have a suboptimal response to vaccinations, it is important to update transplant candidates' immunizations before transplantation. These immunizations should be given as early as possible in the disease course because vaccines are often less effective in patients with severe end-organ dysfunction.

B. Immunosuppressed patients are more vulnerable to infection with organisms that are relatively avirulent (in immunocompetent individuals) or at lower inoculum.

C. Diagnosis of infection in transplant recipients may be difficult due to the following:
   1. Muted inflammatory response
   2. Presence of dual infections
   3. Advanced infection at time of presentation
   4. Simultaneous toxic side effects of medications
   5. Anatomic alterations secondary to transplant surgery

D. For patients whose source of infection is linked to an anatomical or technical abnormality, surgical correction of the abnormality is mandatory; otherwise, antimicrobial therapy will fail.

E. Antimicrobial therapy often is not prescribed for "fixed" courses but rather is based on microbial burden. The greater the burden, the longer and more intense the therapy. Therapy is continued until clinical and laboratory evidence demonstrates that active infection has been eradicated.

F. In general, pathogen-specific antimicrobial therapy is preferred over broad-spectrum, empiric antibiotics.

G. Certain antimicrobial agents can significantly interact with cyclosporine and tacrolimus and/or cause additive nephrotoxicity (see Table 5-9). Macrolide and azoles, in particular, should be avoided whenever possible, because they elevate levels of calcineurin inhibitors. If unavoidable, close monitoring of calcineurin inhibitor levels should be implemented.

REFERENCES

1. Green M. Introduction: infections in solid organ transplantation. *Am J Transplant.* 2013;13(suppl 4):3–8.
2. Blumberg EA, Danziger-Isakov L, Kumar D, et al. Foreword: guidelines 3. *Am J Transplant.* 2013;13(suppl 4):1–2.
3. Fischer SA, Lu K. Screening of donor and recipient in solid organ transplantation. *Am J Transplant.* 2013;13(suppl 4):9–21.
4. Danziger-Isakov L, Kumar D. Vaccination in solid organ transplantation. *Am J Transplant.* 2013;13(suppl 4):311–317.
5. Ison MG, Grossi P. Donor-derived infections in solid organ transplantation. *Am J Transplant.* 2013;13(suppl 4):22–30.
6. Ison MG, Nalesnik MA. An update on donor-derived disease transmission in organ transplantation. *Am J Transplant.* 2011;11:1123–1130.
7. Greenwald MA, Kuehnert MJ, Fishman JA. Infectious disease transmission during organ and tissue transplantation. *Emerg Infect Dis.* 2012;18(8):e1.

8. Seem DL, Lee I, Umscheid CA, et al. Excerpt from PHS guideline for reducing HIV, HBV and HCV transmission through organ transplantation. *Am J Transplant.* 2013;13(8):1953–1962.

9. Organ Procurement and Transplantation Network. Available at http://optn.transplant.hrsa.gov/ContentDocuments/OPTN_Policies#nameddest=Policy_15. Accessed January 9, 2015.

10. Jani AA. Infections after solid organ transplantation. *Medscape.* 2014. Available at http://emedicine.medscape.com/article.430550-overview. Accessed August 26, 2015.

11. Pappas PG, Alexander BD, Andes DR, et al. Invasive fungal infections among organ transplant recipients: results of the transplant-associated infection surveillance network (TRANSNET). *Clin Infect Dis.* 2010;50(8):1101–1111.

12. Dubberke ER, Burdette SD. Clostridium difficile infections in solid organ transplantation. *Am J Transplant.* 2013;13(suppl 4):42–49.

13. Fever in Organ Transplant Recipients. Available at http://www.antimicrobe.org/e54.asp#r184. Accessed January 9, 2015.

14. Morris MI, Fischer SA, Ison MG. Infections transmitted by transplantation. *Infect Dis Clin North Am.* 2010;24(2):497–514.

15. Chong PP, Razonable RR. Diagnostic and management strategies for donor-derived infections. *Infect Dis Clin North Am.* 2013;27(2):253–270.

16. Avery RK, Michaels MG. Strategies for safe living after solid organ transplantation. *Am J Transplant.* 2013;13(suppl 4):304–310.

17. Razonable R. Management of viral infections in solid organ transplant recipients. *Expert Rev Anti Infect Ther.* 2011;9(6):685–700.

18. Razonable R. Human herpesviruses 6,7 and 8 in solid organ transplant recipients. *Am J Transplant.* 2013;13:67–78.

19. Ramanan P, Razonable R. Cytomegalovirus infections in solid organ transplantation: a review. *J Infect Chemother.* 2013;45(3):260–271.

20. Kotton D, Kumar D, Caliendo A, et al. International consensus guidelines on the management of cytomegalovirus in solid organ transplantation. *Transplantation.* 2010;89:779–795.

21. Vella J, Bennett W, Brennan D. Cytomegalovirus in renal transplant recipients. In: Murphy B, ed. *Up to Date.* Waltham, MA: Wolters Kluwer; 2015. Available at http://www.uptodate.com/contents/cytomegalovirus-infection-in-renal-transplant-recipients. Accessed September 7, 2015.

22. Fishman J. Infection in the solid organ transplant. In: Marr K, ed. *Up to Date.* Waltham, MA: Wolters Kluwer; 2015. Available at http://www.uptodate.com/contents/infection-in-the-solid-organ-transplant-recipient#H5. Accessed August 1, 2015.

23. Vallet-Pichard A, Fontaine H, Mallet V, et al. Viral hepatitis in solid organ transplantation other than liver. *J Hepatol.* 2011;55:474–482.

24. Levitsky J, Doucette K. Viral hepatitis in solid organ transplantation. *Am J Transplant.* 2013;13:147–168.

25. Hirsch H, Randhawa P. BK polyomavirus in solid organ transplantation. *Am J Transplant.* 2013;13:179–188.

26. Brennan D, Ramos E. Management of BK virus-induced (polyomavirus-induced) nephropathy in kidney transplantation. In: Murphy B, ed. *Up to Date.* Waltham, MA: Wolters Kluwer; 2015. Available at http://www.uptodate.com/contents/management-of-bk virus-induced-polyomavirus-induced-nephropathy-in-kidney-transplantation. Accessed August 20, 2015.

27. Manuel O, Lopez-Medrano F, Kaiser L, et al. Influenza and other respiratory virus infections in solid organ transplant recipients. *Clin Microbiol Infect.* 2014;20(suppl 7):102–108.

28. Renaud C, Campbell A. Changing epidemiology of respiratory viral infections in hematopoietic cell transplant recipients and solid organ transplant recipients. *Curr Opin Infect Dis.* 2011;24(4):333–343.

29. Clark NM, Reid GE; AST Infectious Diseases Community of Practice. Nocardia infections in solid organ transplantation. *Am J Transplant.* 2013;13:83–92.

30. Zaas A, Zaas D, Palmer S. Bacterial infections following lung transplantation. In: Trulock E, Marr K, eds. *Up to Date.* Waltham, MA: Wolters Kluwer; 2013. Available at http://www.uptrodate.com/contents/bacterial-infections-following-lung-transplantation. Accessed June 20, 2015.

31. Miller R, Assi M; AST Infectious Diseases Community of Practice. Fungal infections in solid organ transplantation. *Am J Transplant.* 2013;13:250–261.

32. Li XF, Liu ZP. Aspergillus in solid organ transplant. *Transplant Proc.* 2010;13(suppl 4):228–241.

33. Khan A, El-charobaty E, El-Sayegh S. Fungal infection in renal transplant patients. *J Clin Med Res.* 2015;7(6):371–378.

34. Kaufman CA, Freifeld AG, Andes DR, et al. Endemic fungal infections in solid organ and hematopoietic cell transplant recipients enrolled in the Transplant-Associated Infection Surveillance Network. *Transpl Infect Dis.* 2014;16(2):213–224.

35. Neofytos D, Fishman JA, Hom D, et al. Antifungal prophylaxis in solid organ transplant recipients: epidemiology and outcome. *Transpl Infect Dis.* 2010;39(suppl 4):S200–S206.

36. Choi YI, Hwana S, Park BC, et al. Clinical outcomes of Pneumocystis carinii pneumonia in adult liver transplant. *Transplant Proc.* 2013;45(8):3057–3060.

37. Iriart X, Challan Belval T, Fillaux J, et al. Risk factors of pneumocystis pneumonia in solid organ recipients in the era of the common use of posttransplantation prophylaxis. *Am J Transplant.* 2015;15(1):190–199.

38. Assi M, Martin S, Wheat LJ, et al. Histoplasmosis after solid organ transplant. *Clin Infect Dis.* 2013;57(11):1542–1549.

39. Munoz P, Verio M. Parasitic infections in solid organ transplant recipients. *Curr Opin Organ Transplant.* 2011;16(6):565–575.

40. Hernando Martinez AF, Beckham JD. Cryptococcosis in solid organ recipients. *Curr Opin Infect Dis.* 2015;28(4):300–307.

41. Mani B, Mathur M, Clauss H, et al. Strongyloides stercoralis and organ transplantation. *Case Rep Transplant.* 2013;2013:549038. doi: 10.1155/2013/549038.

42. Garfin PM. Posttransplant lymphoproliferative disorder. *Medscape.* 2015. Available at http://emedicine.medscape.com//article/431364-overview. Accessed August 26, 2015.

43. Allen UD, Preiksitis JK; AST Infectious Disease Community of Practice. Epstein-Barr and post transplant lymphoproliferative disease in solid organ transplant recipients. *Am J Transplant.* 2013;(13):107–120.

44. Chin-Hong P, Lough J, Robies J. Human papillomavirus in transplant recipients. *Infectious Disease & Antimicrobial Agents.* Available at http://www.antimicrobe.org/new/t18_dw.html. Accessed August 26, 2015.

45. Grim SA, Clark NM. Management of infectious complications in solid-organ transplant recipients. *J Clinic Pharm Ther.* 2011;90(2):333–342.

46. Garzoni C, Vergidis P; AST Infectious Disease Community of Practice. Methicillin-resistant vancomycin-intermediate and vancomycin-resistant Staphylococcus aureus infections in solid organ transplantation. *Am J Transplant.* 2013;13:50–58.

47. Sousa D, Justo I, Domingues A, et al. Community-acquired pneumonia in immunocompromised older patients: incidence, causative organisms and outcome. *Clin Microbiol Infect.* 2013;19(2):187–192.

48. Honda H, Dubberke ER. Clostridium difficile in solid organ transplant recipients. *Curr Opin Infec Dis.* 2014;37(4):336–341.

49. Angarone M, Ison MG. Diarrhea in solid organ recipients. *Curr Opin Infec Dis.* 2015;28(4):308–316.

50. Bilal M, Khehra R, Strahotin C, et al. Long-term follow-up of fecal microbiota transplantation for treatment of recurrent Clostridium difficile infection in a dual solid-organ transplant recipient. *Case Rep Gastroenterol.* 2015;9(2):156–159.

51. Patel G, Snydman DR; AST Infectious Disease Community of Practice. Vancomycin resistant *Enterococcus* infections in solid organ transplantation. *Am J Transplant.* 2013;13:59–67.

52. Van Duin D, van Delden C; AST Infectious Diseases Community of Practice. Multi-drug resistant gram-negative bacterial infections in solid organ transplantation. *Am J Transplant.* 2013;13:31–41.

53. Shohham S, Marr KA. Invasive fungal infections in solid organ transplant recipients. *Future Microbiol.* 2012;7(5):639–655.

54. Park BJ, Pappas PG, Wannemuenker M, et al. Invasive non-Aspergillus mold infections in transplant recipients—United States 2001–2006. *Emerging Infect Dis.* 2011;17(10):1855–1864.

55. Coster LO. Parasitic infections in solid organ transplant recipients. *Infect Dis Clin North Am.* 2013;27(2):395–427.

56. Visvesvara GS, Arrowood MJ, Qvarnstrom Y, et al. Concurrent parasitic infections in a renal transplant patient [letter]. *Emerg Infect Dis.* 2013;19(12):2044–2045.

57. Rubin L, Levin M, Ljungman P, et al. 2013 IDSA clinical practice guideline for vaccination in the immunocompromised host. *Clin Infect Dis.* 2014;58(3):309–318.

SELF-ASSESSMENT QUESTIONS

1. Which of the following statements regarding transplant immunizations is FALSE?
   a. Transplant candidates and recipients are at increased risk for complications due to end-organ failure and immunosuppression.
   b. It is more appropriate to immunize patients in the latter phases of diseases that lead to organ failure.
   c. It is critical to update immunizations prior to transplant to minimize risk of a suboptimal response.
   d. The ideal time frame in which to administer posttransplant vaccinations is unknown.

2. Which of the following potential organ donors would be considered as at increased risk for transmission of hepatitis, HIV, or other infectious diseases?
   a. A person who has had sex with a person who has injected drugs by IV, IM, or SQ route for nonmedical reasons in the preceding 12 months
   b. A person who has been in jail or prison for more than 72 hours in the preceding 12 months
   c. A person who has been diagnosed with or has been treated for syphilis, gonorrhea, *Chlamydia*, or genital ulcers in the preceding 12 months
   d. All of the above

3. You are caring for a 39-year-old heart transplant recipient in the intermediate/transplant step-down unit who has been admitted for assessment and treatment for possible cryptococcal meningitis. Which of the following manifestations would you expect to observe in your patient?
   a. Mental status changes
   b. Stiff neck
   c. Headache
   d. All of the above

4. Which transplant recipients are most likely to develop CMV?
   a. Recipient CMV seropositive, donor CMV seropositive
   b. Recipient CMV seropositive, donor CMV seronegative
   c. Recipient CMV seronegative, donor CMV seropositive
   d. Recipient CMV seronegative, donor CMV seronegative

5. Approximately 50% of recipients with HBV infection will have end-stage liver disease and/or hepatocellular carcinoma at 10 years posttransplant.
   a. True
   b. False

6. Which of the following statements regarding polyomaviruses (BK and JC) is TRUE?
   a. Approximately 80% of the general adult population is seropositive for the BK and JC viruses.
   b. Viruses tend to persist in the kidneys, ureters, brain, and spleen.
   c. Both (a) and (b).
   d. Neither (a) or (b).

7. Pancreas transplant recipients are particularly susceptible to candidiasis due to:
   1. underlying diabetes mellitus.
   2. indwelling urinary catheters.
   3. poor nutritional status.
   4. drainage of exocrine secretions into the bladder.
   a. 1, 2, and 3
   b. 1, 2, and 4
   c. 2, 3, and 4
   d. 1, 3, and 4

8. All of the following are risk factors for the development of multidrug-resistant gram-negative bacteria in transplant recipients EXCEPT:
   a. shortened hospital length of stays.
   b. surgery.
   c. antibiotic therapy.
   d. intensive care unit admissions.

9. The most common portal of entry for fungal infection in a transplant recipient is:
   a. gastrointestinal tract.
   b. skin.
   c. donor transmission.
   d. respiratory tract.

10. A 40-year-old female presents to the ED approximately 8 weeks status post kidney transplantation with complaints of severe pain at the surgical graft site. On admission, her temperature is 102.6°F (39.2°C), white blood cell count is 15,000/μL, and urinary sediment is present. She denies urinary frequency, urgency, or dysuria. Which of the following are suspected diagnoses for this patient?
    1. Acute cellular rejection
    2. Acute pyelonephritis
    3. Urinary tract infection
    4. Humoral rejection
    a. 1 and 2 only
    b. 2 and 3 only
    c. 1 and 3 only
    d. 2 and 4 only

11. You are caring for a liver transplant recipient on the intermediate (step-down) care unit on postoperative day 10. Your patient has had a complicated postoperative course. Your patient was colonized with vancomycin-resistant *Enterococcus* (VRE) prior to transplant. There are two other patients on the unit who are colonized with VRE. Which of the following statements is LEAST accurate?
    a. You should not be assigned to take care of one of the other VRE-colonized patients.
    b. You should observe the abdominal incision for signs of infection.
    c. Your patient may not develop a fever in response to an infection.
    d. Because he was colonized with VRE prior to transplantation, your patient is less likely to develop a VRE infection.

12. The major protozoal pathogens affecting transplant recipients are:
    a. CMV and *Enterococcus.*
    b. *Toxoplasma gondii* and *Cryptosporidium parvum.*
    c. *Histoplasma* and *Pseudomonas.*
    d. *Legionella* and *Nocardia.*

Correct Answers:
1.b   2.d   3.d   4.c   5.a   6.c   7.b   8.a   9.d   10.b   11.d   12.b

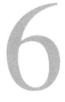

C H A P T E R

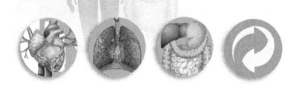

Transplant Complications: Noninfectious Diseases

Vicki McCalmont, RN, MS, ANP-BC, CNS, CCTC

Kristi Ortiz, RN, MS, ANP-BC, CNS

 ## I. INTRODUCTION

A. Several factors have increased short- and long-term transplant survival rates:

1. The development of potent immunosuppression regimens that have reduced graft loss and death from acute rejection
2. Individualized immunosuppressive therapies
3. Earlier detection and treatment of infection

B. Survival rates are also influenced by the emergence of long-term medical complications posttransplant.

C. This chapter will provide an overview of the following major (noninfectious, nonrejection) long-term complications following transplantation:

1. Cardiovascular disease
2. Renal insufficiency (RI)
3. Hyperlipidemia
4. Metabolic syndrome
5. Diabetes mellitus (DM)
6. Obesity
7. Malignancy
8. Bone disease
9. Gastrointestinal (GI) dysfunction
10. Gout
11. Gingival hyperplasia
12. Sexual dysfunction
13. Neurocognitive impairment

D. Monitoring of recipients for posttransplant complications:
   1. While each transplant organ group may have unique posttransplant complications, the amount of evidence for posttransplant complications is highest in the renal transplantation population.
   2. The American Society for Transplantation (AST) has developed guidelines for routine surveillance of kidney transplant recipients in the outpatient setting.[1]
      a. These detection and prevention guidelines, which include specific recommendations, strength of evidence, and pertinent reviews of the scientific literature, are designed to be used as a reference by health care professionals.
      b. Given the similarities across organ transplant groups, many of the AST renal transplant guidelines are applicable to other types of solid organ transplant recipients.

 II. CARDIOVASCULAR DISEASE (CVD)

A. For the purposes of this discussion, CVD refers to a wide range of vascular and heart-related diseases, disorders, and events that include
   1. Hypertension (HTN)
   2. Arteriosclerosis
   3. Atherosclerosis
   4. Coronary artery disease (CAD)
   5. Myocardial infarction (MI)
   6. Congestive heart failure (CHF)
   7. Peripheral vascular disease (PVD)
   8. Cerebral vascular disease
   9. Stroke

B. A discussion of each of these CVDs is beyond the scope of this chapter. Given, however, that HTN is the most common disorder across all organ types, it will be discussed in detail below.

C. Cardiovascular complications have been emerging as the major cause of late morbidity and mortality in all solid organ transplant groups.[2]
   1. For example, from 2007 to 2011, CVD was the leading cause of death in renal transplant recipients and accounted for 31% of all deaths.[3]
   2. Approximately 40% of renal transplant recipients have a cardiovascular event within the first 3 years posttransplant.[4]

D. There is some evidence that mortality rates due to CVD in transplant recipients are greater than in the general population; for example:
   1. The annual risk of a fatal or nonfatal CVD event is 3.5% to 5% in kidney transplant recipients; this is 50-fold higher than the general population.[5]

E. Risk factors for CVD
   1. Transplant recipients may have CVD risk factors that are common to the general population as well as risk factors that are unique to transplantation.
   2. Risk factors common to the general population[5,6]:
      a. Male gender
      b. Older age
      c. Family history of premature CVD

        d. Elevated serum lipid concentrations

        e. Obesity

        f. Diet high in fat and cholesterol content

        g. Sedentary lifestyle

        h. Cigarette smoking

        i. Excessive alcohol consumption

        j. Prothrombic factors

        k. Left ventricular hypertrophy

3. Transplant-specific risk factors:

        a. Maintenance immunosuppressive therapy—particularly calcineurin inhibitors (CNI), mammalian target of rapamycin (mTOR) inhibitors, and corticosteroids.[7]

        b. Treatment of acute rejection episodes requiring increased dosing of immunosuppression.

        c. Chronic rejection.

        d. CKD with or without proteinuria.

        e. Anemia.

        f. Please refer to organ-specific chapters for additional information on risk factors.

F. Given the prevalence of CVD in the transplant population, pre- and posttransplant screening for CVD is imperative. Examples of screening tools include the following:

1. Framingham Heart Study Risk Assessment Tool: estimates 10-year risk of myocardial infarction or coronary death in adults who do not have heart disease or diabetes[8] (available at http://cvdrisk.nhlbi.nih.gov/calculator.asp)

2. German Prospective Cardiovascular Munster (PROCAM) study score: considers sex, age, low-density lipoprotein (LDL) cholesterol, high-density lipoprotein (HDL) cholesterol, triglycerides, systolic blood pressure (BP), smoking, diabetes mellitus (DM), and family history[9] (PROCAM is available at http://www.chd-taskforce.com/coronary_risk_assessment.html)

3. Systematic Coronary Risk Evaluation Project (SCORE) risk chart: estimates 10-year risk of fatal CVD; considers age, gender, smoking status, systolic blood pressure, and total cholesterol.[10]

G. Risk factors for coronary heart disease (CHD)[11,12]:

1. Nonmodifiable risk factors:

        a. Age:

           i. Males: ≥45 years

           ii. Females: ≥55 years

        b. Male gender

        c. Family history of premature CHD:

           i. MI or sudden death before age 55 in father or other male first-degree relative

           ii. MI or sudden death before age 65 in mother or other female first-degree relative

2. Modifiable risk factors:

        a. Hypertension

        b. Elevated LDL cholesterol

        c. Cigarette smoking

        d. Thrombogenic/hemostatic state

        e. DM

   f. Obesity

   g. Sedentary lifestyle

   h. Atherogenic diet

  3. Negative (protective) risk factor: HDL cholesterol >60 mg/dL (>1.5 mmol/L)

  4. Emerging risk factors:

   a. Lipid risk factors:

    i. Triglycerides

    ii. Lipoprotein remnants

    iii. Elevated lipoprotein(a)

    iv. Small LDL particles

    v. HDL subspecies

    vi. Apolipoprotein B

    vii. Total cholesterol/HDL cholesterol ratio

   b. Nonlipid risk factors:

    i. Elevated homocysteine level

    ii. Thrombogenic/hemostatic factors

    iii. Inflammatory markers (e.g., elevated high-sensitivity C-reactive protein)

    iv. Homocysteine (if elevated, may indicate a lack of folic acid, vitamin B_6, and vitamin B_{12}).

    v. Prothrombotic factors (fibrinogen)

    vi. Subclinical atherosclerotic disease

    vii. Impaired fasting glucose (110 to 125 mg/dL) (2.85 to 3.24 mmol/L)

 H. Guidelines for primary and secondary prevention of cardiovascular disease and stroke are shown in Table 6-1.[12]

TABLE 6-1 Guidelines for Primary and Secondary Prevention of Cardiovascular Disease and Stroke

Parameter	Goals		
	Primary Prevention		**Secondary Prevention**
Smoking	Cessation of smoking		Cessation of smoking
	No exposure to environmental smoke or secondhand smoke		No exposure to environmental smoke or secondhand smoke
	Avoid smokeless tobacco		Avoid smokeless tobacco
Blood pressure control	<140/90 mm Hg		<140/90 mm Hg
Diet	Heart-healthy diet		Heart-healthy diet
	Optimize weight—reduce calories		Optimize weight—reduce calories
	if overweight		if overweight
	Saturated fat <10% of total calories		Saturated fat: <7% of total calories
	Cholesterol <300 mg/d		Cholesterol: <200 mg/d
	Salt intake <6 g/d		Limit *trans*-fatty acids
	Limit *trans*-fatty acids (<5% total calories)		
	Limit alcohol intake		

(continued)

TABLE 6-1 Guidelines for Primary and Secondary Prevention of Cardiovascular Disease and Stroke (Continued)

Parameter	Goals		
	Primary Prevention		**Secondary Prevention**
Lipid management *Primary goals: (risk factors*: HTN, smoking, HDL<40, family Hx of premature) CHD (CHD in male first degree relatives <55, men ≥45; women ≥55)	≤1 risk factor: ≥2 risk factors + 10 y risk <20%: ≥2 risk factors + 10 y risk ≥20% or in setting of DM, CHD	LDL <160 mg/dL LDL <130 mg/dL LDL <100 mg/dL	LDL <100 mg/dL or <70 mg/dL
Secondary goals if LDL is at target goal and triglycerides are >200 mg/dL (2.26 mmol/L)	≤1 risk factor ≥2 risk factors + 10 y risk ≤ 20% ≥2 risk factors + 10 y risk ≥20%	Non-HDL <190 mg/dL Non-HDL <160 mg/dL Non-HDL <130 mg/dL	
Triglycerides (Tg)	<150 mg/dL—normal 150–199 mg/dL—borderline high 200–499—high >500—very high (risk for pancreatitis if untreated)	For triglycerides ≥200 mg/dL), non-HDL should be <130 mg/dL *Non-HDL = total cholesterol minus HDL* For triglycerides 200–499 mg/dL ; non-HDL based on risk factors All abnormal Tg need diet, exercise and weight control + meds >200	
HDL	Men: >40 mg/dL Women: >50 mg/dL	Men: >40 mg/dL Women: >50 mg/dL	
Physical activity	30 min of moderately intense exercise on most, if not all, days of the week	30 min 7 d/wk, minimum: 5 d/wk	

Weight	Optimize weight
	BMI: 18.5–24.9 kg/m²
	Waist circumference:
	  Men: <40 inches
	  Women: <35 inches
	Waist-to-hip ratio:
	  Men >9.0
	  Women >8.5
	Overweight/obese patients: 10% ↓ in weight during first year of therapy
		BMI: 18.5–24.9 kg/m²
		Waist circumference:
		  Men: <40 inches
		  Women: <35 inches
		Waist-to-hip ratio:
		  Men <9.0
		  Women <8.5
		Initial goal: 10% ↓ in weight from baseline	

Management of DM	Normal fasting blood glucose: <110 mg/dL HgbA$_{1c}$ <7%	HgbA$_{1c}$ <7% Preprandial BG 90–130 Postprandial BG <180 Bedtime glucose 100–140	
Anticoagulation/ antiplatelet therapy	In setting of chronic AF: anticoagulation with warfarin to goal INR between 2.0 and 3.0 (target: 2.5)	INR 2.0–3.0 for patients with AF or flutter and as indicated in MI patients Aspirin and/or clopidogrel as indicated Newer anticoagulants: rivaroxaban (Xareltro); dabigatran (Pradaxa) will increase cyclosporine drug levels, dose needs adjusted and follow levels; no INR monitoring is needed for the newer drugs.	

TABLE 6-1 Guidelines for Primary and Secondary Prevention of Cardiovascular Disease and Stroke (*Continued*)

Parameter	Goals		Secondary Prevention
	Primary Prevention		
RAA system blockers (unless otherwise contraindicated)		ACEI	Indefinitely in setting of: EF ≤ 40% Hypertension DM Chronic kidney disease Consider in other settings
		ARBs	In setting of ACEI intolerance and HF or MI with EF ≤ 40%
		Aldosterone blockade	In combination with therapeutic ACEI and β-blocker doses for status post-MI patients with potassium level <5.0 mEq/L and creatinine <2.5 mg/dL (men) or <2.0 mg/dL (women) and with EF ≤40% and DM or HF
β-Blocker therapy (unless otherwise contraindicated)		Indefinitely in patients with MI, ACS, or LV dysfunction with or without HF symptoms Consider for other patients in setting of CHD, DM, or vascular disease	In combination with therapeutic ACEI and β-blocker doses for status post-MI patients with potassium level <5.0 mEq/L and creatinine <2.5 mg/dL (men) or <2.0 mg/dL (women) and with EF ≤ 40% and DM or HF
Influenza vaccine			Recommended for all patients with CVD unless otherwise contraindicated Recommended for all transplant patients unless otherwise contraindicated

ACEI, angiotensin-converting enzyme inhibitors; ACS, acute coronary syndrome; AF, atrial fibrillation; ARB, angiotensin receptor blocker; BMI, body mass index; CHD, coronary heart disease; CVD, cardiovascular disease; DM, diabetes mellitus; HDL, high-density lipoprotein; HF, heart failure; HgbA$_{1c}$, hemoglobin A$_{1c}$; Hx, history; INR, international normalized ratio; LDL, low-density lipoprotein; LV, left ventricular; MI, myocardial infarction; NSR, normal sinus rhythm; RAA, renin-angiotensin-aldosterone; RI, renal insufficiency; Tg, triglycerides.
From Kelly SC, Gonzalo R, Petrasko M. A focus on cardiovascular risk modification: clinical significance and implementation of the 2013 ACC/AHA cholesterol guidelines. *S D Med.* 2014;67(8):320–323.

III. HYPERTENSION

A. Overview:
   1. Common complication of all types of solid organ transplantation
   2. May develop as early as the first few days and weeks after transplantation and increase over time or may develop later in the posttransplant course.
   3. Hypertension is the most common complication seen posttransplant (affecting >70% of transplant patients)[11] and can lead to graft loss, MI, heart failure (HF), stroke, renal failure, and death if not treated.

B. Definition of HTN in the general population:
   1. National Institutes for Health (NIH) commissioned a medical committee
      (the Joint National Committee [JNC]) to develop evidence-based consensus
      guidelines for the treatment of HTN (Table 6-2).[13]
   2. Per JNC-8 guidelines published in December 2013[13]:
      a. Hypertension is defined as repeated BP readings >140/90 mm Hg on two
         separate readings.
      b. Blood pressure goals:
         i. Adults under age 60 with no comorbidities: <150/90
         ii. Adults over age 60 with comorbidities (e.g., DM, renal disease):
             <140/90

C. There is no evidence that a BP of 130/80 improves outcomes for the
    general population.[13] Uncontrolled hypertension, however, can lead to
    graft loss, MI, HF, and stroke.

D. Definition of HTN—transplant population:
   1. To date, there is no standard definition of HTN for transplant recipients.
      The AST advocates following the 2013 NIH JNC-8 consensus guidelines for
      treatment:
      a. These guidelines are updated by the JNC every 5 to 10 years.
      b. Current target BP goals include those shown in Table 6-2.[13]

E. Etiology in transplant recipients—general:
   1. Pretransplant HTN
   2. Pretransplant renal disease
   3. Calcineurin inhibitors (CNI)[14-16]:
      a. Produce afferent arteriolar vasoconstriction through enhanced sympathetic
         nervous system activity and up-regulation of renin-angiotensin-aldosterone
         system.
      b. Cause sodium and water retention.
      c. Reduce nitric oxide (a vasodilating prostaglandin).
      d. Mediate elaboration of vasoconstrictor cytokines (e.g., adenosine, platelet-
         derived growth factor, endothelin 1).
      e. Note: Cyclosporine (Neoral, Gengraf) typically causes more HTN than
         tacrolimus (Prograf, Astagraf XL).
      f. Use caution when using CNIs in combination with other CYP3A inhibitors
         or inducers as this will alter the drug metabolism; a dose adjustment is
         strongly advised, and a trough level should be monitored to avoid an
         adverse reaction.

TABLE 6-2 **Hypertension in the General Population**

No Comorbidities		Comorbidities: DM, CKD	
Age	**BP Goal**	**Age**	**BP Goal**
Age ≥60	<150/90 mm Hg	Age ≥60	<140/90 mm Hg
Age <60	<140/90 mm Hg	Age <60	<140/90 mm Hg

DM, diabetes mellitus; CKD, chronic kidney disease.
Adapted from JNC-8 Guidelines, 2013.
From James, PA, Oparil S, Carter BL, et al. 2014 evidenced-based guidelines for the management of high blood pressure in adults:
reports from the panel members appointed to the Eighth Joint National Committee (JNC 8). *JAMA.* 2014;311(5):507–520.

     i. Drugs that are CYP pathway inhibitors (will cause an increase in transplant drug levels when used together) include, but are not limited to, the following:
- Cyclosporine (Neoral, Gengraf)
- Tacrolimus (Prograf, Astagraf XL)
- Alprazolam (Xanax)
- Quetiapine (Seroquel)
- Amlodipine (Norvasc)
- Amiodarone (Cordarone)
- Diltiazem (Cardizem)
- Atorvastatin (Lipitor)
- Hydrocortisone (Prednisone)
- Erythromycin (E-mycin)
- Fluconazole (Diflucan)
- Levofloxacin (Levaquin)
- Glyburide (Diabeta)
- Fluoxetine (Zoloft)

    ii. Drugs that are CYP pathway inducers (will cause a decrease in transplant drug levels when used together) include, but are not limited to
- Tobacco
- Rifampin (Rifadin)
- Phenytoin (Dilantin)
- Carbamazepine (Tegretol)
- Omeprazole (Prilosec)

    iii. If a patient taking tacrolimus is prescribed Diflucan for a fungal infection, the drug-drug interaction (DDI) may increase the tacrolimus level, and therefore, the tacrolimus dose may need to be decreased to avoid any drug toxicities.

    iv. If a patient is taking tacrolimus and is placed on antiseizure medications like phenytoin, the tacrolimus level will decrease, and the tacrolimus dose may need to be increased to avoid rejection.

4. Corticosteroid therapy increases sodium and water retention
5. High body mass index (BMI), chart listed in Table 6-3.[17]
6. Smoking

F. Etiology in transplant recipients: organ specific:
1. Renal transplant recipients[18,19]:
   a. HTN in donor

TABLE 6-3 **Body Mass Index Values**

BMI	Interpretation
<18.5	Underweight
18.5–24.7	Normal
25 ≤ 30	Overweight
≥30	Obesity
≥40	Extreme obesity

From American Heart Association. Body Composition Tests. Available at http://www.heart.org/HEARTORG/GettingHealthy/WeightManagement/BodyMassIndex/Body-Mass-Index-BMI-Calculator_UCM_307849_Article.jsp. Accessed March 5, 2015.

      b. Uncontrolled renin secretion from the remaining kidney
      c. Renal artery stenosis (RAS)
      d. Chronic allograft nephropathy
      e. Recurrence of intrinsic renal disease
  2. Heart transplant recipients:
      a. Abnormal regulation of sodium balance associated with cardiac denervation and renal impairment
      b. Structural changes in resistance arteries
  3. Liver transplant recipients:
      a. Cirrhosis
      b. Portopulmonary hypertension

G. Clinical signs and symptoms of HTN (note: HTN is often asymptomatic):
  1. Headache
  2. Dizziness
  3. Nosebleeds
  4. Visual disturbances

H. Treatment options[14,20]:
  1. Goals:
      a. Prevent damage to the kidneys and heart
      b. Prevent cerebral vascular events
      c. Prevent graft dysfunction or graft loss
  2. Nonpharmacologic therapy:
      a. Used alone, may be successful only if patient's systolic blood pressure (SBP) is within 10 mm Hg of target SBP
      b. Strategies:
         i. Smoking cessation
         ii. Weight reduction
         iii. Salt restriction
         iv. Fluid restriction (as indicated)
         v. Regular exercise
  3. Pharmacologic therapy:
      a. Antihypertensive agents are shown in Table 6-4[13]
      b. Substitution of another immunosuppressive agent for cyclosporine

TABLE 6-4 Antihypertensive Agents/Cardiac Medications

Medication	Advantages	Disadvantages
Specific β1-blockers (e.g., atenolol, metoprolol)	Agents of choice in patients with coronary artery disease (CAD) and good left ventricular function	↓ Cardiac output May ↓ renal blood flow Reflex tachycardia if abruptly stopped
Alpha 1-blocker + nonspecific β-blocker (e.g., labetalol, carvedilol)	May be effective for patients who need both vasodilatation and heart rate control	Bronchospasm Avoid with peripheral vascular disease Possible ↑ risk of cerebrovascular events May exacerbate cyclosporine-induced hyperkalemia ↓ Cardiac output Erectile dysfunction

TABLE 6-4 **Antihypertensive Agents/Cardiac Medications (*Continued*)**

Medication	Advantages	Disadvantages
Alpha1-blockers (e.g., terazosin)	May help in patients with benign prostatic hyperplasia; May ↑ renal blood flow	Orthostatic hypotension Syncope
Calcium channel blockers: dihydropyridines (e.g., nifedipine)	Best agents to prevent cyclosporine A–induced vasoconstriction Does not affect cardiac conduction	Edema (nonsodium retentive) Reflex tachycardia Avoid with active CAD, CHF May exacerbate cyclosporine-induced gingival hyperplasia
Calcium channel blocker: diltiazem	Can prevent cyclosporine A–induced vasoconstriction Effects cardiac conduction (less than verapamil)	↑ Cyclosporine levels ↑ Tacrolimus levels Bradycardia
Calcium channel blocker: verapamil	Can prevent cyclosporine A-induced vasoconstriction Effects cardiac conduction and negative inotrope effect	↑ Cyclosporine levels ↑ Tacrolimus levels ↓ Cardiac output Bradycardia Constipation
Angiotensin-converting enzyme inhibitors (ACEI) (e.g., enalapril)	May be best agents for patient with ↓ left ventricular function or left ventricular dilatation	Hyperkalemia ↓ Renal perfusion (stop if creatinine ↑ 30% over baseline) Dry cough Neutropenia Angioedema (lips)
Angiotensin II blockers (e.g., losartan)	May be best agents to ↓ proteinuria experimentally. May ↓ cyclosporine-mediated renal fibrosis	Deterioration in renal function (particularly in patients with renal artery stenosis) Hyperkalemia Angioedema to lips
Alpha2 agonists (e.g., clonidine)	Effective in many people ↓ Central sympathetic discharge	Drowsiness Dry mouth
Direct vasodilators (e.g., hydralazine, minoxidil)	Hydralazine often used with patients intolerant to ACEI or alpha II blockers with congestive heart failure Minoxidil effective in refractory patients	Reflex tachycardia Sodium retention Headache Lupus syndrome at high doses
Diuretics (e.g., furosemide, bumetanide)	Often necessary in volume overloaded patients	Electrolyte disorders (Na, K, Mag, Ca, Mag) Volume depletion may activate renin-angiotensin II system May exacerbate cyclosporine-induced fibrosis Contraindicated if sulfa allergy

Data from JNC-8 guidelines and Epocrates online.
From James, PA, Oparil S, Carter BL, et al. 2014 evidenced-based guidelines for the management of high blood pressure in adults: reports from the panel members appointed to the Eighth Joint National Committee (JNC 8). *JAMA.* 2014;311(5):507–520.

4. RAS[1,21,22]:
   a. Risk factors for RAS include
      i.   Procurement and operative techniques postrenal transplant (such as suturing or trauma)
      ii. Atherosclerotic disease
      iii. Cytomegalovirus (CMV) infection
      iv. Delayed graft function
   b. Administering an angiotensin-converting enzyme (ACE) inhibitor or angiotensin II receptor blocker (ARB) to the patient with RAS can lead to a rise in creatinine and reversible decline in glomerular filtration rate (GFR). This will aid in the diagnosis of RAS.
   c. Treatment options for RAS include correcting the stenosis with angioplasty, stent, or bypass surgery.

 IV. RENAL INSUFFICIENCY (RI)[21,22]

A. Overview:
   1. Scope of problem: see Table 6-5[23–26]

B. Etiology[22]:
   1. Nonrenal transplant recipients: pretransplant RI (also known as chronic kidney disease [CKD]) is associated with end-stage heart or liver disease related to low perfusion states and chronic high-dose diuretic use:
      a. The degree of chronic kidney disease is staged from one to five (Table 6-6).[27]
   2. Posttransplant nephrotoxicity may be associated with the use of
      a. CNIs (cyclosporine, tacrolimus)
      b. Antibiotics
      c. Certain nonmaintenance immunosuppressants used to treat acute rejection

TABLE 6-5 Scope of the Problem of Renal Insufficiency

Kidney[23]	Heart[24]	Lung[25]	Heart-Lung[25]	Liver[26]
According to the US Renal Data System report, renal graft failure carries a 4% annual rate	Cumulative prevalence: Abnormal Cr ≤2.5: 17%, 35%, and 40% at 1, 5, and 10 y posttransplant, respectively	Cumulative prevalence: Abnormal Cr ≤2.5: 16%, 36%, and 40% within 1, 5, and 10 y posttransplant, respectively	Cumulative prevalence Cr ≤2.5: 12% and 32% within 1 and 5 y posttransplant, respectively	Cumulative prevalence Cr ≤2.5: 22% at 5 y
	Abnormal Cr: >2.5 mg/dL: 6%, 12%, and 17% at 1, 5, and 10 y posttransplant, respectively	Abnormal Cr >2.5 mg/dL: 4%, 5%, 15%, and 20% within 1, 5, and 10 y posttransplant, respectively		

Cr, creatinine.
Messa P, Ponticelli C, Berardinelli L. Coming back to dialysis after kidney transplant failure. *Nephrol Dial Transplant.* 2008;23(9):2738–2742; Lund LH, Edwards LB, Kucheryavaya AY, et al. The registry of the International Society for Heart and Lung Transplantation: thirty-first official adult heart transplant report—2014. *J Heart Lung Transplant.* 2014;33(10):996–1008; International Society for Heart and Lung Transplantation. *The Registry Of The International Society For Heart And Lung Transplantation: Thirty-First Adult Lung And Heart-Lung Transplant Report.* Available at http://www.ishlt.org/registries/slides. asp?slides=heartLungRegistry. Accessed August 8, 2015; Weber ML, Ibrahim HN, Lake JR. Renal dysfunction in liver transplant recipients: evaluation of the critical issues. *Liver Transpl.* 2012;18:1290–1301.

TABLE 6-6 **Definition and Stages of Chronic Kidney Disease**

GFR	Stages of Chronic Kidney Disease	
	Stage	**Description**
>90	1	Normal with ↑ GFR
60–89	2	Mild kidney disease
30–59	3	Moderate kidney disease
15–29	4	Severe kidney disease
<15	5	End-stage renal failure/dialysis

The number represents the stage of kidney disease. Kidney disease is defined as pathologic abnormalities found in tissues, blood, or imaging tests.
Adapted from The National Kidney Foundation. *Kidney Disease Improving Global Outcomes Clinical Practice Guidelines For Chronic Kidney Disease: Evaluation, Classification And Stratification. Part 4: Definition And Classification Of Chronic Kidney Disease. Guideline 1: Definition And Stages Of Chronic Kidney Disease.* Available at http://www2.kidney.org/professionals/KDOQI/guidelines_ckd/p4_class_g1.htm

    C. Risk factors for RI/CKD[28]:
       1. Pretransplant RI/CKD:
          a. Preexisting renal dysfunction
          b. DM
          c. HTN
          d. Older age
          e. Generalized atherosclerosis
       2. Perioperative events:
          a. Hypotension
          b. Use of pressor agents
          c. Sepsis
          d. CMV infection
       3. HTN
       4. Hyperlipidemia
       5. Proteinuria

    D. Posttransplant RI/CKD:
       1. Types of cyclosporine-induced injury:
          a. Acute[29]:
             i. Severe, rapid, and intense vasoconstriction of preglomerular (afferent) arterioles leads to decrease in renal blood flow and GFR; this vasoconstriction is presumably mediated by an increase in sympathetic tone and is activated by the renin-angiotensin system, thereby decreasing production of vasodilator molecules resulting in vasoconstriction.
            ii. Effects are dose related and are often reversed with withdrawal of cyclosporine.
          b. Chronic[29]:
             i. Characterized by structural changes in renal architecture, which cause sustained functional nephrotoxicity and induce:
               • Glomerular ischemia
               • Tubular atrophy
               • Tubulointerstitial fibrosis
               • Glomerulosclerosis
          c. Injury worsens over time and results in permanent renal dysfunction.

E. Assessment[30,31]:

1. Potential clinical manifestations:
   a. Elevated serum creatinine >2 mg/dL:
      i. Calcium channel blockers (CCB) have been used to reduce cyclosporine-induced nephrotoxicity by reducing afferent arteriolar tone. Administering a CCB with cyclosporine may reduce the accumulation of cyclosporine within the renal tubule cells.
      ii. Renal-sparing protocols involve substituting sirolimus for the calcineurin inhibitor.
   b. Decreased creatinine clearance/GFR
   c. Proteinuria
   d. Increased serum potassium level
   e. Increased serum uric acid level
   f. Decreased sodium excretion
   g. HTN
   h. Fluid retention
   i. Anemia
   j. Hypomagnesemia:
      i. Common after transplant due to calcineurin-induced down-regulation of renal expression of magnesium channel TRPM6.
      ii. Signs and symptoms include weakness, muscle spasms, nausea, vomiting, diarrhea, and cardiac arrhythmias.
2. Monitor trough levels of cyclosporine (Sandimmune, Neoral, Gengraf) or tacrolimus (Prograf, Astagraf XL).
   a. Nephrotoxicity typically occurs with high trough levels but may occur at low trough levels.[29]
3. Assess patient's volume status to determine if dehydration is contributing to RI.
4. Review patient's medication profile to identify other medications that may be contributing to nephrotoxicity, such as:
   a. Antibiotics
   b. Antihypertensive medications
   c. Diuretics
   d. Nonsteroidal anti-inflammatory drugs (NSAIDs)

F. Interventions:

1. Target patients who have a significant increase in serum creatinine during the first 6 months posttransplant[28]
2. Immunosuppression management:
   a. If possible, reduce dose of CNI: cyclosporine or tacrolimus.
   b. Consider changing patient's CNI from cyclosporine to tacrolimus.
3. BP control:
   a. Diastolic HTN has been linked to severe RI.
   b. Antihypertensive agents (see Table 6-4).[13]
   c. Screen for secondary causes: sleep apnea, primary aldosteronism, and RAS.
4. Aggressive treatment of hyperlipidemia

 V. HYPERLIPIDEMIA

A. Overview[32]:

1. Hyperlipidemia is a significant posttransplant problem (Table 6-7).[24,25,33-35]
   a. The terms "hyperlipidemia" and "dyslipidemia" are used interchangeably. This disease process involves abnormally elevated levels of any or all lipid proteins.

TABLE 6-7 **Hyperlipidemia**

Type of Transplant	Scope of Problem
Kidney	Hyperlipidemia and hypertriglyceridemia have been reported in 50%–90% of kidney transplant recipients.[33,35]
Heart	Cumulative prevalence in survivors at 1 and 5 posttransplant: 60%, 88%, respectively[24]
	Total cholesterol, LDL, apolipoprotein B, and triglyceride levels may increase during the first 3 mo posttransplant
Lung	Cumulative prevalence in survivors during first posttransplant year: 27% cumulative prevalence in survivors within five posttransplant: 59%[25]
Heart-lung	Cumulative prevalence in survivors within 1 and 5 y: 26.7% and 70%, respectively (per ISHLT 2014 database)[25]
Liver	May affect up to 45% of recipients[34]

From Lund LH, Edwards LB, Kucheryavaya AY, et al. The registry of the International Society for Heart and Lung Transplantation: thirty-first official adult heart transplant report—2014. *J Heart Lung Transplant.* 2014;33(10):996–1008; International Society for Heart and Lung Transplantation. *The Registry Of The International Society For Heart And Lung Transplantation: Thirty-First Adult Lung And Heart-Lung Transplant Report.* Available at http://www.ishlt.org/registries/slides.asp?slides=heartLungRegistry. Accessed August 8, 2015; Razeghi E, Shafipour M, Ashraf H, et al. Lipid disturbances before and after renal transplant. *Exp Clin Transplant.* 2011;9(4):230–235; Charlton M. Obesity, hyperlipidemia and metabolic syndrome. *Liver Transpl.* 2009;15(suppl 2):S83–S89; Gosmanova EO, Tangpricha V, Gosmanov AR. Endocrine-metabolic pathophysiologic conditions and treatment approaches after kidney transplantation. *Endocr Pract.* 2012;18(4):579–589.

    b. Hypercholesterolemia is referencing cholesterol levels that are higher than normal.

    c. Hypertriglyceridemia is referencing triglyceride levels that are higher than normal.

  2. Hyperlipidemia in the transplant patient may be related to high fat diets, genetic predisposition and immunosuppressive medications.

B. Etiology: risk factors associated with hypercholesterolemia:

  1. History of pretransplant hyperlipidemia and/or obesity

  2. Genetic factors

  3. Male gender

  4. Older age

  5. Posttransplant medications[36]:

    a. Immunosuppressive agents:

      i. Cyclosporine: decreases bile acid synthesis from cholesterol, thus increasing serum cholesterol, LDL cholesterol levels and triglyceride levels.

      ii. Corticosteroids can cause hyperlipidemia. They increase in LDL, total cholesterol, and triglycerides and a decrease in HDL levels by:

- Increasing acetyl coenzyme A (CoA) carboxylase activity and free fatty acid synthesis.
- Increasing hepatic synthesis of very-low-density lipoproteins.
- Increasing the 3-hydroxy-3-methyglutaryl coenzyme A (HMG-CoA) reductase enzyme that is used for "statin therapy." *Of note, statins are used to inhibit this enzyme and normalize the lipid profile.*
  - There is a risk for myopathy or rhabdomyolysis when both cyclosporine (Neoral, Gengraf) and pravastatin (Pravachol) are taken concurrently. Tacrolimus (Prograf) and sirolimus (Rapamune) are not metabolized the same as cyclosporine and do not carry a drug-drug interaction risk for rhabdomyolysis.
  - Any patient taking a "statin" medication is at risk for myopathy.
- Inhibiting LDL.

    iii. Tacrolimus is similar to cyclosporine but has less pronounced effects on lipid metabolism.

    iv. Mammalian target of rapamycin (mTOR) inhibitors (everolimus [Zortress] and sirolimus [Rapamune]) are used as potent immunosuppressive agents in solid organ transplant recipients.

        • mTOR inhibitors reduce the catabolism of circulating lipoproteins by inhibiting the activity of lipases, resulting in an increased prevalence of dyslipidemia up to 75% of patients.

        • The risk/benefit ratio should be carefully considered before starting an mTOR inhibitor in patients with preexisting hyperlipidemia.[18]

        • Everolimus (Zortress) carries a 21% to 24% increase in hyperlipidemia.

        • Sirolimus (Rapamune) carries a 30% to 64% increase in hyperlipidemia.

  b. Antihypertensive agents:

    i. Beta-blockers (atenolol [Tenormin]) and diuretics (hydrochlorothiazide [HCTZ]) can elevate LDL and triglycerides.

  c. Effect of posttransplant medications on lipoproteins (Table 6-8)[35]

6. Comorbid conditions:

  a. DM: associated with hypertriglyceridemia and hypercholesterolemia

  b. Proteinuria: associated with elevated LDL and lipoprotein A

  c. Renal dysfunction

  d. Obesity[37]:

    i. Causes excessive production of very-low-density lipoprotein (VLDL) particles

    ii. Increases triglyceride levels

    iii. Increases LDL levels

    iv. Decreases HDL levels

7. Diet high in saturated fat and/or cholesterol

C. Major consequences of posttransplant hyperlipidemia[38]:

1. CVD

2. Chronic cardiac allograft vasculopathy (CAV)[39]

D. Screening for posttransplant hyperlipidemia[40]:

1. Fasting (8 to –12 hours) total cholesterol, LDL, HDL, and triglyceride levels at least twice during the first posttransplant year.

2. Use of fasting lipids may change in the future as the American College of Cardiology (ACC) and American Heart Association (AHA) have recommended moving away from lowering LDL-C to specific target levels and treating with moderate to high-intensity statins in patients with atherosclerotic heart disease. This intensity will reduce LDL-C by 40% to 50% and can be assessed using nonfasting blood samples.[41]

TABLE 6-8 Relative Risk of Adverse Effects of Immunosuppressants Agents on Lipid Metabolism

Cyclosporine	Tacrolimus	Mycophenolate Mofetil	Sirolimus	Everolimus	Corticosteroids	Azathioprine
↑↑	↔	↔	↑↑	↑↑	↑↑	Unknown

↑↑, substantially increased; ↔, unchanged.
Adapted from Gosmanova EO, Tangpricha V, Gosmanov AR. Endocrine-metabolic pathophysiologic conditions and treatment approaches after kidney transplantation. *Endocr Pract.* 2012;18(4):579–589.

a. More frequent screening for recipients with history of pretransplant hyperlipidemia and those at high risk for hyperlipidemia (e.g., patients on rapamycin [Sirolimus]).

b. Using data from the National Health and Nutrition Survey III (NHANES III) elevated LDL or non-HDL levels were linked to higher risk of death.[41]

3. Regular screening throughout the posttransplant course, particularly for recipients with risk factors for CVD.

4. Download the 2013 Prevention Guidelines Tools: Cardiovascular Risk Calculator: http://my.americanheart.org/cvriskcalculator:

   a. This risk calculator estimates 10-year and lifetime risks for atherosclerotic cardiovascular disease (ASCVD) events based upon age, sex, race, total cholesterol, HDL cholesterol, SBP, any BP-lowering medications, DM, and smoking status.

   b. Presence or absence of CHD or other forms of ASCVD:
      i. Acute coronary syndrome
      ii. Prior history of MI
      iii. Stable or unstable angina
      iv. Coronary or other arterial revascularization procedure
      v. Transient ischemic attack (TIA) or stroke
      vi. Peripheral arterial disease

   c. The underlying causes and secondary risks for ASCVD (Table 6-9)[40]:
      i. Very high LDL cholesterol ≥190 mg/dL (≥4.92 mmol/L)
      ii. Age 40 to 75 with DM + LDL 70 to 189
      iii. LDL 70 to 189 + 10-year risk of ASVD >7.5% (use risk calculator above in section IV-C)

TABLE 6-9 **Risk Category for Atherosclerotic Cardiovascular Disease and Therapy**

Risk Category	Type of Dyslipidemia	Goal	Treatment
HIGH Low-density lipoprotein (LDL)	Very high LDL cholesterol ≥190 mg/dL (≥4.92 mmol/L) Age 40–75 with DM + LDL 70–189 LDL 70–189 + 10-y risk of ASCVD >7.5%	First line: high-intensity dose statin to achieve LDL reduction 50% or more	Atorvastatin 40–80 mg daily Rosuvastatin 20–40 mg daily
MODERATE LDL	LDL 70–189 with 10-y risk of 5%–7.5% LDL >160 + genetic risks (CV disease in first-degree male < age 55)	Moderate-dose intensity statin (average LDL reduction about 30% to <50%):	Atorvastatin 10–20 mg daily. Fluvastatin 80 mg (XL) daily Lovastatin 40 mg daily. Pitavastatin 2–4 mg daily Pravastatin 40–80 mg daily. Rosuvastatin 5–10 mg daily
PREVENTION/LOW LDL		Daily dose lowers low-density lipoprotein-cholesterol (LDL-C) on average, by <30%	Simvastatin 10 mg Pravastatin 10–20 mg Lovastatin 20 mg Fluvastatin 20–40
	NONSTATINS	Encourage statin use, lifestyle modification	Do not add Gemfibrozil (Lopid) to any statin

(continued)

TABLE 6-9 **Risk Category for Atherosclerotic Cardiovascular Disease and Therapy (*Continued*)**

Risk Category	Type of Dyslipidemia	Goal	Treatment
ELEVATED TRIGLYCERIDES (Tg)	Elevated serum triglycerides: Normal: <150 mg/dL Borderline-high: 150–199 mg/dL High: 200–499 mg/dL Very high: ≥500 mg/dL SI units: Normal: <1.69 mmol/L Borderline high: 1.69–2.24 mmol/L High: 2.26–5.63 mmol/L Very high: ≥5.65 mmol/L	Borderline-high: • Weight reduction • ↑ physical activity • Drug therapy for high Tg Contributing factors: Overweight Obesity Physical inactivity Smoking Excess alcohol intake High carbohydrate diet Certain disease states (e.g., type 2 DM) Certain drugs (e.g., corticosteroids) Genetic disorders	High: • Intensify therapy to lower LDL or • Add nicotinic acid or fibrate Very high: • Prevent acute pancreatitis with very low-fat diet (≤15% of total intake), weight reduction, ↑ physical activity, and omega-3 fatty acids, fibrate or nicotinic acid • No evidence that adding a nonstatin to a statin will ↓ CV risk
High-density lipoprotein (HDL)	Low HDL cholesterol: <40 mg/dL (<1.03 mmol/L)	Achieve target LDL goal: Strong predictor of coronary heart disease Physical inactivity Type 2 DM/insulin resistance Smoking High carbohydrate intake Certain drugs (e.g., beta-blockers)	When LDL goal is reached: Weight reduction Physical activity Isolated low HDL: Nicotinic acid Fibrates

New lipid guidelines focus on reducing CV risk using the 10-year risk calculator http://my.americanheart.org/cvriskcalculator.
Dyslipidemia is a risk factor for ASCVD. First recommendation is lifestyle modification (diet and exercise). If unsuccessful, then drug therapy. Current guidelines do not recommend titrating statins to an LDL number, they titrate to lower LDL by a set percentage. Drugs are selected to achieve high intensity, moderate intensity, or prevention in the low-risk group for ASCVD events.
Patients at *risk* for atherosclerotic cardiovascular disease (ASCVD) include primary LDL-C >160 mg/dL or evidence of genetic hyperlipidemias, family history of premature ASCVD with onset <55 years in a first-degree male relative or <65 years in a first-degree female relative, and high sensitivity C-reactive protein >2 mg/L.
Patients with **clinical** ASCVD (defined as acute coronary syndromes; prior MI, stable or unstable angina, coronary revascularization, stroke, or TIA believed to be of atherosclerotic origin, and peripheral arterial disease or past revascularization) are at increased risk for recurrent ASCVD and death. These patients should take high-intensity statin therapy to ↓ risk for future ASCVD events and/or death.
DM, diabetes mellitus; MI, myocardial infarction; CV, cardiovascular.
From Stone NJ, Robinson J, Lichtenstein AH, et al. 2013 ACC/AHA guideline on the treatment of blood cholesterol to reduce atherosclerotic cardiovascular risk in adults. A report of the American College of Cardiology/American Heart Association Task Force on Practice Guidelines. *Circulation*. 2013;129(25 suppl 2):S1–S45.

    d. Once risks have been assessed, the patient's risk category is determined and therapy is individualized (Table 6-10).[40]

        i. The CV Risk Calculator (Section IV-C) can be used for all transplant recipients.

        ii. If the 10-year risk calculator score exceeds 7.5, follow treatment guidelines per the ACC/AHA recommendations to reduce ASCVD risks.

E. Treatment: given the multifactorial etiology of hyperlipidemia, a multifaceted and individualized treatment strategy is imperative.[42]

    1. Similar to treatment of hyperlipidemia in the general population

TABLE 6-10 Secondary Causes of Dyslipidemia

Secondary Cause	Elevated LDL-C	Elevated Triglycerides
Diet	Saturated or *trans* fats Weight gain Anorexia	Weight gain, very low-fat diets, ↑intake of refined carbohydrates, excessive alcohol intake
Drugs	Diuretics, cyclosporine, glucocorticoids, amiodarone	Sirolimus, beta-blockers (not carvedilol), thiazide diuretics, steroids (glucocorticoid or anabolic), estrogens, raloxifene, tamoxifen. bile acid sequestrants, protease inhibitors, retinoic acid
Diseases	Transplant (d/t meds and organ function), biliary obstruction, nephrotic syndrome	Transplant (d/t meds and organ function). Nephrotic syndrome, chronic renal failure, lipodystrophies, diabetes
Disorders and altered states of metabolism	Hypothyroidism, obesity, pregnancy	Disorders and altered states of metabolism Diabetes (poorly controlled), hypothyroid, obesity, pregnancy

Adapted from Stone NJ, Robinson J, Lichtenstein AH, et al. 2013 ACC/AHA guideline on the treatment of blood cholesterol to reduce atherosclerotic cardiovascular risk in adults. A report of the American College of Cardiology/American Heart Association Task Force on Practice Guidelines. *Circulation.* 2013;129(25 suppl 2):S1–S45 (2013 ACC/AHA Blood Cholesterol Guideline).

2. Nonpharmacologic interventions:
   a. Optimization of weight
   b. Exercise
   c. Smoking cessation
   d. Diet low in saturated fat and cholesterol
3. Pharmacologic interventions:
   a. Indications for drug therapy vary among transplant populations and transplant centers.
      i. Some heart transplant centers prescribe HMG-CoA reductase inhibitors, also known as statins, for all recipients, even those with normal cholesterol profiles.
         * There is evidence that pravastatin (Pravachol), in addition to lowering cholesterol levels in heart transplant recipients, may have additional beneficial effects.
         * For example, Kobashigawa and colleagues demonstrated that pravastatin also decreased the incidence of rejection associated with hemodynamic compromise, increased 1-year survival, and decreased the development of CAV.[42]
      ii. Heart transplant recipients: ISHLT guidelines for adults[43]:
         * Begin statins 1 to 2 weeks following heart transplantation (regardless of cholesterol levels).
         * Initial dose should be lower than typical dose due the potential drug-drug interactions between statins and cyclosporine for myopathy and rhabdomyolysis.
4. In patients with high risk for ASCVD, new guidelines were developed in 2013. The ACC and AHA convened an expert panel to formulate evidence-based medical practice guidelines.[40]
   a. This group discontinued the use of LDL targets and recommended appropriate statin intensity (based on risk) to reduce risk of ASCVD complications in patients most likely to benefit.

      i. The four high-risk groups that could benefit from statin therapy are
- Patients with known ASCVD
- Patients with LDL-C ≥190 mg/dL (4.9 mmol/L)
- Patients age 40 to 75 with DM
- Patients age 40 to 75 with ≥7.5% risk of developing ASCVD in the next 10 years using the Global Risk Assessment for Primary Prevention: http://my.americanheart.org/professional/StatementsGuidelines/PreventionGuidelines/Prevention-Guidelines_UCM_457698_SubHomePage.jsp

  b. Moderate to high intensity statins are recommended in patients with atherosclerotic heart disease. This intensity will reduce LDL-C by 40% to 50%.

  c. The use of nonstatins was not advised, unless the patient had a statin allergy. Nonstatin therapy did not significantly lower the ASVCD risk upon review.

  d. The 2013 ACC/AHA Cholesterol Guidelines can be accessed online: http://circ.ahajournals.org/content/early/2013/11/11/01.cir.0000437738.63853.7a.full.pdf

5. Drugs that affect lipid metabolism (Table 6-11).[40,44]

6. Drug interactions:

  a. Interactions may occur between cyclosporine and statins such that both serum concentrations (statins and cyclosporine levels) are increased.

  b. Recommendations to follow cyclosporine levels closely and assess for toxicities.

  c. Recommendations to limit pravastatin to 20 mg/d when also receiving cyclosporine due to potential risk for increased statin serum levels and toxic side effects: myalgia, myopathy, and rhabdomyolysis.

  d. Increased serum levels of statins can lead to the development of rhabdomyolysis[45]:

      i. Rhabdomyolysis is a potentially fatal disease that is characterized by the destruction of striated muscle.

      ii. As the muscle breaks down and becomes necrotic, intracellular muscle contents leak into the circulation and extracellular fluid.

      iii. Rhabdomyolysis may be asymptomatic; however, symptoms typically include the classic triad of muscle pain, weakness, and dark urine:
- Muscle pain may be generalized or may involve specific muscle groups such as the thighs, calves, and lower back.[46]
- Symptoms may develop acutely upon initiation of statin therapy or many months or years later.

      iv. Additional risk factors associated with rhabdomyolysis include[45,47]
- Older age
- Female gender
- DM
- Concurrent renal or liver disease
- Concurrent use of fibrate-type agents[14]

      v. Instruct patients to promptly report muscle pain, weakness, or any other untoward symptoms:
- Up to 29% of patients who take statins report muscle aches, myalgias, or weakness.[46,47]
- Approximately 10% of patients have a "true statin intolerance" based upon adverse reactions assessed after taking two different statins.[47]

TABLE 6-11 Drugs that Affect Lipid Metabolism

Drug Class	Dose Range	Effect	Potential Side Effects	Contraindications	Follow-up Monitoring
HMG CoA reductase inhibitors		↓ LDL 18%–55% ↓ Triglycerides 7%–30% ↑ HDL 5%–15%	Myopathy Rhabdomyolysis ↑ liver enzymes	Absolute: Liver disease (acute or chronic)	Advise patient to reports: jaundice, abdominal pain, muscle aches
Lovastatin	20–80 mg	LDL ↓ 21%—42%		Relative: Certain medications that are metabolized through the cytochrome p450 system: Cyclosporine, macrolide antibiotics, some antifungal agents	Monitor patient for:
Pravastatin	20–40 mg	LDL ↓ 22%–37%			Muscle pain, tenderness, soreness
Simvastatin	20–80 mg	LDL ↓ 26%–47%			Onset of therapy: evaluate patient for muscle symptoms; check CK (if ↑ 3× baseline, DC)
Fluvastatin	20–80 mg	LDL ↓ 22%–35%			Subsequent visit:
Atorvastatin	10–80 mg	LDL ↓ 35%–60%			Evaluate patient for muscle symptoms
Rosuvastatin	5–40 mg	LDL ↓ 45%–63%			If patient develops muscle pain, tenderness, or soreness: check CK
					Onset of therapy: monitor ALT and AST
					Monitor ALT and AST immediately after onset of therapy, 4–12 wk after onset of therapy, and annually thereafter or as indicated
					Consider statin dose reduction if LDL <40 on two consecutive lab draws.
Bile acid sequestrants			Mainly GI:	Absolute: Dysbeta-lipoproteinemia Triglycerides >400 mg/dL (4.52 mmol/L)	Monitor patient for side effects at onset of therapy and at each follow-up visit
Cholestyramine	4–24 g	↓ LDL 15%–30%	Indigestion		May interfere with absorption of cyclosporine; check cyclosporine levels
Colestipol	5–30 g	↑ HDL 3%–5%	Bloating	Relative: Triglycerides >200 mg/dL (2.26 mmol/L)	Cyclosporine and other medications should not be taken 1 h before or 4 to 6 h after bile acid sequestrant is taken
Colesevelam	2.6–4.4 g	Triglycerides: ↑ or no change	Constipation		
			Abdominal pain		
			Flatulence		
			Nausea		
			↓ Absorption of other medications		
			Side effects may preclude long-term compliance		

(continued)

TABLE 6-11 Drugs that Affect Lipid Metabolism (Continued)

Drug Class	Dose Range	Effect	Potential Side Effects	Contraindications	Follow-up Monitoring
Nicotinic acid					
Immediate-release	1.5–3 g	↓ LDL 5%–25%	Flushing	Absolute:	Monitor patient for side effects at onset of therapy and at each follow-up visit
Extended-release	1–2 g	↓ Triglycerides 20%–50%	Itching	Chronic liver disease	FBS and uric acid:
Sustained-release	1–2 g	↑ HDL 15%–35%	Tingling	Severe gout	At onset of therapy,
			Headache	Relative:	6–8 wk later;
			Nausea	Diabetes	Annually or as indicated thereafter
			Flatulence	Hyperuricemia	AST and ALT:
			Heartburn	Peptic ulcer disease	At onset of therapy; start dose low and advance slow
			Fatigue	New onset atrial fibrillation	6–8 wk later;
			Rash		At dose of 1,500 mg;
			Hyperglycemia		6–8 wk after reaching maximum dose;
			Hyperuricemia		Annually or as indicated thereafter
			Gout		For patients on cyclosporine: may ↑ LFTs and uric acid
			Hepatotoxicity		
Fibric acid derivatives					
Gemfibrozil	600 mg BID	↓ LDL 5%–20%	Abdominal pain	Absolute:	Monitor patient for side effects at onset of therapy and at each follow-up visit
Fenobibrate	200 mg BID	↓ Triglycerides 20%–50%	Dyspepsia	Severe renal disease	Monitor PT/INR
Clofibrate	1,000 mg BID	↑ HDL 10%–20%	Headache	Severe liver disease	May potentiate effects of warfarin
			Drowsiness		Use with caution in diabetic patients: interacts with insulin and sulfonylureas
			Cholelithiasis		
			Myopathy		

ALT, alanine aminotransferase; AST, aspartate aminotransferase; CK, creatine kinase; GI, gastrointestinal; HDL, high-density lipoprotein; FBS, fasting blood glucose; HMG CoA, 3-hydroxy-3-methylglutaryl coenzyme A; LDL, low-density lipoprotein; LFT, liver function test; PT, prothrombin time; INR, international normalized ratio.

Cyclosporine, macrolide antibiotics, various antifungal agents, and other cytochrome P-450 inhibitors (fibric acid derivatives and nicotinic acid should be used with caution).

From Stone NJ, Robinson J, Lichtenstein AH, et al. 2013 ACC/AHA guideline on the treatment of blood cholesterol to reduce atherosclerotic cardiovascular risk in adults. A report of the American College of Cardiology/American Heart Association Task Force on Practice Guidelines. *Circulation.* 2013;129(25 suppl 2):S1–S45; National Cholesterol Education Program. National Cholesterol Education Program (NECP) expert panel on detection, evaluation, and treatment of high blood cholesterol in adults (Adult Treatment Panel III). Final report. *Circulation.* 2002;106:3143–3421.

        vi. If rhabdomyolysis is suspected, obtain hepatic function tests and a serum creatine kinase (CK).

- CK may be within normal range, but it typically begins to rise within 12 hours of development of rhabdomyolysis, peaks after 1 to 3 days, and then declines over a period of 3 to 5 days after the muscle injury ceases.

    e. Monitor lipid profile, CK, and hepatic function tests:

      i.   When a statin is started.

      ii. Anytime a statin dose is increased.

      iii. Stop the statin:

- If the patient is symptomatic with myalgias or other adverse effects
- If the CK is 10 or more times the upper limit of normal
- If hepatic function is three or more times the upper limit of normal.

    f. Some patients may not tolerate any statins. Others may tolerate one statin; but, not another.

      i.   It is recommended that patients be given a trial of at least two different statins before they are labeled with a statin allergy.

 VI. METABOLIC SYNDROME[10,37]

A. Overeating and the development of obesity may lead to maladaptive cardiovascular and renal disease risk factors that include a cluster of conditions: hypertension, dyslipidemia, abdominal obesity, and insulin resistance.

   1. Metabolic syndrome increases risk for heart disease, renal disease, diabetes, and stroke.[48]

B. Closely related to "insulin resistance"—a condition in which the normal function of insulin is hampered. To rule in for the diagnosis of metabolic syndrome, the patient must have any three of the following risk factors:

   1. Excess body fat, particularly in the abdominal area (commonly seen in patients with insulin resistance).

   2. Physical inactivity/obesity: exercise and weight loss are keys to improving this syndrome and reducing heart disease and diabetes risks.

   3. Genetic predisposition (in certain individuals).

   4. Hypertriglyceridemia: diet and drug therapy.

   5. Low HDL: encourage exercise to increase HDL.

   6. Hypertension: 40% of patients with hypertension have metabolic syndrome.

C. Definitions of metabolic syndrome (Table 6-12)[49]:

   1. World Health Organization (WHO) clinical definition

   2. National Cholesterol Education Program Adult Treatment Panel III

   3. American Heart Association/National Heart, Lung, and Blood Institute (AHA/NHLBI)

   4. International Diabetes Federation (IDF)

   5. Consensus definition: AHA/NHLBI and IDF

D. Management of metabolic syndrome[12,44]:

   1. Control LDL cholesterol.

   2. Weight reduction (WHO estimates 1.6 billion people worldwide are overweight defined as a BMI >25).[12,17]

TABLE 6-12 Definitions of Metabolic Syndrome

	World Health Organization (1998)	NCEP ATP III (2001)	AHA/NHLBI (2004)	International Diabetes Federation (2005)	Consensus Definition: AHA/NHLBI and IDF
Criteria	Insulin resistance (defined as Type 2 DM or IFG (↑ 100 mg/dL) or IGT) plus two of the following:	Any three of the following	Any three of the following	BMI ↑ 30 kg/m² plus two of the following:	Any three of the following:
Abdominal obesity	Waist-to-hip ratio: Men: ↑ 0.9 Women: ↑ 0.85 or BMI ↑ 30 kg/m²	Waist circumference: Men: ↑ than 102 cm Women: ↑ than 88 cm	Waist circumference: Men: 102 cm or ↑ Women: 88 cm or ↑		↑ Waist circumference (according to population and country-specific definitions)
Triglycerides	150 mg/dL or ↑ and/or HDL cholesterol in: Men ↓40 mg/dL Women: ↓ 50 mg/dL	150 mg/dL or ↑	150 mg/dL or ↑	150 mg/dL or ↑	150 mg/dL or ↑
HDL cholesterol		Men: ↓ 40 mg/dL Women: ↓ 50 mg/dL	Men: ↓ 40 mg/dL Women: ↓ 50 mg/dL	HDL cholesterol in: Men: ↓ 40 mg/dL Women: ↓ 50 mg/dL	HDL cholesterol in: Men: ↓ 40 mg/dL Women: ↓ 50 mg/dL
Blood pressure	140/90 mm Hg or ↑	130/85 mm Hg or ↑	130/85 mm Hg or ↑	130/85 mm Hg or ↑	130/85 mm Hg or ↑
Fasting glucose		110 mg/dL or ↑	100 mg/dL or ↑	100 mg/dL or ↑	100 mg/dL or ↑
Microalbuminuria	Urinary albumin secretion rate 20 µg/min or ↑, or albumin-to-creatinine ratio 30 mg/g or ↑				

AHA/NHLBI, American Heart Association/National Heart, Lung, and Blood Institute; IDF, International Diabetes Federation; DM, diabetes mellitus; IFG, impaired fasting glucose; IGT, impaired glucose tolerance; HDL, high-density lipoprotein; NCEP ATP III, National Cholesterol Education Program Adult Treatment Panel III.
Adapted from Kassi E, Pervanidou P, Kaltsas G, Chrousos G. Metabolic syndrome: definitions and controversies. *BMC Med.* 2011;9:48-60.

3. Increase physical activity to
   a. Lower very-low-density lipoprotein (VLDL) levels
   b. Lower LDL levels (in certain patients)
   c. Increase HDL cholesterol
   d. Lower BP
   e. Decrease insulin resistance

 VII. DIABETES MELLITUS

A. Overview:
   1. DM that develops de novo after transplantation is also referred to as new onset diabetes after transplantation (NODAT).[50]
   2. Metabolic syndrome was found in 57% of pretransplant recipients. Recipients with preexisting metabolic syndrome were more likely to develop NODAT compared to recipients without metabolic syndrome (34.4% vs. 27.4%, $p = 0.057$).[51]
   3. Incidence of DM varies from 2% to 53% of all solid organ transplant recipients[52,53]:
      a. Kidney: 30%
      b. Heart: 18.5% of recipients within 1 to 5 years posttransplant
      c. Lung: 18.5% of recipients within 1 to 5 years posttransplant
      d. Liver: 15%
   4. Onset[53]:
      a. Typically occurs early in the posttransplant period or when corticosteroid therapy is augmented to treat rejection.
      b. Carries the same short- and long-term risks as DM in the general population.
      c. Typically diagnosed as per general population guidelines

B. Etiology/risks[14,54]:
   1. Primary cause: immunosuppressive agents (Table 6-13)[54-56]
   2. Overweight/obesity (BMI ≥30)

C. Screening: posttransplant DM[6,54]:
   1. Tests:
      a. Fasting blood glucose (FBG) (Table 6-14)[57,58]
      b. Oral glucose tolerance test: 2-hour plasma glucose (Table 6-15)[57,58]
      c. Hemoglobin A_{1c} (HgbA1c)[59]
         i. Measures average glycemic levels over a period of weeks
         ii. Elevated $HgbA_{1c}$ reflects chronic state of hyperglycemia
         iii. May be more appropriately used to monitor the effectiveness of glycemic therapy rather than diagnose DM
   2. Recommended frequency for testing:
      a. Posttransplant months 1 to 3: FBG weekly
      b. Posttransplant months 2 to 6: FBG every other week
      c. Posttransplant months 6 to 12: FBG monthly
      d. After first year: FBG and/or HgbA1c tested at least yearly

D. Transplant recipients at increased risk for posttransplant DM[14,54,60]:
   1. Immunosuppressive medications, which cause insulin resistance and decreased insulin production are
      a. Calcineurin inhibitor risk (tacrolimus 26% vs. cyclosporine 30%) based on the DIRECT Study (Diabetes Incidence after Renal Transplantation); results may vary based upon study reviewed. All studies report higher risk for DM in the tacrolimus group over the cyclosporine group[60]:

TABLE 6-13 Immunosuppressive Agents

Immunosuppressive Agent	Metabolized	Inhibits Insulin Secretion	Causes Insulin Resistance	Directly Affects Release of Insulin from Islets	Causes Temporary or Permanent Structural Damage to Islets
Cyclosporine*	Liver P450 pathway	X			X (at high doses)
Tacrolimus*,†	Liver P450 pathway	X			X (at high doses)
Mycophenolate mofetil	Liver P450 pathway	X			
Sirolimus	Liver P450 pathway	X			
Corticosteroids	Liver P450 pathway	X	X	X	

*Has additive effect when given in combination with corticosteroids.
†Tacrolimus appears to be more diabetogenic than cyclosporine.
From Kesiraju S, Paritala P, Rao Ch UM, et al. New onset of diabetes after transplantation—an overview of epidemiology, mechanism of development and diagnosis. *Transpl Immunol.* 2014;30(1):52–58; Moini M, Schilsky ML, Tichy EM. Review on immunosuppression in liver transplantation. *World J Hepatol.* 2015;7(10):1355–1368; Adams DH, Sanchez-Fueyo A, Samuel D. From immunosuppression to tolerance. *J Hepatol.* 2015;62(1 suppl):S170–S185.

TABLE 6-14 American Diabetes Association, World Health Organization 2013, Diagnostic Criteria for Diabetes Mellitus

Diagnosis	Fasting Blood Glucose (FBG) Test Results	HgbA1c Results
Normal	<100 mg/dL (<5.6 mmol/L)	<5.7
Prediabetes (Impaired fasting glucose)	100–125 mg/dL (5.6–6.9 mmol/L)	5.7%–6.4%
Diabetes (must be confirmed on a subsequent day)	≥126 mg/dL (7.0 mmol/L)	≥6.5
+ *Symptoms of polyuria, polydipsia, unexplained weight loss*	Random blood glucose	≥200 mg/dL (11.1 mmol/L)

From American Diabetes Association. Diagnosis and classification of diabetes mellitus. *Diabetes Care.* 2013;36(suppl 1): S67–S74; Hughes LD. The transplant patient and transplant medicine in family practice. *J Family Med Prim Care.* 2014;3(4): 345–354.

TABLE 6-15 Oral Glucose Tolerance Test

Diagnosis	2-h Plasma Glucose Test Results
Normal	<140 mg/dL (<7.8 mmol/L)
Impaired glucose tolerance	140–199 mg/dL (7.8–11.0 mmol/L)
Diabetes (2 h after 75 g glucose load)	≥200 mg/dL (≥11.1 mmol/L)

From American Diabetes Association. Diagnosis and classification of diabetes mellitus. *Diabetes Care.* 2013;36(suppl 1): S67–S74; Hughes LD. The transplant patient and transplant medicine in family practice. *J Family Med Prim Care.* 2014;3(4): 345–354.

        i. Tacrolimus is thought to cause insulin resistance leading to hyperglycemia; the exact mechanism is unknown.

    b. mTOR inhibitor risk (sirolimus 6.6%)

    c. corticosteroids

2. Older recipients (>45 years)
3. African American, Afro-Caribbean, or Hispanic ethnicity[60] if taking tacrolimus
4. Age >40
5. Family history of DM among first-degree relatives
6. Impaired glucose tolerance test pretransplant or $HgbA_{1c}$ >6.5 pretransplant
7. Presence of metabolic syndrome:
   a. Hypertriglyceridemia
   b. Elevated LDL
   c. Low HDL:
      i. Men: <40
      ii. Women: <50
   d. Hypertension
   e. Hyperuricemia
8. Recipients of deceased donor kidneys
9. Presence of certain HLA antigen mismatches such as A30, B27, or B42
10. Male recipient of an allograft from a male donor
11. CMV infection
12. Pretransplant polycystic kidney disease
13. Hepatitis C virus infection
14. Acute rejection episodes

E. Treatment of posttransplant DM:
1. Similar to treatment of DM in general population:
   a. Dietary therapy:
      i. Very few transplant recipients can be managed by dietary therapy alone.
   b. Oral hypoglycemic agents:
      i. May be sufficient for some patients with moderate hyperglycemia (FBG <200 mg/dL [<11.1 mmol/L]) or patients with normal FBG but with postprandial hyperglycemia[60]
   c. Insulin therapy:
      i. Required for 40% to 50% of transplant recipients with DM[61]
   d. Weight loss
   e. Exercise
2. Components of Diabetes Control and Complications Trial (DCCT) recommendations[62]:
   a. Strict control of blood glucose levels is essential.
   b. Achieving normal fasting blood sugar and $HgbA_{1c}$ is thought to reduce incidence of rejection in the diabetic transplant recipient.
   c. In the DCCT, a 2% decrease in average $HgbA_{1c}$ was associated with a 60% reduction in the risk of several complications of DM including retinopathy, nephropathy, and neuropathy.
3. Surveillance for complications of DM:
   a. Cardiovascular disease:
      i. Posttransplant DM imposes a greater relative risk for cardiovascular morbidity and mortality than hyperlipidemia or hypertension.

b. Infections
c. Retinopathy
d. Nephropathy
e. Neuropathy

F. Transplant-specific treatment strategies[60]:
1. Decrease dose of steroids and/or calcineurin inhibitors when possible.
2. Withdraw steroids when possible.
3. Change immunosuppression regimens (e.g., from tacrolimus to cyclosporine).
4. Oral medications typically prescribed for transplant patients are listed below by class and in decreasing order of frequency:
   a. Meglitinides (nateglinide [Starlix]):
      i. Combined with cyclosporine, may increase nateglinide levels and increase risk for hypoglycemia.
   b. Sulfonylureas (glipizide [Glucotrol]):
      i. Negligible drug-drug interactions (DDI) with immunosuppressants
      ii. Contraindicated if patient has a sulfa allergy
      iii. Caution: risk for hypoglycemia
   c. Biguanides (metformin [Glucophage]):
      i. Combined with cyclosporine, may decrease metformin efficacy
      ii. Monitor renal function
      iii. Risk for lactic acidosis
      iv. Induces ovulation (consider birth control in females if appropriate).
   d. Thiazolidinediones (pioglitazone [Actos]):
      i. No DDIs with transplant med
      ii. Monitor liver function
   e. Dipeptidyl peptidase-4 inhibitors (sitagliptin [Januvia]):
      i. Monitor renal function
      ii. No DDIs with immunosuppressants
5. When oral medications do not achieve glycemic control (HgbA1c <7) or cause adverse effects, insulin may be needed:
   a. Long-acting basal insulins: (insulin glargine [Lantus])
   b. Premeal short-acting insulins: (insulin aspart [NovoLog] or insulin lispro [Humalog])

G. Patient monitoring:
1. Oral hypoglycemic agents:
   a. Most agents are excreted, at least partially, through the kidneys.
   b. Use with caution in patients with renal impairment.
   c. Monitor renal or hepatic function as indicated.
   d. Encourage patient home blood glucose monitoring.
2. Monitor recipient for rejection in the setting of
   a. Immunosuppression dose reduction
   b. Steroid withdrawal
   c. Changes in immunosuppressive agents

H. DM in specific transplant populations:
1. Cystic fibrosis (CF) patients: the pancreas is the second most commonly affected organ in patients with CF.[63] In CF, pancreatic juice becomes concentrated and thickened secretions lead to obstruction, inflammation, injury to the acini, decreased exocrine enzyme secretion, and pancreatic insufficiency. DM ensues when beta cells are damaged.

2. Kidney transplant recipients: possible contributing factors: adult polycystic kidney disease, hepatitis C infection.[1,64,65]

3. Pancreas[66] transplant recipients:

   a. $HgbA_{1c}$ is typically normal by 1 month posttransplant.[67]

   b. Impaired glucose tolerance posttransplant have poorer pancreas graft survival; testing begins 2 weeks posttransplant.[68]

   c. Once euglycemia has been achieved, recurrent hyperglycemia that requires insulin therapy typically is associated with one or more of the following:

      i.   Graft failure secondary to acute or chronic rejection

      ii. Insulin resistance with new-onset type 2 DM

      iii. Islet cell toxicity secondary to immunosuppression

      iv. Immune-related islet cell destruction

   d. Follow-up screening for glucose intolerance includes a fasting glucose and $HgbA_{1c}$ at every clinic visit:

      i.   An oral glucose tolerance test (with insulin concentrations) is done if there have been no recent rejection episodes (see Table 6-15)[57,58] and

         • The fasting blood glucose level is >100 mg/dL (5.55 mmol/L).

         • $HgbA_{1c}$ is elevated >6.5.

   e. New-onset type 2 DM:

      i.   Typically represents a genetic predisposition to insulin resistance that is exacerbated by immunosuppressive agents and/or considerable weight gain

      ii. Treatment options:

         • Insulin therapy to protect function of islet cells until other treatment strategies become effective (e.g., treatment of rejection, weight loss, oral hypoglycemic agents, or manipulation of immunosuppression regimen).

         • Because posttransplant resumption of insulin therapy constitutes graft failure in pancreas transplant recipients, some centers may be reluctant to reinitiate insulin, preferring instead to use oral hypoglycemic agents.

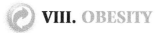 VIII. OBESITY

A. Overview:

1. Obesity is a common problem among solid organ transplant recipients.

2. Assessment of obesity:

   a. Estimation of body fat:

      i.   Waist circumference: high-risk waistline:

         • Females: ≥35 inches

         • Males: ≥40 inches

      ii. Waist-to-hip ratio: measured at smallest area of the waist and largest area around the hip. High risk if ratio is

         • Females: ≥0.85

         • Males: ≥0.9

   b. Body mass index (BMI):

      i.   Assesses weight relative to height

      ii. Two formulas:

         • Weight (in kilograms) divided by height in meters squared

         • Multiply weight in pounds by 703, divide by height in inches, divide by height in inches again

        iii. BMI calculator online: http://www.nhlbi.nih.gov/health/educational/ lose_wt/BMI/bmicalc.htm

        iv. Body mass index values (see Table 6-3)[17]:

B. **Determinants of obesity**[34,69,70]:

   1. Age

   2. Gender

   3. Genetic factors

   4. Environmental factors

C. **Obesity is a major risk factor for CHD and is associated with**[71]:

   1. Dyslipidemia:

     a. Elevated blood cholesterols and triglyceride levels

     b. Decreased HDL levels

   2. Hypertension

   3. DM

D. **Obesity in the pretransplant period:**

   1. Goal: optimize transplant candidate's weight prior to listing and transplantation.

   2. Weight loss guideline: deficit of 500 to 1,000 calories/d depending on the patient's:

     a. Current intake

     b. Anticipated time on transplant waiting list

     c. Ability to exercise[70]

   3. Weight loss medications, supervised programs, or bariatric surgery may be appropriate for certain patients.

   4. Liquid diets are *not* appropriate for the pretransplant patient.

E. **Obesity in the posttransplant period:**

   1. Associated with increased posttransplant morbidity such as[34,70]:

     a. Delayed kidney graft function

     b. Decreased kidney graft survival

     c. Increased incidence of wound infection

     d. Increased incidence of surgical complications (e.g., thrombosis)

     e. Decreased respiratory function and endurance

   2. Contributing factors[34,70]:

     a. Immunosuppressive medications (the average patient will gain 5 to 10 during the first year posttransplant):

       i. Corticosteroids

       ii. Higher rates of weight gain seen with cyclosporine[71]

     b. Excess caloric intake due to

       i. Enhanced appetite secondary to corticosteroid use

       ii. Poor eating habits

       iii. Resolution of pretransplant malabsorption

     c. Caloric intake that exceeds expenditure due to sedentary habits and lack of exercise

     d. Genetic predisposition

     e. Age, gender, and race

F. **Components of healthy posttransplant weight loss program**[34,70]:

   1. Reduction in calories

   2. Behavior modification

3. Exercise
4. Immunosuppressant modifications to consider
   a. Decrease or wean corticosteroids
   b. Substitute tacrolimus (Prograf, Astagraf XL) for cyclosporine (Neoral, Gengraf)

G. Psychological aspects of weight loss[70]:
   1. Assessment of patient's readiness and motivation:
      a. If patient is not willing to embark on weight loss program, identify and remove barriers to weight loss.
   2. Establishment of reasonable goals with respect to desired
      a. Amount of weight loss:
         i. Initial goal: reduce body weight by approximately 10% from baseline (typically over 6 months).
         ii. When this goal is reached, further weight loss, if indicated, can be considered.
            • When target weight is reached, weight maintenance program is initiated.
            • Sustained physical activity is useful in preventing weight regain.
      b. Cholesterol level
      c. Glucose level
      d. BP
   3. Incorporation of behavioral strategies such as[34,70]
      a. Self-monitoring of eating patterns and physical activity
      b. Stress management
      c. Stimulus control
      d. Problem-solving
      e. Contingency management
      f. Cognitive restructuring
      g. Incorporation of social support

H. Weight loss medications:
   1. To date, the three current weight loss medications are orlistat (Alli, Xenical), sibutramine (Meridia), and phentermine hydrochloride. These have not been tested for safety and efficacy in the transplant population.

I. Sibutramine (Meridia) and orlistat (Alli, Xenical) may be safe for transplant recipients, but are metabolized in the P450 3A4 system and thus may interfere with cyclosporine, tacrolimus, or rapamycin metabolism.
   1. Phentermine hydrochloride is contraindicated in setting of CHF, CAD, severe liver or renal impairment, and poorly controlled hypertension.
   2. Medical providers advocate diet and exercise as the best treatment for weight loss in the transplant patient.

J. Bariatric surgery:
   1. Gastric stapling and other types of weight loss surgery carry inherent surgical risks and must first be discussed with the transplant team.
   2. Bariatric surgery may affect the absorption of medications; decreased absorption of immunosuppressive agents may put the patient at increased risk for rejection.

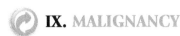 **IX. MALIGNANCY**

A.   Overview:

1. Malignancy is one of the three major causes of death in the posttransplant population (cardiovascular disease and infection are the other two).[72]

2. Data regarding posttransplant malignancies comes from the following sources:

   a. Large tumor registries, for example:

      i.   Australia and New Zealand Dialysis and Transplant Registry: www.anzdata.org.au

      ii. United States Renal Data System (USRDS): www.usrds.org

      iii. Scientific Registry of Transplant Recipients: www.srtr.org

      iv. International Society for Heart and Lung Transplantation Registry: www.ishlt.org

   b. Single center data

3. Factors that contribute to the development of de novo posttransplant malignancy:

   a. Duration of exposure to immunosuppression

   b. Intensity of immunosuppressive agents used

B.   Etiologic factors associated with transplant recipients' increased risk of malignancy include:

1. Impaired immune surveillance caused by chronic immunosuppression therapy (decreased ability to eliminate malignant cells)

2. Mutagenic properties of immunosuppressive agents[72]:

   a. In vitro studies indicate that calcineurin inhibitors (cyclosporine [Sandimmune], cyclosporine modified [Neoral, Gengraf], tacrolimus [Prograf]) are carcinogenic due to the production of cytokine

   b. Azathioprine (Imuran) can damage DNA and RNA.

3. Chronic antigenic stimulation caused by foreign allograft antigens, repeated infections, or transfusions:

   a. May overstimulate immune system and cause PTLD.

   b. Faulty feedback mechanisms may lead to impaired control of immune reactions and uninhibited lymphoid proliferation.

4. Environmental factors (e.g., ultraviolet radiation, particularly in Australia)

5. Genetic factors that alter susceptibility to malignancy by modifying carcinogenic metabolism, interferon secretion, response to viral infections, or major histocompatibility regulation of the immune response:

   a. Pretransplant history of cancer carries a 40% higher risk for cancer over similar patients without a cancer history.[72]

6. Donor history of cancer

7. Chronic viral infections, particularly those shown in Table 6-16[73]:

   a. For example, lymphocyte-depleting antibodies (e.g., antithymocyte globulin: [ATGAM]) may increase the risk of early-onset, EBV-associated posttransplant lymphoproliferative disease (PTLD)[72]

C.   Pathogenesis of posttransplant malignancy[74]:

1. De novo occurrence

2. Recurrent malignancy in recipient

3. Transmission of malignancy from donor:

   a. The following cancers have been transmitted from donor to recipient on at least one occasion: breast, choriocarcinoma, colon, glioblastoma multiforme, liver, lung, lymphoma, melanoma, neuroendocrine, ovarian, pancreatic, prostate, renal cell, and thyroid cancer.[72]

TABLE 6-16 **Viral Infection–Related Malignancies**

Virus	Type of Malignancy
Human Herpes virus 8	Kaposi sarcoma
Epstein-Barr virus	Non-Hodgkin lymphoma Hodgkin lymphoma
Human papillomavirus	Cervical cancer Anogenital cancer
Hepatitis B and hepatitis C virus	Liver cancer

From Grulich AE, Vajdic CM. The epidemiology of cancers in human immunodeficiency virus infection and after organ transplantation. *Semin Oncol.* 2015;42:247–257.

    b. The Organ Procurement and Transplantation Network Disease Transmission Advisory Committee's 2013 report indicated that there were 65 donors reported with potential malignancies. Five were classified as potential/probable transmissions, which affected eight recipients (two deaths).[75]

D.   Characteristics of malignancies in transplant recipients[72]:
    1. Malignancies occur in a relatively short time period following transplantation.
    2. Transplant recipients cancer rates are similar to those of individuals in the general population who are 20 to 30 years older.
    3. The relative risk of developing a posttransplant malignancy is greater in younger transplant recipients compared to transplant recipients over 65 years of age.

E.   Types of malignancies that occur in transplant recipients:
    1. 2011 Transplant Cancer Match Study[76]:
      a. This cohort study used linked data from the US Scientific Registry of Transplant Recipients (175,732 kidney, liver, heart, and lung transplant procedures performed between 1987 and 2008) and 13 state or regional cancer registries.
      b. Key findings:
        i. Four most common malignancies with an elevated risk: non-Hodgkin's lymphoma and cancer of the lung, liver, and kidney:
          • Incidence of these cancers higher in male transplant recipients
          • Except for non-Hodgkin's lymphoma, incidence increased sharply with age
          • Incidence of lung, liver, and kidney malignancy cancers: highest in respective recipients of these organs
        ii. Findings relative to specific types of malignancy are summarized in Table 6-17.[76]
        iii. Carcinomas that are common in the general population (lung, breast, prostate, colon, and invasive uterine cervical cancer) do not occur more frequently in transplant recipients.[72–74]

F.   Skin cancer:
    1. Overview:
      a. The most commonly occurring type of cancer among transplant recipients[74]:
        i. Incidence of skin cancer in Table 6-18.[74]
      b. Risk factors[74]:
        i. Skin type (Fitzpatrick I to III)
        ii. Cumulative exposure to sun

TABLE 6-17 Transplant Cancer Match Study

Non-Hodgkin Lymphoma	Lung Cancer	Liver Cancer	Kidney Cancer
Most common malignancy	Risk highest among lung transplant recipients, possibly due to smoking history	Liver recipients: 95% of malignancies were diagnosed in first 6 mo posttransplant; this may represent cancer that was present in the explanted liver	Risk highest in kidney transplant recipients but also elevated in liver and heart recipients
Most common subtype: Large B-cell lymphoma	Lung recipients: • Most cancers occurred in the native lung • Risk increased over time • Risk for lung transplant recipients was greatest in the first 6 mo posttransplant • Excluding the first 6 mo posttransplant, lung recipients had a 5.5-fold increased risk (compared to general population)	Increased risk noted only in liver recipients	Bi-modal pattern among all recipients: • Early peak during first transplant year • Second peak: 4–15 y posttransplant
Incidence: Highest in lung recipients Lowest in kidney recipients			
Cohorts at highest risk: Young recipients: due to their ↑ susceptibility to primary EBV infection Lung transplant recipients: possibly because of high level of immunosuppressants and large amount of lymphoid tissue in lung allograft			

EBV, Epstein-Barr virus.
From Engels EA, Pfeiffer RM, Fraumeni JF, et al. Spectrum of cancer risk among U.S. solid organ transplant recipients: the Transplant Cancer Match Study. *JAMA.* 2011;306(17):1891–1901.

TABLE 6-18 Incidence of Skin Cancer Compared to General Population

Type of Cancer	Incidence Compared to General Population	Comment
Squamous cell carcinoma	Increased 65-fold	Most common type of skin cancer in transplant recipients Risk increases with time since transplant More aggressive in transplant recipients than in general population Tend to occur in sun-exposed skin
Basal cell carcinoma	Increased 10-fold	
Melanoma	Increased 3- to 5-fold	Risk factors: multiple nevi; fair complexion Mean time to development: 5 y posttransplant
Merkel cell carcinoma	Increased 5- to 10-fold	Tend to develop 7–8 y posttransplant

From Zwald FO, Brown M. Skin cancer in solid organ transplant recipients: advances in therapy and management. *J Am Acad Dermatol.* 2011;65(2):253–261.

     iii.   Older age at time of transplant

     iv.   Duration and intensity of immunosuppression

     v.   Type of transplant

        • Incidence is highest in heart and lung transplant recipients, followed in decreasing order by kidney and liver transplant recipients

     vi.   Retransplantation

     vii.   Pre- or posttransplant history of lymphoma or leukemia

     viii.   Pretransplant history of skin cancer, rheumatoid arthritis, systemic lupus erythematosus, and autoimmune hepatitis

     ix.   History of biologic therapy and phototherapy

2. Basal cell and squamous cell carcinoma[74]:

   a. Squamous cell and basal cell carcinoma: account for 95% of all skin cancers in solid organ transplant recipients.

   b. 75% of squamous and basal cell carcinomas occur on the head, neck, or dorsal surface of the hands.

   c. Squamous cell carcinoma (SCC) seen more frequently than basal cell carcinoma (BCC):

     i.   In the general population, the opposite is true: BCCs are more frequently seen than SCCs.

3. Evolution of cutaneous carcinomas in transplant recipients; compared to the general population, in transplant recipients[73]:

   a. Skin lesions are more aggressive.

   b. Multiple squamous cell carcinomas develop more frequently.

   c. Basal cell carcinomas are more likely to

     i.   Occur in younger males

     ii.   Occur in non–sun-exposed sites

     iii.   Recur or metastasize

4. Characteristics of skin lesions (Table 6-19)[73,77–80]

TABLE 6-19 Characteristics of Skin Lesions

Lesion	Tend to Occur in	Potential Treatment Options	Other
Premalignant cutaneous lesions: Warts	Sun-exposed areas of skin Individuals with light skin	Topical keratolytic agents or retinoic acid Resistant warts: Imiquimod cream (5%) Recalcitrant warts: Topical cidofovir (1%); consider conversion to mTOR inhibitors	Lesions tend to be multiple Generally caused by HPV High frequency of recurrence
Actinic keratosis (premalignant cutaneous lesion)	Areas exposed to light (e.g., forehead, ears, scalp, forearm)	Mild (isolated lesions): Sun protection; cryotherapy; laser, curettage, possibly with topical treatment Moderate: Photodynamic therapy; small areas: diclofenac in hyaluronic acid gel; modify immunosuppression. Severe: Modify immunosuppression; Systemic retinoids for diffusely spreading forms	May be associated with warts; sign that lesion is transforming into squamous cell carcinoma: infiltrate in lesion; rapid recurrence of lesion

(continued)

TABLE 6-19 Characteristics of Skin Lesions (*Continued*)

Lesion	Tend to Occur in	Potential Treatment Options	Other
Squamous cell	Sun-exposed areas of skin; Often develops on warts and lesions of keratosis	Not aggressive: Sun protection; treat actinic keratosis; surgical excision Modify Immunosuppression Clinically aggressive: Sentinel lymph Node biopsy; systemic retinoids as indicated Histologically aggressive: Sentinel lymph node biopsy; Systemic retinoids as indicated	Characterized by: small lesions; small growth; edges well-demarcated No ulceration Characterized by: extensive, rapidly growing lesions; poorly demarcated edges and ulceration Characterized by: poor differentiation; invasion of subcutaneous fat; perineural involvement
Basal cell carcinoma	Sun-exposed areas of skin	Superficial: Sun protection; excision; confirm margins; photodynamic therapy if indicated. Nodular or other: Excision, confirm margins; modify immunosuppression	Most common type of skin cancer in immunosuppressed patients
Melanoma Four types: 1. Superficial spreading 2. Nodular 3. Lentigo maligna 4. Acral lentiginous	Areas exposed to acute, intense exposure to ultraviolet radiation (via sunburn)	Surgical excision Sentinal lymph node biopsy Adjuvant therapy	Overall risk in transplant recipients: 2.4 times the risk compared to general population Characteristics of lesion: "A, B, C, D, E" **A**symmetry of nevus **B**orders: notched, irregular **C**olor: varies from light to dark; may be dark black or blue-black blue-gray, brown or reddish **D**iameter >0.6 mm **E**volving—lesion is changing in size, shape, color or spreading (new lesions appearing)
Kaposi's sarcoma	Trunk and extremities	Reduction in immunosuppression Substituting mTOR inhibitor for calcineurin inhibitor Focal lesions: Cryotherapy Laser therapy Radiotherapy Topical antiviral agent (imiquimod cream—5%) Systemic Kaposi's sarcoma: Chemotherapy	Reported mortality range: 8%–14% involvement: Stage 1: single limb; localized skin lesions Stage 2: >1 limb with skin lesions Stage 3: 1 or more viscera or lymph nodes Stage 4: Life-threatening infection or other neoplasia associated with Stage 1, 2, or 3

From Grulich AE, Vajdic CM. The epidemiology of cancers in human immunodeficiency virus infection and after organ transplantation. *Semin Oncol.* 2015;42:247–257; Ulrich C, Arnold R, Ulrich F, et al. Skin changes following organ transplantation. *Dtsch Arztebl Int.* 2014;111(11):188–194; Ponticelli C, Bencini PL. Nonneoplastic mucocutaneous lesions in organ transplant recipients. *Transpl Int.* 2011;24:1041–1050; Wilkerson BL. Malignant melanoma. *Plast Surg Nurs.* 2011;31(3):105–107; Hosseini-Moghaddam SM, Soleimanirahbar A, Mazzulli T, et al. Post renal transplantation Kaposi's sarcoma: a review of its epidemiology, pathogenesis, diagnosis, clinical aspects, and therapy. *Transpl Infect Dis.* 2012;14:338–345.

G. PTLD:
   1. Overview[81,82]:
      a. Involves a wide spectrum of disorders that range from benign polymorphic B-cell hyperplasia to malignant lymphomas.[81]
      b. Incidence varies from 1% in kidney transplant recipients, 10% in combined heart-lung transplant recipients, and as high as 33% in intestinal or multiorgan transplant recipients.[83]
      c. Often extranodal; may initially involve the gastrointestinal (GI) tract, lung, or kidney.[14]
      d. May involve single or multiple organs.
      e. More common in nonrenal allograft recipients[72]:
         i. This is most likely due to the intense antirejection therapy that may be required in nonrenal allograft recipients as a life-saving mechanism.
   2. Risk factors[72,81,83]:
      a. Intense immunosuppression: for example, polyclonal (antithymocyte globulin [Atgam]) or monoclonal antibody therapy (basiliximab [Simulect])
      b. Primary Epstein-Barr virus (EBV) infection (recipient EBV seronegative; donor EBV seropositive):
         i. EBV infection is considered a secondary malignancy in a transplant recipient due to the high risk for EBV-associated PTLD.[81]
      c. CMV infection
      d. CMV mismatch (recipient CMV seronegative; donor CMV seropositive)
      e. Type of transplant (lung; heart-lung)
   3. Clinical presentation (Note: PTLD may be asymptomatic.):
      a. Symptoms that resemble infectious mononucleosis
      b. Fever
      c. Night sweats
      d. Upper respiratory infection
      e. Weight loss
      f. Diarrhea
      g. Abdominal pain
      h. Lymphadenopathy
      i. Tonsillitis
      j. GI tract involvement: intestinal perforation and peritonitis
      k. Lung lesion or visceral mass
   4. Treatment options[81,83]:
      a. Reduction or withdrawal of immunosuppression
      b. Switching to or adding an mTOR inhibitor due the antineoplastic properties of mTOR inhibitors (sirolimus [Rapamune], everolimus [Zortress])
      c. Rituximab (Rituxan)
      d. Intravenous immunoglobulin (IVIG)
      e. Antiviral therapy
      f. Surgery for localized disease
      g. Cytotoxic chemotherapy
         i. R-CHOP: rituximab, cyclophosphamide, doxorubicin, vincristine, and prednisone
      h. Radiotherapy
      i. Interferon-α

5. Prevention of PTLD[81]:
   a. EBV replication inhibitors (antiviral drugs such as ganciclovir [Cytovene, Valcyte])
   b. IVIG

H. Prevention of cancer[72,84]:
   1. Smoking cessation
   2. Routine self-examination of skin
   3. Hepatitis B vaccination in nonimmune recipients (may help to prevent hepatitis B virus–related hepatocellular carcinoma)
   4. Sun precautions:
      a. Avoiding undue exposure to sunlight
      b. Avoiding tanning beds
      c. Wearing protective clothing:
         i.   Broad-brimmed hats
         ii. Long-sleeve shirts and pants
      d. Wearing sunglasses and sun visors
      e. Using sunscreen lotion that provides protection against ultraviolet-B rays (minimum sun protection factor [SPF] = 50)
   5. Routine cancer screening per American Cancer Society guidelines (Table 6-20)[84]:
      a. These are minimum guidelines. Depending on the patient's family history, personal history, posttransplant course, and current medical status, more aggressive screening tests and/or more frequent screening intervals may be required.
      b. Posttransplant cancer–screening guidelines have been developed for renal transplant recipients and are applicable to most transplant recipients[1] (Table 6-21).[85]

TABLE 6-20   American Cancer Society Routine Cancer Screening Guidelines for General Population

Males and Females	Males	Females
Over 50 y: Routine sigmoidoscopy every 5 y or colonoscopy every 10 y Fecal occult blood test, or fecal immunohistochemical test (FIT) annually	Starting at age 50: Annual prostate-specific antigen test Annual digital rectal examination	Age 20 and over: Monthly self-breast examination Age 40 and over: Annual mammogram Clinical breast examination:
Note: colonoscopy is typically preferred for transplant recipients Annual skin examination by dermatologist Semiannual examination for oral cancer by dentist		Age 20–39: every 3 y Age 40 and over: yearly Pelvic examination with Papanicolaou (PAP) test: • 21–29 every 3 y • 30–65 every 5 y • >65 no testing unless prior abnormal PAP test and then continue to 20 y after the last positive PAP test. • Annual exam/PAP testing is recommended for transplant patients (ACOG)

These are guidelines recommended for patients with normal test results. Increased screening will be done by the doctor as appropriate for cancer or other abnormal findings.
Based upon American Cancer Society 2014 Guidelines. American College of Obstetrics and Gynaecology (ACOG); American Cancer Society. *American Cancer Society Guidelines for the Early Detection of Cancer.* Available at http://www.cancer.org/healthy/findcancerearly/cancerscreeningguidelines/american-cancer-society-guidelines-for-the-early-detection-of-cancer. Accessed July 15, 2015.

TABLE 6-21 Posttransplant Cancer–Screening Guidelines for Renal Transplant Recipients

Type of Carcinoma	Minimum Screening Recommendations
Anogenital	Yearly examination of anogenital area; pelvic examinations for women with cytologic studies Follow-up biopsy of suspicious lesions Prompt treatment of warts
Kaposi's sarcoma	Monthly self-skin checks
Squamous cell	Dermatologist skin check every 6–12 mo to assess total body skin examination, conjunctiva, oropharyngeal mucosa; and receive a biopsy of suspicious lesions
Basal cell	More frequent examination for high-risk patients (those of Arab, Italian, Greek or Jewish ethnicity; those living in Africa or Middle East; those with HHV-8 infection)
PTLD	History and physical examination with particular attention to any symptoms suggestive of disseminated or localized PTLD every 3 mo during first posttransplant year and yearly thereafter
Hepatobiliary	High-risk patients (e.g., those with chronic hepatitis): α-fetoprotein levels may assist in early detection along with liver sonography every 6–12 mo Annual Pap tests and pelvic examination for all women ≥21 y of age and for women <21 y of age who are sexually active
Uterine cervix	Women age 50–69: screening mammography every 1–2 y, with or without clinical breast examinations
Breast	Women age 40–49: may opt for screening mammography every 1–2 y, with or without clinical breast examinations Women ≥age 70 with reasonable life expectancies: may opt for screening mammography every 1–2 y with or without clinical breast examinations High-risk women < age 50: screening mammography every 1–2 y with or without clinical breast exams Patients ≥50 y of age: annual fecal occult blood testing
Colorectal	Flexible sigmoidoscopy every 5 y or colonoscopy every 10 y More frequent screening for patients at higher risk Men ≥50 y with at least 10-y life expectancy: annual digital rectal examination and prostate-specific antigen test
Prostate	Men at higher risk (e.g., family history of prostate screening): start screening at younger age Men at higher risk (e.g., family history of prostate screening): start screening at younger age

Wong G, Chapman JR, Craig JC. Cancer screening in renal transplant recipients: what is the evidence. *Clin J Am Soc Nephrol.* 2008;3(suppl 2):S87–S100.

X. BONE DISEASE

A. Osteoporosis:

1. Definition: condition characterized by loss of bone mass and deterioration of bone tissue such that patients are at risk for bone fragility and fractures[86]
2. Terms to know:
   a. Osteoblasts stimulate bone formation (builds bone).
   b. Osteoclasts stimulate resorption of old bone (breaks down bone).
   c. Bones should be continuously remodeling to renew and maintain healthy bones. This remodeling slows with aging and can be affected by diseases or medications.

3. World Health Organization (WHO) diagnostic criteria for postmenopausal women:
   a. Osteopenia: Bone mineral density (BMD) between 1 standard deviation (SD) and 2.5 SD below the mean BMD of young adult women
   b. Osteoporosis: BMD greater than 2.5 SD below the mean BMD of adult women
4. Bone mass has been shown to be consistently lower in transplant recipients than in age- and sex-matched controls.
5. Vertebral bone loss is typically highest in first 6 to 12 months posttransplant and continues at a lower rate depending on immune suppression.
6. Etiology[86]:
   a. General pretransplant factors that predispose patient to low bone density:
      i.   Chronic renal failure
      ii.   Prolonged use of loop diuretics
      iii. Prerenal azotemia
      iv.   Uncontrolled DM
      v.   Abnormal thyroid function
      vi.   Liver congestion
      vii. Smoking history
      viii. Hypogonadism
      ix.   Severe HF (New York Heart Association [NYHA] Class III–IV)
      x.   Secondary hyperparathyroidism
      xi.   Insufficient intake of dietary calcium and/or vitamin D
      xii. Decreased mobility; lack of weight-bearing exercise
   b. Organ-specific pretransplant risk factors and posttransplant fracture risk[86,87]:
      i.   Cardiac transplant candidates:
         • Severe HF
         • Rapid bone loss the first year posttransplant (BMD ↓ 3% to 10% in the spine and 6% to 11% in the hip)
         • Vertebral fractures: 14% to 36% the first years posttransplant
         • Overall fracture risk: 22% to 35% over lifetime
      ii. Lung transplant candidates:
         • Hypoxemia
         • Prior glucocorticoid therapy
         • CF patients:
            ○ Calcium malabsorption
            ○ Delayed puberty
            ○ Pancreatic insufficiency with vitamin D deficiency
         • 18% to 37% risk for fracture posttransplant
      iii. Pancreas transplant candidates[88,89]:
         • Uncontrolled DM
      iv. Renal transplant candidates:
         • Metabolic abnormalities.
         • Hypercalcemia.
         • Hyperphosphatemia.
         • Hypovitaminosis D (serum levels <30 ng/mL).
         • 10% to 25% of all renal transplants will suffer a fracture over their lifetime.[87]

v.   Liver transplant candidates:
  * 12% to 55% of patients have osteoporosis pretransplant due to chronic liver disease.
  * Low bone turnover pretransplant.
  * Fracture risk during the first year posttransplant: 24% to 65%.
  * Treatment with calcium, vitamin D and bisphosphonates prior to transplant prevents bone loss and lowers fracture risk.

c. Posttransplant factors:
  i.   Corticosteroid therapy—particularly high corticosteroid doses in early transplant period or following episodes of acute rejection; corticosteroid therapy is associated with
    * Increased urinary calcium secretion
    * Decreased intestinal absorption of calcium
    * Increased parathyroid hormone level
    * Decreased skeletal growth factors, including synthesis of androgen and estrogen
    * Increased bone resorption—osteoclasts (rapid bone loss during first year posttransplant)
    * Decreased bone formation by osteoblasts
    * Risk for osteonecrosis through direct and indirect effects on bone effector cells, decreased bone turnover from increasing osteoclasts and decreasing osteoblasts.
  ii. Cyclosporine and tacrolimus may be associated with high rates of bone resorptions—stimulates osteoclasts.
  iii. Sirolimus decreases bone resorption by inhibiting osteoclasts.
  iv. Hyperparathyroidism.
  v.   Postmenopausal females and hypogonadism in males.
  vi. Progressive aging.
  vii. Kidney transplant recipients: persistent metabolic acidosis associated with chronic allograft dysfunction.

7. Assessment:
  a. Dual-energy x-ray absorptiometry (DEXA) of the lumbar spine and hip:
    i.   Pretransplant baseline assessment
    ii. Six months posttransplant
    iii. Periodically thereafter to monitor bone density and effectiveness of therapy
  b. Laboratory tests:
    i.   Calcium
    ii.   25-Hydroxy vitamin D
    iii. Osteocalcin
    iv.   Intact parathyroid hormone
    v.   Alkaline phosphatase
    vi.   Chemistry levels
    vii. Urinary calcium
    viii. Markers of resorption
    ix.   Urinary pyridinoline cross-links
    x.   N-telopeptides

8. Therapeutic options[86,87]:
  a. Calcium supplements: 1,500 mg/d
  b. Vitamin D supplements: 800 to 1,000 mg/d.
    i.   Hypovitaminosis D affects 59% to 91% of all transplant patients.[87]

c. Antiresorptive agents include bisphosphonates, for example, etidronate (Didronel), risedronate (Actonel), ibandronate (Boniva):
   i.   May be administered on daily, weekly, or monthly basis.
   ii. To optimize absorption: medication must be taken with 8 oz of plain water 30 minutes prior to ingesting any food or liquid.
   iii. Medication cannot be taken with mineral water, coffee, tea, juice, or any other liquids.
   iv. To prevent esophageal irritation: patient must remain fully upright for 30 minutes after taking this medication (standing, sitting, or walking).
   v.   Instructions to patients:
       • Take medications exactly as directed.
       • Promptly report any chest pain, new or worsening heartburn, or difficult or painful swallowing.
       • Stop taking medication if above symptoms occur; notify physician.
d. Calcitonin: subcutaneous injections or nasal spray
e. RANK-ligand inhibitor: denosumab (Prolia)[87]:
   i.   Reduces osteoclastic resorption of trabecular structures
   ii. Typically used for the treatment of postmenopausal osteoporosis
   iii. Use in the treatment of osteonecrosis
f. Minimizing steroid dose
g. Withdrawing steroids in patients at high risk for osteoporosis
9. Prevention and treatment of osteopenia/osteoporosis[6,86,87] (Figure 6-1)

B. Avascular necrosis (AVN)[86]:
   1. Often associated with corticosteroid therapy
   2. Typical site in 90% of cases: femoral head
   3. Clinical presentation:
      a. Hip or groin pain that worsens with weight bearing
      b. Pain may be referred to knee
   4. Diagnosis: magnetic resonance imaging
   5. Treatment options:
      a. Core decompression (prior to collapse of femoral head)
      b. Total hip arthroplasty

XI. GASTROINTESTINAL COMPLICATIONS

A. Overview:
   1. 5% to 50% of patients with primary immunodeficiencies may have GI disorders, due to the fact that the GI tract:
      a. Is the largest lymphoid organ
      b. Contains the majority of lymphocytes
      c. Produces a large quantity of immunoglobulin[90] lymphoid tissues
   2. Gastroenterologists classify GI diseases into four etiologic categories:
      a. Adverse drug effect
      b. Infection
      c. Inflammation
      d. Malignancy
   3. Most immunosuppressive agents are associated with some type of GI complication.
   4. Corticosteroids may mask certain clinical manifestations of GI complications such as leukocytosis, abdominal guarding, and rebound.

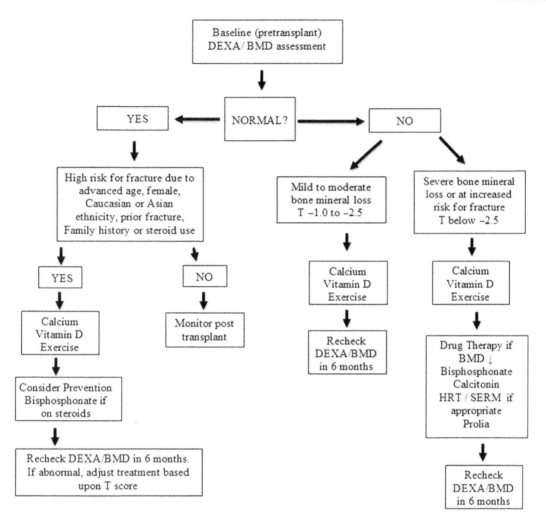

DEXA/BMD = Dual-energy X-ray absorptiometry/Bone mineral density.
HRT = hormone replacement therapy. SERM = Selective estrogen receptor modulator

FIGURE 6-1 Prevention of osteopenia/osteoporosis. (From Kasiske BL, Zeier MG, Chapman JR, et al. KIDGO clinical practice guideline for the care of kidney transplant recipients: a summary. *Kidney Int.* 2010;77(4):299–311; Beckman S, Ivanovic N, Drent G, et al. Weight gain, overweight and obesity in solid organ transplantation—a study protocol for a systematic review. *Syst Rev.* 2015;4(2):2–10; Reichman TW, Therapondos G, Serrano M-S, et al. Weighing the risk: obesity and outcomes following liver transplantation. *World J Hepatol.* 2015;7(11):1484–1493.)

5. The most common posttransplant GI disturbances include[90]
   a. Infections
   b. Mucosal injury, ulceration, or perforation
   c. Biliary tract diseases
   d. Diverticular disease
   e. Pancreatitis
   f. Malignancy
6. The common signs and symptoms associated with these GI disturbances include
   a. Anorexia
   b. Nausea, vomiting, and/or diarrhea
   c. Elevated liver function tests (LFTs)

B. Infections (see chapter on Infectious Diseases for additional information):

1. Chronic immunosuppression can lead to localized GI infections.
2. Infections may occur in one or more portions of the gut between the mouth and the anus.
3. Types of infections[91]:
   a. Viral
   b. Bacterial
   c. Fungal
   d. Parasitic
4. Viral infections[92,93]:
   a. CMV[94,95]:
      i. Enteric and/or gastric infections are common, especially in the first 6 to 12 posttransplant months.
      ii. Any portion of the GI tract can be affected by CMV infection; clinical manifestations depend on the segment of the GI tract that is affected.
      iii. Common symptoms associated with CMV infections of the GI tract include
         • Dysphagia (inability to swallow or difficulty swallowing)
         • Odynophagia (pain with swallowing)
         • Nausea, vomiting, and diarrhea
         • Abdominal pain
         • GI bleeding
         • GI perforation
      iv. Diagnosis of CMV infection
         • Endoscopy and biopsy to rule out CMV gastritis
         • Direct detection of CMV in blood by antigenemia or polymerase chain reaction (PCR)
      v. Prompt investigation of symptoms such as vomiting, diarrhea, leukopenia, and/of elevated LFTs are imperative, particularly in the following settings:
         • The early posttransplant phase
         • Intense immunosuppression to treat rejection
         • CMV mismatch: Recipient is CMV seronegative and received an allograft from a CMV seropositive donor
         • Recent discontinuation of antiviral therapy
      vi. Undetected CMV infection in the GI tract can lead to
         • Spread of the infection to other organs
         • Perforation of the affected viscus
         • Death
      vii. Potential treatment options:
         • Antiviral agents such as ganciclovir (Valcyte; Cytovene)
         • IVIG
   b. Herpes simplex virus (HSV)[96]:
      i. Typically presents as reactivation of a latent HSV infection.
      ii. Transplant patients previously infected with HSV have reactivation rates of up to 50%.
      iii. More common during the first 6 weeks posttransplant.

        iv. Common sites:
- Mild, ulcer-like lesions in the oral cavity and pharynx
- Esophagus

        v. Common symptoms:
- Dysphagia
- Odynophagia
- Orocutaneous lesions
- Fever and malaise

        vi. Prompt investigation of symptoms, particularly in patients who are undergoing intense immunosuppression therapy for rejection, is imperative:
- Untreated ulcers may lead to hemorrhage and esophageal perforation. Potential treatment options:
- Antiviral agents such as ganciclovir (Cytovene), valganciclovir (Valcyte), acyclovir (Zovirax) or valacyclovir (Valtrex)

5. Bacterial infections:
   a. Common pathogens:
      i. *Clostridium difficile*
      ii. *Yersinia enterocolitica*
   b. Bacterial infections may occur more often in recipients who have a concurrent CMV infection.
   c. Common presenting symptoms:
      i. Diarrhea
      ii. Abdominal tenderness
   d. *Helicobacter pylori*:
      i. May cause gastritis and peptic ulcer disease
      ii. Diagnosis:
- Endoscopy and biopsy
- Serum for *H. pylori*

      iii. Potential treatment options include a combination of omeprazole, amoxicillin, and clarithromycin for 10 days.

6. Fungal infections:
   a. Recipients are at greater risk during the first few months posttransplant.
   b. Risk factors for fungal infections include
      i. Antibiotic therapy
      ii. Corticosteroid therapy
      iii. Hyperglycemia
      iv. Indwelling catheters
      v. Recent treatment of rejection
   c. Candida infection is the most common posttransplant GI infection:
      i. Risk factors for candida infection in GI tract:
- Use of broad-spectrum antibiotics
- Recent rejection therapy, particularly with high-dose steroids or antibodies
- Liver transplant recipients: Roux-en-Y choledochojejunostomy

      ii. Symptoms:
- Oral thrush
- Esophagitis: odynophagia, dysphagia (with or without oral thrush), fever, heartburn, epigastric pain, and perforation

iii. Common pathogens:
- *Candida albicans*
- *Candida tropicalis*

d. Diagnosis of fungal infections:
  i. Histopathologic examination
  ii. Cultures
e. Fungal infections may occur concurrently with CMV infection.
f. Potential treatment options include clotrimazole (Mycelex) or nystatin (Mycostatin).

7. Parasitic infections (protozoal or metazoal):
a. Types of parasites:
  i. Protozoa (e.g., microsporidia)
  ii. Metazoa
  iii. Nematodes (e.g., *Strongyloides stercoralis*):
    - Endemic areas for *S. stercoralis*: West Indies, Far East.
    - Living donors with history of *S. stercoralis* infection should have stool and urine tested for larvae.

b. Potential treatment options for *Strongyloides stercoralis* infections include anthelmintic agents such as thiabendazole (Mintezol) or ivermectin (Stromectol)

C. Mucosal injury and perforation[90,97]:
1. Diarrhea:
a. Potential etiology:
  i. Infection
  ii. Immunosuppressive agents (e.g., tacrolimus [Prograf], mycophenolate mofetil [CellCept])
b. Management strategies if etiology is due to immunosuppressive agents:
  i. Reduction in total daily dose (as indicated)
  ii. Dose splitting (e.g., giving medication four times daily instead of two times daily)
  iii. Changing immunosuppressive agents, that is, changing CellCept to Myfortic

2. Ulceration:
a. Potential etiology:
  i. Stress associated with surgery.
  ii. Corticosteroid therapy:
    - Ironically, corticosteroid therapy may also mask symptoms of ulceration.
  iii. Medication-induced: (e.g., azathioprine [Imuran] or mycophenolate mofetil [CellCept]) slowing of intestinal cell turnover, which may lead to impairment of normal gastroduodenal cytoprotection.
  iv. Sequelae associated with posttransplant dialysis:
    - Increased secretion of gastric acid
    - Heparin-induced ulcers
    - Increased levels of histamine and gastrin
  v. Use of NSAIDs.
  vi. Use of calcium channel blockers (CCBs) lowers esophageal sphincter tone and can increase patients' risk for reflux.
b. Symptoms (may also be asymptomatic):
  i. Abdominal pain
  ii. GI bleeding

c. Prophylaxis:
  i. Purpose:
   - Decrease acid secretion
   - Protect GI mucosa from effects of excessive acid secretion
  ii. Types of preventive medications:
   - H_2 receptor antagonists, for example, famotidine (Pepcid) and ranitidine (Zantac)
   - Proton pump inhibitors: for example, omeprazole (Prilosec), pantoprazole (Protonix), and esomeprazole (Nexium)
   - Coating agents, for example, sucralfate (Carafate)
   - Prostaglandins, for example, misoprostol (Cytotec)
  iii. Potential problems with prophylactic medications:
   - H_2 receptor antagonists and coating agents may alter cyclosporine levels; monitor cyclosporine levels carefully.
   - H_2 receptor antagonists and proton pump inhibitors may
     - Decrease acid secretion and thus alter flora in the upper gut.
     - As a result, the patient may be at increased risk for colonization with pathogens; monitor patient for infections such as fungal esophagitis and *C. difficile* colitis.
   - Coating agents may block the absorption of cyclosporine; monitor cyclosporine levels carefully.
 d. Diagnosis: endoscopy
 e. Treatment options for bleeding ulcers:
  i. Injection of epinephrine or alcohol
  ii. Heater probes
  iii. Vicaps electrodes
  iv. Surgical intervention

D. Perforations[97,98]:
 1. Can occur in any segment of the GI tract.
 2. Etiology is typically multifactorial; perforations in lower GI tract have been associated with
  a. Diverticular disease or malignancy
  b. Medications that compromise the integrity of the GI tract (e.g., corticosteroids and other immunosuppressants, NSAIDs)
  c. Infections such as CMV and *H. pylori*
 3. Prevention:
  a. Steroid-sparing immunosuppression regimen
  b. Prompt treatment of infections
  c. Early diagnosis of GI complications
 4. Management: aggressive surgery

E. Biliary tract disease[74-76]:
 1. Types reported in literature:
  a. Biliary calculi:
   i. Transplant recipients are at high risk for biliary calculi.
   ii. Posttransplant cholecystectomy is often required; mortality rate associated with this procedure is high, particularly in heart and liver transplant recipients.[99]
  b. Dilated bile ducts

        c. Cholelithiasis

        d. Gallbladder hydrops

   2. Etiology:

        a. Multifactorial

        b. May be due to cyclosporine-induced cholestasis and decreased bile flow

F. Acute pancreatitis[100,101]:

   1. A rare but serious complication with published mortality rates that range from 50% to 100% in liver and kidney transplant recipients, respectively.

   2. Precipitating factors in liver and kidney transplant recipients include

        a. Liver transplantation:

           i.   Biliary manipulation

           ii. Alcohol use

           iii. Hepatitis B infection

           iv. Malignancy in area around pancreas

        b. Renal transplantation:

           i.   CMV infection

           ii. Hypercalcemia

           iii. Alcohol use

           iv. Cholelithiasis

   3. A possible association between azathioprine and acute pancreatitis has been reported.[102]

   4. Diagnosis:

        a. Computed tomography

   5. Treatment options:

        a. If drug induced, discontinuation of drug

        b. Fasting

        c. Administration of intravenous (IV) fluids

        d. Parenteral nutrition

        e. Surgery if indicated

G. Malignancy (also see section on Malignancy above):

   1. Posttransplant lymphoproliferative disease (PTLD):

        a. Diagnosis: endoscopy

        b. Late sequelae:

           i.   Perforation[39]

           ii. Obstruction

           iii. Bleeding

   2. Low-grade gastric mucosa-associated lymphoid tissue–type lymphomas:

           i.   Occurrence is rare.

           ii. May be associated with *H. pylori*.

H. GI complications in specific transplant populations (Table 6-22)[90,103,104]

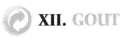

XII. GOUT

A. Pathogenesis of hyperuricemia[39,105,106]:

   1. Adverse effects of calcineurin inhibitors, particularly cyclosporine, on renal excretion of uric acid secondary to vasoconstriction in the renal vasculature; results in decreased secretion of uric acid into urine

   2. RI

   3. Volume contraction secondary to diuretic use

TABLE 6-22 Gastrointestinal Complications in Specific Transplant Population

Type of Transplant	Gastrointestinal Complication

Pancreas	Pancreatitis: Bladder drained procedure:
	• Reflux pancreatitis may cause acute inflammation of graft
	• May mimic rejection
	• Clinical manifestations: Pain; ↑ serum amylase levels
	• Potential etiology
	  – Reflux of urine through ampula and into pancreatic ducts
	  – In older males: hypertrophy of prostate gland
	• Management:
	  – Foley catheter
	  – Resolution of bladder dysfunction
	Pancreatitis: Enteric-drained procedure:
	• Gastrointestinal (GI) bleeding
	• Potential etiology:
	  – Preoperative anticoagulation
	  – Bleeding from duodenoenteric anastomosis

Liver	Types of GI complications:
	• Bile leakage
	• Biliary tract stricture
	• Cholangitis
	• Obstruction of ampullae
	• Biliary obstruction due to sludge or calculi
	Most common complications:
	• Biliary tract stricture
	• Bile leakage
	Clinical manifestations:
	• Vary with type of complication
	• Fever and jaundice are common
	• Biliary obstruction:
	  – ↑ bilirubin
	  – ↑ alkaline phosphatase
	  – ↑ gamma glutamyl transpeptidase (γ-GTP)
	Diagnosis:
	• Cholangiography (gold standard)
	• Endoscopic retrograde cholangiography (ERCP)
	• Magnetic resonance cholangiopancreatography (MRCP)
	Anastomotic leaks:
	• May occur in early postoperative period
	• May result in localized or general peritonitis
	• Monitor biliary output from drains and serum bilirubin
	Etiology of leaks:
	• Technical problems with surgery
	• Ischemic bile duct secondary to hepatic artery thrombosis
	Treatment:
	• Surgical revision
	• ERCP and sphincterotomy with stenting of the leak

(continued)

TABLE 6-22 Gastrointestinal Complications in Specific Transplant Population (*Continued*)

Type of Transplant	Gastrointestinal Complication
	Biliary casts and stones:
	• Long-standing T-tubes may lead to the formation of biliary casts and stones and subsequent biliary obstruction that may necessitate ERCP intervention
	Recurrence of hepatitis B—Prevention and treatment
	• Human hepatitis B immunoglobulin (HBIG) during anhepatic phase then daily for a period of time (e.g., 1 wk)
	• Subsequent HBIG dosing as needed to maintain adequate hepatitis B antibody titer
	• Lamivudine
	Recurrence of hepatitis C—Treatment
	• Interferon and ribavirin
Intestine	Most common GI complication: bleeding
	• May be due to rejection or infection
	• Requires prompt assessment via endoscopy and biopsy and initiation of appropriate treatment
	Leaks from anastomoses: more common
	• May occur during first postoperative week
	• Etiology: surgical technique, poor wound healing secondary to immunosuppression and/or malnutrition
	• Clinical presentation: peritonitis, abdominal distention, fever
	• Treatment: surgical revision and removal of peritoneal contaminants
	Hypermotility
	• Potential etiology
	– Alteration in baseline motility of denervated graft
	– Infection
	– Rejection (particularly in setting of fever and/or abdominal distention)
	• Management
	– Antidiarrheal agents, fiber
	– Treatment of rejection or infection
Kidney	Diverticular disease and colonic perforation
	• Increased incidence reported in kidney transplant recipients with polycystic kidney disease
Heart	Most common GI complications:
	• Diarrhea: most common
	• Bleeding, intestinal perforation—higher risk than other solid organ transplants
	• Heartburn/dyspepsia, constipation, nausea, vomiting, reflux anorexia—lower risk.
	– Many of these patients could be helped by adjusting/changing immune suppression medications

From Agarwal S, Mayer L. Diagnosis and treatment of gastrointestinal disorders in patients with primary immunodeficiency. *Clin Gastroenterol Hepatol.* 2013;11(9):1050–1063; Grass F, Schafer M, Cristaudi A, et al. Incidence and risk factors of abdominal complications after lung transplantation. *World J Surg.* 2015;39(9):2274–2281; Ko GY, Sung KB. Section 11: radiological intervention approaches to biliary complications after living donor liver transplantation. *Transplantation.* 2014;97(suppl 8):S43–S46.

B. Diagnosis:
1. Aspiration of affected joint is required for definitive diagnosis.
   a. Polymorphonuclear leukocytes contain uric acid crystals.

C. Treatment options[106]:
1. Colchicine (Colcryx):
   a. Is given during an acute gout attack to decrease or stop inflammation
   b. May cause GI toxicity
   c. May be administered on an alternate day schedule
2. Glucocorticoids:
   a. Prednisone: oral bolus followed by gradual taper
   b. Adrenocorticotrophic hormone (ACTH)
3. Allopurinol (Zyloprim):
   a. An older xanthine oxidase inhibitor that decreases the synthesis of uric acid and is given only after an acute gout attack has subsided.
   b. Allergic reactions may occur with chronic use:
      i. Note: Rarely given in conjunction with azathioprine (Imuran)
         • Allopurinol potentiates myelosuppression associated with azathioprine (Imuran) by inhibiting the metabolism of the active metabolite of azathioprine (mercaptopurine); this can result in mercaptopurine toxicity.
         • Concurrent administration of allopurinol and azathioprine requires:
            ○ Reduction in azathioprine dose by 75%
            ○ Decrease in the initial allopurinol dose to 50 mg daily
            ○ Careful monitoring of white blood cell count
   c. If allopurinol is to be used, mycophenolate mofetil (CellCept) is often substituted for azathioprine to decrease the risk of leukopenia.
4. Febuxostat (Uloric) is a new–nonpurine selective xanthine oxidase inhibitor that is well tolerated in transplant patients, even within the setting of moderate renal impairment. This medication is often used instead of allopurinol and has no known drug interactions with transplant medications.[107]
5. NSAIDs should be avoided as they may precipitate RI.

 XIII. GINGIVAL HYPERPLASIA

A. Overview[108]:
1. Definition: excessive proliferation of gingival tissue
2. Clinical presentation:
   a. Can affect labial, buccal, palatal, and lingual tissues in all areas of mouth[109,110]
   b. Hyperplasia typically more severe in the anterior maxillary and mandibular regions of the mouth
   c. Overgrowth of soft tissue begins between the teeth and spreads in all directions:
      i. Tissue becomes thick and lobulated.
      ii. Overgrowth may encroach upon the tooth surface, including the chewing surface.
3. Incidence: average incidence in solid organ transplant recipients varies with
   a. Genetic factors
   b. Duration of drug therapy (incidence increases with length of therapy)
   c. Drug dose (higher incidence with higher drug doses)
   d. Immunosuppressant serum drug levels
   e. Salivary concentrations
   f. Oral hygiene

      g. Age (incidence tends to be higher in older patients)

      h. Gender (higher incidence in males)

B. Etiology: known side effect of certain mediations:

   1. Major causative agents[111,112]:

      a. Cyclosporine

      b. CCBs (e.g., amlodipine [Norvasc], diltiazem [Cardizem, felodipine [Plendil], nicardipine [Cardene], nifedipine [Procardia], verapamil [Calan]):

         i. CCBs in combination with cyclosporine increases risk for cyclosporine toxicity and may increase drug levels.

      c. Anticonvulsants (e.g., phenytoin [Dilantin])

C. Pathophysiology[110]:

   1. The mechanism by which hyperplasia is localized in the gingiva, as opposed to other tissues, is unknown.

   2. Proposed mechanisms include higher concentration of drugs (e.g., cyclosporine, CCBs, phenytoin) in gingival tissues directly through gingival blood supply or from the oral cavity itself.

   3. Drug-mediated expression of cytokines and growth factors may affect the growth and function of gingival fibroblasts and epithelial cells.

D. Potential sequelae of gingival hyperplasia:

   1. Interference with normal oral function:

      a. In certain patients, may lead to alveolar bone loss and tooth loss

   2. Difficulty in maintaining oral hygiene with subsequent bacterial overgrowth and secondary inflammatory response

   3. Altered appearance; poor self-image

   4. Noncompliance with medical therapy

E. Treatment options[110,113,114]:

   1. Plaque control

   2. Removal of local irritants

   3. Periodontal surgery:

      a. As with any dental cleaning or procedure, heart transplant recipients with cardiac valvulopathy require preprocedure dental prophylaxis per American Heart Association guidelines (Table 6-23).[113]

      b. Depending upon the extent of the surgery, postprocedure antibiotics may also be indicated.

   4. Laser therapy

   5. Changing immunosuppression regimen (e.g., from cyclosporine to tacrolimus)

TABLE 6-23 Preprocedure Dental Prophylaxis in the Transplant Recipient

Standard adult prophylaxis	Amoxicillin 2 g orally 30–60 min before procedure
If allergic to amoxicillin, ampicillin, or penicillin	Clindamycin 600 mg orally 30–60 min before procedure
	OR
	Cephalexin 2 g orally 30–60 min before procedure
	OR
	Azithromycin or clarithromycin 500 mg orally 30–60 min before procedure

Indicated for patients with the "highest risk for infective endocarditis:" postcardiac transplant *with* posttransplant prosthetic valves or tissue repair valves/rings, previous endocarditis, congenital heart disease.
Adapted from 2008 AHA Prevention of Infective (Bacterial) Endocarditis recommendations.
From American Heart Association. *Endocarditis Prophylaxis Information.* Available at http://www.heart.org/idc/groups/heart-public@ wcm/@hcm/documents/downloadable/ucm_307684/pdf. Accessed March 10, 2015.

F. Prevention:
1. Pretransplant:
   a. Optimization of oral hygiene
   b. Regular dental examinations
   c. Periodontal prophylaxis as indicated
   d. Treatment of dental disease
2. Posttransplant:
   a. Meticulous oral hygiene
   b. Regular dental examinations
   c. Removal of plaque and calculus deposits

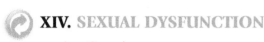

XIV. SEXUAL DYSFUNCTION

A. Overview:
1. Definition of sexual health:
   a. WHO definition of sexual health[115]:
      i. Sexual health is defined as a state of physical, emotional, mental and social well-being in relation to sexuality. It is not simply the absence of disease, dysfunction or illness. Sexual health requires a positive and respectful approach to both sexuality and sexual relationships, as well as the possibility of having pleasurable and safe sexual experiences, free of coercion, discrimination and violence. For sexual health to be attained and maintained, the sexual rights of all persons must be respected, protected and fulfilled.
      ii. Medical definition of erectile dysfunction (ED) as a hemodynamic condition that relies on the intactness of neurological, vascular, endocrinological, tissutal (corpus cavernosuma), psychological and relational factors. Any imbalance or disease state with these systems can lead to ED.[116]

B. Etiologic factors associated with sexual dysfunction[115,117,118]:
1. Pretransplant factors: sexual dysfunction associated with
   a. Comorbidities:
      i. Aging
   b. Medical conditions:
      i. Chronic debilitating illness such as:
         • Renal failure and dialysis
         • Hepatic failure
         • Alcohol abuse
   c. Endocrine disorders:
      i. DM
      ii. Hyperthyroidism or hypothyroidism
      iii. Hypogonadism
   d. Cardiovascular disease:
      i. Arteriosclerosis
      ii. Peripheral vascular disease
      iii. Low cardiac output (CO)
   e. Neurologic disorders:
      i. Peripheral neuropathy
      ii. Nerve injury secondary to prostate surgery
      iii. Stroke

  f. Chronic fatigue
  g. Loss of libido
  h. Medications:
     i. Types of pharmacologically induced sexual dysfunction:
         • Erectile dysfunction
         • Ejaculatory disorder
         • Loss of libido
         • Orgasmic disorder
         • Priapism
     ii. Medications associated with sexual dysfunction (Table 6-24)[117,118]
  2. Posttransplant factors:
     a. Residual pretransplant fears about sexual activity, particularly in heart transplant recipients
     b. Side effects of medications:
        i. Immunosuppressive agents:
            • Calcineurin inhibitors and mTOR inhibitors can lower testosterone levels, which can lead to loss of libido and erectile dysfunction. These levels should be monitored.
        ii. Medications associated with erectile dysfunction (Table 6-24)[117,118]
     c. Loss of libido
     d. Irregular menstrual cycles
     e. Onset of menopause
     f. Vaginal dryness secondary to medications, low estrogen levels, or vascular damage due to poorly controlled DM
     g. Vaginal yeast infections due to elevated blood glucose levels
     h. Fear of infection and pregnancy
     i. Loss of intimacy
     j. Poor body image secondary to
        i.   Weight gain
        ii. Acne
        iii. Hirsutism
        iv. Hair loss
        v.   Surgical scars
     k. Altered roles and relationships
     l. Depression
     m. Partner's fears about safety of resuming sexual activity

C. Treatment options following thorough history and physical examination:
  1. Manipulation of medication regimen as indicated and tolerated
  2. Referral to urology, gynecology, or mental health provider as indicated
  3. Medications to treat erectile dysfunction (e.g., phosphodiesterase 5 [PDE-5] inhibitors such as sildenafil [Viagra, Revatio], vardenafil [Levitra], or tadalafil [Cialis]) have been used in selected transplant recipients.[118]
     a. Approximately 60% of transplant recipients responded to sildenafil treatment if taken correctly:
        i. Take 30 to 60 minutes prior to sexual activity
        ii. Do not take on a full stomach
     b. Metabolism of sildenafil:
        i. Metabolized via the same pathway as cyclosporine (the cytochrome P450 isozyme 3A4 enzymatic pathway)
     c. PDE-5 inhibitors in setting of CVD:
        i. Many transplant recipients have CVD.

TABLE 6-24 **Medications Associated with Sexual Dysfunction**

Category	Medication
Antihypertensive agents	β-Blockers
	Calcium channel blockers
	α-Adrenoceptor antagonists
	ACE inhibitors
	Central acting: Clonidine, Methyldopa
	Hydralazine
	Thiazide diuretics
	Loop diuretics
	Spironolactone
Psychotherapeutic agents	Antidepressants
	Heterocyclic agents
	MAOIs
	SSRIs
	Tricyclic antidepressants
	Lithium carbonate
	Neuroleptics
	Thioridazine
	Anxiolytics
	Clonazepam, Valium
H_2-antagonists	Cimetidine
Anticonvulsants	Phenytoin
	Carbamazepine
	Phenobarbital
Antiparkinson	Primidone
Antispasmodic	Levodopa (Sinemet)
	Cyclobenzaprine (Flexeril)
Lipid-lowering agents	Fibrates
	Statins
5-α-Reductase inhibitor	Finasteride
Prostate cancer	Leuprolide (Lupon)
Drugs of abuse	Nicotine
	Alcohol
	Anabolic steroids
	Heroin, cocaine
	Marijuana
	Amphetamines
	Barbiturates, opiates, methadone

ACE, angiotensin-converting enzyme; MAOI, monoamine oxidase inhibitors; SSRI, selective serotonin reuptake inhibitors.
From Nehra A, Jackson G, et al. The Princeton III Consensus recommendations for the management of erectile dysfunction and cardiovascular disease. *Mayo Clin Proc.* 2012;87(8):766–778; Pastuszak AW. Current diagnosis and management of erectile dysfunction. *Curr Sex Health Rep.* 2014;6(3):164–176.

TABLE 6-25 Cardiovascular Risk Stratification and Recommendations for Treatment with PDE-5 Inhibitors for General Population

Level of Risk	Description	Recommendation
Low	Asymptomatic with less than three major risk factors for CAD	Can be treated with PDE-5 inhibitor without further CV diagnostic evaluation
	Controlled hypertension with ≥1 antihypertensive medication	
	Mild, stable angina (not treated with nitrates)	*Exception*: Patients taking nitrates in any form
	Successful coronary revascularization (3–4 wk)	
	Uncomplicated post-MI (>6–8 wk), no exercise-induced ischemia	
	Mild valvular disease	Require noninvasive evaluation before treatment with PDE-5 inhibitor
	LV dysfunction/CHF (NYHA Class I)	
Intermediate	Asymptomatic, ≥3 major risk factors for CAD, excluding gender	Require further cardiac testing (stress test) before restratification into low- or high-risk category
	Moderate, stable angina (not treated with nitrates)	
	Recent MI (>2 wk and <6 wk); if patient underwent revascularization post-MI; do stress test to assess risk	
	Asymptomatic LV dysfunction/CHF (NYHA Class II); EF <40%	
	Noncardiac sequelae of atherosclerotic disease (peripheral arterial disease, history of stroke or TIAs)	
High	Unstable or refractory angina	Require cardiac assessment and treatment and must be deemed "stable" before considering use of PDE-5 inhibitors and sexual activity
	Uncontrolled hypertension	
	LV disease/CHF (NYHA Class III/IV)	
	Recent MI (<2 wk)	
	High-risk arrhythmias	
	Obstructive hypertrophic cardiomyopathy	
	Moderate/severe valvular disease, particularly AS	
Unknown	Men with ED and no known CVD	If multiple risk factors present:
	• Use RF to assess need for formal CV evaluation	Require noninvasive evaluation before treatment with PDE-5 inhibitor
	• RF include: age <50, presence of abdominal obesity, HTN, dyslipidemia, DM, OSA, family history of CVD (father age <55 or mother age <65), lifestyle factors (high caloric with excess fat, inactivity, excessive ETOH use, smoking)	*may use Framingham risk score to aid stratification of risk.*

AS, aortic stenosis; CAD, coronary artery disease; CHF, congestive heart failure; CV, cardiovascular; CVD, cardiovascular disease; LV, left ventricular; MI, myocardial infarction; NYHA, New York Heart Association; PVD, peripheral vascular disease; TIA, transient ischemic attack; RF, risk factors; HTN, hypertension; DM, diabetes mellitus; OSA, obstructive sleep apnea; ETOH, alcohol. Adapted from Nehra A, Jackson G, et al. The Princeton III Consensus recommendations for the management of erectile dysfunction and cardiovascular disease. *Mayo Clin Proc.* 2012;87(8):766–778.

    ii. For the general population, see Table 6-25[117] for cardiovascular risk stratification and recommendations for treatment with PDE-5 inhibitors.

- Need to ensure each man's CV health will tolerate the physical demands of sexual activity prior to starting treatment for ED.
- Sexual activity is equal to walking 1 mile on a level surface in 20 minutes or briskly climbing two flights of stairs in 10 seconds.[117]

   iii. Caution patient against:
- Taking any nitrate medications within 24 hours of a PDE-5 inhibitor due to risk of severe hypotension, syncope or myocardial infarction
- Taking any alpha-blocker (tamsulosin [Flomax]) within 4 hours of a PDE-5 inhibitor due to hypotension

4. Patient education[117,118]:
   a. Clinicians may be reluctant to discuss sexual issues with patients and their partners. It is important to identify and resolve potential barriers such as:
      i. Viewing topic as irrelevant to nursing practice
      ii. Embarrassment
      iii. Lack of knowledge
      iv. Lack of time
      v. Lack of privacy
      vi. Fear of offending patient and/or partner
   b. Create an environment in which patients and their partners feel comfortable in discussing sexual concerns.
   c. Convey to patients and their partners that posttransplant sexual dysfunction is common.
5. Extended PLISSIT Model[119-121]:
   a. Four levels of nursing interventions (Table 6-26)[119-121]
   b. Permission-giving is a core aspect of each level:
      i. At each level, nurses should begin with reflection and review.
      ii. Seek the patient's perspective by asking questions such as[119 (p. 40)]:
         - "What do you think about that?"

TABLE 6-26 Extended PLISSIT Model: Levels of Nursing Interventions

Level		Description	Example
P	Permission	Inform patient and partner that sexual concerns are an important component of the nursing assessment Introduce topic and give patient permission to think about the impact of his or her illness/transplant on his or her sexuality	"Transplant recipients often experience sexual problems such as a loss of desire. What has been your experience?" "Tell me about any sexual changes you have experienced since your transplant"
LI	Limited information	Provide information about the impact of transplant on sexuality and the effects of medications on sexual function	Discuss the sexual side effects of patient's medications Provide limited educational materials.
SS	Specific suggestions	Employ problem-solving approach; suggest specific solutions to patient's particular problem. Address all aspects of sexuality rather than just sexual behavior	Use of lubricants for discomfort or pain associated with intercourse If a female transplant recipient is concerned about her femininity and body image, discuss what femininity means to her and identify specific strategies to enhance femininity
IT	Intensive therapy	Refer patients to additional resources as indicated	Individuals who require psychosexual counseling should be referred to a mental health provider

From Annon J. The PLISSIT model: a proposed conceptual scheme for the behavioral treatment of sexual problems. *J Sex Educ.* 1976;2:1–15; Davis S, Taylor B. From PLISSIT to Ex-PLISSIT. In: Davis S, eds. *Rehabilitation: The Use of Theories and Models in Practice.* Edinburgh, UK: Elsevier; 2006; Taylor B, Davis S. Using the Extended PLISSIT model to address sexual healthcare needs. *Nurs Stand.* 2006;21:35–40.

- "Are there any other things that you might have thought of?"
- "What have we not covered fully?"

iii. This review process further validates permission-giving, which in turn encourages patients/partners to further discuss problems and concerns.

iv. At each level, review interactions with patients/partners.

XV. NEUROCOGNITIVE IMPAIRMENT

A. Overview:
1. Neurocognitive function is a dynamic process that involves the ability to perceive, retain, reason, and flexibly respond to information in the environment.
2. Four major classes of neurocognitive function:
   a. Receptive functions: ability to select, acquire, integrate, and classify information
   b. Memory and learning: ability to store and retrieve information
   c. Thinking: ability to mentally organize and reorganize information
   d. Expressive functions: ability to communicate or act upon information
3. Each class is distinct but the functions are interdependent.
4. Neurocognitive impairment is a deficit or dysfunction in one or more of the four neurocognitive functions.
5. Biological, psychological, and social factors affect both the pattern and severity of neurocognitive impairment.
6. Neurocognitive function can be measured using the Montreal Cognitive Assessment Battery (MoCA) found at http://www.mocatest.org.[122]
7. In-hospital delirium can be measured using the Confusion Assessment Method (CAM) found at http://www.hospitalelderlifeprogram.org/delirium-instruments.

B. Pretransplant neurocognitive impairment:
1. Occurs in a significant number of patients with end-stage organ disease
2. Examples of organ-specific etiologic factors:
   a. End-stage renal disease: uremia, hyperphosphatemia, and metabolic abnormalities
   b. End-stage heart disease: decreased CO
   c. End-stage lung disease: hypoxia
   d. End-stage liver disease: encephalopathy, metabolic abnormalities, and nutritional deficits

C. Posttransplant neurocognitive impairment:
1. The precise prevalence of neurocognitive impairment among transplant recipients is unknown; however, subsets of patients in each transplant population have significant posttransplant neurocognitive dysfunction.
2. Etiologic factors:
   a. Medications[123]:
      i. Immunosuppressive agents
      ii. Antimicrobial agents:
         - Antivirals
         - Antifungal agents
         - Antibiotics
   b. Iatrogenic factors: for example, effects of cardiopulmonary bypass

       c. Comorbidities such as
         i.   Infections
         ii. Severe illness
         iii. Prolonged hospitalizations
         iv. Cerebrovascular events
         v.   Psychiatric illness
         vi. Dehydration
       d. Substance abuse
       e. Acute rejection

D. Medications:
   1. Immunosuppressants:
      a. Can cause neurocognitive impairment through
         i.   Direct effects on central nervous system (CNS)
         ii. Indirect effects through
             • Infections that involve CNS
             • Neoplasms that cause neurological impairment
      b. Neurotoxicity can occur in setting of immunosuppressant blood levels within the therapeutic range.
      c. Neuropsychiatric side effects of common immunosuppressive agents (Table 6-27).[123]
   2. Side effects of antimicrobial agents are listed in the following tables[123]:
      a. Antiviral agents (Table 6-28)[123]
      b. Antifungal agents (Table 6-29)
      c. Antibacterial agents (Table 6-30)

TABLE 6-27 Neuropsychiatric Side Effects of Common Immunosuppressive Agents

Medication	Reported Neuropsychiatric Side Effects	Comments
Cyclosporine	Fine tremors	40%–60% of patients on CNI's experience side effects.
	Confusion	
	Paresthesias	Symptoms are typically mild in most patients but may be more pronounced in liver transplant recipients due to advanced liver insufficiency and subsequent blood-brain barrier abnormalities
	Hyperesthesias/dysasthesias	
	Headache	
	Insomnia	
	restlessness	Predisposing factors:
	Anxiety/agitation	Hypomagnesemia
	Blurred vision	Hypocholesterolemia <120 mg/dL)
	Apathy	High-dose corticosteroids
	Delirium	Aluminium overload
	Vivid dreams	Fever
	Photophobia	Infection
	Seizures	Intravenous administration of cyclosporine
	Stupor/coma	Advanced liver failure
	Psychosis	Malignant hypertension
	Encephalopathy	Renal insufficiency
	Sensorimotor disturbances	Drug interactions that ↑ cyclosporine levels
	Cerebrovascular events	

(continued)

TABLE 6-27 **Neuropsychiatric Side Effects of Common Immunosuppressive Agents** (*Continued*)

Medication	Reported Neuropsychiatric Side Effects	Comments
Tacrolimus	Tremulousness Sleep disturbance Restlessness Headache Dysesthesia Mood changes Visual symptoms Vivid dreams/nightmares	Predisposing factors: Intravenous administration of tacrolimus Drug interactions that ↑ tacrolimus levels
Corticosteroids	Cognitive (↓memory, concentration Attention, mental speed and easily distracted) Affective (anxiety, depression, mania, labile emotions) Psychotic (Obsessional thoughts, Hallucinations, delirium) Behavioral (Irritability, restless, aggressive) Encephalopathy	Females may be at higher risk for side effects. Side effects may be dose related (side effects more severe with dose >40 mg/d) Alternate day dosing may ↓ risk and severity of side effects Dose must be gradually tapered in order to avoid rebound psychiatric symptoms or relapse in medical condition Side effects may occur months after continuous treatment; however, most side effects occur within first 3 wk
Mycophenolate Mofetil Azathioprine	Tremor Insomnia Anxiety Depression Hypertonia Paraesthesia Somnolence None reported AA AA a	Adverse effects are higher with dose of 3 g/d

From Heinrich TW, Marcangelo M. Psychiatric issues in solid organ transplantation. *Harv Rev Psychiatry.* 2009;17:398–406.

E. Infections:

1. Polymicrobial and multiorgan infections are common in transplant recipients.
2. CNS infections are particularly serious.
    a. CNS infections are difficult to treat due to reduced penetration of antimicrobial agents.
    b. The CNS does not tolerate inflammation or pressure effects.
    c. The CNS has minimal capacity for regeneration.
    d. Progressive multifocal leukoencephalopathy is a rare infection in the brain caused by from the JC virus.
        i.   Transplant patients are more likely to get this disease due to the weakened immune system.
        ii. Patients with this disease have symptoms similar to stroke: trouble speaking, visual changes, and decline in mental function and balance.

TABLE 6-28 Antiviral Agents

Medication	Reported Neuropsychiatric Side Effects	Comments
Acyclovir	Tremor/myoclonus Confusion Agitation Lethargy Hallucinations Clouding of consciousness Extrapyramidal symptoms Unilateral focal symptoms Seizures Psychotic depression	Symptoms typically develop within first 24 to 72 h of treatment. Symptoms are typically reversible. Renal failure is associated with ↑ risk of neurotoxicity.
Ganciclovir	Nightmares Visual hallucinations Agitation Delirium Headache	Renal insufficiency is a risk factor for side effects. Reduce dose in setting of renal insufficiency. Side effects may occur immediately or 2 wk after administration has been started. Side effects typically resolve after dose reduction or stopping medication. For amelioration of side effects: temporarily stop medication and then reintroduce at a lower dose.
Alpha-Interferon	Delirium Anxiety Irritability Depression with affective lability Initial dose associated with: Headache Lethargy ↓ Concentration Insomnia Fatigue-induced psychomotor retardation and dulled cognition	Used in liver transplant population in setting of chronic hepatitis C infection Side effects are dose related

From Heinrich TW, Marcangelo M. Psychiatric issues in solid organ transplantation. *Harv Rev Psychiatry*. 2009;17:398–406.

TABLE 6-29 Antifungal Agents

Medication	Reported Neuropsychiatric Side Effects	Comments
Amphotericin	Delirium Confusion Restlessness Headache Tremor	Does not cross blood-brain barrier; therefore, central nervous system (CNS) toxicity is low CNS toxicity associated with intrathecal administration
Metronidazole	Sensory peripheral neuropathy Ataxia Seizures Hallucinations Depression Agitation	Peripheral neuropathy reversed by discontinuing medication Side effect: Metallic taste

From Heinrich TW, Marcangelo M. Psychiatric issues in solid organ transplantation. *Harv Rev Psychiatry*. 2009;17:398–406.

TABLE 6-30 Antibacterial Agents

Medication	Reported Neuropsychiatric Side Effects	Comments
Penicillins Cephalosporins	Seizures Delirium	Side effects ↑ in setting of renal insufficiency
Quinolones	Ciprofloxacin: visual hallucinations, disorientation, impaired thinking	Side effects typically uncommon but ↑ when nonsteroidal anti-inflammatory agents are administered
Aminoglycosides	Delirium Neuromuscular blockade: hypoactive deep tendon reflexes, flaccid paralysis, mydriasis Gentamicin: delirium, particularly with intrathecal administration	Side effects ↑ in setting of renal insufficiency

From Heinrich TW, Marcangelo M. Psychiatric issues in solid organ transplantation. *Harv Rev Psychiatry.* 2009;17:398–406.

   iii. The best treatment is stopping immune suppression if possible.
   iv. This disease carries a 30% to 50% risk of mortality.
   v. Hexadecyloxypropyl-cidofovir (CMX001) is currently under investigation by the National Institutes of Health as a possible treatment option.[124]

 F. Stroke: Etiology:
   1. Angioinvasive infections:
    a. Invade intracranial vessels directly
    b. Result in in situ thrombosis or hemorrhage
   2. Vasculitis:
    a. Example: intracranial extension of varicella zoster along trigeminovascular network
   3. Endocarditis with subsequent cerebral embolization:
    a. Example: virulent organisms (*Aspergillus;* pseudomonas) associated with friable vegetation
   4. Accelerated atherosclerotic disease associated with DM, hypertension, or hypercholesterolemia

 G. Acute rejection:
   1. Can precipitate encephalopathy
   2. Immunosuppressant levels must be carefully monitored.
    a. Rejection can lead to decreased drug clearance.
    b. Decreased drug clearance can lead to toxic immunosuppression levels even with standard doses.

 H. Potential indications of neurocognitive impairment:
   1. Impairment in attention/memory/processing speed:
    a. Inability to focus and resist distractions
    b. Slowness in learning new information
    c. Difficulty in remembering critical information
    d. Failure to comprehend multistep directions
    e. Inability to carry out instructions
   2. Frontal/executive deficits:
    a. Failure to generalize information to new situations
    b. Mental inflexibility
    c. Deficient self-awareness about cognitive problems
    d. Lack of initiation when a problem is recognized

I. Potential consequences of unrecognized neurocognitive impairment:
   1. Noncompliance with medical regimen
   2. Graft rejection
   3. Infections
   4. Failure to inform health care clinicians about important symptoms and side effects
   5. Depression/anxiety
   6. Feelings of loss of control
   7. Conflict between patient and staff

J. Assessment and treatment of neurocognitive impairment:
   1. Formal neurocognitive assessment (consider using MoCA) to[122]
      a. Identify presence of cognitive impairment and potential etiology
      b. Establish differential diagnosis
      c. Determine impact of neurocognitive impairment on patient's ability to cope with demands of transplant process
      d. Prevent negative outcomes by
         i. Teaching patient compensatory strategies
         ii. Modifying demands placed on patient
      e. Intervene as indicated to
         i. Ameliorate negative effects of previously unrecognized neurocognitive impairment
         ii. Address newly developed neurocognitive problems
         iii. Refer patient to formal rehabilitation program

K. Strategies to manage neurocognitive impairment:
   1. Optimize organization, structure, and ease of use of all educational materials.
   2. Begin transplant teaching early in transplant process.
      a. Break information up into small, manageable units.
      b. Provide short educational sessions.
      c. Use multimodal cues (words, colors, symbols) as indicated.
      d. Individualize teaching according to patient's needs.
   3. Strategies for specific disorders:
      a. Memory disorders:
         i. Provide patient with log book for medication list and other important medical information.
         ii. Provide pill dispensers to minimize demands on memory.
         iii. Develop alarm system to cue patient to perform daily tasks.
         iv. Provide deliberate reminders for nonroutine tasks (via postcards, email, phone calls).
         v. Involve patient's family and friends.
      b. Executive disorders:
         i. Don't expect patient to spontaneously report critical information; deliberately check for important symptoms.
         ii. Enlist the assistance of another person to provide cues and directions for the patient.
   4. For all intervention and prevention strategies:
      a. Verify the effectiveness of these strategies with the patient/family member.
      b. Ask patient/family members what works best for them.
      c. Each transplant team member must implement and reinforce strategies.

XVI. SUMMARY: STRATEGIES TO PREVENT LONG-TERM COMPLICATIONS[26,33,57,85]

A. Tailor immunosuppression therapy to decrease the risk of CVD, cancer, and infection.

1. Maintain patient on minimum amount of immunosuppression that is needed to prevent acute rejection.
   a. Consider individual recipient's risk factors.
      i. Recipients who *may* require more immunosuppression:
         - Recipients of prior transplants
         - Younger recipients
         - African American recipients
         - Female recipients, particularly those who have had one or more pregnancies
         - Recipients with history of severe vascular rejection
         - Recipients with history of more than one acute rejection episode
         - Kidney transplant recipients with more than one major histocompatibility mismatch
      ii. Recipients who *may* require less immunosuppression:
         - De novo transplant recipients
         - Older recipients
         - White recipients
         - Male recipients
         - Recipients with history of no or mild cellular rejection
         - Recipients with no or only one acute rejection episodes
         - Kidney transplant recipients with zero major histocompatibility mismatches
2. Select the most effective and least toxic immunosuppressants.
3. Adapt immunosuppression regimen to patient's risk profile and/or most bothersome adverse side effects; for example:
   a. In patients with severe hyperlipidemia: avoid use of or minimize dose of cyclosporine (Sandimmune) or cyclosporine modified (Neoral, Gengraf), tacrolimus (Prograf, Astagraf XL), prednisone, or sirolimus (Rapamune).
   b. In patients with hypertension: reduce dose of cyclosporine, tacrolimus or prednisone as indicated and tolerated.
   c. In patients with DM: wean or minimize prednisone dose; change patient from tacrolimus (Prograf, Astagraf XL) to cyclosporine.[26]
   d. In patients with diarrhea: consider changing mycophenolate mofetil (CellCept) to mycophenolate acid (Myfortic); for intolerable diarrhea, consider changing sirolimus (Rapamune) to another medication.

B. Adopt strategies to prevent medication nonadherence.

1. Use medications that can be dosed once daily whenever possible.
2. Maintain regular contact with patients and members of their support system:
   a. Ask patients about potential barriers to medication adherence such as side effects and financial constraints.
   b. Collaborate with interdisciplinary team members to develop solutions for financial problems associated with the cost of medications.
3. Educate patients and family members.

    4. Help patients to develop a system that reminds them to take their medications.

    5. Identify patients who are at high risk for nonadherence.

    6. Develop targeted risk factor interventions for patients who are at high risk for nonadherence.

C. Monitor renal function at regular intervals.

    1. Identify patients at risk for RI.

    2. Develop targeted interventions.

D. Monitor graft function closely for acute and chronic rejection.

    1. Biopsies and lab work per protocol.

    2. Monitor patient for signs and symptoms of rejection.

E. Treat hyperlipidemia aggressively:

    1. Assess lipid profile.

       a. Elevated total cholesterol levels are typically associated with elevated LDL cholesterol and triglycerides.

       b. In the general population, treatment of elevated LDL levels has been shown to decrease the risk for ischemic events and reduce mortality.

    2. Treat specific dyslipidemia(s).

    3. Monitor patient's response with regard to

       a. Improvement in lipid profile

       b. Side effects of medications

F. Treat hypertension aggressively.

    1. Assess patient's risk factors.

    2. Monitor response to antihypertensive therapy with regard to

       a. BP

       b. Side effects of antihypertensive agents

G. Encourage a healthy lifestyle.

    1. Regular aerobic exercise to

       a. Optimize weight

       b. Counteract effects of corticosteroid therapy

       c. Improve mood state

    2. Smoking cessation

    3. Heart-healthy diet:

       a. The AHA/ACC diet and exercise guidelines are summarized in Table 6-31.[57,85,125]

H. Screen for cancer routinely

I. Prevent infection:

    1. Infection prophylaxis during periods of antirejection therapy

    2. Annual influenza vaccination unless otherwise contraindicated

    3. Strict control of blood glucose levels in patients with DM

J. Preserve bone health:

    1. Screen for decreased bone mineral density with DEXA scan of the lumbar spine and hip:

       a. Baseline (pretransplantation)

       b. Six months posttransplant

       c. Every 12 or 24 months thereafter to assess bone health

       d. Recheck 6 months after initiating a new drug treatment to assess effectiveness

TABLE 6-31 **Therapeutic Lifestyle Changes—Diet and Exercise**

Nutrient	Recommended Intake Goals
Saturated fat	5%–6% of total calories
Polyunsaturated fat	7% of total calories
Monounsaturated fat	10% of total calories
Total fat	<30% of total calories
Carbohydrate	50%–60% of total calories
Fiber	20–30 g/d
Protein	15%–18% of total calories
Total calories	Balance energy intake and expenditure to maintain desirable body weight or prevent weight gain
Exercise	Adults 18–65: 150 min of moderate intensity of 75 min of high-intensity exercise per week and 2 d of muscle strengthening exercise per week
	Adults >65: 150 min of any activity a week, based on ability. Focus on maintaining balance, strength, and endurance

Expert panel recommends: Encouraging a dietary pattern that emphasizes intake of fruits, vegetables, and whole grains; low-fat dairy products, poultry, fish, legumes, nontropical vegetable oils, and nuts; and limiting intake of sweets, sugar-sweetened beverages, and red meats.
This dietary pattern can be adapted to the appropriate calorie requirements if weight loss/gain is the goal, for personal and cultural food preferences, and for medical conditions: diabetes, gout, renal disease, etc.
Adapted from Eckel RH, Jakicic JM, Anderson JL, Haperin JL, et al. 2013 AHA/ACC guideline on lifestyle management to reduce cardiovascular risk. *J Am Coll Cardiol.* 2014;63(25-PA):2960–2984.
From American Diabetes Association. Diagnosis and classification of diabetes mellitus. *Diabetes Care.* 2013;36(suppl 1):S67–S74; Wong G, Chapman JR, Craig JC. Cancer screening in renal transplant recipients: what is the evidence. *Clin J Am Soc Nephrol.* 2008;3(suppl 2):S87–S100.

2. Prevent or treat osteopenia/osteoporosis:
   a. Calcium and vitamin D supplements
   b. Bisphosphonates to reverse bone loss and increase bone mass
   c. Calcitonin (Miacalcin nasal)
   d. Denosumab (Prolia)
   e. Hormone replacement therapy in carefully selected patients
   f. Exercise

REFERENCES

1. Kasiske BL, Zeier MG, Chapman JR, et al. KIDGO clinical practice guideline for the care of kidney transplant recipients: a summary. *Kidney Int.* 2010;77(4):299–311.
2. Gillis KA, Patek RK, Jardine AG. Cardiovascular complications after transplantation: treatment options in solid organ recipients. *Transplant Rev.* 2014;28(2):47–55.
3. U.S. Renal Data System (USRDS). *Annual Data Report: Atlas of Chronic Kidney Disease and End-Stage Renal Disease in the United States.* Bethesda, MD: National Institutes of Health, National Institute of Diabetes and Digestive and Kidney Diseases; 2013.
4. Glicklish D, Vohra P. Cardiovascular risk assessment before and after kidney transplantation. *Cardiol Rev.* 2014;22(4):153–162.
5. Lentine KL, Costa SP. Cardiac disease evaluation and management among kidney and liver transplantation candidates. *J Am Coll Cardiol.* 2012;60(5):434–480.
6. Chandraker A. Overview of care of the adult kidney transplant recipient. In: Post TW, eds. *UpToDate.* Waltham, MA: UpToDate; 2014. Accessed October 8, 2014.
7. Diekmann F. Immunosuppressive minimization with mTOR inhibitors and belatacept. *Transpl Int.* 2015;28(8):921–927.

8. National Cholesterol Education Program Risk Assessment Tool for Estimating 10-year Risk of Developing Hard CHD (Myocardial Infarction and Coronary Death). Available at http://cvdrisk.nhlbi.nih.gov/calculator.asp. Accessed October 8, 2014.
9. Uthoff H, Staub D, Socrates T, et al. PROCAM-, FRAMINGHAM-, SCORE- and SMART-risk score for predicting cardiovascular morbidity and mortality in patients with overt atherosclerosis. *Vasa.* 2010;39(4):325–333.
10. SCORE (Systematic Coronary Risk Evaluation) Risk Charts. Available at http://www.escardio.org/communities/EACPR/toolbox/health-professionals/Pages/SCORE-Risk-Charts.aspx. Accessed October 10, 2014.
11. Eckel RH, Cornier MA. Update on the NCEP ATP-III emerging cardiometabolic risk factors. *BMC Med.* 2014;12:115–124.
12. Kelly SC, Gonzalo R, Petrasko M. A focus on cardiovascular risk modification: clinical significance and implementation of the 2013 ACC/AHA cholesterol guidelines. *S D Med.* 2014;67(8):320–323.
13. James, PA, Oparil S, Carter BL, et al. 2014 evidenced-based guidelines for the management of high blood pressure in adults: reports from the panel members appointed to the Eighth Joint National Committee (JNC 8). *JAMA.* 2014;311(5):507–520.
14. Kaplan B, Qazi Y, Wellen JR. Strategies for the management of adverse events associated with mTOR inhibitors. *Transplant Rev.* 2014;28(3):126–133.
15. Adamczak M, Gazda M, Gojowy D, et al. Hypertension in patients after liver transplantation. *J Hypertens.* 2015;33(suppl 1):e32.
16. Castrogudin JF, Molina E, Vara E. Calcineurin inhibitors in liver transplantation: to be or not to be. *Transplant Proc.* 2011;43(6):2220–2223.
17. American Heart Association. Body composition tests. Available at http://www.heart.org/HEARTORG/GettingHealthy/WeightManagement/BodyMassIndex/Body-Mass-Index-BMI-Calculator_UCM_307849_Article.jsp. Accessed March 5, 2015.
18. Dobrowolski LC, Bemelman FJ, Ineke JM, et al. Renal denervation of the native kidneys for drug-resistant hypertension after kidney transplantation. *Clin Kidney J.* 2015;8(1):79–81.
19. Birdwell KA, Jaffe G, Bian A, et al. Assessment of arterial stiffness using pulse wave velocity in tacrolimus users the first year post kidney transplantation: a prospective cohort study. *BMC Nephrol.* 2015;16:93.
20. American Heart Association. *American Heart Association Recommended Blood Pressure Levels.* Available at www.americanheart.org. Accessed October 8, 2014.
21. Behzadi AH, Kamali, K, et al. Obesity and urologic complications after renal transplantation. *Saudi J Kidney Dis Transpl.* 2014;25(2):303–308.
22. Bahirwani R, Forde KA, et al. End-stage renal disease after liver transplantation in patients with pre-transplant chronic kidney disease. *Clin Transplant.* 2014;28(2):205–210.
23. Messa P, Ponticelli C, Berardinelli L. Coming back to dialysis after kidney transplant failure. *Nephrol Dial Transplant.* 2008;23(9):2738–2742.
24. Lund LH, Edwards LB, Kucheryavaya AY et al. The registry of the International Society for Heart and Lung Transplantation: thirty-first official adult heart transplant report—2014. *J Heart Lung Transplant.* 2014;33(10):996–1008.
25. International Society for Heart and Lung Transplantation. *The Registry Of The International Society For Heart And Lung Transplantation: Thirty-First Adult Lung And Heart-Lung Transplant Report.* Available at http://www.ishlt.org/registries/slides.asp?slides=heartLungRegistry. Accessed August 8, 2015.
26. Weber ML, Ibrahim HN, Lake JR. Renal dysfunction in liver transplant recipients: evaluation of the critical issues. *Liver Transpl.* 2012;18:1290–1301.
27. The National Kidney Foundation. *Kidney Disease Improving Global Outcomes Clinical Practice Guidelines For Chronic Kidney Disease: Evaluation, Classification And Stratification. Part 4: Definition And Classification Of Chronic Kidney Disease. Guideline 1: Definition And Stages Of Chronic Kidney Disease.* Available at http://www2.kidney.org/professionals/KDOQI/guidelines_ckd/p4_class_g1.htm. Accessed August 8, 2015.
28. Diaz G, O'Connor M. Cardiovascular and renal complications in patients receiving a solid-organ transplant. *Curr Opin Crit Care.* 2011;17:382–389.
29. Issa N, Kukla A, Ibrahim HN. Calcineurin inhibitor toxicity: a review and perspective of the evidence. *Am J Nephrol.* 2013;37(6):602–612.
30. Soderlund C, Radegran G. Immunosuppressive therapies after heart transplantation—the balance between under- and over-immunosuppression. *Transplant Rev.* 2015;29(3):181–189.
31. Asrani AK, Leise MD, West CP, et al. Use of sirolimus in liver transplant recipients with renal insufficiency: systematic review and meta-analysis. *Hepatology.* 2010;52(4):1360–1370.
32. Rosenson RR. Treatment of lipids (including hypercholesterolemia) in secondary prevention. In: Post TW, ed. *UpToDate.* Waltham, MA: UpToDate; 2014. Accessed October 8, 2014.
33. Razeghi E, Shafipour M, Ashraf H, et al. Lipid disturbances before and after renal transplant. *Exp Clin Transplant.* 2011;9(4):230–235.
34. Charlton M. Obesity, hyperlipidemia and metabolic syndrome. *Liver Transpl.* 2009;15(suppl 2):S83–S89.
35. Gosmanova EO, Tangpricha V, Gosmanov AR. Endocrine-metabolic pathophysiologic conditions and treatment approaches after kidney transplantation. *Endocr Pract.* 2012;18(4):579–589.

36. Maryam M, Schilsky ML, Tichy EM. Review on immunosuppression in liver transplantation. *World J Hepatol.* 2015;7(10):1355–1368.
37. Pederson SD. Metabolic complications of obesity. *Best Pract Res Clin Endocrinol Metab.* 2013;27(2):179–193.
38. Salvadori M, Bertoni E. What's new in clinical solid organ transplantation by 2013. *World J Transplant.* 2014;4(4):243–266.
39. Kittleson MM, Kobashigawa JA. Long-term care of the heart transplant recipient. *Curr Opin Organ Transplant.* 2014;19(5):515–524.
40. Stone NJ, Robinson J, Lichtenstein AH, et al. 2013 ACC/AHA guideline on the treatment of blood cholesterol to reduce atherosclerotic cardiovascular risk in adults. A report of the American College of Cardiology/American Heart Association Task Force on Practice Guidelines. *Circulation.* 2013;129(25 suppl 2):S1–S45.
41. Doran B, Guo Y, Xu J, et al. Prognostic value of fasting versus nonfasting low-density lipoprotein cholesterol levels on long-term mortality: insight from the National Health and Nutrition Examination Survey III (NHANES-III). *Circulation.* 2014;130(7):546–553.
42. Kobashigawa JA, Moriguchi JD, Laks H, et al. Ten-year follow-up of a randomized trial of pravastatin in heart transplant patients. *J Heart Lung Transplant.* 2005;24(11):1736–1740.
43. Costanza MR. The International Society for Heart and Lung Transplantation guidelines for the care of heart transplant recipients. *J Heart Lung Transplant.* 2010;29(8):914–956.
44. National Cholesterol Education Program. National Cholesterol Education Program (NECP) expert panel on detection, evaluation, and treatment of high blood cholesterol in adults (Adult Treatment Panel III). Final report. *Circulation.* 2002;106:3143–3421.
45. Torres PA, Helmstetter JA, Kaye AM, et al. Rhabdomyolysis: pathogenesis, diagnosis, and treatment. *Ochsner J.* 2015;15(1):58–69.
46. Stroes ES, Thompson PD, Corsini A, et al. Statin-associated muscle symptoms: impact on statin therapy—European Atherosclerosis Society Consensus Panel Statement on Assessment, Aetiology and Management. *Eur Heart J.* 2015;36(17):1012–1022.
47. Jacobson TA. NLA Task Force on statin safety—2014 update. *J Clin Lipidol.* 2014;8(3 suppl):S1–S4.
48. Whaley-Connell A, Sowers JR. Basic science: pathophysiology: the cardiorenal metabolic syndrome. *J Am Soc Hypertens.* 2014;8(8):604–606.
49. Kassi E, Pervanidou P, Kaltsas G, et al. Metabolic syndrome: definitions and controversies. *BMC Med.* 2011;9:48–60.
50. Tobin ST, Klein CL, Brennan DC. New-onset diabetes after transplant (NODAT) in renal transplant recipients. In: Post TW, ed. *UpToDate.* Waltham, MA: UpToDate; 2014. Accessed March 5, 2015.
51. Bayer ND, Cochetti PT, Kumar A, et al. Association of metabolic syndrome with development of new onset diabetes after transplantation. *Transplantation.* 2010;90(8):861–866.
52. McCaughan JA, McKnight AJ, Maxwell AP. Genetics of new-onset diabetes after transplantation. *J Am Soc Nephrol.* 2014;25(5):1037–1049.
53. Palepu S, Prasad GV. New-onset diabetes mellitus after kidney transplantation: current status and future directions. *World J Diab.* 2015;6(3):445–455.
54. Kesiraju S, Paritala P, Rao Ch UM, et al. New onset of diabetes after transplantation—an overview of epidemiology, mechanism of development and diagnosis. *Transpl Immunol.* 2014;30(1):52–58.
55. Moini M, Schilsky ML, Tichy EM. Review on immunosuppression in liver transplantation. *World J Hepatol.* 2015;7(10):1355–1368.
56. Adams DH, Sanchez-Fueyo A, Samuel D. From immunosuppression to tolerance. *J Hepatol.* 2015;62(1 suppl):S170–S185.
57. American Diabetes Association. Diagnosis and classification of diabetes mellitus. *Diabetes Care.* 2013;36(suppl 1):S67–S74.
58. Hughes LD. The transplant patient and transplant medicine in family practice. *J Family Med Prim Care.* 2014;3(4):345–354.
59. Pham PT, Pham PC, Lipshutz GS, et al. New onset diabetes mellitus after solid organ transplantation. *Endocrininol Metab Clin N Am.* 2007;36:873–890.
60. Pham PT, Pham PM, Pham SV, et al. New onset diabetes after transplantation (NODAT): an overview. *Diabetes Metab Syndr Obes.* 2011;4:175–186.
61. Alberti KG, Eckel RH, Grundy SM, et al. Harmonizing the metabolic syndrome. A joint interim statement of the International Diabetes Federation Task Force on Epidemiology and Prevention; National Heart, Lung, and Blood Institute; American Heart Association; World Heart Federation, International Atherosclerosis Society, International Association for the study of Obesity Diagnosis and management of the metabolic syndrome. *Circulation.* 2009;120:1640–1645.
62. Wilkinson A, Davidson J, Dotta F, et al. Guidelines for the treatment and management of new onset diabetes after transplantation. *Clin Transplant.* 2005;19:291–298.
63. Kelly T, Buxbaum J. Gastrointestinal manifestations of cystic fibrosis. *Dig Dis Sci.* 2015;60(7):1903–1913.
64. Stevens KK, Patel RK, Jardine AG. How to identify and manage diabetes mellitus after renal transplantation. *J Ren Care.* 2012;38(suppl 1):125–137.

65. Luan FL, Steffick DE, Ojo AO. New-onset diabetes mellitus in kidney transplant recipients discharged on steroid-free immunosuppression. *Transplantation.* 2011;91(3):331–341.
66. White SA, Shaw JA, Sutherland DE. Pancreas transplantation. *Lancet.* 2009;373(9677):1808–1817.
67. Davis NF, Burke JP, Kelly R, et al. Predictors of 10-year pancreas allograft survival after simultaneous pancreas and kidney transplantation. *Pancreas.* 2014;43(5):750–754.
68. Mittal S, Gough SC. Pancreas transplantation: a treatment option for people with diabetes. *Diabet Med.* 2014;31(5):512–521.
69. American Heart Association. *Obesity: Impact on Cardiovascular Disease.* Available at http://www.heart.org/HEARTORG/GettingHealthy/WeightManagement/Weight-Management_UCM_001081_SubHomePage.jsp. Accessed March 5, 2015.
70. Beckman S, Ivanovic N, Drent G, et al. Weight gain, overweight and obesity in solid organ transplantation—a study protocol for a systematic review. *Syst Rev.* 2015;4(2):2–10.
71. Reichman TW, Therapondos G, Serrano M-S, et al. Weighing the risk: obesity and outcomes following liver transplantation. *World J Hepatol.* 2015;7(11):1484–1493.
72. Chapman JR, Webster AC, Wong G, et al. Cancer in the transplant recipient. *Cold Spring Harb Perspect Med.* 2013;3(7):1–16.
73. Grulich AE, Vajdic CM. The epidemiology of cancers in human immunodeficiency virus infection and after organ transplantation. *Semin Oncol.* 2015;42:247–257.
74. Zwald FO, Brown M. Skin cancer in solid organ transplant recipients: advances in therapy and management. *J Am Acad Dermatol.* 2011;65(2):253–261.
75. Green M, Covington S, Taranto S, et al. Donor-derived transmission events in 2013: a report of the Organ Procurement Transplant Network Ad Hoc Disease Transmission Advisory Committee. *Transplantation.* 2015;99(2):282–287.
76. Engels EA, Pfeiffer RM, Fraumeni JF, et al. Spectrum of cancer risk among U.S. solid organ transplant recipients: the Transplant Cancer Match Study. *JAMA.* 2011;306(17):1891–1901.
77. Ulrich C, Arnold R, Ulrich F, et al. Skin changes following organ transplantation. *Dtsch Arztebl Int.* 2014;111(11):188–194.
78. Ponticelli C, Bencini PL. Nonneoplastic mucocutaneous lesions in organ transplant recipients. *Transpl Int.* 2011;24:1041–1050.
79. Wilkerson BL. Malignant melanoma. *Plast Surg Nurs.* 2011;31(3):105–107.
80. Hosseini-Moghaddam SM, Soleimanirahbar A, Mazzulli T, et al. Post renal transplantation Kaposi's sarcoma: a review of its epidemiology, pathogenesis, diagnosis, clinical aspects, and therapy. *Transpl Infect Dis.* 2012;14:338–345.
81. Jiminez S. Epstein-Barr virus-associated post-transplantation lymphoproliferative disorder. *Clin J Oncol Nurs.* 2015;19(1):94–98.
82. Singavi AK, Harrington AM, Fenske T. Post-transplant lymphoproliferative disorders. *Cancer Treat Res.* 2015;165:307–327.
83. Ashrafi F, Shahidi S, Zeinab E, et al. Outcome of rapamycin therapy for post-transplant lymphoproliferative disorder after kidney transplant: case studies. *Int J Hematol Oncol Stem Cell Res.* 2015;9(1):26–32.
84. American Cancer Society. *American Cancer Society Guidelines for the Early Detection of Cancer.* Available at http://www.cancer.org/healthy/findcancerearly/cancerscreeningguidelines/american-cancer-society-guidelines-for-the-early-detection-of-cancer. Accessed July 15, 2015.
85. Wong G, Chapman JR, Craig JC. Cancer screening in renal transplant recipients: what is the evidence. *Clin J Am Soc Nephrol.* 2008;3(suppl 2):S87–S100.
86. Dounousi E, Leivaditis K, Eleftheriadis T, et al. Osteoporosis after renal transplantation. *Int Urol Nephrol.* 2015;47(3):503–511.
87. Kulak CA, Borba VZ, Junior JK, et al. Bone disease after transplantation: osteoporosis and fracture risk. *Arq Bras Endocrinol Metabol.* 2014;58(5):484–492.
88. Schwartz AV. Epidemiology of fractures in type 2 diabetes. *Bone.* 2016;82:2–8.
89. Khan TS, Fraser LA. Type 1 diabetes and osteoporosis: from molecular pathways to bone phenotype. *J Osteoporos.* 2015;2015:174–186.
90. Agarwal S, Mayer L. Diagnosis and treatment of gastrointestinal disorders in patients with primary immunodeficiency. *Clin Gastroenterol Hepatol.* 2013;11(9):1050–1063.
91. Yun JH, Lee SO, Jo KW. Infections after lung transplantation: time of occurrence, sites and microbiologic etiologies. *Korean J Intern Med.* 2015;30(4):506–514.
92. Piaserico S, Sandini E, Peserico A, et al. Cutaneous viral infections in organ transplant patients. *G Ital Dermatol Venereol.* 2014;149(4):409–415.
93. Azevedo LS, Pierrotti LC, Abdala E, et al. Cytomegalovirus infection in transplant recipients. *Clinics (Sao Paulo).* 2015;70(7):515–523.
94. Kobashigawa J, Ross H, Bara C, et al. Everolimus is associated with a reduced incidence of cytomegalovirus infection following de novo cardiac transplantation. *Transpl Infect Dis.* 2013;15(2):150–162.

95. Fallatah SM, Marquez MA, Bazerbachi F, et al. Cytomegalovirus infection post-pancreas-kidney transplantation—results of antiviral prophylaxis in high-risk patients. *Clin Transplant.* 2013;27(4):503–509.

96. Netchiporouk E, Tchervenkov J, Paraskevas S, et al. Evaluation of herpes simplex virus infection morbidity and mortality in pancreas and kidney-pancreas transplant recipients. *Transplant Proc.* 2013;45(9):3343–3347.

97. Park CS, Hwang S, Jung DH, et al. Pneumatosis intestinalis after adult living donor liver transplantation: report of three cases and collective literature review. *Kor J Hepatobiliary Pancreat Surg.* 2015;19(1):25–29.

98. Kutsch E, Kreiger P, Consolini D, et al. Colonic perforation after rituximab treatment for posttransplant lymphoproliferative disorder. *J Pediatr Gastroenterol Nutr.* 2013;56(6):e41.

99. Vernadakis S, Sotiropoulos GC, Fouzas I, et al. Cholecystectomy due to symptomatic gallbladder disease after orthotopic liver transplantation: report of three cases. *Transplant Proc.* 2012;44(9):2757–2758.

100. Tabakovic M, Salkic NN, Bosnjic J, et al. Acute pancreatitis after kidney transplantation. *Case Rep Transplant.* 2012;2012:768193.

101. Martins FP, Kahaleh M, Ferrari AP. Management of liver transplantation biliary stricture: results from a tertiary hospital. *World J Gastrointest Endosc.* 2015;25(7):747–757.

102. Tenner S. Drug induced acute pancreatitis: does it exist? *World J Gastroenterol.* 2014;20(44):16529–16534.

103. Grass F, Schafer M, Cristaudi A, et al. Incidence and risk factors of abdominal complications after lung transplantation. *World J Surg.* 2015;39(9):2274–2281.

104. Ko GY, Sung KB. Section 11: radiological intervention approaches to biliary complications after living donor liver transplantation. *Transplantation.* 2014;97(suppl 8):S43–S46.

105. Weiler S, Aellig N, Fauchere I, et al. Treatment of gout in a renal transplant patient leading to severe thrombocytopenia. *J Clin Pharm Ther.* 2014;39(5):571–572.

106. Becker M. Hyperuricemia and gout in renal transplant recipients. In: Post TW, eds. *UpToDate.* Waltham, MA: UpToDate; 2014. Accessed on October 8, 2014.

107. Sofue T, Inui M, Hara T, et al. Efficacy and safety of febuxostat in the treatment of hyperuricemia in stable kidney transplant recipients. *Drug Des Devel Ther.* 2014;8:245–253.

108. Moffitt ML, Bencivenni D, Cohen RE. Drug-induced gingival enlargement: an overview. *Compend Cont Educ Dent.* 2013;334(5):330–336.

109. Weng RR, Foster CE, Hsieh LL, et al. Oral ulcers associated with mycophenolate mofetil use in a renal transplant recipient. *Am J Health Syst Pharm.* 2011;68(7):585–588.

110. Georgakopoulou EA, Achtari MD, Afentoulide N. Dental management of patients before and after renal transplantation. *Stomatologija.* 2011;13(4):107–112.

111. Livada R, Shiloah J. Calcium channel blocker-induced gingival enlargement. *J Hum Hypertens.* 2014;28:10–14.

112. Comacchio AL, Bumeo JG, Aragon CE. The effects of antiepileptic drugs on oral health. *J Can Dent Assoc.* 2011;71:b140.

113. American Heart Association. *Endocarditis Prophylaxis Information.* Available at http://www.heart.org/idc/groups/heart-public@wcm/@hcm/documents/downloadable/ucm_307684/pdf. Accessed March 10, 2015.

114. Fornaini C, Rocca JP. CO_2 laser treatment of drug-induced gingival overgrowth—case report. *Laser Ther.* 2012;21(1):39–42.

115. World Health Organization. *Brief Sexuality-Related Communication: Recommendations for a Public Health Approach.* Geneva: World Health Organization; 2015:15–17.

116. Caretta N, Feltrin G, Tarantini G, et al. Erectile dysfunction, penile atherosclerosis, and coronary artery vasculopathy in heart transplant recipients. *J Sex Med.* 2013;10:2295–2302.

117. Nehra A, Jackson G, et al. The Princeton III Consensus recommendations for the management of erectile dysfunction and cardiovascular disease. *Mayo Clin Proc.* 2012;87(8):766–778.

118. Pastuszak AW. Current diagnosis and management of erectile dysfunction. *Curr Sex Health Rep.* 2014;6(3):164–176.

119. Annon J. The PLISSIT model: a proposed conceptual scheme for the behavioral treatment of sexual problems. *J Sex Educ.* 1976;2:1–15.

120. Davis S, Taylor B. From PLISSIT to Ex-PLISSIT. In: Davis S, eds. *Rehabilitation: The Use of Theories and Models in Practice.* Edinburgh, UK: Elsevier; 2006.

121. Taylor B, Davis S. Using the Extended PLISSIT model to address sexual healthcare needs. *Nurs Stand.* 2006;21:35–40.

122. Tiffin-Richards FE, Costa AS, et al. The Montreal cognitive assessment (MoCA)—a sensitive screening instrument for detecting cognitive impairment in chronic hemodialysis patients. *PLoS One.* 2014;9(10):e106–e115.

123. Heinrich TW, Marcangelo M. Psychiatric issues in solid organ transplantation. *Harv Rev Psychiatry.* 2009;17:398–406.

124. Gosert R, Rinaldo CH, Wernli M, et al. CMX001 (1-O-hexadecyloxypropyl-cidofovir) inhibits polyomavirus JC replication in human brain progenitor-derived astrocytes. *Antimicrob Agents Chemother.* 2011;55(5):2129–2136.

125. Eckel RH, Jakicic JM, Anderson JL, et al. 2013 AHA/ACC guideline on lifestyle management to reduce cardiovascular risk. *J Am Coll Cardiol.* 2014;63(25-PC):2960–2984.

SELF-ASSESSMENT QUESTIONS

1. You are caring for a 52-year-old male who is 7 months postrenal transplant who is reporting severe generalized myalgias. You review his medication list and see that he is taking tacrolimus, mycophenolate mofetil, prednisone, pravastatin, lisinopril, folic acid, and a multivitamin. What blood test would you anticipate to be ordered?
   a. Tacrolimus level
   b. Creatinine kinase (CK)
   c. Blood urea nitrogen (BUN)
   d. Random cortisol level

2. Metabolic syndrome risk factors include:
   1. abdominal obesity
   2. dyslipidemia
   3. hypotension
   4. renal insufficiency
   5. hyperglycemia
   a. 1, 2, and 5
   b. 1, 2, and 3
   c. 2, 3, and 4
   d. 1, 2, and 4

3. Solid organ transplant recipients have a 50 to 100 times increased risk of nonmelanoma skin cancer.
   a. True
   b. False

4. Which viral illness carries the greatest risk for PTLD?
   a. CMV
   b. HSV
   c. EBV
   d. PCP

5. You are teaching a recent transplant recipient about the risks of steroid use. When explaining the risk of osteoporosis you explain that vertebral bone loss is typically highest:
   a. in the first 5 years posttransplant.
   b. as long as the patient is on steroids.
   c. after 5 years posttransplant.
   d. in the first 6 to 12 months posttransplant.

6. The goal blood pressure for the transplant recipient is <140/90
   a. True
   b. False

7. Your patient is prescribed a bisphosphonate for osteoporosis. You explain that the patient should:
   1. take this medication with 8 oz of plain water prior to ingesting any food.
   2. take this medication with carbonated beverage to help with absorption.
   3. remain upright for 30 minutes after taking this medication.
   4. take this medication at the same time you take your calcium supplement.
   a. 1 and 2
   b. 2 and 3
   c. 3 and 4
   d. 1 and 3

8. Your pretransplant patient has a history of gout. Now posttransplant, you are aware that the patient has an increased risk of gout due to use of:
   1. prednisone.
   2. diuretics.
   3. statins.
   4. calcineurin inhibitors.
   a. 1 and 4
   b. 2 and 4
   c. 1 and 3
   d. All of the above

9. Your patient is 12 months posttransplant and presents with leukopenia, nausea, vomiting, diarrhea, and fever. The probable diagnosis with this presentation is:
   a. HSV infection.
   b. posttransplant lymphoproliferative disease.
   c. CMV gastritis.
   d. *Clostridium difficile* colitis.

10. Which of the following medications are typically associated with the development of gingival hyperplasia?
    1. Cyclosporine
    2. Diuretics
    3. Anticonvulsants
    4. Antihyperlipidemic agents
    5. Calcium channel blockers
    a. 1, 3, and 5
    b. 1, 4, and 5
    c. 2, 3, and 4
    d. 1, 2, and 5

11. Which medications can be associated with sexual dysfunction?
    a. Beta-blockers
    b. Immunosuppressants
    c. Antidepressants
    d. Lipid-lowering agents
    e. All of the above

12. Which of the following cancers is the most common in solid organ transplant recipients?
    a. Breast
    b. Colon
    c. Prostate
    d. Squamous cell carcinoma
    e. Basal cell carcinoma

Correct Answers:
1.b   2.a   3.a   4.c   5.d   6.a   7.d   8.b   9.c   10.a   11.e   12.d

C H A P T E R

7

Care of Living Donors

Dianne LaPointe Rudow, ANP-BC, DNP, CCTC

I. INTRODUCTION

A. **The history of living organ donation**

1. The first successful living donor transplant was performed in 1954 in Boston, Massachusetts, United States, between identical twin brothers.[1]
   a. The hospital created a separate live donor team to advocate on the live organ donor's behalf.
2. The advent of immunosuppressant drugs in the 1970s facilitated transplantation from nonidentical family members and a subsequent increase in organ transplantation from deceased donors.
3. As more candidates met transplantation criteria and the number of deceased donors declined, the number of live kidney donors exceeded the number of deceased donor transplants in 2004. Currently, the number of live donors is slowly declining.[2]
4. Numerous studies have shown that kidney donation is safe and that most donors lead normal lives with a single kidney and have minimal risk of end-stage renal disease (ESRD) providing they lead a healthy lifestyle.[3-5]
5. Live liver donation has been performed for children since the late 1980s and adults since 1998. The largest volume of procedures occurs in centers where there are limited numbers of deceased donors. This may be due to donor shortages in certain areas of the world or certain countries' who do not utilize deceased donors at all. Medical outcomes have been studied, and although liver donation portends a higher risk than kidney donation, it is still believed to be safe enough to perform at experienced centers.[6,7]
6. The benefits for the recipient of a living donor transplant are clear.
   a. The organ is from a (typically) young healthy person who has undergone an intense medical evaluation.
   b. Data indicate that patients with ESRD benefit significantly with pre-emptive kidney transplantation and less time on dialysis.[8]
   c. The surgery can be planned when the recipient's medical status is stable and, in the case of liver donation, before a liver transplant candidate becomes too sick to undergo transplantation.

      d. The cold ischemic time is reduced, as the time the organ is without a blood supply is very short compared to the time involved in deceased donor transplantation.

  7. The negative aspects of live donation for the recipient include

      a. Having a family member or close friend undergo major surgery, which they themselves do not medically require or benefit from, on behalf of the recipient

      b. In the case of liver donation, receiving a partial graft that is often initially smaller than needed

B. Ethical issues in living donor transplantation

  1. The following ethical principles may be applied to the living donor[9]:

      a. Autonomy: The right to act intentionally, with understanding and without internal or external controlling influences

      b. Beneficence: The duty to provide benefits to others and to balance benefits, risks, and costs so as to obtain the best overall results.

      c. Nonmaleficence: The duty not to intentionally create a harm or injury through acts of either commission or omission

      d. Justice: The duty to act fairly, including the allocation of scarce resources

  2. Each duty is a *prima facie* duty, which means that it is binding or obligatory unless it is overridden by another moral duty.

  3. In clinical practice, an ethics consult can facilitate complex decision making when ethical conflicts arise.

  4. The risks and benefits of living donor transplantation need to be carefully balanced as many ethical issues may be raised.

      a. The act of living donation is a unique situation—exposing one individual to potential harm for the benefit of another.[10]

      b. The potential living donor is considering a surgery and subsequent risk that is not medically necessary, will temporarily disable him or her, and will expose him or her to some risk of morbidity and mortality.

      c. The Hippocratic Oath, which states *primum non nocere*—"firstly, do no harm"[11]—must be considered when determining donor suitability. Additionally, donor benefits may need to be considered, that is, saving a loved one's life.

      d. A broader ethical view may be argued that an increase in living donation reduces the number of individuals waiting on the transplant list.

  5. Informed consent. Respect for an individual's autonomy is the central reason that each person has the right to consent to or refuse living donation.

      a. Individuals must be given the necessary information about the choices available and understand the potential consequences of each course of action, hence the term "informed consent."

      b. While potential donors may be given an appropriate, detailed description of the benefits and risks of donation, it is unclear how much information is actually retained and how this plays in the decisions to choose to move forward with donation. Studies on successful approaches to informed consent are needed.

      c. There is a well-described tendency for some people to decide at an early stage, even before presenting to the transplant program, that they wish to donate and then to be impervious to any suggestion that they should make a more informed decision in the light of further education about the process, risks, and long-term outcomes.[12]

d. Knowing that the potential recipient has end-stage organ failure and can die can be, in fact, coercive and interfere with true informed consent.

6. Key principles of informed consent

   a. Potential living donors should be approached "neutrally," in other words in an unbiased manner.

   b. Education about the risks and benefits should be provided at an appropriate educational and health literacy level; cultural background must be taken into consideration.

   c. Potential donors should be fully informed about risks, benefits, and alternatives as early as possible.

   d. Coercive internal and external pressures should be probed for and detected wherever possible.

   e. The potential living donor should be provided an opportunity to discreetly withdraw from further consideration.

7. The clinical team caring for the living donor must incorporate ethical principles into practice as well. The living donor team must

   a. Ensure that "The person who gives consent to be a live organ donor should be competent, willing to donate, free from coercion, medically and psychosocially suitable, fully informed of the risks and benefits as a donor, and fully informed of the risks, benefits, and alternative treatment available to the recipient."[13]

   b. Maintain the confidentiality of the donor and ensure that medical records are not accessible to the recipient.

   c. Support a donor who decides not to donate; assist the donor to remove him- or herself from further consideration.

   d. Ensure that donors who are found to be unsuitable for donation for medical or psychosocial reasons receive support and appropriate referrals for care.

8. Payment for organs

   a. Per the World Health Assembly resolution WHA63.22, "cells, tissues, and organs should only be donated freely, without any monetary payment or other reward of monetary value. Purchasing, or offering to purchase, cells, tissues, or organs for transplantation, or their sale by living persons or by the next of kin for deceased persons, should be banned."[14]

   b. The Declaration of Istanbul defines "transplant commercialism" as "a policy or practice in which an organ is treated as a commodity, including by being bought or sold or used for material gain."[15]

   c. It is illegal in the United States and most countries worldwide to pay for or receive any financial benefit from being a live organ donor. All donors considering living donation must be informed that, if it is determined that they received any financial compensation, they may be criminally prosecuted.

C. **Regulatory oversight of living donor practices**

1. As both the number of living donor kidney transplants and the number of extrarenal transplants increased, much national and global attention was given to the care and regulatory oversight of the living organ donor. Previous live donors expressed dissatisfaction with their care and follow-up and transplant centers' practice and resources varied. Many consensus conferences were held to standardize the approach to live donor care and various regulatory bodies gained oversight to the care of the living donor.

2. In November 2002, the Advisory Council on Organ Transplant (ACOT) made recommendations to the Secretary of Health and Human Services that each institution that performs living donor transplantation provide an independent donor advocate (ILDA) to ensure that informed consent standards are adhered to and ethical principles are applied to practice.[16]

3. Effective June 28, 2007, the Center for Medicare Services (CMS) Conditions of Participation regulated live donor care for the first time.[17] These regulations include the following:

   a. Living donor selection must be consistent with the general principles of ethics.

   b. Assurance that a prospective living donor receives a medical and psychosocial evaluation prior to donation.

   c. Documentation in the living donor's medical records the living donor's suitability for donation.

   d. Documentation that the living donor has given informed consent.

   e. Specification of components of informed consent required during the education process.

   f. Blood type verification for living donor transplantation immediately before removal of the organ and prior to implantation.

   g. Centers must have a live donor postoperative management policy.

   h. An ILDA or team must evaluate all live donors.

   i. Policies surrounding aspects of paired kidney donation.

   j. Live donor program Quality Assurance Process Improvement Program.

4. In September 2007, the Organ Procurement and Transplantation Network (OPTN) was given oversight of living donation in the United States. The OPTN has developed policies that transplant programs that perform living donation are required to follow.[18] Policies currently exist in the following areas:

   a. Requirements for protocols that hospitals who recover live donor organs must follow

   b. ILDA requirements

   c. Informed consent requirements

   d. Medical evaluation requirements

   e. Psychosocial evaluation requirements

   f. Registration and blood type verification of living donors before donation

   g. Placement of living donor organs

   h. Packaging, labeling, and transporting living donor organs, vessels, and tissue-typing material.

   i. Reporting requirements including 2-year live donor follow-up

5. The initial regulatory requirements continue to evolve as evidence in the literature changes and the transplant community analyzes practice and provides suggestions for improvement. Recent revisions to policies surrounding the care of the living organ donor have been made based on significant contributions from worldwide consensus conferences and published in the literature.[19-26] These include the following topics:

   a. Care of the kidney donor

   b. Care of the extrarenal donor

   c. Ethical issues in live donation

   d. Psychosocial evaluation of living donors

   e. Transplant program quality and surveillance

   f. Paired kidney donation

   g. Living donor follow-up

   h. Best practices in living kidney donation

II. THE LIVING DONOR EVALUATION

The living donor evaluation typically involves many phases including the referral or screening process, the evaluation process, and the live donor team decision process. A multidisciplinary team of health care professionals experienced in living donation is involved in the entire process. Care must be taken that potential donors are not pressured or coerced by the recipient or other family members. The donor should be seen separately, in the absence of the prospective recipient and the family, and should be reassured that his or her views with respect to donation, as well as his or her medical and social history, will be kept confidential.

A. **The Interdisciplinary Team Utilized to Care for the Living Organ Donor**

1. The physician is a trained transplant nephrologist/hepatologist (depending on organ being donated) who is responsible for the medical evaluation of the potential living donor and carefully evaluates the donor, assists in the donor decision-making process, and may be available for postoperative care. This physician
   a. Performs a full history and physical for potential donors
   b. Determines the need for additional testing for risk stratification, the identification of systemic disease, or likelihood of developing systemic disease
   c. Interprets diagnostic tests results
   d. Assists with the education of potential and actual donors
   e. Follows donors postoperatively as needed
2. A board-certified surgeon who has successfully completed training and has experience in the living donor organ procurement. The surgeon's role is to
   a. Assess the potential living donor for surgical suitability
   b. Determine surgical feasibility given the donor and recipient anatomy
   c. Participate in the live donor team meetings to determine suitability
   d. Consider the ILDA's recommendation regarding the donor's suitability
   e. Participate in the education process for all potential donors
3. The live donor coordinator is a licensed registered nurse who coordinates the care of the live organ donors. The coordinator is responsible for
   a. Structuring the process of the evaluation, education, and consent for living donation
   b. Screening potential donors by telephone
   c. Obtaining consent for the donor evaluation
   d. Determining blood type compatibility
   e. Ensuring confidentiality of the donor record
   f. Assisting in the coordination of the medical evaluation
   g. Facilitating additional medical testing of the potential donor
   h. Explaining medical information in terms that the donor can understand
   i. Educating the donor about the process of evaluation, the risks involved, organ allocation, and the intended recipient's medical condition
   j. Participating in the living donor team meetings to determine candidacy
   k. Supporting the donor if they choose not to donate or if they are declined by the medical team
   l. Providing pre-, peri-, and postoperative care and education.
4. The social worker is involved in the evaluation and care of potential and actual live organ donors. The social worker's role is to
   a. Conduct a clinical psychosocial assessment of the living donor and his/her support system

b. Participate in living donor team's collaborative decision-making process regarding the appropriateness of the candidate with the living donor team

c. Educate and counsel the candidate about living donation with written information and through individual, family, and group meetings

d. Provide advocacy and emotional and concrete support to the donor and his/her family during the inpatient stay

e. Coordinate discharge planning orders of the medical team

f. Offer postdischarge counseling and donor recognition

5. The financial coordinator counsels the donor regarding the finances of living donation, particularly with regard to insurance coverage. Specifically, the financial coordinator

a. Verifies available benefits for living donation with the intended recipient's insurance company and obtains any preauthorizations required for the comprehensive donor evaluation

b. Explores alternative options in the event that coverage for living donation is denied by the recipient's insurance company

c. Informs the living donor of the possibility of future health problems related to donation that may not be covered by the recipient's insurance

d. Provides education regarding the living donor's potential difficulty in obtaining health, life, or disability insurance and risk of increased costs of health, life, or disability insurance.

6. The ILDA ensures protection of the rights of living donors and prospective living donors.[17,18,27-31] The role of the ILDA can be performed by one person or by a team. The ILDA

a. Functions independently of the candidate's team and must not be involved in transplantation activities on a routine basis.

b. Must demonstrate knowledge of living organ donation, transplantation, medical ethics, informed consent, and the potential impact of family and external pressures on the living donor's decision to donate.

c. May be a nurse, social worker, physician, clergy, ethicist, or psychologist. Some programs use nonclinicians in this role.[31]

d. Must follow the transplant program's written protocols and grievance process when necessary to protect the rights and best interests of the living donor.[17,18]

e. Must determine whether the living donor has received information on each of the following areas and assist the donor in obtaining additional information from other professionals as needed about[18,27-30]:

    i. The informed consent process

    ii. The evaluation process

    iii. The surgical procedure

    iv. Potential medical risks

    v. Potential psychosocial risks

    vi. Follow-up requirements and the benefit and need for obtaining follow-up care

7. The psychiatrist/psychologist is often involved in the assessment of the living organ donor, especially those with a psychiatric history, questionable competence, and distant relationship with the recipient or questionable motives. The psychiatrist/psychologist will

a. Screen for underlying psychiatric illness

b. Determine how pre-existing psychiatric illness may impact donation

  c. Make recommendation for pre- and postdonation mental health interventions

  d. Assess the potential donor's understanding of the risks and benefits of donation

  e. Assess the potential donor's ability to give informed consent

  f. Assess for any internal and/or external coercion

B. **The Referral Process**

 1. Potential living donors may learn about the opportunity to be a live donor from many sources, including

  a. The potential recipient

  b. The potential recipient's medical team or dialysis center

  c. The potential recipient's friends or family members

  d. The Internet/social media (Facebook, Twitter, etc.)

  e. Donor solicitation websites (e.g., matchingdonors.com)

  f. Billboards/media campaigns

 2. Regardless of how potential donors learn about living donation, they should be encouraged to make the first inquiry to the transplant center to start the donation evaluation process. This can help ensure that the donor is making an independent choice to be evaluated.

 3. The referral process involves the following:

  a. A medical screening questionnaire done in person, by phone, in writing, or via the Internet. This can rule out any obvious contraindications to donation.

  b. Blood type and, in kidney donation, histocompatibility testing.

  c. Basic vital signs, height, weight, and blood pressure.

  d. Basic education about the donation process and risks/benefits of donation.

C. **Types of Living Donors**

 1. Traditionally, living donors were biologically related to the recipient, for example siblings, parents, children, and cousins. Over the past decade, as surgical innovations developed, laparoscopic kidney donation was introduced and immunosuppression agents improved, and the relationship of the donor and recipient became less important.

 2. Transplant programs now consider both emotionally and nonemotionally related individuals as potential donors, that is, spouses, life partners, friends, and strangers.

 3. Certain religious and community groups are working together to pair donors and recipients.

 4. Increased participation in social media has fostered the development of relationships based on the purpose of living donation.

  a. This is more common with kidney donation than extrarenal donation and is likely related to

   i. The availability of long-term data on kidney donation

   ii. The minimal invasiveness of laparoscopic nephrectomy

   iii. The lower morbidity and mortality of live kidney donation compared to liver or lung donation

 5. Paired kidney donation (PKD) is an option that is increasing for ABO-incompatible pairs and transplant candidates who are highly sensitized.[32]

  a. PKD can be done with either one or two recipient/donor pairs who exchange donors or with more participants (i.e., longer "chains").

    b. PKD procedures can be done internally (between/among one program's patients) or through a paired exchange program in which multiple transplant programs participate.

D. **Selection of the Living Donor**[18]

1. Age >18 years old
2. Completed a comprehensive medical and surgical evaluation
3. Completed a psychosocial evaluation by a qualified health care professional
4. Education about all elements of donation and transplant; informed consent obtained

E. **Exclusion Criteria for Living Donor**

1. Transplant center protocols vary in terms of inclusion and exclusion criteria based on center culture, experience, and amount of risk the center is willing to accept. That being said, per OPTN policy, all live donor programs must exclude all donors with any of the following exclusion criteria[18]:
   a. A donor who is both <18 years old and mentally incapable of making an informed decision
   b. HIV infection
   c. Active malignancy or incompletely treated malignancy
   d. High suspicion of donor coercion
   e. Belief that an illegal financial exchange has occurred between the donor and recipient
   f. Evidence of acute symptomatic infection (until resolved)
   g. Uncontrolled, diagnosable psychiatric conditions requiring treatment before donation, including any evidence of suicidality
   h. Kidney donor exclusion criteria:
      i. Uncontrollable hypertension or hypertension with evidence of end-organ damage
      ii. Diabetes mellitus
   i. Liver donor exclusion criteria:
      i. Hepatitis C virus RNA positive
      ii. Hepatitis B surface antigen positive
      iii. Donors with ZZ, Z-null, null-null, and S-null alpha-1 antitrypsin phenotypes and untypable phenotypes
      iv. Expected donor remnant volume <30% of native liver volume (based on radiological imaging)
      v. History of previous living liver donation

F. **Elements Included in Education and Informed Consent Process**[17,18,33]

1. The donor must confirm (typically in writing) that he or she
   a. Is willing to donate
   b. Is free from inducement and coercion
   c. Has been informed that he or she can decline to donate at any time
   d. Understands that it is a federal crime to offer to donate any human organ for anything of value including, but not limited to, cash, property, and vacations
2. The clinicians educating the donor must disclose
   a. Any alternate procedures or treatment for the recipient, including deceased donor transplantation
   b. The fact that deceased donor organ may become available for the candidate before the living donor's evaluation occurs

3. There should be a disclosure that any transplant candidate may have risk factors for increased morbidity or mortality that are not disclosed to the donor.
4. The donor's personal health information obtained during the donor evaluation is subject to the same regulations as all medical records and could reveal conditions that must be reported to local, state, or federal public health authorities.
5. The transplant program that performs the donor nephrectomy is responsible for reporting living donor follow-up information specifically to the OPTN.[34]
6. As part of the predonation education and consent process, the donor must commit to postoperative follow-up testing coordinated by the live donor program.
7. Any infectious disease or malignancy pertinent to acute recipient care that is discovered during the donor's first 2 years of follow-up care.
   a. May need to be reported to local, state, or federal public health authorities
   b. Will be disclosed to the recipient's transplant center
   c. Will be reported through the OPTN Improving Patient Safety Portal
8. Any transplant program may refuse a living donor. If this occurs, the donor must be informed that different transplant programs may have different selection criteria and the donor can seek a second opinion elsewhere.
9. The live donor should be informed that there are risks to the donor evaluation. They include[18]
   a. Allergic reactions to contrast dye
   b. Identification of reportable infections
   c. Diagnosis of serious medical conditions
   d. Identification of adverse genetic findings unknown to the donor
   e. Discovery of certain abnormalities that will require more testing at the donor's expense
10. Potential medical or surgical risks[2,5,18]:
    a. Death
    b. Scars, hernia, wound infection, blood clots, pneumonia, nerve injury, pain, fatigue, and other consequences typical of any surgical procedure.
    c. Abdominal symptoms such as bloating and nausea and potential bowel obstruction.
    d. Donor morbidity and mortality may be impacted by obesity, hypertension, or other pre-existing donor-specific conditions.
11. Potential psychosocial risks include[17,18,35-38]
    a. Problems with body image
    b. Postdonation depression or anxiety
    c. Chronic pain
    d. Lifestyle changes
    e. Feelings of emotional distress or grief if the transplant recipient dies, has complications, or has an otherwise unanticipated adverse outcome
12. Donors need to understand the potential financial impact of living donation, these including[17,18,34,35]
    a. Direct costs:
       i. Medical expenses (although the evaluation and surgery are covered by the recipient's insurance).
       ii. Personal expenses such as travel, housing, and child care costs.
       iii. Resources might be available to defray some donation-related costs.

    b. Indirect costs:
       i. Lost wages related to donation that might not be reimbursed
    c. Need for lifelong follow-up at the donor's expense.
    d. Potential loss of employment or income.
    e. Potential difficulty obtaining future employment.
    f. Potential negative impact on the ability to obtain, maintain, or afford health insurance, disability insurance, or life insurance.
    g. Future health problems experienced by living donors following donation may not be covered by the recipient's insurance.
    h. The Medicare status of program should be disclosed so that donor is aware of the ability of recipients to pay for immunosuppression posttransplant.
13. Transplant programs are required to disclose to the potential donor program-specific recipient patient and graft survival rates and how these rates compare to national data from the Scientific Registry of Transplant Recipients (SRTR).
14. Disclosures specific to kidney donors include[3-5,18,39]
    a. Education about expected postdonation kidney function and how chronic kidney disease (CKD) and ESRD might potentially impact the living donor in the future.
       i. On average, living donors may have a 25% to 35% permanent loss of kidney function after donation.
       ii. Baseline risk of ESRD for living kidney donors does not exceed that of the general population with the same demographic profile.
       iii. Living donor risks must be interpreted in light of the known epidemiology of both CKD and ESRD. When CKD or ESRD occur, CKD generally develops in midlife (40 to 50 years old) and ESRD generally develops after age 60. The medical evaluation of a young living donor cannot predict lifetime risk of CKD or ESRD.
       iv. Living donors may be at a higher risk for CKD if they sustain damage to the remaining kidney. The development of CKD and subsequent progression to ESRD may be faster with only one kidney.
       v. Dialysis is required if the donor develops ESRD.
    b. In the United States, current practice is to prioritize prior living kidney donors who subsequently become kidney transplant candidates.
    c. Surgical complications can be transient or permanent.
15. Disclosures specifically for liver donors[7,18]
    a. Surgical risks may be transient or permanent and include but are not limited to
       i. Acute liver failure with need for liver transplant.
       ii. Transient liver dysfunction with recovery. This typically depends upon the amount of the total liver removed for donation.
       iii. Risk of bleeding and need for blood product transfusions.
       iv. Biliary complications, including leak or stricture that may require additional intervention including reoperation.

G. The Medical Evaluation

A careful and comprehensive medical and psychosocial evaluation should be performed by an experienced live donor transplant team.

1. The goals of the live donor evaluation are to determine donor suitability[18]:
    a. Assess immunological compatibility:
       i. Although incompatibility no longer excludes transplantation of some organs, appropriate treatment of the recipient or enrollment in

a paired exchange program may be required to overcome potential incompatibility and acute rejection.

b. Assess general health of the donor to exclude comorbidities that may increase the risk of the surgery and put the donor at risk for long-term consequences of donation.

c. Assess surgical risk for the donor to determine if donor characteristics make the surgery more complex or at high risk for complications.

d. Identify if there are any diseases present that may be transmitted from the donor to the recipient.

e. Assess anatomy and function of intended organ for donation to ensure the donor has adequate organ reserve for both the short and long term and that the recipient receives a suitable organ for transplant.

f. Educate the donor on individual risks (perioperative and long term) based on assessment and existing data.

2. Both recipient and donor criteria must be considered when assessing the risk/benefit balance.

3. Key components of the medical evaluation are shown in Table 7-1[17-19,21,26,39]

a. Medical history:

i. Existing medical conditions or a personal history of any of the following medical conditions:

- Hypertension
- Diabetes
- Lung disease
- Heart disease
- Gastrointestinal disease
- Autoimmune disease
- Neurological disease
- Genitourinary disease
- Hematologic disorders
- Bleeding/clotting disorders
- History of cancer including melanoma
- Infectious disease

TABLE 7-1 Components of the Medical Evaluation

Key Components of the Live Donor Medical Evaluation

- Medical and psychosocial history
- Physical exam
- Laboratory testing
- Radiological testing
- Health maintenance
- Age-appropriate screening tests
- Organ-specific testing

From Center for Medicare Services Conditions of Participation; CMS COP42 CFR, Part 405, 482,488 and 498. *Federal Register.* 2007;72(61). Available at http://www.cms.gov/CFCsAndCoPs/downloads/trancenterreg2007.pdf. Accessed February 22, 2015; Living donor policies of the Organ Procurement and Transplantation Network. Available at http://optn.transplant.hrsa.gov/ContentDocuments/OPTN_Policies.pdf#nameddest=Policy_14. Accessed February 22, 2015; Delmonico F. A report of the Amsterdam Forum on the Care of the Live Kidney Donor: data and medical guidelines. *Transplantation.* 2005;79(6 suppl):S53–S66; Barr ML, Belghiti J, Villami FG, et al. A report of the Vancouver Forum on the care of the live organ donor: lung, liver, pancreas, and intestine data and medical guidelines. *Transplantation.* 2006;81(10):1373–1385; LaPointe Rudow D, Hays R, Baliga P, et al. Consensus Conference on Best Practices in Live Kidney Donation: recommendations to optimize education, access, and care. *Am J Transplant.* 2015;15(4):914–922; Moore DR, Feurer ID, Zaydfudim V, et al. Evaluation of living kidney donors: variables that affect donation. *Prog Transplant.* 2012;22(4):385–392.

    ii. Kidney donors:
- Genetic renal disease
- Kidney disease
- Proteinuria
- Hematuria
- Kidney injury
- Kidney cancer
- Nephrolithiasis
- Gestational diabetes

    iii. Current or past medications used that are toxic to the organ intended for donation (nephrotoxic/hepatotoxic)

    iv. Use of pain medication

    v. Allergies

b. Family history:
    i. Liver/kidney disease
    ii. Coronary artery disease
    iii. Diabetes
    iv. Hypertension
    v. Cancer
    vi. Clotting/bleeding disorders

c. Psychosocial history:
    i. History of mental illness including depression, anxiety, abuse, and suicide attempts
    ii. Active or past smoking and illicit drug use/abuse
    iii. Public Health Service (PHS) high-risk behavior[40]
    iv. Occupation, employment status, insurance status, and social stability

d. Comprehensive physical exam:
    i. Height, weight, and body mass index (BMI)
    ii. Blood pressure:
- Kidney donors may need to record blood pressure on more than one occasion or have 24-hour blood pressure monitoring.

    iii. Examination for evidence of organ disease

e. Laboratory testing includes general health screening, infectious disease screening, and organ-specific testing (Table 7-2).[18,19,21]

f. Radiological testing: The imaging modality utilized varies based on center preference and expertise, but typically, computed tomography (CT) angiograms or magnetic resonance imaging (MRI) is used.
    i. Kidney: assessment of
- Size of each kidney
  - Determine if kidneys are equal size.
- Evidence of mass, stone, or cyst
- Arterial and venous structures
- Collecting system

    ii. Liver: assessment of
- Projected graft volume (transplanted portion)
- Donor's remnant volume (remains with donor)
- Vascular anatomy
- Presence of steatosis

g. Age-appropriate health screening tests

h. Organ-specific testing based on history

TABLE 7-2 **Live Donor Evaluation Tests**

General Health Screening	Organ-Specific Testing

• ABO and subtype if necessary
• Complete blood cell count with platelets
• Comprehensive metabolic panel
• Prothrombin time, international normalized ratio, partial thromboplastin time
• Chest radiograph
• Electrocardiogram
• Hypercoagulability workup
• Metabolic testing
  – Lipids
  – Glucose tolerance
• Evaluation for coronary artery disease and need for further testing
• Evaluation for pulmonary disease for smokers and need for further testing
	Kidney
	• Urinalysis
	• Urinary protein and albumin secretion
	• Measurement of glomerular filtration rate
	• Screening for polycystic kidney disease per policy
	• Screen for nephrolithiasis
	Liver
	• Screen for hepatitis
	• Autoimmune liver disease
	• Metabolic liver disease
	• Steatosis
	• Need for biopsy based on history, test results, or body mass index

Infectious Disease Screening	**Age-Appropriate Cancer Screening**
Detailed history of infectious disease and travel as well as Public Health Service screening • CMV (cytomegalovirus) antibody • EBV (Epstein-Barr virus) antibody • HIV 1, 2 (human immunodeficiency virus) antibody testing • HepBsAg (hepatitis B surface antigen) • HepBcAB (hepatitis B core antibody) • HCV (hepatitis C virus) antibody testing • Nucleic acid testing as indicated for HBV, HIV, HCV (based on PHS guidelines) • Syphilis testing • Tuberculosis screening • Testing for diseases prevalent in endemic areas such as Chagas disease, Strongyloides, West Nile virus	Cervical cancer Breast cancer Prostate cancer Colon cancer Skin cancer Lung cancer

From Living donor policies of the Organ Procurement and Transplantation Network. Available at http://optn.transplant.hrsa.gov/ContentDocuments/OPTN_Policies.pdf#nameddest=Policy_14. Accessed February 22, 2015; Delmonico F. A report of the Amsterdam Forum on the Care of the Live Kidney Donor: data and medical guidelines. *Transplantation*. 2005;79(6 suppl):S53–S66; Barr ML, Belghiti J, Villami FG, et al. A report of the Vancouver Forum on the care of the live organ donor: lung, liver, pancreas, and intestine data and medical guidelines. *Transplantation*. 2006;81(10):1373–1385.

H. **The Psychosocial Evaluation**

1. Per OPTN and CMS requirements, the living donor psychosocial evaluation must be performed by a psychiatrist, psychologist, masters-prepared social worker, or licensed clinical social worker.[17,18] The assessment should include *all* of the following components:

   a. An evaluation for any psychosocial issues, including mental health issues, that can put a donor at increased risk for poor psychosocial outcome.

   b. Determination if the donor has behaviors that may increase risk for disease transmission as defined by the *U.S. Public Health Service (PHS) Guideline*.[40]

    c. Identification of a history of smoking, alcohol, and drug use, abuse, and dependency.

    d. Identification of factors that warrant intervention prior to the final donation decision.

        i.   Intervention can include additional education or counseling.

    e. Ensure that the living donor understands the short- and long-term medical and psychosocial risks for both themselves and the recipient.

    f. An assessment of whether the decision to donate is free of inducement, coercion, and other undue pressure.

    g. Determination of the living donor's ability to make an informed decision.

    h. Assessment of the donor's ability to cope with the major surgery and related stress. This includes evaluating whether the donor has a realistic plan for donation and recovery, with social, emotional, and financial support available as recommended.

    i. Identification of the living donor's occupation, employment status, health insurance status, living arrangements, and social support and confirmation that these factors are sufficient to minimize harm.

 III. LIVING DONOR SURGERY, POSTOPERATIVE MANAGEMENT, AND LONG-TERM OUTCOMES

  A. **The Surgical Procedure**

    1. Typically, there is a surgical team focused on the living donor and one focused on the recipient, including an anesthesiologist for each team.

      a. It is important for both the donor and the recipient to be assessed by the medical team prior to beginning either surgery. This ensures that no unforeseen issues have arisen since last assessment that would prohibit the transplant from moving forward.

      b. Having resources to start the recipient surgery soon after the donor surgery is underway in a separate but nearby operating room can help enhance team communication and minimize cold ischemic time. If a kidney paired donation will occur with another center, the team must be experienced with packing and shipping the donor kidney in an efficient manner to minimize cold ischemia time.

      c. Successful ABO verification protocols according to CMS and OPTN policies require effective team communication before and during surgical procedures.[17,18]

    2. Surgical Approach to Living Kidney Donation

      a. The most common surgical procedure for living kidney donation is the laparoscopic nephrectomy.

        i.   It has been shown that donors who undergo laparoscopic nephrectomy have reduced analgesic requirements, a shorter hospital stay, and an earlier return to normal activity.[41]

        ii. The left kidney is frequently the preferred kidney for donation, unless there is some anatomic reason to use the right, such as number of vessels or size.

        iii. The surgeon makes three or four small incisions for the instruments and camera; the kidney is removed through an extraction site typically a Pfannenstiel incision.[41]

        iv. Various techniques can be used, including hand-assisted or robot-assisted laparoscopic nephrectomy and use of a single port.

3. Surgical Approach to Living Liver Donation
   a. Living donor liver transplantation was initially performed only in the pediatric setting, usually a parent donating the left lateral segment of the liver to his or her child.[42]
   b. Adults require increased liver volume, and therefore, the right lobe is typically donated; however, a full left lobe can be used in certain circumstances.[42]
   c. Liver donation is successful due to the organ's innate ability to regenerate itself in both the donor and recipient after transplantation.[43,44]
   d. The surgical approach is more complex than kidney donation requiring a midline incision and complex dissection of the hepatic artery, hepatic vein, portal vein, and bile ducts.
   e. A few transplant programs have incorporated the laparoscopic approach to this surgery, more commonly in the setting of left lateral and left lobe donation.[43]
   f. Morbidity and mortality for liver donors are higher than that of kidney donors. Given the increased risk and complexity of the surgery, smaller numbers of live liver donor procedures are performed worldwide.

B. **Complications of Living Organ Donation**
1. Living donation is not without risk, despite careful selection of suitable candidates.
2. Complications typical of any surgery can occur as well as organ-specific adverse events.
3. Regardless of the organ donated, there are possible psychiatric complications that occur, including, but not limited to, the following:
   a. Problems with altered body image
   b. Postoperative depression or anxiety
   c. Feelings of emotional distress or bereavement
   d. Exacerbation of a pre-existing mental illness.
4. Financial hardship can occur as well, especially if complications develop and the length of disability is longer than expected.
5. A critical role of the live donor team is to support the donor and assess and intervene should complications occur.
6. Kidney donation
   a. Kidney donation has a very low morbidity rate compared to liver donation. However, there are risks associated with anesthesia and the surgical procedure itself and patients require careful monitoring perioperatively (see Table 7-3).[4,18,41,45,46]
   b. The incidence of serious complications of donor nephrectomy is low and includes, but is not limited to, the following:
      i. Complications associated with general anesthesia
      ii. Risk of bleeding and blood transfusion
      iii. Conversion from a laparoscopic to open procedure
      iv. Return to the operating room
      v. Pulmonary embolism
      vi. Death[4,18,41]
   c. More common, short-term complications include, but are not limited to, the following:
      i. Pulmonary problems such as atelectasis and pneumonia
      ii. Abdominal distention

TABLE 7-3 Complications of Kidney Donation

Complications of Kidney Donation
• General anesthesia
• Risk of bleeding and blood transfusion (~1%)
• Conversion from laparoscopic to open surgery (~1%)
• Return to the operating room (<1%)
• Abdominal distention and bloating (ileus) (~4%)
• Pneumonia, blood clots, wound infection
• Risk of dying: 3.1 per 10,000 (0.03%)
• Nerve damage, numbness, pain
• Damage to other organs (<1%)
• Unknown risks

From Segev DL, Muzzaale AD, Mehta SH, et al. Perioperative mortality and long-term survival following live kidney donation. *JAMA.* 2010;303(10):959–966; Living donor policies of the Organ Procurement and Transplantation Network. Available at http://optn. transplant.hrsa.gov/ContentDocuments/OPTN_Policies.pdf#nameddest=Policy_14. Accessed February 22, 2015; Rocca JP, Davis E, Edye M. Live donor nephrectomy. *Mt Sinai J Med.* 2012;79(3):330–341; Muzaale AD, Massie AB, Wang MC, et al. Risk of end-stage renal disease following live kidney donation. *JAMA.* 2014;311(6):579–586; Mjoen G, Hallan S, Hartmann A, et al. Long-term risks for kidney donors. *Kidney Int.* 2014;86(1):162–167.

      iii. Ileus
      iv. Blood clots
      v. Wound infection
      vi. Urinary tract infection
      vii. Shoulder discomfort and neurologic symptoms, probably due to phrenic nerve irritation[4,41]
    d. The spleen, adrenal gland, and other organs can sometimes be damaged during the removal of the kidney
    e. Unknown risks
  7. Liver donation
    a. Morbidity and mortality associated with liver donation are directly related to the volume of liver removed.[6,7,18,21,42-44] Common complications are shown in Table 7-4.[6,7,18,21,27,42-44,47]
    b. The incidence of complications of liver donation is estimated at 40%, but most complications are minor and temporary, and serious complications remain at under 5% in most studies.[7]
    c. Severe complications have occurred, including
      i. Death
      ii. Acute liver failure (resulting in the need for liver transplant)
      iii. Vascular thrombosis
      iv. Pulmonary emboli
      v. Bleeding requiring transfusion
      vi. Need for reoperation
    d. Additional complications can include, but are not limited to, the following:
      i. Biliary complications including leak or stricture that may require additional intervention such as endoscopic retrograde cholangiopancreatography (ERCP) or stenting
      ii. Aborted procedures
      iii. Hernia
      iv. Wound infection
      v. Blood clots

TABLE 7-4 Complications of Liver Donation

Complications of Liver Donation

- Death (risk is 1–5 in 1,000 transplants, likely relative to the amount of liver tissue removed)
- Acute liver failure with need for liver transplant
- Transient liver dysfunction with recovery
- Biliary complications including leak or stricture that may require additional intervention
- Risk of red cell transfusions or other blood products
- Hernia, wound infection, scars, blood clots, pneumonia, nerve injury, pain, fatigue, and other consequences typical of any surgical procedure
- Abdominal or bowel symptoms such as bloating, nausea, and development of bowel obstruction

From Olhtoff KM, Abecassis MM, Emond JC, et al.; Adult-to-Adult Living Donor Liver Transplantation Cohort Study Group. Outcomes of adult to adult living donor transplantation: comparison of the adult-to adult living donor liver transplantation cohort study and national experience. *Liver Transpl.* 2011;17(7):789–797; Abecassis MM, Fisher RA; A2ALL Study Group, et al. Complications of living donor hepatic lobectomy- a comprehensive report. *Am J Transplant.* 2012;12(5):1208–1217; Living donor policies of the Organ Procurement and Transplantation Network. Available at http://optn.transplant.hrsa.gov/ContentDocuments/OPTN_Policies.pdf#nameddest=Policy_14. Accessed February 22, 2015; Barr ML, Belghiti J, Villami FG, et al. A report of the Vancouver Forum on the care of the live organ donor: lung, liver, pancreas, and intestine data and medical guidelines. *Transplantation.* 2006;81(10):1373–1385; Rudow DL. The living donor advocate: a team approach to educate, evaluate, and manage donors across the continuum. *Prog Transplant.* 2009;19(1):64–70; Lobritto S, Kato T, Emond J. Living-donor liver transplantation: current perspective. *Semin Liver Dis.* 2012;32(4):333–340; Song GW, Lee SG. Living donor liver transplantation. *Curr Opin Organ Transplant.* 2014;19(3):217–222; Olthoff KM, Emond JC, Shearon TH, et al. Liver regeneration after living donor transplantation: adult-to-adult living donor liver transplantation cohort study. *Liver Transpl.* 2015;21(1):79–88; Cheah YL, Simpson MA, Pomposelli JJ, et al. Incidence of death and potentially life-threatening near-miss events in living donor hepatic lobectomy: a world-wide survey. *Liver Transpl.* 2013;19(5):499–506.

      vi.   Pneumonia

      vii.   Bowel obstruction

      viii. Nerve injury

      ix.   Chronic pain

      x.   Fatigue

      xi.   Other consequences typical of any surgical procedure

C. **Postoperative Nursing Care of the Live Organ Donor**

1. The immediate postoperative care of living organ donors should be the same as that of any routine surgical patient.
2. It is important to note that despite the fact that donors are prescreened and determined to be healthy, postoperative complications can occur due to immobility, anesthesia, and the removal of a whole or portion of a vital organ.
3. Additionally, the hospitalization for donation may be the donor's first experience with surgery and pain. Consequently, the living donor may be overwhelmed and frightened and require additional support and reassurance.
4. Continuous monitoring of vital signs, laboratory values, and pain is critically important. Hypertension or hypotension must be reported to the surgical team immediately and promptly addressed.
5. The pulmonary status of the donor should be monitored carefully.
   a. The patient has had general anesthesia and is at risk for pulmonary complications.
   b. Careful monitoring of the oxygen saturation, especially in the immediate postoperative period, is imperative.
   c. The chest should be auscultated to identify any abnormalities such as rales or rhonchi.

d. Early ambulation and encouragement of deep breathing exercises and/or incentive spirometer exercises are important to prevent atelectasis.

6. The living donor must be monitored for bleeding, wound drainage, and evidence of complications.

7. Upon arrival to the unit, the wound should be inspected and any abnormalities should be reported. Daily wound care should be performed according to the physician's recommendations.

8. Prophylactic antibiotics are routinely administered for the first 24 hours after surgery. Prompt identification and reporting of a rise in temperature or any signs of infection is critical.

9. The live donor has received intravenous fluids in the operating room; therefore, maintenance of accurate intake and output is critical.

10. A deep vein thrombosis (DVT) prevention protocol should be followed. This may or may not include heparin, but early ambulation and compression stockings or devices are used to ensure lower extremity circulation.

11. Assess for pain and document response to medications. Depending on the surgical approach and organ donated, patients may receive epidural medication, patient-controlled analgesia, or intravenous pain medications. Prompt transition to oral agents is recommended once the patient is tolerating food.

    a. It is not uncommon for the donor to experience more pain than the organ recipient. This may be due to the fact that the recipient is receiving steroids and pain perception is diminished.

       i. The kidney recipient may not have as extensive surgery as the donor due to placement of the kidney in the abdominal cavity.

    b. The application of cold/heat therapy may be beneficial in helping with pain control.

    c. Splinting the incision or applying an abdominal binder may decrease pain.

12. Diet is advanced as tolerated.

    a. It is not uncommon for the live donor to have a poor appetite, nausea from the anesthetics and pain medications, and constipation.

    b. The nurse must observe for prolonged nausea, dehydration, and the development of an ileus.

    c. Management is determined by symptoms and response to medication. Routinely, patients are advanced to regular diet within 1 to 2 days.

    d. Treatment for an ileus may be needed in 17% of donor patients.[48] Care consists of initial bowel rest, reduced opioid use, and early ambulation followed by a slow advancement of diet as the ileus resolves.

13. The interdisciplinary team must also address the emotional well-being of the living donor and family.

    a. Exploring the donor's feelings and keeping the lines of communication open are very important during the recovery period.

    b. Donors are concerned about the recipient but may also have feelings of neglect if the family does not recognize the contribution and sacrifice the donor has made.

D. Organ-Specific Postoperative Nursing Care of the Living Donor

1. Kidney donors

    a. Kidney donors who undergo laparoscopic nephrectomy typically recover quite quickly and have length of stay of 1 to 2 days.

b. Nephrotoxic medications should be avoided.

c. Meticulous attention to recording of intake and output is mandatory.

d. Because there has been a reduction in kidney function, elevations from baseline creatinine are common; intravenous fluids are given to hydrate and flush the remaining kidney.

e. Postoperative laboratory studies such as serum electrolytes, blood urea nitrogen (BUN), and creatinine will be ordered to monitor the donor's recovery from the surgical procedure. It is not uncommon for the creatinine to be 25% to 50% higher than baseline.[18] This improves over months as the remaining kidney hypertrophies.

f. The live donor can be discharged to home if
  i. Their pain is controlled with oral agents.
  ii. They are tolerating a diet.
  iii. They are voiding on their own.

2. Liver donor

a. Liver donors who donate the right lobe may require 24 hours in the intensive care unit for monitoring.

b. Daily laboratory testing will be ordered to monitor hepatic and renal function including
  i. Aspartate aminotransferase (AST)
  ii. Alanine aminotransferase (ALT)
  iii. Total bilirubin
  iv. Complete blood cell count
  v. Electrolytes
  vi. BUN
  vii. Creatinine
  viii. Prothrombin time (PT)
  ix. International normalized ratio (INR)

c. The indicators of liver function, the values of AST, ALT, total bilirubin, and PT/INR, will peak abnormally high 1 to 2 days postoperatively and then fall quite rapidly and approach normal levels by days 7 to 14 if the liver is recovering and growing.[7,42]

d. The nurse should monitor the liver donor for change in mental status because subtle signs of encephalopathy can indicate liver failure.
  i. It is very important to assess the donor's mental status because the liver metabolizes opioids and liver function may be decreased.
  ii. The physician must be notified immediately if there is a change in mental status.

e. A Doppler ultrasound may be ordered on postoperative day 1 to assess the hepatic blood flow and ensure vessel patency.

f. A drain may be placed in the operative site to drain any bile that leaks from the cut surface of the liver.
  i. Drainage should be assessed for color, consistency, and amount.
  ii. A biliary tube may also be placed to prevent a stricture of the bile ducts and to assess the function of the liver.
  iii. If there is no drain, the patient should be monitored for right shoulder pain, chills, fever, and elevated white blood cell count, which also could indicate a bile leak.

g. The liver donor is typically hospitalized for 5 to 7 days.

h. The remaining portion of the liver will regenerate over weeks to months postdonation.[44]

E. **Discharge Teaching for Living Donors**
   1. The donor must be given verbal and written discharge instructions regarding postoperative care. These instructions may vary from center to center.
   2. The nurse caring for the donor should ensure that the living donor has been educated prior to discharge and understands the following:
      a. Pain management regimen.
      b. Activity restrictions including lifting, exercise, travel, and return to work.
      c. Heart healthy diet to promote healing:
         i.   If the gall bladder was removed (common in right lobe donation), liver donors may need to avoid fatty foods.
         ii. Pain medication can be constipating; therefore, instructions on diet related to constipation should be given.
      d. Wound assessment; the nurse should instruct the donor to call if they have any redness, foul smell, or discharge from the incision.
      e. What to expect during the healing process (e.g., fatigue is common).
      f. When to call the living donor team; the donor should call the live donor team if they
         i.   Develop a fever
         ii. Have pain that is not controlled with the pain medication
         iii. Experience shortness of breath
         iv. Have any questions or concerns
      g. Emergency contact numbers.
      h. Importance of follow-up: follow-up appointments and instructions.
   3. Follow-up care
      a. Follow-up care is very important to ensure that the donor recovers without complications.
      b. Typically, the donor returns to see the surgeon or transplant team within a few weeks of surgery.
      c. Communication with the donor's primary care physician is very important for continuity of care.
      d. Following discharge, the nurse should call the donor to determine if the patient is recovering as expected, to answer any questions the donor might have, and to provide support and reassurance.

F. **Long-Term Outcomes**
   1. The long-term outcomes of living organ donation can range from an uncomplicated, short-term recovery to rare instances of disability, chronic organ failure, or even death.
   2. Most donors recover and resume their normal quality of life, are happy with their donation experience, and would do it again if possible.[35,38] However, there can be long-term medical and psychological effects of living organ donation.
   3. Recent studies[45,46,49] suggest that the incidence of ESRD in previous kidney donors is higher than originally predicted although the absolute number remains low.
      a. ESRD is more prevalent in kidney donors whose relative had a genetic kidney disease[46] and are African American, obese, or smokers.[45]
      b. These emerging data indicate the importance of long-term health promotion and healthy living for previous living donors.
      c. The nurse's role in educating and monitoring donors so that they know how to maintain a healthy life is crucial to their long-term health.

    d. Living kidney donors should be encouraged to establish care with a primary care physician for lifelong monitoring.

4. Liver donors tend to do very well in the long term, once they recover from the initial surgery and/or complications.[7]

    a. This is likely because the liver will regenerate to its presurgical size.

    b. Some liver donors experience chronic gastrointestinal distress because the gall bladder is often removed at the time of donation. Therefore, there may be some fat absorption delays in the gut.

    c. Other long-term effects may include pain or discomfort along the abdominal scar and adhesions.[38]

5. The psychological health of all living donors is very important and all donors should be assessed postdonation for any signs of mental illness or depression, especially if this was part of their medical history prior to donation.

    a. There have been several reported suicides in living donors.[47]

    b. Living donors have experienced grief in adjusting to a new body image and may actually mourn the loss of an organ.[35,37]

    c. When the transplant outcome is poor, dissatisfaction with the donation process can occur.

    d. Severe postdonation complications may impact the donor's quality of life and lead to resentment and regret. Therefore, it is important that psychological counseling be available to the donor to facilitate emotional healing postdonation.

6. Women liver and kidney donors have successfully carried pregnancies without developing organ failure. The risk of pre-eclampsia is slightly higher in previous kidney donors.[18]

7. Live donor care by designated experts in the field of living donation should be provided to all potential and actual living donors to ensure that they make informed choices about donation, are carefully evaluated to ensure that donation is safe for them, and meticulously monitored and counseled postdonation to promote long-term health. The nurse plays a critical role in this process.

REFERENCES

1. Murray JE, Merril JP, Harrison JH. Kidney transplantation between seven pairs of identical twins. *Ann Surg.* 1958;148(3):343–359.

2. Organ Procurement and Transplant Network. Available at http://optn.transplant.hrsa.gov/converge/latestData/step2.asp. Accessed February 22, 2015.

3. Ibrahim HN, Foley MB, Tan L, et al. Long-term consequences of kidney donation. *N Engl J Med.* 2009;360(5):459–469.

4. Segev DL, Muzzaale AD, Mehta SH, et al. Perioperative mortality and long-term survival following live kidney donation. *JAMA.* 2010;303(10):959–966.

5. Lentine KL, Schnitzler MA, Xiao H, et al. Racial variation in medical outcomes among living kidney donors. *N Engl J Med.* 2010;363(8):724–732.

6. Olhtoff KM, Abecassis MM, Emond JC, et al. Adult-to-Adult Living Donor Liver Transplantation Cohort Study Group. Outcomes of adult to adult living donor transplantation: comparison of the adult-to adult living donor liver transplantation cohort study and national experience.. *Liver Transpl.* 2011;17(7):789–797.

7. Abecassis MM, Fisher RA; A2ALL Study Group, et al. Complications of living donor hepatic lobectomy- a comprehensive report. *Am J Transplant.* 2012;12(5):1208–1217.

8. Grams ME, Massie AB, Coresh J, et al. Trends in the timing of pre-emptive kidney transplantation. *J Am Soc Nephrol.* 2011;22(9):1615–1620.

9. Testa G. Ethical issues regarding related and nonrelated living organ donors. *World J Surg.* 2014;38(7):1658–1663.

10. Reese PP, Boudville N, Garg AX. Living kidney donation: outcomes, ethics, and uncertainty. *Lancet.* 2015;385(9981):2003–2013.
11. Bakker D. Living related and living unrelated organ donation: a clinician's view of the ethical aspects. In: Price DPT, Akveld H, eds. *Living Organ Donation in the Nineties: European Medico-Legal Perspectives.* Leicester, UK: University of Leicester; 1996:25–31.
12. LaPointe Rudow D. Experiences of the live organ donor: lessons learned pave the future. *Narrat Inq Bioeth.* 2012 Spring;2(1):45–54.
13. Abecassis M, Adams M, Adams P, et al. The US Live Organ Donor Consensus Group: consensus statement on the live organ donor. *JAMA.* 2000;284(22):2919.
14. World Health Organization Guiding Principles on Human Cell, Tissue, and Organ Transplantation. Available at www.tts.org/education/news/legislative-news. Accessed July 20, 2015.
15. Declaration of Istanbul. Available at www.declarationofistanbul.org. Accessed July 20, 2015.
16. Consensus Report: Secretary Tommy G. Thompson's Advisory Committee on Organ Transplantation (ACOT). Available at http://organdonor.gov/legislation/acotrecs118.html. Accessed August 20, 2015.
17. Center for Medicare Services Conditions of Participation; CMS COP42 CFR, Part 405, 482,488 and 498. *Federal Register.* 2007;72(61). Available at http://www.cms.gov/CFCsAndCoPs/downloads/trancenterreg2007.pdf. Accessed February 22, 2015.
18. Living donor policies of the Organ Procurement and Transplantation Network. Available at http://optn.transplant.hrsa.gov/ContentDocuments/OPTN_Policies.pdf#nameddest=Policy_14. Accessed February 22, 2015.
19. Delmonico F. A report of the Amsterdam Forum on the Care of the Live Kidney Donor: data and medical guidelines. *Transplantation.* 2005;79(6 suppl):S53–S66.
20. Pruett T, Tibell A, Alabdulkareem A, et al. The ethics statement of the Vancouver Forum on the live lung, liver, pancreas and intestine donor. *Transplantation.* 2006;81(10):1386–1387.
21. Barr ML, Belghiti J, Villami FG, et al. A report of the Vancouver Forum on the care of the live organ donor: lung, liver, pancreas, and intestine data and medical guidelines. *Transplantation.* 2006;81(10):1373–1385.
22. Dew M, Jacobs CL, Jowsey SG, et al. Guidelines for the psychosocial evaluation of living unrelated donors in the United States. *Am J Transplant.* 2007;7:1047–1054.
23. Living Kidney Donor Follow-Up Conference Writing Group; Leichtman A, Abecassis M, et al. Living kidney donor follow-up: state-of-the-art and future directions, conference summary and recommendations. *Am J Transplant.* 2011;11(12):2561–2568.
24. Kasiski BL, McBride MA, Cornell DL, et al. Report of a Consensus Conference on Transplant Program Quality and Surveillance. *Am J Transplant.* 2012;12(8):1988–1996.
25. Melcher M, Blosser CD, Baxter-Lowe LA, et al. Dynamic challenges inhibiting optimal adoption of kidney paired donation: findings of a consensus conference. *Am J Transplant.* 2013;13(4):851–860.
26. LaPointe Rudow D, Hays R, Baliga P, et al. Consensus Conference on Best Practices in Live Kidney Donation: recommendations to optimize education, access, and care. *Am J Transplant.* 2015;15(4):914–922.
27. Rudow DL. The living donor advocate: a team approach to educate, evaluate, and manage donors across the continuum. *Prog Transplant.* 2009;19(1):64–70.
28. Sites AK, Freeman JR, Harper MR, et al. A multidisciplinary program to educate and advocate for living donors. *Prog Transplant.* 2008;18(4):284–289.
29. Hays RE, LaPointe Rudow D, Dew MA, et al. The Independent Living Donor Advocate: a Guidance Document from the American Society of Transplantation's Living Donor Community of Practice (LDCOP). *Am J Transplant.* 2015;15(2):518–525.
30. Steel JL, Dunlavy A, Friday M, et al. The development of practice guidelines for ILDAs. *Clin Transplant.* 2013;27(2):178–184.
31. Steel JL, Dunlavy A, Friday M, et al. A national survey of independent living donor advocates: the need for practice guidelines. *Am J Transplant.* 2012;12(8):2141–2149.
32. Segev DL, Gentry SE, Warren DS, et al. Kidney paired donation and optimizing the use of live donor organs. *JAMA.* 2005;293:1883–1890.
33. Gordon EJ. Informed consent for living donation: a review of key empirical studies, ethical challenges and future research. *Am J Transplant.* 2012;12:2273–2280.
34. Living Donor Follow-up Policies of the Organ Procurement and Transplantation Network. Available at http://optn.transplant.hrsa.gov/media/1200/optn_policies.pdf#nameddest=Policy_18. Accessed October 14, 2015.
35. Dew MA, Myaskovsky L, Steel JL, et al. Managing the psychosocial and financial consequences of living donation. *Curr Transpl Rep.* 2014;1(1):24–34.
36. Jowsey SG, Jacobs C, Gross CR, et al. Emotional well-being of living kidney donors: findings from the RELIVE study. *Am J Transplant.* 2014;14(11):2535–2544.
37. Lentine KL, Schnitzler MA, Xiao H, et al. Depression diagnoses after living kidney donation: linking U.S. Registry data and administrative claims. *Transplantation.* 2012;94(1):77–83.
38. Ladner DP, Dew MA, Forney S, et al. Long-term quality of life after liver donation in the adult to adult living donor livers transplantation cohort study (A2ALL). *J Hepatol.* 2015;62(2):346–353.

39. Moore DR, Feurer ID, Zaydfudim V, et al. Evaluation of living kidney donors: variables that affect donation. *Prog Transplant.* 2012;22(4):385–392.

40. Public Health Service Guideline for Reducing Human Immunodeficiency Virus, Hepatitis B Virus, and Hepatitis C Virus Transmission Through Organ Transplantation. Available at http://www.publichealthreports.org/issue-open.cfm?articleID=2975. Accessed February 22, 2015.

41. Rocca JP, Davis E, Edye M. Live donor nephrectomy. *Mt Sinai J Med.* 2012;79(3):330–341.

42. Lobritto S, Kato T, Emond J. Living-donor liver transplantation: current perspective. *Semin Liver Dis.* 2012;32(4):333–340.

43. Song GW, Lee SG. Living donor liver transplantation. *Curr Opin Organ Transplant.* 2014;19(3):217–222.

44. Olthoff KM, Emond JC, Shearon TH, et al. Liver regeneration after living donor transplantation: adult-to-adult living donor liver transplantation cohort study. *Liver Transpl.* 2015;21(1):79–88.

45. Muzaale AD, Massie AB, Wang MC, et al. Risk of end-stage renal disease following live kidney donation. *JAMA.* 2014;311(6):579–586.

46. Mjoen G, Hallan S, Hartmann A, et al. Long-term risks for kidney donors. *Kidney Int.* 2014;86(1):162–167.

47. Cheah YL, Simpson MA, Pomposelli JJ, et al. Incidence of death and potentially life-threatening near-miss events in living donor hepatic lobectomy: a world-wide survey. *Liver Transpl.* 2013;19(5):499–506.

48. Kim MJ, Min GE, Yoo KH, et al. Risk factors for postoperative ileus after urologic laparoscopic surgery. *J Korean Surg Soc.* 2011;80(6):384–389.

49. Steiner RW, Ix JH, Rifkin DE, et al. Estimating risks of de novo kidney diseases after living kidney donation. *Am J Transplant.* 2014;14(3):538–544.

SELF-ASSESSMENT QUESTIONS

1. An important part of the donor evaluation includes all of the following EXCEPT:
   a. assessment of immunological compatibility.
   b. assessment of competence.
   c. assessment of financial ability to pay for surgery.
   d. assessment of medical history.

2. An important part of the consent process is:
   1. understanding the risks of the surgery.
   2. disclosure that it is a federal crime to be paid for donation.
   3. disclosure of the recipient patient and graft survival at the transplant program.
   4. ensuring the confidentiality of the process
   a. 1, 2, and 3
   b. 1, 2, and 4
   c. 2, 3, and 4
   d. All of the above

3. Which of the following may be a sign of a bile leak in the liver donor?
   1. Black stools
   2. Right shoulder pain
   3. Left lower quadrant pain
   4. Disorientation
   a. 1 and 3
   b. 3 and 4
   c. 2 only
   d. All of the above

4. Which of the following patients may be at increased risk for ESRD post kidney donation?
   1. African American male
   2. Caucasian male with a history of inguinal hernia
   3. Female with a body mass index of 36
   a. 1 and 2 only
   b. 1 and 3 only
   c. 2 and 3 only
   d. All of the above

5. Which of the following severe complications have been reported in living liver donors?
   1. Liver failure resulting in a donor needing a liver transplant
   2. Death of the donor
   3. Pulmonary emboli
   a. 1 and 2 only
   b. 1 and 3 only
   c. 2 and 3 only
   d. All of the above

6. Which of the following can be a complication of kidney donation?
   1. Bleeding
   2. Ileus
   3. Deep vein thrombosis
   a. 1 and 2 only
   b. 2 and 3 only
   c. 1 and 3 only
   d. All of the above

7. The donor and recipient operations are undertaken on the same day at similar times in parallel operating rooms staffed by two full teams of OR personnel. This is done for which of the following reason(s)?
   1. Convenience of the families and staff
   2. Ensure there are no unforeseen problems with the recipient that prevent transplantation
   3. Minimize warm ischemic time
   4. Minimize cold ischemic time
   a. 1 and 2
   b. 2 and 3
   c. 3 and 4
   d. 2 and 4

8. The role of the living donor advocate includes determining that a live donor is:
   1. mentally competent and willing to donate.
   2. free from coercion.
   3. medically and psychosocially suitable.
   4. fully informed of the risks and benefits as a donor.
   5. fully informed of the risks, benefits, and alternative treatment available to the recipient.
   a. 1, 2, and 3
   b. 1, 2, 3, and 4
   c. 1, 2, 3, and 5
   d. All of the above

9. Upon discharge, the nurse should ensure the donor has been given instructions on:
   a. wound care.
   b. diet information.
   c. information on when to call the transplant team.
   d. all of the above.

10. For living liver donation in pediatric transplantation, which of the following lobes is used?
    a. Right lateral segment
    b. Right frontal segment
    c. Left lateral segment
    d. Left posterior segment

Correct Answers:
1.c   2.d   3.c   4.b   5.d   6.d   7.d   8.d   9.d   10.c

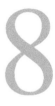

CHAPTER 8

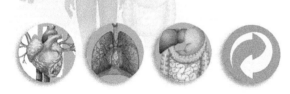

Professional Issues

Rebecca P. Winsett, RN, PhD

Cynthia L. Russell, RN, PhD, FAAN

 I. INTRODUCTION

Professionalism is fundamental to nursing practice, and the behavior that underpins professionalism is civil behavior. In this chapter, we elucidate professional behaviors in scope and practice of transplant nursing. Professionalism embodies the values of altruism, autonomy, human dignity, integrity, and social justice. However, when working in a highly charged atmosphere such as transplantation, these behaviors must be built into the culture of the organization.

 II. TRANSPLANT EDUCATION

   A. Education of self

      1. The field of transplantation is constantly changing. Examples of change include xenotransplantation, pharmacogenomics, transplantation of extremely young and old individuals, use of technology to enhance transplantation procedures, larger transplant databases, and use of computers to manage transplantation. Consequently, transplant nurses must continuously update their knowledge and skills. The 2011 Institute of Medicine Report, *The Future of Nursing: Leading Change, Advancing Health*, provides an action-oriented blueprint for nurses suggesting that nurses should practice to the full extent of their education and training and should achieve higher levels of education and training through an improved education system that promotes seamless academic progression.[1]

      2. Educational opportunities for transplant nurses may be formal or informal.

         a. Formal options may include the following:

            i. Completing formal degree-supporting coursework from colleges or universities where interprofessional education is increasingly more common

           ii. Attending professional transplant conferences where continuing education programs are offered

          iii. Reading and discussing peer-reviewed journals

b. Informal learning opportunities include the following:
  i. Attending lectures and/or educational rounds
  ii. Observing and/or participating in teaching at the patient's bedside
3. Staffing and economic constraints are changing transplant nursing education. It is becoming increasingly more difficult for transplant nurses to take time away from work, and travel funds provided by employers are greatly limited. To enhance accessibility, formal and informal education programs are offered through online learning and webinar formats. These approaches allow the transplant nurse to participate in relatively low-cost educational opportunities at convenient times. Many programs provide continuing education units for participants who are required by many states for maintaining licensure.
4. Continued education, coupled with successful clinical practice, enables the transplant nurse to progress from a "novice" to "expert" practitioner and engage in increasingly complex clinical decision-making processes involving clinical reasoning and judgment.[2]
5. Certification in the specialty of transplant nursing indicates that a transplant nurse has met a high level of competence and has the knowledge and skills needed to provide quality care for transplant donors, recipients, and families in specialty practice.
  a. Through the American Board for Transplant Certification,[3] a transplant nurse may be certified as a Procurement Coordinator, a Transplant Nurse Coordinator, and/or a Clinical Transplant Nurse.
  b. A certification is also offered for Transplant Preservationists.

B. Education of other health care providers
1. Transplant nurses have a responsibility to educate other health care providers, particularly new staff nurses and nursing students, about organ donation and transplantation.
2. Education about organ donation
  a. Hospitals are required to implement specific protocols to assist in the identification and evaluation of potential donors and ensure that every potential donor family is informed of the option to donate.[4]
  b. Health care providers' lack of knowledge about organ donation, including reticence regarding donation after circulatory death, may contribute to the limited availability of donor organs.
  c. Health care professionals are the critical link in the organ procurement process, because they are the first individuals who establish rapport with a potential donor's family and consequently have the opportunity to discuss the option of organ donation.[5]
  d. Education of all health care workers, particularly those who work in emergency departments and inpatient units (including intensive care and transplant units), is an essential component of any transplant program.
3. Education about transplantation
  a. Transplant nurses must continually educate new transplant staff members and students about the complex and ever-changing field of transplantation. Education should be provided as transplant care is delivered, in a highly interprofessional manner. Interprofessional education is an effective method for simulating "real-life" situations to improve patient, family, and community outcomes.[6]
  b. Given the growing number of transplant recipients in the general population and their increasing longevity, transplant nurses must

also educate nontransplant staff members who care for recipients upon readmission to the hospital, in an outpatient setting, or in the community.

    c. Transplant standards of care are a valuable resource and should be used to educate and guide all health care providers caring for transplant patients, families, and communities.

C. Education of the general public

1. There continues to be a gap between the number of patients needing an organ transplant and the number of organs available to transplant. Transplant nurses are active in efforts to narrow this gap.

2. Transplant nurses facilitate organ donation by educating the public about the following:

    a. The benefits and procedures of organ donation

    b. Living donation

    c. The need for individuals who wish to be organ donors to communicate this intention to their families

    d. The concept of brain death

3. Education of the public may be formal or informal. Transplant staff may have opportunities to provide this education in academic and community settings or via the media.

4. There are many patient and family resources about organ donation. The transplant nurse can support the patient, family, and the community with resources such as those available at the following:

    a. United Network for Organ Sharing: www.unos.org

    b. National Kidney Foundation: www.kidney.org

5. Transplant nurses are involved in influencing public policy related to organ donation, recognizing that policy changes are necessary for improving public health. Transplant nurses are also cognizant of unethical approaches to increase the donor pool through such efforts as organ trafficking and payment for organ donation.[7]

 III. PROFESSIONAL PRACTICE EVALUATION

A. Professional nursing practice includes periodic self-evaluation. The goal of this process is to determine if the transplant nurse's practice meets the appropriate standards or if there are opportunities for improvement.

1. A thorough self-evaluation should include evaluations from superiors, professional peers, peers from other professions, as well as patients, families, and the community. The professional transplant nurse must be accountable to those receiving care and also to colleagues.

2. Evaluation of transplant nursing competence occurs through periodic employer-based evaluations using established tools. A 360-degree evaluation involves input from supervisors, peers, and patients, families, and communities. Transplant Nurse Coordinator competency-based evaluation tools are available through the International Transplant Nurses Society.[8]

3. Several important standards in general nursing practice include the following:

    a. *Scope and Standards of Nursing*[9]

    b. *Nursing's Social Policy Statement*[10]

    c. *Code of Ethics for Nursing*[11]

4. In the specialty of transplant nursing, the following documents delineate the standards, accountabilities, and competencies for both transplant specialists and generalists:
   a. *Scope and Standards of Transplant Nursing Practice*[12]
   b. *Core Competencies for Transplant Nursing*[13]
5. Worldwide variation in transplant nursing practice influences practice evaluation. Consequently, local, state, or regional standards, guidelines, statutes, rules, and/or regulations should also be considered when conducting a practice self-evaluation.

B. If opportunities for practice improvement are identified, appropriate steps should be taken to remedy the practice-standard gap. This might include formal or informal didactic or practice educational strategies.
   1. A plan for remediation of the identified gap should include the following:
      a. Dates for remediation
      b. Steps that will be taken for remediation
      c. Date when a repeat evaluation will be conducted to determine if remediation was successful
   2. If remediation is not successful, the process is repeated until the standard is met.

 IV. QUALITY/PERFORMANCE IMPROVEMENT

A. Transplant programs are required to implement performance improvement plans to improve patient, family, and community outcomes.[14] The transplant nurse participates in the program's performance improvement plan and is able to verbalize the transplant unit's performance improvement plan goals, processes, and outcomes.

B. The role of the transplant nurse in performance improvement depends upon his/her level of transplant nursing knowledge, skills, and education. For example, the novice transplant nurse may attend unit performance improvement meetings, collect quality data, summarize data, and/or follow performance improvement committee recommendations. The expert transplant nurse may lead unit performance improvement meetings, identify outcomes for improvement, analyze data, make recommendations for action, and share findings across the organization through facility-wide programs.
   1. Quality of transplant nursing care achieves the best outcome for the patient that is safe, effective, and timely. Consistent unit performance is a team effort.
   2. The interdisciplinary transplant team strives to achieve excellent transplant outcomes. As a member of this team, it is important that the transplant nurse should do the following:
      a. Participates in the governance structure of the unit
      b. Understands performance improvement methodology
      c. Promotes the culture of high accountability

C. Chapter 19 addresses quality assurance and performance improvement in more detail.

V. COLLEGIALITY

A. Collegiality is the relationship of colleagues working together toward a mutual goal. A collegial relationship is crucial for ensuring quality and safety and for maintaining professional standards.[15] Transplant nurses must work on interprofessional teams and share transplant knowledge and skills with peers and colleagues to improve patient, family, and community outcomes.

B. Collegiality and professional practice evaluation are mutually linked. Transplant nurses must support each other by giving and receiving feedback on nursing practice. This process improves transplant nursing role performance and contributes to a productive and healthy work environment.

C. One aspect of collegiality is mentoring. Mentorship involves someone who is more experienced guiding a less experienced person through a learning process.[16] The goal of the mentoring process is career development and professional enhancement. The mentor and mentee have a commitment to the relationship, which often lasts over an extended period of time. The mentor supports and nurtures the mentee in professional growth.

 VI. ENVIRONMENTAL HEALTH

A. The connection between air pollution, home energy, water quality, and sanitation is a focus of global environmental health. It is defined by the World Health Organization as "physical, chemical and biological factors" that have an influence in the health of a community or individuals.[17]

B. Nurses must practice in an evidence-based manner that reduces environmental health risks for all colleagues, health care consumers, families, and communities. The *Scope and Standards for Nurses* purports that nurses must be educated about environmental health concepts, strategies, and practices.[18] Efforts can be health care facility focused and/or community focused.

   1. Health care facility–focused efforts: Nurses must assess the practice environment for factors such as sound, odor, noise, and light that threaten health. The nurse should support the use of appropriate products in health care.

   2. Community-focused efforts: In the community, commonly encountered hazardous materials risks include chemicals used for sterilization and/or compounds found in medical devices. Single-use devices may decrease perceived use of infections but also contribute to landfill waste. Reprocessing single-use devices may reduce waste but must be balanced with occupational, ethical, and quality of care concerns. All nurses, including transplant nurses, must be knowledgeable about environmental health risks and strategies to reduce risks while preserving the environment.

 VII. COLLABORATION

A. Collaboration is defined as working with others to do a task and to achieve shared goals. Transplant nurses should consider the following factors in regard to communicating and collaborating with patients, peers, colleagues, within and between departments, and within and between organizations.

1. What behaviors indicate that the nurse listens and hears what colleagues are actually communicating?
2. What behaviors, both verbal and nonverbal, indicate that the nurse is respectful toward others?
3. How can the nurse's behaviors be adapted or modified based on the patient and family with whom he/she is interacting?
4. What structures and processes are used to identify learning styles of patients?
5. When responsible for the education of others, what type of teaching/learning styles ensures that the message is understood?
6. How does the nurse match education and understanding level to learning style and teaching?
7. What strategies help the nurse understand the cultural and ethnic values of patients, families, and colleagues?
8. How does the nurse communicate to others that he/she respects cultural and ethnic diversity?
9. How does the organization recognize and appreciate the cultural and ethnic diversity of associates and patients?

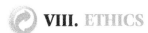 VIII. ETHICS

A. Moral and ethical responsibilities of the transplant nurse include advocating for vulnerable populations in the practice environment and demonstrating ethical and moral behaviors in the research.

B. Ethics and morals are interrelated and often used interchangeably.

1. *Morals* are the principles of personal behavior upon which right and wrong are based. Morals are embedded within the culture in which one lives.
   Ethics is defined as the social system in which morals are applied. This chapter addresses both moral behavior and the ethical conduct within the organization and within transplantation.
2. The American Nurses Association *Code of Ethics*[11] is the document that outlines ethical conduct for US nurses. The document outlines the following nine provisions:
   a. Respect for persons regardless of their socioeconomic status, personal attributes, or health problems
   b. Commitment to the patient
   c. Patient advocacy
   d. Responsibility and accountability for individual nursing practice
   e. Professional competency and personal and professional growth
   f. Establishing, maintaining, and improving the health care environment
   g. Advancement of the nursing profession
   h. Collaboration with other health care professionals and the public
   i. Responsibility of the profession to articulate nursing values, maintain the integrity of the profession, and shape social policy

C. The Code of Ethics and Conduct for European Nursing[19] and the *International Council of Nurses Code of Ethics for Nurses*[20] are similar documents for nurses outside the United States.

D. Transplant nurses have a responsibility to do the following:
1. Maintain donor and recipient confidentiality
2. Address any discrepancies between their personal values and difficult candidate/recipient situations

E. The major ethical principles that underpin ethical decision making are listed below[21]:
1. Autonomy: A competent individual's independence, self-reliance, and ability to decide
   a. The principle of autonomy and self-determination supports the informed consent process with respect to decision making regarding therapeutic options and participation in research.
   b. Informed consent means that the patient has the following:
      i. The legal capacity to provide consent
      ii. The ability to exercise free power of choice without any form of constraint or coercion
      iii. Sufficient knowledge and comprehension to make an enlightened decision
2. Nonmaleficence: the principle that one must "do no harm"
   a. Prohibits intentional harm
   b. Requires the justification of risks by probable benefits
   c. Requires that agents exercise due care and meet the legal and moral standards regarding knowledge, skills, and diligence
3. Beneficence: the principle to provide benefits and balance benefits and harms
   a. More altruistic and far-reaching than the principle of nonmaleficence
   b. Requires positive acts to prevent harm, remove harmful conditions, confer benefits, and balance benefits and harms
4. Justice: principle that one has been treated justly when one has been given what one is due or owed—that is, what one deserves and can legitimately claim
   a. Comparative and noncomparative justice
      i. Comparative justice is determined by balancing the competing claims of others (e.g., transplant eligibility criteria).
      ii. Noncomparative justice is judged by a standard that is independent of others' claims (e.g., innocent individuals do not deserve punishment).
   b. Distributive justice refers to the distribution of benefits under conditions of scarcity (e.g., scarcity of donor organs).
      i. Macroallocation issues involve decisions regarding social justice and public health policy (e.g., equality and rights in health care, the ability to pay and access to organ transplantation).
      ii. Microallocation issues involve decisions regarding who shall live when not all can live (e.g., the allocation of scarce lifesaving medical resources such as donor organs, listing criteria, behaviors that may lead to organ failure such as alcoholism, substance abuse).

F. Many situations in transplantation often pose moral and ethical conflict. It is important that transplant nurses and interprofessional teams facilitate appropriate moral and ethical decisions. When thinking about clinical ethical dilemmas, the goal is to do the following:

1. Facilitate clinical decision making that focuses on the patient and respects the patient's rights and interests
2. Promote the participation of all relevant professionals (e.g., transplant physicians, surgeons, coordinators, staff nurses, advanced practice nurses, social workers, chaplains, ethicists, and so forth)
3. Enhance organizational commitment and cooperation such that all involved parties develop and implement plans in support of the patient

G. Clinical ethics extend across the entire life span continuum. Examples in the field of transplantation include the following:

1. Prepregnancy (the pros and cons of pregnancy in transplant recipients)
2. During pregnancy (the pros and cons of terminating a pregnancy that is endangering the life of the transplant recipient)
3. Infancy (the pros and cons of transplantation in an infant with multiple congenital anomalies)
4. Childhood and adolescence (the extent to which children and adolescents should be involved in making decisions about transplantation)
5. Adulthood (the pros and cons of retransplantation)
6. Old age (the pros and cons of transplantation in the older adult)

H. Resources for ethics consultations

1. Many situations in the field of transplantation present ethical dilemmas and can benefit from ethics consultations.
2. Key elements of ethics consultations include the following[22]:
   a. Identification of individuals who can initiate ethics consultations (e.g., health care providers, clinicians, patients, family members)
   b. Identification of individuals who should be notified that the ethics consultation has been initiated
   c. Complete and accurate documentation in the patient's record
   d. Promotion of accountability through case review or quality improvement process

I. Written informed consent

1. Informed consent is "the knowing consent of an individual or his/her legally authorized representative, under circumstances that provide the prospective subject or representative sufficient opportunity to consider whether or not to participate without undue inducement or any element of force, fraud, deceit, duress, or other forms of constraint or coercion."[23(p. 9–10)]
2. The written informed consent for a procedure or to participate in research is not merely getting the patient to sign the form to put in the chart. Rather, it is a *continuing process* that involves providing information to patients and families so that they understand the procedure or research study and have enough information to make an informed decision regarding whether or not they want to participate.
3. Table 8-1 delineates the differences between the procedural consent and the research consent.

TABLE 8-1 Differences in Informed Consent for Invasive Procedures and Research Studies

Invasive Procedure Requiring Written Informed Consent	Research Study Requiring Written Informed Consent
The decision to undergo a procedure is based on a perceived health need.	Participation is not based on a health need.
Risks and benefits are presented, and the patient may choose to undergo procedure even if there are great risks.	Risks and benefits are weighed against current and future risks and benefits. These risks include psychological, physical, and financial risks to participating. The patient does not have to participate in research study to have ongoing health care.
Patient expects to have improved health based on procedure.	Patient expects not to have health compromised by participating in the study.
Patient is provided enough information to be able to make an informed decision. If patient is not able to make an informed decision due to health status, next of kin is provided with information and gives consent according to local or state laws.	Patient is provided with enough information to make an informed decision. In the case where an experimental procedure is planned, there is additional oversight with a medical ethics committee or institutional review board (IRB).
The consent process is a hospital-based procedure and is considered a legal document. The patient has the right to cancel participation at any time; however, if the consent is for a procedure that will improve his or her health, revoking the consent may be difficult for the patient and difficult for the health care provider to accept the patient canceling the procedure.	The IRB or ethics committee oversees the consent process; approval from this body must be obtained before approaching a potential subject about participation. The informed consent document itself must be approved by this body. The consent is a legal document; the participant has the right to withdraw participation at any time.

 IX. EVIDENCE-BASED PRACTICE AND RESEARCH

The transplant professional is able to describe the difference between evidence-based practice and research.

    A.   Evidence-based practice

        1. Evidence-based practice results from the synthesis of multiple research studies. It may also include internal outcomes of performance improvement projects. Integrating evidence into practice also considers practice experts and patient values.[15]

        2. Web-based resources for evidence-based practices include the following:

            a. Cochrane Collaboration International: A nonprofit, independent organization dedicated to making up-to-date, accurate information about the effects of health care readily available worldwide through the Cochrane Database of Systematic Reviews: www.cochrane.org/reviews/index.htm

            b. The National Institute for Health and Care Evidence: a complementary organization supported by the U.K. Health System: www.nice.org.uk

            c. Johanna Briggs Institute: An arm of the School of Translational Science within the University of Adelaide, South Australia: http://joannabriggs.org

            d. McMaster Health Information Research Unit: http://hiru.mcmaster.ca/hiru/HIRU_McMaster_PLUS_projects.aspx

        3. Several taxonomies are available to evaluate the evidence associated with a particular practice.

            a. The highest level of evidence is the meta-analysis or evidence-based practice guidelines.

    b. The lowest level of evidence is the nonresearch expert opinion article. This type of article is important and may guide future research. However, it would not be part of the synthesis of research that changes practice.

B. Transplant Research

  1. Research is the systematic collection of information in order to increase generalizable knowledge.[24]

  2. Research with human subjects is overseen by the institution's institutional review board (IRB) or ethics review committee.

    a. A human subject is defined as a living person. The definition of "living person," however, may be more complex in organ procurement research. For example, if the research uses data from a living person prior to organ donation or after the organ has been transplanted, the research may be considered human subjects research. Oversight of the review board is required to determine whether the study constitutes human subject research.

  3. Three principles from the 1979 Belmont Report[21] guide research: respect for persons, beneficence, and justice. It is important for transplant nurses to know what these principles mean as they pertain to biomedical research.

    a. Respect for persons

      i.   This principle is grounded in the belief that subjects participate in research voluntarily and with adequate information.

      ii. This principle states that investigators must give sufficient and accurate information on the purpose of the research, its risks and benefits, in a manner so that a person can choose to either refuse or agree to participate.

      iii. Transplant nurses have the responsibility to provide accurate, clear, and comprehensive information about the research study and to maintain confidentiality about the data collected during the course of the study.

      iv. Transplant nurses are often perceived by patients/families to hold positions of power and authority. Therefore, it is essential that transplant nurses refrain from any actions or statements that might in any way influence a patient's decision regarding participation in a research study.

    b. Beneficence

      i.   Beneficence requires a balancing benefits and harms.

      ii. Researchers must make every effort to maximize the benefits and minimize the risks that may be associated with a research study.

      iii. Transplant professionals have a responsibility to inform patients/families when risk/benefit considerations change so that the patient/family can decide whether to continue their participation in the research study.

    c. Justice

      i.   Justice requires that all persons have an equal opportunity to participate in research so that no one specific gender, ethnic, or cultural group bears the burden of research participation.

      ii. This principle requires that researchers refrain from using a particular group of potential research subjects solely because that group is easily accessible.

  4. The Research Consent

    a. The research consent is a document that explains the risks and benefits of the research as well as what the subject is asked to do as a research subject. Informed consent is a continuing process that involves providing information to patients and their families so that they understand the research study and have enough information to make an informed decision regarding whether or not they want to participate in the research study.

   b. Transplant nurses should know the following:
      i.   The circumstances that are perceived as coercion or undue influence during the consent process
      ii. As the patient advocate, how to ensure that the consent process is provided in an environment that is not coercive, where the patient and family can consider the research and have enough knowledge to volunteer participation
5. Even though a transplant nurse may not be the researcher, he/she can facilitate the principles of respect, beneficence, and justice by
   a. Creating an environment conducive to listening, so that the consenter can explain the research study
      i.   This includes, but is not limited to, making certain that
           • The room is quiet and that interruptions are minimized
           • The patient is free from pain, fatigue, anxiety, etc.
      ii. See Table 8-2 for additional factors that may influence a patient's understanding on the purpose of the research and impact the capacity to volunteer to participate
   b. Assessing the patient's understanding of the procedure so that the nurse and the patient are confident that an *informed* decision was made
   c. Notifying the consenter if the patient/family has questions
   d. Verifying that informed consent was obtained *before* initiating a research protocol
   e. Obtaining research data per protocol (e.g., drawing laboratory samples, documenting vital signs, administering medications)
   f. Notifying the principal investigator or study coordinator of any patient-related factors that may impact the study protocol
   g. Completing administrative responsibilities such as
      i.   Placing copies of the research study and IRB approval in the designated location
      ii. If multiple studies are being conducted simultaneously, creating a chart that lists each study, the investigators and/or study coordinators, and their contact information
      iii. Placing the signed informed consent document in the designated area of the medical record

TABLE 8-2 Factors That Influence a Patient's Ability to Volunteer for Research Study

Factor	Example
Development related	Cognitive status; external factors that may inhibit patients' ability to make decisions in concordance with their developmental stage (e.g., pain, stress, mental acuity, disease process)
Illness related	Past and current illness history; past experiences with health care system
Psychological issues, cultural and religious values	Desire to "please" health care providers
External pressures	Lack of insurance coverage, threat of catastrophic health events, family pressure
Investigator related	Consent language above reading level. Conciseness of language. Overuse of acronyms. Lack of validation of understanding

From Montalvo W, Larson E. Participant comprehension of research for which they volunteer: a systematic review. *J Nursing Scholarship*. 2014;46(6):423–431, Ref.[25]; Roberts LW. Informed consent and the capacity for voluntarism. *Am J Psychiatry*. 2002;159(5):705–712, Ref.[26]

X. RESOURCE UTILIZATION

A. Resource utilization is a way to evaluate the type and amount of resources used to achieve the planned outcome. For example, what is the cost of treatment for delayed graft function? Once this cost is known, the organization can use this information to compare costs for prevention with the treatment costs. Is it worth the cost of pulsatile perfusion to reduce delayed graft function?

1. Transplant nurses should be able to identify the following:
   a. The structures and processes that are used to streamline processes and improve efficiency (e.g., LEAN, Six Sigma, all cost analysis)
   b. The unit, departmental, or organizational teams that evaluate and address transplant resource utilization
   c. The cost containment methods that are used in the department
   d. The manner in which cost containment interventions impact the quality of care provided to transplant patients and families
   e. Methods that the unit and department use to share information relative to cost and cost-effectiveness
   f. Professional development activities that can assist in augmenting resource utilization
   g. Strategies that the transplant team uses to ensure that quality of care and cost containment are balanced

 XI. LEADERSHIP

All nurses have leadership capabilities. The terms "leader" and "manager" are often used interchangeably, but there are some distinct differences.[27]

A. A manager is the formal role for a nurse who has responsibility for a specific group and thus has concomitant authority. A leader, on the other hand, may not have any delegated authority, but, because of certain characteristics such as good communication skills, expertise, and knowledge, is able to guide others. Managers can be great leaders, but all nurses have the potential to be leaders.

B. In evaluating their leadership potential, transplant nurses should do the following:

1. Compare and contrast the characteristics of a good leader and those of a good manager
2. Evaluate their skills relative to the following:
   a. Communicating with others (e.g., patients, families, the interprofessional team)
   b. Conflict resolution
   c. Facilitating coordination of care for patients
3. Assess the structures and processes that are in place in their units, departments, or organization that do the following:
   a. Promote a healthy work environment
   b. Recognize and reward scholarly work
   c. Recognize and reward advanced certification or professional development
4. Identify activities that demonstrate a commitment to transplant nursing

REFERENCES

1. Institute of Medicine. *The Future of Nursing: Leading Change, Advancing Health.* Washington, DC: The National Academies Press; 2011.
2. Benner P. *From Novice to Expert: Excellence and Power in Clinical Nursing Practice.* Commemorative Edition. Upper Saddle River, NJ: Prentice Hall; 2001.
3. American Board for Transplant Certification. 2014. Available at http://www.abtc.net/Pages/default.aspx. Accessed September 10, 2014.
4. Health Resources and Services Administration. *Organ Procurement and Transplant Network.* 42 CFR Part 121. Vol 98-HRSA-01. 1998.
5. Bastami S, Matthes O, Krones T, et al. Systematic review of attitudes toward donation after cardiac death among healthcare providers and the general public. *Crit Care Med.* 2013;41(3):897–905.
6. Reeves S, Zwarenstein M, Goldman J, et al. Interprofessional education: effects on professional practice and health care outcomes. *Cochrane Database Syst Rev.* 2009;1:1–23.
7. Chapman J, Capron AM, Levin A, et al. Organ trafficking and transplant tourism: the role of global professional ethical standards-the 2008 Declaration of Istanbul. *Transplantation.* 2013;95(11):1306–1312.
8. International Transplant Nurses Society. *ITNS Home Page.* 2014. Available at http://www.itns.org/. Accessed February 4, 2015.
9. American Nurses Association. *Scope and Standards of Practice: Nursing.* 2nd ed. Silver Spring, MD: American Nurses Association; 2010.
10. American Nurses Association. *Nursing's Social Policy Statement: The Essence of the Profession.* Silver Spring, MD: American Nurses Association; 2010.
11. American Nurses Association. *Code of Ethics for Nurses with Interpretive Statements.* Silver Spring, MD: American Nurses Association; 2015.
12. American Nurses Association; International Transplant Nurses Society. *Transplant Nursing: Scope and Standards of Practice.* Silver Spring, MD: Nursesbooks.org; 2009.
13. Cupples SA, ed. *Introduction to Transplant Nursing Core Competencies.* St. Louis: Mosby-Elsevier; 2008.
14. Centers for Medicare & Medicaid Services. 2014. Available at http://www.cms.hhs.gov/CFCsAndCoPs/downloads/Trancenterreg2007.pdf. Accessed September 13, 2014.
15. Padgett S. Professional collegiality and peer monitoring among nursing staff: an ethnographic study. *Int J Nurs Stud.* 2013;50(10):1407–1415.
16. Hodgson A, Scanlan J. A concept analysis of mentoring in nursing leadership. *Open J Nursing.* 2013;3:389–394.
17. World Health Organization. *Environmental Health.* 2014. Available at http://www.who.int/topics/environmental_health/en/. Accessed October 13, 2014.
18. American Nurses Association. *Environmental Health.* 2014. Available at http://www.nursingworld.org/Environmental-Health. Accessed October 13, 2014.
19. Sasso L, Stievano A, González Jurado M, et al. Code of ethics and conduct for European nursing. *Nurs Ethics.* 2008;15(6):821–836.
20. International Council of Nurses. *The ICN Code of Ethics for Nurses.* Geneva, Switzerland: International Council of Nurses; 2012.
21. National Commission for the Protection of Human Subjects of Biomedical and Behavioral Research. *The Belmont Report: ethical principles and guidelines for the protection of human subjects of research.* Washington, DC: US Department of Health, Education, and Welfare; 1979:GPO 887–809.
22. Molter NC. Professional caring and ethical practice. In: Alspach JG, ed. *Core Curriculum for Critical Care Nursing.* St. Louis, MO: Saunders Elsevier; 2006:1–44.
23. Department of Health and Human Services. *Protection of Human Subjects.* Title 45 Part 46. Washington, DC: Code of Federal Regulations; 2009.
24. Department of Health and Human Services. Common Rule. *Federal Register.* 1991;56. Vol 45 CFR Part 46 subpart A:28002–28032.
25. Montalvo W, Larson E. Participant comprehension of research for which they volunteer: a systematic review. *J Nurs Scholarsh.* 2014;46(6):423–431.
26. Roberts LW. Informed consent and the capacity for voluntarism. *Am J Psychiatry.* 2002;159(5):705–712.
27. Kouzes JM, Posner BZ. *The Leadership Challenge: How to Make Extraordinary Things Happen in Organizations.* New York: John Wiley & Sons; 2012.

SELF-ASSESSMENT QUESTIONS

1. Certification is available for which of the following practice areas?
   1. Procurement Coordinator
   2. Transplant Nurse Coordinator
   3. Clinical Transplant Nurse
   4. Transplant Preservationists
   a. 1, 2, and 3
   b. 1, 3, and 4
   c. 2, 3, and 4
   d. All of the above

2. Which of the following guide transplant nursing evaluation?
   1. Scope and Standards of Nursing
   2. American Nurses Association. Guide to the Code of Ethics for Nurses
   3. Scope and Standards of Transplant Nursing Practice
   4. Core Competencies for Transplant Nursing
   a. 1 and 2
   b. 1 and 3
   c. 3 and 4
   d. All of the above

3. Novice transplant nurses typically lead unit performance improvement meetings, identify outcomes for improvement, analyze data, and make recommendations for action and sharing findings across the organization through facility-wide programs.
   a. True
   b. False

4. Collegiality is important for (choose all that apply):
   1. Interprofessional team work
   2. Quality and safety in practice
   3. Mentoring
   4. Giving and receiving feedback
   5. Maintaining professional standards
   a. 1, 3, and 4
   b. 2, 3, and 5
   c. 1, 4, and 5
   d. All of the above

5. Environmental health and safety is defined as all the physical, chemical, and biological factors external to a person and all the related factors impacting behaviors.
   a. True
   b. False

6. Novice transplant nurses can improve the quality of care by:
   a. becoming familiar with their patients' preferred learning styles.
   b. leading a conference on leadership and its impact on nursing.
   c. knowing the unit's goals and how the care they provide impacts those goals.
   d. a and c.
   e. b and c.

7. When transplant nurses discuss a procedure or a research study with a patient/family and provide information in a way that the patient family will understand and give them enough information to make an informed decision, they are practicing the principle of:
   a. autonomy.
   b. beneficence.
   c. justice.
   d. beneficence and justice.

8. Informed consent is defined as obtaining the patient's signature on the consent form.
   a. True
   b. False

9. The goals of clinical ethics are to:
   1. facilitate decision making that focuses on the patient.
   2. promote collaboration with all relevant professionals.
   3. enhance organizational commitment and cooperation such that all involved parties develop and implement plans in support of the patient.
   a. 1 and 2
   b. 2 and 3
   c. 1 and 3
   d. 1, 2, and 3

10. Transplant nurses at the bedside should have no voice in unit decisions.
    a. True
    b. False

CHAPTER 9

Heart Transplantation

Vicki McCalmont, RN, MS, ANP-BC, CNS, CCTC

Angela Velleca, RN, BSN, CCTC

 ## I. INTRODUCTION

The topics in this chapter are discussed generally in the order presented in the American Board for Transplant Certification (ABTC) candidate handbook for the Certified Clinical Transplant Nurse (CCTN) examination (available at www.abtc.net).

 ## II. OVERVIEW OF HEART FAILURE (HF)

A. Definition: Heart failure (HF) is a complex clinical syndrome resulting from a structural or functional cardiac disorder impairing left ventricular (LV) filling or ejection. Left ventricular dysfunction can progress to left ventricular failure causing symptoms of shortness of breath and fatigue. When right ventricular (RV) failure is present, patients report peripheral and/or abdominal swelling; the ventricles can fail together or separately.[1]

B. HF is an important cause of morbidity and mortality worldwide. In the United States, congestive heart failure affects 5.7 million people and there are 700,000 new diagnoses annually.[2]

C. End-stage heart disease (ESHD) is a common end point for which heart transplantation, mechanical circulatory support (MCS), and hospice care are the three main therapeutic options.

III. PATHOPHYSIOLOGY OF HEART FAILURE

A. The heart cannot pump blood at a rate commensurate with the body's metabolic needs and/or can pump effectively only if the diastolic volume is abnormally elevated.[3]

B. Left versus right heart failure[3,4] (Table 9-1)

1. Overview

a. HF may be described in terms of the ventricle that is initially impaired.

i. Fluid accumulates behind (upstream to) the affected chamber.

TABLE 9-1 **Clinical Findings in Heart Failure**

Left-Sided Heart Failure		Right-Sided Heart Failure
Systolic	**Diastolic**	
Anxiety	Exercise intolerance	Dependent pitting edema
Sudden light-headedness	Orthopnea	Fatigue, weakness
Fatigue, weakness, lethargy	Dyspnea, dyspnea on exertion	↓ exercise tolerance
Orthopnea	Paroxysmal nocturnal dyspnea	Weight gain or loss
Dyspnea, dyspnea on exertion	Cough with frothy white or pink sputum (in pulmonary edema)	Anorexia
Paroxysmal nocturnal dyspnea		Ascites
Tachypnea (on exertion)	Tachypnea (on exertion)	Cachexia
Cheyne-Stokes respirations (if severe)	Basilar crackles, rhonchi, wheezes	Nausea, vomiting
Diaphoresis	CXR: pulmonary edema	Abdominal pain (from liver congestion)
Palpitations	Hypoxia	Hepatomegaly
Sacral edema, pitting of extremities	Respiratory acidosis: ↑ pH and ↑ $PaCO_2$	Hepatojugular reflux
Basilar rales, rhonchi, crackles, wheezes	↑ pulmonary artery diastolic pressure	Venous distention
Cool, moist, cyanotic skin	↑ pulmonary capillary wedge pressure	Splenomegaly
Hypoxia		Hypotension
Respiratory acidosis: ↑ pH and ↑ $PaCO_2$	S_3, S_4 heart sounds	Bounding pulses
↑ pulmonary artery diastolic pressure	Holosystolic murmur (if tricuspid, mitral regurgitation)	S_3, S_4 heart sounds
↑ pulmonary capillary wedge pressure	Symptoms of right-sided heart failure	Murmur of tricuspid insufficiency
Nocturia		↑ CVP, RA, and RV pressures
Mental confusion		CXR: enlarged RA, RV
↓ pulse pressure		Dysrhythmias
Pulsus alternans		Oliguria
Lateral displacement of point of maximal impulse		Nocturia (secondary to ↑ renal perfusion when patient is lying in bed)
S_3, S_4 heart sounds		Kussmaul's sign (constrictive cardiomyopathy):
Murmur of mitral insufficiency		paradoxical ↑ in venous distention and pressure during inspiration

CXR, chest x-ray; CVP, central venous pressure; $PaCO_2$, arterial partial pressure of carbon dioxide; RA, right atrium; RV, right ventricle. Adapted from Lessig ML. The cardiovascular system. In: Alspach JG, ed. *Core Curriculum for Critical Care Nursing*. 6th ed. Philadelphia, PA: Elsevier; 2006:185–380; Garg A, Vignesh C, Singh V, Ray S. Acute right heart syndrome: rescue treatment with inhaled nitric oxide. *Indian J Crit Care Med*. 2014;18(1):40–42; Jaski B. *The 4 Stages of Heart Failure*. Minneapolis, MN: Cardiotext Publishing, 2015:6–8, 21–31, 86–95, 103–110.

> ii. LV failure: Fluid accumulates in the pulmonary capillary bed.
> iii. RV failure: Fluid accumulates in the systemic venous circulation.

C. HF with preserved or reduced ejection fraction (EF)[5-7] (Table 9-2)
  1. Overview
    a. HF can also be characterized by abnormalities in systolic and/or diastolic function—based on whether the dysfunction stems from an inability of the ventricle to contract normally and pump sufficient blood (systolic HF) or an inability of the heart to relax and fill normally (diastolic HF).
    b. Heart failure with preserved ejection fraction (HFpEF) is a form of diastolic dysfunction. Heart failure with reduced ejection fraction (HFrEF) is characterized by systolic dysfunction.[5]

TABLE 9-2 **Etiology of Heart Failure**

Cardiomyopathy	Infection	Metabolic Disorders	Electrolyte Deficiency	Nutritional Disorders	Systemic Diseases	Toxins
Dilated (idiopathic)	Chagas' disease	**Endocrine**:	Hypokalemia	Kwashiorkor anemia	**Connective tissue disorders**	Alcohol
Hypertrophic	Infection	Diabetes mellitus	Hypomagnesemia	Thiamine deficiency (beriberi)	Systemic lupus erythematosus	Cocaine
Restrictive	Viral	Thyroid disease		Selenium deficiency	Scleroderma	Radiation therapy
Ischemic	Bacterial	Adrenal insufficiency		Carnitine deficiency	Sarcoidosis	Chemotherapeutic agents (e.g., anthracyclines)
Valvular:	Fungal	Pheochromocytoma			Rheumatoid arthritis	Chemicals (e.g., hydrocarbons, lead)
Obstruction		Acromegaly			Polyarteritis nodosa	
Insufficiency		**Familial storage disease**:			Polymyositis	
Hypertensive		Hemochromatosis			**Connective tissue disorders**	
Infective (viral)		Glycogen storage disease			Systemic lupus erythematosus	
Peripartum					Scleroderma	
Familial					Sarcoidosis	
					Rheumatoid arthritis	
					Polyarteritis nodosa	
					Polymyositis	
					Amyloidosis	

From Kallikazaros I. Heart failure with preserved ejection fraction. *Hellenic J Cardiol.* 2014;55:265–266; Komamura K. Review article. Similarities and differences between the pathogenesis and pathophysiology of diastolic and systolic heart failure. *Cardiol Res Pract.* 2013;2013:Article ID 824135; Blair J, Huffman M, Shah S. Heart failure in North America. *Curr Cardiol Rev.* 2013;9:128–146.

2. HFpEF or diastolic dysfunction[5]
   a. A patient with HFpEF will usually have one or more disease processes: diastolic dysfunction from the impaired LV relaxation and/or increased LV diastolic stiffness, enlarged LV size, increased LV volume, increased arterial and ventricular stiffness, and abnormal systolic function.[6]
   b. Diagnosis of this clinical syndrome requires that these three criteria be fulfilled:
      i.   Signs and symptoms of HF
      ii. EF > 45%
      iii. Evidence of diastolic dysfunction echocardiographically or hemodynamically or equivalent (concentric left ventricular hypertrophy, increased LV size, atrial fibrillation, or elevated brain natriuretic peptide [BNP] levels).[6]
3. Restrictive cardiomyopathy, hypertrophic cardiomyopathy, constrictive pericarditis, and valvular cardiomyopathy are common diagnoses/disease pathologies in the majority of patients with HFpEF (Table 9-2).
   a. Restrictive (the heart is stiff and unable to relax correctly); this can be caused by
      i.   *Radiation therapy* causing scarring to the heart.
      ii. *Amyloidosis* causes abnormal protein fibers to accumulate in the heart muscle.
      iii. *Sarcoidosis* produces lumps (called granulomas) in the heart and other organs.
      iv. *Hemochromatosis* is a genetic condition that causes iron to build up in the heart and other parts of the body.
      v.   *Post–heart transplant restrictive cardiomyopathy* is associated with the development of diffuse small vessel transplant coronary artery disease.
4. Hypertrophic (enlarged heart)—ventricular walls get thicker and the heart chamber becomes smaller, thereby limiting the filling and pumping ability. It may be congenital (hypertrophic cardiomyopathy) or acquired (e.g., hypertensive heart disease, aortic stenosis).
5. Valvular (caused by structural defects to the heart valves altering flow within the heart and circulation. Can lead to enlarged chambers and decreased function).
   a. Clinical features of HFpEF (diastolic failure)[5,7,8]
      i.   Defined as pulmonary or systemic venous congestion in the setting of near normal systolic function
   b. Hemodynamically, the principal abnormality of diastolic failure is the inability of the ventricles to relax and fill adequately. This leads to elevated left ventricular end-diastolic pressure (LVEDP) and may be associated with
      i.   Systemic hypertension
      ii. S_4 gallop
      iii. Normal or increased EF
      iv. Small LV cavity, concentric LV hypertrophy
6. HFrEF or systolic dysfunction[7]
   a. HF can occur with reduced ejection fraction (HFrEF) as defined by an EF < 40% or systolic HF.[8] The patient with HFrEF may have a low cardiac output (CO) state whereby the LV cannot pump oxygen-rich blood to the systemic circulation. The weakened LV remodels and dilates, thereby enlarging the chamber, increasing LV volume and pressure. This further weakens the LV and may dilate the mitral valve annulus leading to a backup of blood (functional mitral regurgitation).

b. Left atrial (LA) pressure and volume increase when blood inadequately empties into the LV. This volume backs up into the lungs via the pulmonary venous system. As pulmonary pressures increase (pulmonary hypertension) and pulmonary capillary wedge pressure (PCWP) exceeds 24 mm Hg (oncotic pressure), the ensuing pulmonary congestion symptomatically causes an increased work of breathing, dyspnea, cough, pleural effusions, and respiratory failure if left untreated.[7,8]

c. Nonischemic, idiopathic, viral, ischemic, familial, valvular, and postpartum are common cardiomyopathy diagnoses/disease pathologies in the majority of patients with HFrEF (see Table 9-2).

   i. **Ischemic** (caused by loss of blood supply to the heart, typically related to coronary artery disease)

   ii. **Nonischemic**—heart failure with reduced EF, with normal coronaries. Variety of possible causes are listed below:

- Idiopathic (unknown cause)
- Viral (bacterial or viral infections can inflame and damage the heart muscle [myocarditis])
- Familial: Inherited genes in the family that may be responsible for the cardiomyopathy
- Valvular (caused by structural defects to the heart valves altering flow within the heart and circulation. Can lead to enlarged chambers and decreased function)
- Postpartum (can occur during last trimester or within 6 months after pregnancy)
- Congenital: born with a structural heart defect
- Alcohol (resulting from chronic alcohol use)
- Drug abuse (causing irreversible damage to the heart, e.g., cocaine, methamphetamines)

d. Other causes of HFrEF include the following:

   i. Long-standing uncontrolled hypertension

   ii. Tachycardia-related cardiomyopathy

   iii. Hyperthyroidism

   iv. Advanced infiltrative diseases (sarcoid, amyloid, hemochromatosis)

   v. Hypertrophic cardiomyopathy[9]

e. Clinical features of HFrEF[5,8,9]

   i. Impaired myocardial contractility leads to weakened systolic contraction.

   ii. Hemodynamically, HFrEF is associated with

- Normal or low blood pressure (BP).
- S_3 gallop.
- Decreased CO.
- Reduced stroke volume (SV).
- Increased ventricular diastolic pressure.
- Decreased EF: the amount of blood ejected in a single heartbeat relative to the total LV volume; normal EF is approximately 60%.
- Large, dilated heart on chest radiograph.

7. RV failure[1,4,8]

a. May be caused by a primary RV injury/abnormality or increased pressure in the pulmonary vasculature leading to elevated right heart pressure and eventually failure.

b. The RV is not able to pump blood into the pulmonary system.

c. As the RV fails, there is systemic venous congestion and hypoperfusion.

d. LV failure is the most common cause of RV failure.

e. LV failure typically precedes RV failure except in the setting of

   i. RV infarct

   ii. Arrhythmogenic RV dysplasia

   iii. Certain primary pulmonary disease processes (chronic pulmonary arterial hypertension, acute respiratory distress syndrome [ARDS], or pulmonary emboli [PE])

IV. EVALUATION OF OBJECTIVE MEASURES OF END-STAGE HEART DISEASE: POTENTIAL FINDINGS[1,9–11]

A. Vital signs/weights

1. Heart rate (HR)

  a. May be increased in an attempt to maintain CO

    i. With systolic and diastolic dysfunction, stroke volume (SV) is decreased; this may precipitate a compensatory increase in HR ($CO = SV \times HR$).

  b. May be decreased due to effects of β-blockers or ivabradine (Corlanor)

2. Heart rhythm

  a. May be irregular due to atrial fibrillation, atrial flutter, or supraventricular tachycardia with variable atrioventricular block.

  b. Pulsus alternans: Pulse has normal rate, but you can feel (or see on an arterial line tracing) strong beats alternating with weak beats. This is associated with an alternating impairment in LV preload.

3. Blood pressure

  a. Assess for hypotension and hypertension.

  b. Typically maintained as low as tolerable (without causing symptoms such as light-headedness or dizziness), so as to decrease myocardial workload.

  c. May be low in right-sided HF.

4. Weight

  a. Think of weight as an HF vital sign.

  b. Always check daily weights in the hospital and ask the patient to continue daily weights at home and report this information to the doctor upon every encounter.

  c. Weigh patients in the morning using the same scale and technique for accuracy.

  d. On admission, check height and weight and calculate a body mass index (BMI). A BMI > 30 has been correlated with poor transplant outcomes and is a relative contraindication to transplantation.[10]

5. Fluid balance

  a. Carefully record and monitor all daily fluid input and output. HF patients typically require fluid restriction (<1.5 L/day).

6. Heart failure lethal triad[4]

  a. Hypotension (systolic BP < 100).

  b. Activation of sympathetic nervous system (indicated by heart rate [HR] > 100).

  c. Activation of renin-angiotensin system (indicated by serum sodium [Na+] < 130). Hyponatremia can be due to volume overload or sodium depletion from diuretic use.

TABLE 9-3 **Heart Failure: Potential Abnormal Findings**

Finding	Comment
Jugular venous distention	When patient is reclining at 45-degree angle, jugular veins are distended.
	Indicates ↑ right atrial and right ventricular filling pressures (right-sided heart failure)
S_3 (ventricular gallop)	Related to early diastolic filling; can be normal in young adults
	Typically indicative of severely ↑ left ventricular end-diastolic pressure; common in patients with restrictive or constrictive disease; may be associated with left- or right-sided HF, ischemia, and fluid overload
S_4 (atrial gallop)	Related to late diastolic filling; associated with ischemia or infarction, systemic and pulmonary hypertension, ventricular failure
S_3 and S_4 (summation gallop)	Associated with tachycardia (due to shortened diastole) and HF
Splenomegaly	May be associated with right-sided heart failure
Hepatomegaly	Common in right-sided heart failure
Hepatojugular reflux	Upper right abdomen is compressed for ~10 s; this results in ↑ venous return to the heart from the liver; hepatojugular reflux: jugular pulses are prominent; level of filling of neck veins ↑; this ↑ is associated with the inability of the right side of the heart to manage added volume
Peripheral cyanosis	Bluish discoloration of the lips, nose, earlobes, extremities: indicative of poor peripheral perfusion associated with ↓ cardiac output or pronounced vasoconstriction
Dependent edema	Ambulatory patients: typically localized in lower extremities
	Bedridden patients: typically localized in sacral and presacral areas
Cachexia	State of malnutrition, wasting, and loss of skeletal muscle mass; associated with severe heart failure
Ascites	Accumulation of fluid in peritoneal cavity; associated with right-sided heart failure
Cough or wheeze	Cough may be associated with pulmonary venous congestion or intolerance of angiotensin-converting enzyme (ACE) inhibitor therapy
	Wheeze may be associated with intolerance of β-blocker therapy
Crackles	May present initially in dependent lung fields; as pulmonary congestion ↑, crackles become more diffuse
Altered mental status	Cognitive dysfunction (e.g., confusion, memory impairment, inability to focus) may be associated with ↓ cardiac output and ↓ perfusion to the brain
Cool peripheries	Low cardiac output state

From Jaski B. *The 4 Stages of Heart Failure*. Minneapolis, MN: Cardiotext Publishing; 2015:6–8, 21–31, 86–95, 103–110; Blair J, Huffman M, Shah S. Heart failure in North America. *Curr Cardiol Rev*. 2013;9:128–146; McMurray JJ, Adamopoulos S, Anker SD, et al. European Society of Cardiology (ESC) Guidelines for the diagnosis and treatment of acute and chronic heart failure 2012. The Task Force for the Diagnosis and Treatment of Acute and Chronic Heart Failure 2012 of the European Society of Cardiology. Developed in collaboration with the Heart Failure Association (HFA) of the ESC. *Eur Heart J*. 2012;33:1787–1847.

B. Heart failure physical exam (Table 9-3)[4,7,9]

Use a systematic approach to determine the type and severity of HF. A head to toe examination begins at the head assessing temporal wasting and ends at the ankles/toes assessing edema and capillary refill.

1. Head exam:
   a. Assess temples for temporal wasting (look for a pronounced indentation in the appearance of the muscles covering the temporal bones). This is present in cases of advanced HF and is a sign of malnutrition.

    b. Look at the sclera for jaundice indicating liver disease from passive congestion, hepatitis, or possibly cirrhosis.

2. Neck veins:
    a. Place the patient at a 30-degree incline. Jugular venous pressure (JVP) is estimated by placing a ruler on the patient's sternum at the level of the second intercostal space (angle of Louis).
    b. Turn the patient's head to the side to better visualize the neck veins.
    c. Measure to the top of the visible distended internal jugular neck vein and add 5 cm.
    d. If there are no visible neck veins, take your other hand and compress the middle of the abdomen. If the neck vein now distends and remains elevated, the patient has a positive abdominal jugular reflex (AJR). This is a positive sign for fluid volume overload even though the neck veins appeared normal.

3. Heart sounds:
    a. A third heart sound (S_3) or ventricular gallop results from a reduced EF and impaired diastolic function.
    b. A fourth heart sound (S_4) or atrial gallop reflects a lack of ventricular compliance due to ischemic heart disease, hypertension, or hypertrophy.

4. Pulmonary assessment:
    a. Pulmonary crackles can be auscultated if fluid is leaking from the capillaries into the alveolar spaces. Over time, crackles increase and effusions can develop. However, patients with chronic HF may not have crackles.
    b. Pulmonary hypertension is assessed with pulmonary artery catheter monitoring.
    c. All patients with HF should complete a sleep apnea screening questionnaire because sleep apnea is a risk factor that can lead to HF if undiagnosed. Some programs use the STOP-BANG© questionnaire to screen patients (Table 9-4).[11,12]

5. Gastrointestinal (GI) assessment:
    a. Review liver function and viral hepatitis tests.
    b. Palpate liver for enlargement.

6. Skin and hair assessment: The condition of the skin and hair will reveal the state of the HF, perfusion, oxygenation, and nutrition. It can also unveil underlying diseases such as thyroid disorders, diabetes, neuropathies, and vascular disorders.
    a. Color (cyanosis, jaundice, hyperpigmentation)
        i. Cyanosis is a bluish color in the skin that can indicate reduced CO, peripheral vascular disease, or anemia.
        ii. Jaundice is a yellowing of the skin that can indicate passive liver congestion secondary to heart failure or underlying liver disease.
        iii. Hyperpigmentation (skin that has changed from normal to bronze) can result from sun damage, inflammation, or a variety of diseases. Excess iron or hemochromatosis should be considered.
    b. Temperature: Cool, lower extremities with delayed capillary refill may indicate a low CO or PVD.
    c. Moisture: Clammy, moist skin can be related to hypoperfusion, low cardiac output state.

TABLE 9-4 **STOP-BANG© Questionnaire**

This yes/no questionnaire is used to assess if the patient has potential for obstructive sleep apnea (OSA).

Do you **Snore** Loudly (loud enough to be heard through closed doors or loud enough that your bed partner wakes you)?	Yes or No
Do you often feel **Tired, Fatigued, or Sleepy** during the **daytime** (do you fall asleep during usual activities, work, driving, etc.)?	Yes or No
Has anyone Observed you Stop Breathing, Choking, or Gasping during your sleep?	Yes or No
Do you have or are you being treated for High Blood Pressure?	Yes or No
Is your Body Mass Index more than 35 kg/m²	Yes or No
Are you age 50 or older?	Yes or No
Do you have a large neck size? (measured around Adam's apple) For male, is your shirt collar 17 inches/43 cm or larger? For female, is your shirt collar 16 inches/41 cm or larger?	Yes or No
Are you a Male?	Yes or No

Scoring the STOP-BANG for the general population
OSA—low risk: yes to 0 to 2 questions
OSA—intermediate risk: yes to 3 to 4 questions
OSA—high risk: yes to 5 to 8 questions
or yes to 2 or more of 4 STOP questions + male gender
or yes to 2 or more of 4 STOP questions + BMI > 35 kg/m²
or yes to 2 or more of 4 STOP questions + neck circumference 17 inches/43 cm in male or 16 inches/41 cm in female
Adapted from the STOP-BANG Questionnaire and reprinted with the permission of the Toronto Western Hospital University Health Network.
From Luo J, Huang R, et al. Value of STOP-BANG questionnaire in screening patients with obstructive sleep hypopnea syndrome in sleep disordered breathing clinic. *Chin Med J (Engl).* 2014;127(10):1843–1848; Mehra R. Sleep apnea ABCs: airway, breathing, circulation. *Cleve Clin J Med.* 2014;81(8):479–489.

    d. Edema or swelling in the legs, abdomen, or areas around the eyes.

    e. Hair thinning

       i. Hair follicles survive by the blood flowing through veins and arteries; when this is reduced, hair loss can occur.

    f. Hairless legs, feet, or toes are a red flag for malnutrition and thyroid or vascular disease, which can lead to stroke and myocardial infarction.

C. Hemodynamic parameters: see "Clinical Findings in Heart Failure"[4,13] (see Table 9-1)

D. Radiologic tests

    1. Chest radiograph may be normal in some patients.

    2. Abnormal chest radiograph findings may include the following:

       a. Pulmonary vasculature: Pulmonary edema or congestion associated with left-sided HF.

       b. Cardiac silhouette: Heart may be enlarged.

       c. Enlarged right atrium (RA) or RV: Indicative of right-sided HF.

       d. Pleural effusions: May be associated with left-sided failure.

       e. Valve calcifications: May be associated with valvular disease.

       f. Placement of any lines and pacemakers or indications of past cardiac surgeries, such as sternal wires.

       g. Presence of any coexisting mediastinal, thoracic, or pulmonary diseases, nodules, or tumors.

E. Electrocardiogram
   1. May indicate nonspecific changes
      a. LV hypertrophy
      b. Q waves from old myocardial infarction (MI)
   2. Atrial dysrhythmias and bundle-branch blocks common.
      a. High incidence (70% to 80%) of atrial fibrillation.[6]
      b. Atrial fibrillation often is secondary to LA enlargement.
   3. Dysrhythmias may be associated with ischemic heart disease, conduction abnormalities, electrolyte imbalances, and other factors.
   4. Increased QRS voltage may indicate LV enlargement.
   5. QRS duration > 120 ms and left bundle-branch block (LBBB) morphology may indicate need for biventricular pacing.

F. Echocardiogram
   1. The echocardiogram allows the cardiologist to visualize all valves and chambers of the heart, estimate right and left heart filling pressure, and assess systolic and diastolic function to more accurately diagnose the specific type of cardiomyopathy. Different cardiomyopathies will have distinguishing features reflected in the appearance of the ventricular wall chamber size, thickness, and function.
   2. Chamber size:
      a. Dilated cardiomyopathy: As myocardial fibers degenerate and become fibrotic, atria and ventricles dilate.
      b. The etiology of the damaged myocardium may be due to the following etiologies: Idiopathic, viral, ischemic, toxic (alcohol, drugs), pregnancy, genetic, myocarditis (human immunodeficiency virus [HIV] infection, Chagas' disease), chemotherapy, or stress (Takotsubo).
   3. Wall thickness:
      a. LV dilatation and hypertrophy are common in hypertrophic cardiomyopathy.
   4. Ejection fraction (EF):
      a. Left ventricular EF varies depending on the pathology and is not used as criteria for transplantation; it is used to assess decompensation and treatment response.[10]
   5. Thrombus formation:
      a. Atrial fibrillation: Potential for thrombi formation in atria (requires anticoagulation therapy); typically detected by transesophageal echocardiography
      b. LV hypokinesis, systolic dysfunction, and aneurysm: Potential for thrombi formation in the LV due to stasis of blood flow contributing to clot formation
         i. If thrombus is noted, anticoagulation is required.
   6. Valve function:
      a. Dilatation of mitral annulus may occur secondary to LV dilatation.
      b. Primary valvular disease may be the cause of cardiomyopathy.
   7. Systolic and diastolic function:
      a. Diastolic function can be measured by echocardiography using a number of parameters including color flow Doppler, myocardial strain, and tissue Doppler.

8. Pericardial effusion: Abnormal amount of fluid collecting inside the heart sac located between the heart and pericardium

   a. Pericardial effusions: Potential etiologies include, but are not limited to,

      i. Infection

      ii. Myocardial infarction

      iii. Injury to the pericardium during a surgery or medical procedure

      iv. Uremia

      v. Autoimmune diseases (lupus, rheumatoid arthritis)

   b. Large pericardial effusions can result in cardiac tamponade (hypotension, JVD, and muffled heart sounds), which is a medical emergency.

G. Cardiac catheterization: purposes

1. Right heart catheterization:

   a. To assess right heart pressures and volume status: See "Clinical Findings in Left-Sided and Right-Sided Heart Failure."

   b. To assess CO and perfusion state in patients who may require inotropic support.

   c. To assess PVR and transpulmonary gradient.

      i. If the PVR > 5 woods unit or the TPG >15 are irreversible, the patient may not be a candidate for heart transplantation.[10]

   d. To perform endomyocardial biopsy (EMB) if myocarditis or an infiltrative disease process is suspected and diagnosis will guide treatment.

2. Left heart catheterization:

   a. Assess coronary artery anatomy and determine potential for coronary revascularization.

   b. Measure left ventricular pressures.

3. Determine ventricular size and contractility (i.e., EF).

4. Evaluate valve function.

5. Detect structural defects.

H. Electrophysiology study: purpose

1. To diagnose and treat supraventricular and ventricular arrhythmias

I. Cardiopulmonary exercise testing: VO_2 max

1. VO_2 max is a measurement of oxygen consumption at peak exercise.

2. The failing heart does not have the ability to provide sufficient oxygen to meet the aerobic needs of the peripheral tissues, thus increasing CO_2 and lactic acid production during anaerobic metabolism.

3. An VO_2 max <14 mL/kg/min or <50% predicted for age is typically used to determine transplant candidacy.[10]

J. Laboratory tests (Table 9-5)[14]

K. New York Heart Association (NYHA) Classification of Heart Failure (Table 9-6)[15,16]

L. Heart failure progression: American College of Cardiology/American Heart Association Stages of Heart Failure (Table 9-7)[16-20]

M. Heart failure staging (Figure 9-1)

N. Monitoring of subjective and objective signs of worsening HF (Box 9-1)[10,16,20-22]

(*text continues on page 321*)

TABLE 9-5 Laboratory Tests

Liver function tests	Total bilirubin and liver enzymes may be ↑ due to ↓ CO and ↑ liver congestion
Renal function tests	Serum creatinine and BUN may be ↑ due to: ↓ CO and subsequent ↓ perfusion to kidneys Nephrotoxic side effects of medications such as calcineurin inhibitors and certain diuretics
BNP	↑ may reflect myocyte stretch and ↑ ventricular pressures
NT proBNP	Note: falsely low levels may occur in obese patients because adipose tissue removes BNP from circulation; falsely elevated levels may occur in elderly and female patients and in the setting of hypertension and treatment with nesiritide. The NT proBNP is a more sensitive marker to diagnose severity of heart failure, levels ↑ when LVEF <40%, and with increasing age
C-reactive protein	↑ indicates inflammation
Cardiac troponin I and troponin T	Sensitive markers of myocyte injury ↑ in acute MI
Creatine kinase	MB isoenzyme sensitive for cardiac tissue; ↑ creatine kinase MB may be associated with myocardial muscle damage (cardiomyopathy, congestive heart failure, myocardial infarction)
ABG	To assess patient for hypoxemia: O_2 pressure and/or O_2 saturation in arterial blood is lower than normal; generally defined as PaO_2 < 55 mm Hg or SaO_2 below 88% on room air (a sea level) Cardiogenic shock: metabolic acidosis on ABGs (↓ pH; ↓ HCO_3)

	Electrolyte Imbalance	**Potential Etiology**	**CV signs and symptoms**
Serum electrolytes	Hyponatremia	Inadequate Na intake Excessive Na loss Certain loop or thiazide diuretics	Dehydration, concurrent hypovolemia: weak, rapid pulse, ↓ CVP, ↓ PAWP, ↓ PA pressures Concurrent hypervolemia: rapid, bounding pulse, ↑ CVP, ↑ PA pressure, ↑ jugular venous pressure, SOB
Serum electrolytes	**Electrolyte Imbalance** Hypernatremia	**Potential Etiology** Retention of Na Impaired renal function Osmotic diuretics Osmotic diuresis associated with DM	**CV signs and symptoms** ↑ ECF: weak, thready pulse; hypertension ↓ ECF: tachycardia often → bradycardia; hypotension (may or may not be associated with postural changes)
	Hypokalemia	Excessive K loss via GI fluid loss Certain diuretics	Weak, irregular pulses; palpitations Orthostatic hypotension: dysrhythmias (PACs, PVCs, sinus bradycardia, PAT, AV blocks, AV, or ventricular tachycardia) EKG changes (flat or inverted T wave, ST segment depression, U wave) Digoxin toxicity

TABLE 9-5 Laboratory Tests (*Continued*)

	Hyperkalemia	Renal failure (↓ K excretion)	Irregular pulse, ↓ CO, hypotension
		ACE inhibitors	EKG changes (tall peaked T waves, flat P wave, prolonged PR interval, wide QRS interval, depressed ST segment)
			Dysrhythmias (bradycardia, heart block, ventricular dysrhythmias, asystole)
	Hypomagnesemia	Malabsorption of Mg	Irregular pulse
		Excessive loss of Mg via GI loss (emesis/diarrhea)	Hypotension in some patients
		Loop or thiazide diuretics	Dysrhythmias (tachycardia, atrial fibrillation, heart block, torsades de pointes, PAT, PVCs, SVT, VT, VF)
		Osmotic diuresis associated with DM	
			EKG changes (prolonged PR interval, wide QRS, prolonged QT interval, depressed ST segment, U wave, flat T wave)
	Hypermagnesemia	Overuse of Mg supplements	Dysrhythmias (bradycardia, heart block)
		Overuse of antacids or laxatives that contain Mg	EKG changes (prolonged PR interval, wide QRS complex, tall T wave)
		Impaired Mg excretion due to renal failure	Hypotension due to ↓ myocardial contractility may → cardiac arrest
	Hypophosphatemia	Hyperglycemia, Thiazide or loop diuretics	Hypotension
		↓ absorption of PO_4 due to diarrhea, prolonged use of PO_4-binding antacids or laxatives	Tachycardia
			↓ CO
	Hyperphosphatemia	Impaired renal excretion of PO_4	Irregular HR
		Excessive use of PO_4-containing laxatives	

ABG, arterial blood gas; ACE, angiotensin-converting enzyme; AV, atrioventricular; BNP, brain natriuretic peptide; BUN, blood urea nitrogen; CO, cardiac output; CVP, central venous pressure; DM, diabetes mellitus; ECF, extracellular fluid; EKG, electrocardiogram; GI, gastrointestinal; HCO_3, bicarbonate; HR, heart rate; K, potassium; LVEF, left ventricular ejection fraction; Mg, magnesium; MI, myocardial infarction; Na, sodium; O_2, oxygen; PA, pulmonary artery; PACs, premature atrial contractions; PaO_2, arterial partial pressure of oxygen; PAT, paroxysmal atrial tachycardia; PO_4, phosphorous; PAWP, pulmonary artery wedge pressure; PVCs, premature ventricular contractions; SaO_2, arterial oxygen saturation; SVT, supraventricular tachycardia; VF, ventricular fibrillation; VT, ventricular tachycardia.
From Malarkey LM, McMorrow ME. *Nursing Guide to Laboratory and Diagnostic Tests.* Saunders; 2005.

TABLE 9-6 New York Heart Association Classification of Heart Failure

Functional Capacity	Objective Assessment
Class I. Patients with cardiac disease but without resulting limitation of physical activity. Ordinary physical activity does not cause undue fatigue, palpitation, dyspnea, or anginal pain.	**A.** No objective evidence of cardiovascular disease
Class II. Patients with cardiac disease resulting in slight limitation of physical activity. They are comfortable at rest. Ordinary physical activity results in fatigue, palpitations, dyspnea, or anginal pain.	**B.** Objective evidence of minimal cardiovascular disease
Class IIIA. Patients with cardiac disease resulting in marked limitation of physical activity. They are comfortable at rest. Less than ordinary activity causes fatigue, palpitations, dyspnea, or anginal pain.	**C.** Objective evidence of moderately cardiovascular disease
Class IIIB. Patients with cardiac disease resulting in marked limitation of physical activity. They are comfortable at rest. Mild physical activity causes fatigue, palpitations, dyspnea, or anginal pain.	**D.** Objective evidence of moderately severe cardiovascular disease
Class IV. Patients with cardiac disease resulting in inability to carry on any physical activity without discomfort. Symptoms of heart failure or the anginal syndrome may be present even at rest. If any physical activity is undertaken, discomfort is increased	**E.** Objective evidence of severe cardiovascular disease

From American College of Cardiology/American Heart Association, *ACC/AHA Guidelines for the Evaluation and Management of Chronic Heart Failure in the Adult*. American College of Cardiology/American Heart Association; 2001; Heart Failure Society of America. *The Stages of Heart Failure—NYHA Classification*. Heart Failure Society of America; 2006.

TABLE 9-7 Heart Failure Progression

Stage	Description	Example
A	Patients at high risk for developing heart failure but no structural heart disorder	Hypertension Coronary artery disease Diabetes mellitus
B	Patients with structural heart disorders who does not have symptoms of heart failure	Previous myocardial infarction Left ventricular (LV) hypertrophy LV dilatation or hypocontractility Asymptomatic valvular heart disease
C	Patients with current or past symptoms of heart failure associated with underlying structural heart disease	Known structural heart disease, symptomatic Dyspnea or fatigue secondary to LV systolic dysfunction Reduced exercise capacity
D	Patients with end-stage heart disease requiring advanced therapy	Marked symptoms at rest despite maximal medical/CRT therapy Patients who are frequently hospitalized for HF and cannot be safely discharged without advanced therapies: Hospitalized patients awaiting heart transplantation Patients at home who are receiving continuous intravenous support for symptom relief Patients on mechanical circulatory assist device Patients in hospice setting for HF management

Adapted from Hunt SA, Abraham WT, Chin MH, et al. *American College of Cardiology/American Heart Association 2005 Guideline Update for the Diagnosis and Management of Chronic Heart Failure in the Adult: A Report of the American College of Cardiology/American Heart Association Task Force on Practice Guidelines (Writing Committee to Update the 2001 Guidelines for the Evaluation and Management of Heart Failure)*; 2005; Heart Failure Society of America. *The Stages of Heart Failure—NYHA Classification*. Heart Failure Society of America; 2006; Starling R. Medical grand rounds advanced heart failure transplant, LVADs, and beyond. *Cleve Clin J Med*. 2013;80(1):33–40; Fang KC, Ewald GA, Allen LA, et al. Advanced (stage d) heart failure: a statement from the heart failure society of America guidelines committee. *J Card Fail*. 2015;21(6):519–534; Reed BN, Rodgers JE, Sueta, CA. Polypharmacy in heart failure: drugs to use and avoid. *Heart Fail Clin*. 2014;10(4):577–590.

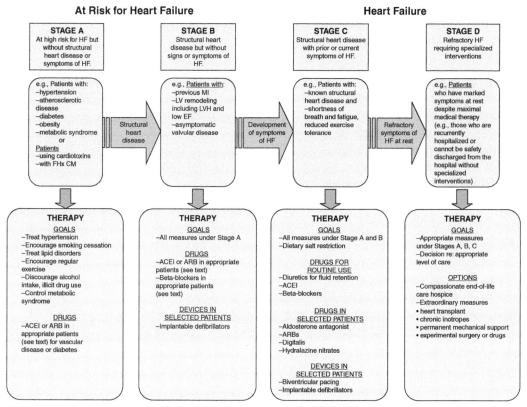

FIGURE 9-1   Stages in the evolution of HF and recommended therapy by stage.

 V. TREATMENT OF HEART FAILURE

A.   Patients with end-stage HF may be on a medical regimen that includes the following[20–22]:

1.   Hypertension and lipid disorders should be controlled to lower HF risk (level of evidence A [Table 9-8]).[18,20]

2.   HF education to facilitate self-care should include symptom monitoring, daily weights, heart-healthy diet low in sodium, fluid restriction, safe medication practices, and routine physical exercise to increase exercise tolerance (level of evidence B).

3.   Cardiac rehabilitation may reduce mortality and hospitalization and improves functional capacity, exercise duration, and quality of life (level of evidence B).

4.   Treatment of sleep disorders with continuous positive airway pressure can increase left ventricular ejection fraction (LVEF) and functional status in patients with HF and sleep apnea (level of evidence B).

5.   Other conditions that may contribute to HF, such as obesity, diabetes mellitus (DM), tobacco use, and any cardiotoxic drug abuse (cocaine, methamphetamines), should be avoided or controlled (level of evidence C).

6.   Sodium restriction (e.g., ≤2 g/day) is recommended for HF patients to prevent fluid accumulation or facilitate diuresis (level of evidence C).

7.   Fluid restriction (e.g., ≤ 2 L/day) to help prevent fluid accumulation.

BOX 9-1   Subjective and Objective Signs of Worsening Heart Failure[20]

Subjective:
- ↑ dyspnea at rest or with exertion
- ↑ orthopnea
- ↑ paroxysmal nocturnal dyspnea
- ↑ weakness, fatigue
- ↓ appetite and/or early satiety
- ↑ abdominal fullness
- Difficulty sleeping
- Development of chest pain/pressure or ↑ in angina

Objective:
- ↑ edema (abdominal, peripheral)
- New-onset or worsening dysrhythmias
- Weight gain >3 lb for more than 2 consecutive days
- Vomiting
- Development of cardiac cachexia
- New onset or increasing frequency of syncope
- ↑ serum creatinine >2.0 mg/dL (may be secondary to use of diuretics and ACE inhibitors)
- ↑ blood urea nitrogen >50 mg/dL (unless patient has intrinsic renal disease)
- Serum sodium <134 mEq/L
- ↑ liver enzymes and bilirubin over baseline
- Diuretic unresponsiveness
- ↑ brain natriuretic peptide level over baseline level *in certain patients*

Note: Brain natriuretic peptide (BNP) increases with age and is higher in women than in men. Research has shown that BNP may be related to a number of other factors such as weight, kidney function, and indicators of cardiovascular damage such as hypertension, previous myocardial infarction or stroke, angina, and diabetes mellitus. Serum BNP levels may parallel the severity of heart failure (HF); however, at this time, there is insufficient clinical evidence to warrant the use of BNP levels as targets for the adjustment of therapy in individual patients. Patients on optimal HF medications may have markedly increased BNP levels, and patients with advanced HF may have normal BNP levels. Further clinical trials are needed to determine the role of BNP measurement in diagnosing and managing HF.

---

8. Pharmacologic therapy with one or more of the medications shown in Table 9-9.[18-22]
   a. The American Heart Association (*Get with the Guidelines*) recommends the following for treatment as a standard of care for patients with LVEF≤ 40%, unless contraindicated:
      i. Angiotensin-converting enzyme inhibitors (ACE)/angiotensin II receptor blockers (ARB)
      ii. Beta-blockers
      iii. Aldosterone antagonists
      iv. Hydralazine/nitrates (for African Americans with LV dysfunction)
   b. ICD if EF is <35%; or cardiac resynchronization therapy-defibrillation (CRT-D) device therapy is indicated when the EF < 35% and the QRS duration is 120 ms or greater with LBBB.
   c. The following beta-blockers, bisoprolol (Zebeta), carvedilol (Coreg), and metoprolol succinate (Toprol-XL), but *not* metoprolol tartrate (Lopressor), have evidence to show reduced morbidity and mortality in patients with systolic HF.

B. Patients with refractory HF who fail to respond to inotropic therapy may require mechanical circulatory support (MCS) to maintain CO and prevent irreversible failure of other organs (Figure 9-2). See chapter Mechanical Circulatory Support for additional information.

TABLE 9-8 **Medical Evidence Scale**

Levels of Evidence:

IA	Evidence obtained from meta-analysis of randomized control trial or one properly designed randomized control trial
IIA	Evidence from at least one controlled study without randomization or quasi-experimental study
III	Evidence from uncontrolled trials: nonexperimental descriptive studies, comparative studies, correlation studies, and case-control studies
IV	Evidence from expert committee reports or opinions, based on clinical experience of respected authorities, or both

Grades of Recommendations:

A	Good scientific evidence suggests that the benefits of the treatment substantially outweigh the potential risks. Clinicians should discuss the treatment with eligible patients based on level 1 evidence.
B	At least fair/consistent scientific evidence suggests that the benefits of the treatment outweigh the potential risks. Clinicians should discuss the treatment with eligible patients based on level 2 or 3 evidence.
C	At least fair but inconsistent scientific evidence suggests that there are potential benefits provided by the proposed treatment, but the balance between benefits and risks is too close for making this recommendation. Clinicians should not offer it unless there are individual considerations, level 3 or 4
D	Little or no scientific evidence suggests that the risks of the treatment outweigh potential benefits. Clinicians should not routinely offer the service to asymptomatic patients, level 4

Adapted from Reed BN, Rodgers JE, Sueta, CA. Polypharmacy in heart failure: drugs to use and avoid. *Heart Fail Clin.* 2014;10(4):577–590; Starling R. Medical grand rounds advanced heart failure transplant, LVADs, and beyond. *Cleve Clin J Med.* 2013;80(1):33–40.

 VI. HEART TRANSPLANTATION

A. Historical perspective

1. First heart transplant: December 3, 1967, Cape Town, South Africa, by Dr. Christiaan Barnard[23]
   a. Confirmed that heart transplantation was technically possible and that a transplanted heart could indeed sustain life.
2. This early success gave rise to the worldwide development of heart transplant centers in the late 1960s and early 1970s. However, without effective immunosuppression, heart transplantation outcomes were poor, and therefore, heart transplantation was not deemed a viable therapeutic option.
3. In the 1970s, two important advances revolutionized the field of heart transplantation: The development of the EMB procedure[24] and the discovery of cyclosporine.[25,26] These advances improved survival, and since 2000, approximately 3,000 heart transplant procedures per year have been reported to the International Society for Heart and Lung Transplantation (ISHLT).

B. Goals of heart transplantation: To extend survival and improve quality of life

C. Indications: Heart transplantation is considered in the setting of[10,17,18,20]

1. Terminal HF that is unresponsive to optimal medical therapy
2. Refractory HF requiring inotropic or MCS with reversible end-organ damage
3. Refractory angina, not amenable to revascularization, on optimal medical therapy

TABLE 9-9 Pharmacologic Therapy for Heart Failure

Medication	Action(s)
Diuretics	↓ intravascular and extravascular fluid volume, thereby ↓ preload
Angiotensin-converting enzyme (ACE) inhibitors	↓ afterload by blocking the formation of angiotensin II and inhibiting the release of aldosterone, thereby ↓ sodium retention ↓ preload via vasodilation
Angiotensin II receptor blockers (ARBs)	↓ blood pressure by blocking the vasoconstrictor and aldosterone-secreting effects of angiotensin II
β-Adrenergic receptor antagonists (β-blockers)	↓ preload
Aldosterone antagonists (spironolactone)	↓ preload by ↑ excretion of sodium and water
Direct-acting vasodilators (hydralazine/nitrates)	↓ preload
Nitrates	↓ preload via dilatation of systemic veins and by ↓ venous return, thereby ↓ LV filling pressure ↓ afterload by vasodilation of systemic arteries
Anticoagulants	↓ risk of thromboembolism associated with atrial fibrillation, LV hypokinesis, or systolic dysfunction
Digitalis glycosides	↓ preload May be used for rate control in setting of atrial fibrillation or atrial flutter
Inotropic agents: milrinone	↑ myocardial contractility without ↑ heart rate ↓ afterload and preload via arterial and venous smooth muscle relaxation and by ↑ peripheral vasodilation
Inotropic agents: dobutamine	↑ myocardial contractility ↑ stroke volume and cardiac output ↓ systemic vascular resistance
Nesiritide (human B-type natriuretic peptide)	↑ vasodilation, ↓ pulmonary capillary wedge pressure, ↑ renal blood flow, and ↑ urinary output
Vasopressors: dopamine	Dose: 2–10 mcg/kg/min (β-adrenergic effects): ↑ vasoconstriction, ↑ blood pressure, and ↑ renal and cerebral perfusion Dose: > 10 mcg/kg/min: α-adrenergic effects: peripheral vasoconstriction; ↑ systemic vascular resistance, ↑ afterload and blood pressure; may possibly ↓ cardiac output
Vasopressors: phenylephrine hydrochloride	↑ blood pressure via arteriolar vasoconstriction; ↑ stroke volume; may ↓ heart rate

Starling R. Medical grand rounds advanced heart failure transplant, LVADs, and beyond. *Cleve Clin J Med.* 2013;80(1):33–40; Fang KC, Ewald GA, Allen LA, et al. Advanced (stage d) heart failure: a statement from the heart failure society of America guidelines committee. *J Card Fail.* 2015;21(6):519–534; Reed BN, Rodgers JE, Sueta, CA. Polypharmacy in heart failure: drugs to use and avoid. *Heart Fail Clin.* 2014;10(4):577–590; Yancy CW, Jessup M, et al. 2013 ACCF/AHA Guideline for the Management of Heart Failure: a Report of the American College of Cardiology Foundation/American Association Task Force on Practice Guidelines. *J Am Coll Cardiol.* 2013;62(16):147–239.

4. Refractory, life-threatening dysrhythmias
5. Congenital heart disease with progressive ventricular failure not amenable to conventional surgical repair
6. Any NYHA Class 4 HF where the transplant selection team deems that the cardiomyopathy is associated with a poor short-term prognosis without transplantation

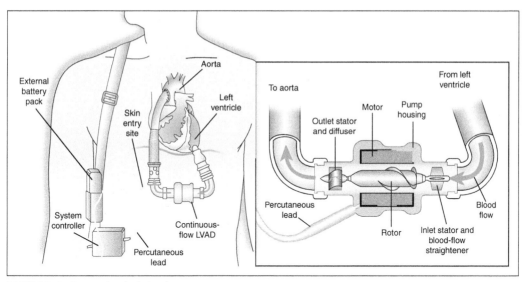

FIGURE 9-2 Mechanical circulatory support.

a. Types of cardiomyopathies leading to heart transplant may include the following:
  i. Ischemic, nonischemic, idiopathic, viral, valvular, restrictive, postpartum, familial, congenital, hypertrophic, and arrhythmogenic right ventricular dysplasia (ARVD)

D. Selection process: Patients undergo a comprehensive, interdisciplinary pretransplant evaluation to identify the following[10,27] (Table 9-10):
  1. Severity of the patient's functional impairment
  2. Prognosis
  3. Physiologic or psychological comorbidities
  4. Likelihood that the patient will be able to resume an active and relatively normal lifestyle following transplantation
  5. Potential to comply with the posttransplant regimen
  6. Level of psychosocial support

E. ISHLT recommendations: Listing criteria and contraindications are shown in Table 9-11.[10]
  1. Patients with completed transplant evaluations are presented to a multidisciplinary selection committee for heart transplant listing consideration. If accepted, the team confirms insurance approval and then places the patient on the transplant waiting list.
  2. Comprehensive education is provided to the patient and care partner at the time of listing.

F. Reassessment of patients while on the waiting list
  1. While on the waiting list, patients undergo periodic reassessment.
  2. The ISHLT-recommended schedule for heart transplant evaluation is shown in Table 9-10.[10]

G. Listing status
  1. Patients awaiting heart transplantation are assigned a status, which corresponds to how medically urgent it is that the candidate receive a transplant (Table 9-12).

(*text continues on page 331*)

TABLE 9-10 ISHLT-Recommended Schedule for Heart Transplant Evaluation and Waitlist Management

Test	Baseline	Repeat			
		3 Months	6 Months	9 Months	12 Months (and Yearly)
Complete H & P					
• Follow-up assessment	X	X	X	X	X
• Weight/BMI	X	X	X	X	X
Immunocompatibility					
• ABO	X				
• Repeat ABO	X				
HLA tissue typing	Only at transplant				
PRA and flow cytometry:	X				
• >10%	Every 1–2 mo				
• VAD	Every 1–2 mo				
• Transfusion	2 wk after transfusion then per protocol				
Assessment of heart failure severity					
• MVO$_2$ with RER	X				X
• Echocardiogram	X				X
• RHC (vasodilator challenge as indicated)	X		X		X
• ECG	X				X
Evaluation of multiorgan function					
Routine lab work (BMP, CBC, LFT)	X	X	X	X	X
PT/INR more frequently per protocol if on VAD or Coumadin	X	X	X	X	X
Urinalysis	X	X	X	X	X
GFR (MDRD quadratic equation)	X	X	X	X	X
Urine sample for protein excretion	X	X	X	X	X
PFT with arterial blood gases	X				
CXR (PA and lateral)	X				X

Abdominal ultrasound	X	
Carotid Doppler (if indicated or > 50 y)	X	
ABI (if indicated or > 50 y)	X	
DEXA scan (if indicated or > 50 y)	X	
Dental examination	X	X
Ophthalmologic examination (if diabetic)	X	X
Infectious serology and vaccination		
Hep B surface Ag	X	
Hep B surface Ab	X	
Hep B core Ab	X	
Hep C Ab	X	
HIV	X	
RPR	X	
HSV IgG	X	
CMV IgG	X	
Toxoplasmosis IgG	X	
EBV IgG	X	
Varicella IgG	X	
PPD	X	
Flu shot (yearly)	X	
Pneumovax (every 5 y)	X	
Hep B immunizations 1, 2, and 3	X	
Hep B surface Ab (immunity)	6 wk after third immunization	
Preventive and malignancy		
Stool for occult blood × 3	X	X
Colonoscopy (if indicated or > 50 y)	X	
Mammography (if indicated or > 40 y)	X	X
Gyn/PAP (if indicated ≥18 y sexually active)	X	X
PSA and digital rectal exam (men >50 y)	X	X

(continued)

TABLE 9-10 ISHLT-Recommended Schedule for Heart Transplant Evaluation and Waitlist Management (*Continued*)

Test	Baseline		Repeat			
		3 Months	6 Months	9 Months	12 Months (and Yearly)	
General consultations						
Social work	X					
Psychiatry	X					
Financial	X					
Neurologic/psychiatric (if applicable)	X					

ABI, ankle-brachial index; BMI, body mass index; BMP, basic metabolic panel; CBC, complete blood count; CMV, cytomegalovirus; CXR, chest x-ray; DEXA, dual-energy x-ray absorptiometry; EBV, Epstein-Barr virus; ECG, electrocardiogram; GFR, glomerular filtration rate; GYN, gynecology; H & P, history and physical; Hep B core Ab, hepatitis B core antibody; Hep B surface Ab, hepatitis B surface antibody; Hep B surface Ag, hepatitis B surface antigen; Hep C Ab, hepatitis C antibody; HIV, human immunodeficiency virus; HLA, human leukocyte antigen; HSV, herpes simplex virus; INR, international normalized ratio; LFT, liver function test; MDRD, modification of diet in renal disease; PA, posterior-anterior; PAP, Papanicolaou; PFT, pulmonary function test; PPD, purified protein derivative; PRA, panel reactive antibody; PSA, prostate-specific antigen; PT, prothrombin time; RER, respiratory exchange ratio; RPR, rapid plasma reagin; VAD, ventricular assist device.
Adapted from Mehra MR, Kobashigawa J, Starling R, et al. Listing criteria for heart transplantation: International Society for Heart and Lung Transplantation Guidelines for the care of cardiac transplant candidates—2006. *J Heart Lung Transplantation.* 2006;25(9):1024–1042.

TABLE 9-11 **International Society for Heart and Lung Transplantation (ISHLT) Recommendations: Listing Criteria and Contraindications**

Parameter	Recommendation
Maximal Cardiopulmonary Exercise Test MVO_2 (on optimal medical therapy) with respiratory exchange ratio (RER) >1.05 and achievement of anaerobic threshold	Patients intolerant of β-blocker: Use cutoff for peak VO_2 of ≤14 mL/kg/min to guide listing decision. In presence of β-blocker: Use cutoff for peak VO_2 of ≤12 mL/kg/min to guide listing decision. Patients <50 y and women: Consider use of alternate standards in addition to peak VO_2 to guide listing decision, including percent of predicted peak VO_2 (≤50%). If MVO_2 is submaximal (RER < 1.05), consider use of ventilation equivalent of carbon dioxide (V_E/V_{CO2}) slope of > 35 to guide listing decision in obese patients (body mass index [BMI] > 30 kg/m²), consider adjusting VO_2 to lean body mass. Lean body mass–adjusted peak VO_2 of < 19 mL/kg/min can serve as an optimal threshold to guide prognosis.
Heart Failure Survival Score (HFSS)	When CPX VO_2 is ambiguous (e.g., peak VO_2 > 12 and <14 mL/kg/min), consider HFSS as adjunct to guide listing decision for ambulatory patients. (The HFSS is a multivariable predictive index that includes seven measurements: resting heart rate, mean blood pressure, ejection fraction, serum sodium level, peak VO_2, intraventricular conduction delay, and presence of ischemic cardiomyopathy.)
Right heart catheterization	Right heart catheterization (RHC) should be performed on all candidates in preparation for listing for cardiac transplantation and annually until transplantation. RHC should be performed at 3- to 6-month intervals in listed patients, especially in the presence of reversible pulmonary hypertension or worsening heart failure symptoms. A vasodilator challenge should be administered when the pulmonary artery systolic pressure is ≥50 mm Hg and either the transpulmonary gradient (TPG) is ≥15 or the pulmonary vascular resistance is > 3 Wood units while maintaining a systolic arterial blood pressure > 85 mm Hg. When an acute vasodilator challenge is unsuccessful, hospitalization with continuous hemodynamic monitoring should be performed, as often, the PVR will decline after 24–48 h of treatment consisting of diuretics, inotropes, and vasoactive agents. If medical therapy fails to achieve acceptable hemodynamics and if the left ventricle cannot be effectively unloaded with mechanical adjuncts including an intra-aortic balloon pump (IABP) and/or left ventricular assist device (LVAD), it is reasonable to conclude that pulmonary hypertension is irreversible. Patients intolerant of β-blocker: Use cutoff for peak VO_2 of ≤14 mL/kg/min to guide listing decision. In presence of β-blocker: Use cutoff for peak VO_2 of ≤12 mL/kg/min to guide listing decision. Patients <50 y and women: Consider use of alternate standards in addition to peak VO_2 to guide listing decision, including percent of predicted peak VO_2 (≤50%). If CPX is submaximal (RER <1.05), consider use of ventilation equivalent of carbon dioxide (V_E/VCO_2) slope of >35 to guide listing decision in obese patients (body mass index [BMI] >30 kg/m²) and consider adjusting VO_2 to lean body mass. Lean body mass–adjusted peak VO_2 of <19 mL/kg/min can serve as an optimal threshold to guide prognosis.
Heart Failure Survival Score (HFSS)	When CPX VO_2 is ambiguous (e.g., peak VO_2 >12 and < 14 mL/kg/min), consider HFSS as adjunct to guide listing decision for ambulatory patients. (The HFSS is a multivariable predictive index that includes seven measurements: resting heart rate, mean blood pressure, ejection fraction, serum sodium level, peak VO_2, intraventricular conduction delay, and presence of ischemic cardiomyopathy.)

(continued)

TABLE 9-11 **International Society for Heart and Lung Transplantation (ISHLT) Recommendations: Listing Criteria and Contraindications (*Continued*)**

Parameter	Recommendation
Right heart catheterization	Right heart catheterization (RHC) should be performed on all candidates in preparation for listing for cardiac transplantation and annually until transplantation.
	RHC should be performed at 3- to 6-month intervals in listed patients, especially in the presence of reversible pulmonary hypertension or worsening heart failure symptoms.
	A vasodilator challenge should be administered when the pulmonary artery systolic pressure is $\geq$50 mm Hg and either the transpulmonary gradient (TPG) is $\geq$15 or the pulmonary vascular resistance is >3 Wood units while maintaining a systolic arterial blood pressure >85 mm Hg.
	When an acute vasodilator challenge is unsuccessful, hospitalization with continuous hemodynamic monitoring should be performed, as often, the PVR will decline after 24–48 h of treatment consisting of diuretics, inotropes, and vasoactive agents.
	If medical therapy fails to achieve acceptable hemodynamics and if the left ventricle cannot be effectively unloaded with mechanical adjuncts including an intra-aortic balloon pump (IABP) and/or left ventricular assist device (LVAD), it is reasonable to conclude that pulmonary hypertension is irreversible.
Pulmonary artery hypertension and elevated PVR	Should be considered as a relative contraindication to cardiac transplantation when the PVR is >5 Wood units or the PVR index is > 6 or the TPG exceeds 16–20 mm Hg.
	If the pulmonary artery systolic pressure exceeds 60 mm Hg in conjunction with any of the preceding three variables, the risk of right heart failure and early death is increased.
	If the PVR can be reduced to $\leq$2.5 with a vasodilator but the systolic pressure falls < 85 mm Hg, the patient remains at high risk of right heart failure and mortality after heart transplantation.
Age	Patients should be considered for cardiac transplantation if they are $\leq$70 y of age.
	Carefully selected patients >70 y of age may be considered for cardiac transplantation. For centers considering these patients, the use of an alternate-type program (e.g., use of older donors) may be pursued.
Cancer	Patients with preexisting neoplasms: Collaboration with oncologists is recommended to stratify each patient with regard to risk of tumor recurrence. Cardiac transplantation should be considered when tumor recurrence is low based on tumor type, response to therapy, and negative metastatic workup. The specific amount of time to wait to transplant after neoplasm remission will depend on the aforementioned factors and no arbitrary time period for observation should be used.
Obesity	Pretransplant BMI >30 kg/m^2 or percent ideal body weight (PIBW) >140% are associated with poor outcome after cardiac transplantation. For obese patients, weight loss is recommended to achieve a BMI of <30 kg/m^2 or PIBW of <140% before listing for cardiac transplantation.
Diabetes	Diabetes with end-organ damage other than nonproliferative retinopathy or poor glycemic control (glycosylated hemoglobin [HbA$_{1c}$] > 7.5) despite optimal effort is a relative contraindication for transplant.
Renal dysfunction	Renal function should be assessed using estimated glomerular filtration rate (eGFR) or creatinine clearance under optimal medical therapy. Evidence of abnormal renal function requires further investigation, including renal ultrasonography, estimation for proteinuria, and evaluation for renal artery disease, to exclude intrinsic renal disease. It is reasonable to consider the presence of irreversible renal dysfunction (eGFR < 40 mL/min) as a relative contraindication for heart transplantation alone.

TABLE 9-11 International Society for Heart and Lung Transplantation (ISHLT) Recommendations: Listing Criteria and Contraindications (*Continued*)

Parameter	Recommendation
Cerebrovascular disease	Clinically severe cerebrovascular disease, which is not amenable to revascularization, may be considered a contraindication to transplantation.
Peripheral vascular disease (PVD)	PVD may be considered as a relative contraindication to transplantation when its presence limits rehabilitation and revascularization is not a viable option.
Tobacco use	Education on the importance of tobacco cessation and reduction in environmental or secondhand exposure should be performed before the transplant and continue throughout the pre- and posttransplant periods.
	It is reasonable to consider active tobacco smoking as a relative contraindication to transplantation. Active tobacco smoking during the previous 6 mo is a risk factor for poor outcomes after transplantation.
Substance abuse	A structured rehabilitation program may be considered for patients with recent (24 mo) history of alcohol abuse if transplantation is being considered.
	Patients who remain active substance abusers (including alcohol) should not receive heart transplantation.
Psychosocial assessment	Psychosocial assessment should be performed before listing for transplantation. Evaluation should include an assessment of the patient's ability to give informed consent and comply with instruction including drug therapy, as well as assessment of the support systems in place at home or in the community.
	Mental retardation or dementia may be regarded as a relative contraindication to transplantation.
	Poor compliance with drug regimens is a risk factor for graft rejection and mortality. Patients who have demonstrated an inability to comply with drug therapy on multiple occasions should not receive transplantation.

Adapted from Mehra MR, Kobashigawa J, Starling R, et al. Listing criteria for heart transplantation: International Society for Heart and Lung Transplantation guidelines for the care of cardiac transplant candidates—2006. *J Heart Lung Transplantation.* 2006;25(9):1024–1042.

2. There are four statuses for patients on the heart transplant waiting list:
   a. **Status 1A** patients are typically admitted to the listing transplant center hospital (with the exception for 1A(b) candidates) and has at least one of the following devices or therapies in place:
      i. Who are in the intensive care unit on life support (ventilator, intra-aortic balloon pump) and/or high-dose intravenous (IV) medications with a pulmonary artery catheter use to titrate therapy to optimize heart function.
      ii. Who have had a ventricular assist device (VAD) or ECMO to support their heart function or have a device-related complication.
      iii. An exception may be the outpatient with a VAD who is allotted 30 days of 1A time following the VAD implant.
         • Another exception is the electrically unstable patient deemed appropriate for the 1A status following a regional United Network for Organ Sharing (UNOS) board review.
   b. Examples of **Status 1B** patients include patients who are
      i. Receiving non-ICU or home continuous IV inotropic therapy
      ii. On a VAD (not using the 30 days of status 1A time)
   c. **Status 2** patients are patients who do not meet the criteria for status 1A or Status 1B. Most often, these patients are waiting at home for a donor heart and are taking oral heart failure medications.

TABLE 9-12 Heart Transplantation Status: Organ Procurement and Transplantation Network Definitions/Criteria

1A A patient listed as status 1A is admitted to the listing transplant center hospital (*with the exception for 1A(b) candidates*) and has at least one of the following devices or therapies in place:

(a) **Mechanical circulatory support** for acute hemodynamic decompensation that includes at least one of the following:

  (i) **Left and/or right ventricular assist device** implanted. Candidates listed under this criterion may be listed for **30 d** at any point after being implanted as status 1A once the treating physician determines that they are clinically stable. Admittance to the listing transplant center hospital is not required.

  (ii) **Total artificial heart**

  (iii) **Intra-aortic balloon pump**

  (iv) Extracorporeal membrane oxygenator (**ECMO)**

Qualification for status 1A under criterion 1A(a)(ii), (iii), or (iv) is valid for **14 d** and must be recertified by an attending physician every **14 d** from the date of the candidate's initial listing as status 1A to extend the status 1A listing.

(b) **Mechanical circulatory support** with objective medical evidence of **significant device-related complications** such as thromboembolism, device infection, mechanical failure, and/or life-threatening ventricular arrhythmias. Other complications: Pump thrombus, persistent hemolysis, persistent bleeding, RV failure can petition using a regional board review. (Candidate sensitization is not an appropriate device-related complication for qualification as status 1A under this criterion). *Admittance to the listing center transplant hospital is not required.* Qualification for status 1A under this criterion is valid for 14 d and must be recertified by an attending physician every 14 d from the date of the candidate's initial listing as status 1A to extend the status 1A listing.

(c) **Continuous mechanical ventilation.** Qualification for status 1A under this criterion is valid for 14 d and must be recertified by an attending physician every 14 d from the date of the candidate's initial listing as status 1A to extend the status 1A listing.

(d) **Continuous infusion** of a single high-dose intravenous **inotrope** (e.g., **dobutamine ≥ 7.5 mcg/ kg/min or milrinone ≥ 0.50 mcg/kg/min) or multiple intravenous inotropes, in addition to continuous hemodynamic monitoring of left ventricular filling pressures**; qualification for status 1A under this criterion is **valid for 7 d** and may be renewed for an additional 7 d for each occurrence of a status 1A listing under this criterion for the same patient. VASODILATOR (nitroglycerine/Nipride) infusions do not qualify as inotropes.

1B A patient listed as status 1B has at least one of the following devices or therapies in place:

(a) Left and/or right **ventricular assist device** implanted

(b) Continuous infusion of **intravenous inotropes**

A patient who does not meet the criteria for status 1A or 1B may be assigned to any desired status upon application by his/her transplant physician(s) and justification to the applicable Regional Review Board that the candidate is considered, using accepted medical criteria, to have an urgency and potential for benefit comparable to that of other candidates in this status as defined above. The justification must include a rationale for incorporating the exceptional case as part of the status criteria. A report of the decision of the Regional Review Board and the basis for it shall be forwarded for additional review by the Thoracic Organ Transplantation and Membership and Professional Standards Committees to determine consistency in application among and within all regions and continued appropriateness of the candidate status criteria.

2 A patient who does not meet the criteria for status 1A or 1B is listed as status 2.

7 A patient listed as status 7 is considered **temporarily unsuitable to receive a thoracic organ transplant (on-HOLD).**

Adapted from OPTN policy 3.7.3.

    d. **Status 7** patients are temporarily inactive on the heart transplant waiting list. An example of a status 7 patient would be one who
  i. Is too sick to undergo transplantation (e.g., a patient who develops an infection and cannot undergo transplant surgery until the infection has cleared)
  ii. Is too well for transplantation

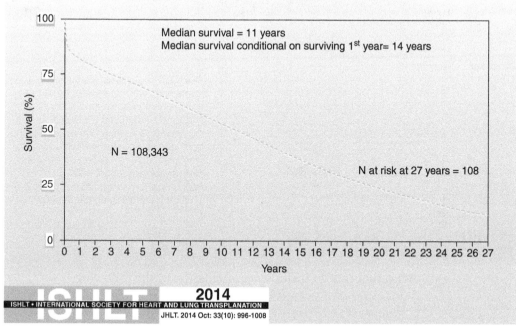

FIGURE 9-3 Adult heart transplantation survival by era January 1982 through June 2012. (Lund L, Edwards L, Kucheryavaya A, et al. The registry of the International Society for Heart and Lung Transplantation: thirty-first official adult heart transplant report—2014. *International Society Heart Lung Transplant.* 2014;33 (10):996–1008. Accessed September 10, 2015.)

      iii. Has lost health care insurance

      iv. Requests temporary inactive status

   3. Patients status on the waiting list may change over time—depending on their medical condition and current needs.

H. Survival rates:

   1. Per the Scientific Registry of Transplant Recipients (SRTR) 2012 Annual Data Report, patient survival rates for adult US patients undergoing heart transplantation are as follows[28]:

      a. 1-year patient survival from 2005 to 2007: 88%

      b. 3-year patient survival from 2007 to 2010: 81%

      c. 5-year patient survival from 2005 to 2010: 75%

      d. 10-year patient survival from 2000 to 2010: 56.6%

      e. Median overall patient survival from 1982 to 2012: 11 years or 14 years if the patient survives beyond the first-year posttransplant (*n* = 108,343; Figure 9-3).

   2. Current 1- and 5-year ISHLT Registry patient survival rates are approximately 84.5% and 72%, respectively, for adult patients undergoing transplantation between 2006 and June 2011 (*n* = 18,896)[28]

I. Diagnoses: ISHLT diagnoses for patients who underwent heart transplantation between January 2006 and 2013 are shown in Figure 9-4.[28]

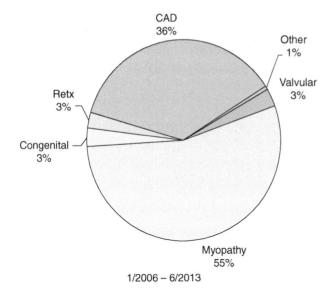

FIGURE 9-4   ISHLT diagnoses for patients who underwent heart transplantation between January 2006 and June 2012. (Lund L, Edwards L, Kucheryavaya A, et al. The registry of the International Society for Heart and Lung Transplantation: thirty-first official adult heart transplant report—2014. *Int Soc Heart Lung Transplant.* 2014;33(10):996–1008. Accessed September 10, 2015.)

VII. EDUCATION FOR PATIENTS/CAREGIVERS AWAITING HEART TRANSPLANTATION

A.   Education should include an explanation of the following:

1. Description of and rationale for preoperative tests and procedures
2. Postoperative course (e.g., length of stay in intensive care unit [ICU] and intermediate care unit, progressive ambulation, use of incentive spirometer)
3. Lines that will be inserted (e.g., intravenous [IV] lines, pulmonary artery catheter, arterial line, urinary catheter, chest tubes, drains, pacing wires, endotracheal tube, naso- or orogastric tube)
4. Incisional care
5. Pain management plan
6. Activity limitations, lifestyle, and body image changes
7. Medications and side effects: with extra emphasis on the triple immune suppression medications
8. Importance of compliance with posttransplant medical regimen (e.g., EMB, follow-up lab work, vital sign monitoring, principles of infection and rejection with prompt reporting of symptoms of illness)[24,25]

VIII. PREPARATION OF PATIENT FOR SURGERY[26]

Preoperative protocols differ among transplant centers. Typical preoperative procedures follow.

A.   Obtain preoperative tests and results in timely manner.

1. Chest radiograph
2. Laboratory tests: Complete blood cell (CBC) count, complete metabolic profile (renal and hepatic function tests, electrolyte panel), coagulation tests, urinalysis, panel reactive antibodies (PRA), viral serologies
3. Recipient/donor prospective crossmatch (if required)[29]
   a. A crossmatch may be indicated if the potential recipient's PRA is >10% before transplant, indicating a higher risk for rejection if the recipient has unacceptable antibodies to the donor's HLA antigens. See the Basics in Transplant Immunology chapter for additional information.

      b. Accepting a graft from a donor that has antigens to which the recipient has antibodies could result in a positive crossmatch and may cause antibody-mediated rejection.

      c. Several bioassays are used to detect circulating donor-specific antibodies (DSA) before or after transplant with the following sensitivities:

         i. Multiplex bioassay using magnetic beads and lasers to identify unacceptable antigens or donor-specific antibodies: 93%

         ii. Complement-dependent cytotoxicity: 43%

         iii. Basic flow cytometry uses cell surface stains to detect antibodies: 43%

         iv. Enzyme-linked immunosorbent assay: 21%

      d. Studies have shown that recipients who are highly sensitized prior to transplantation are more likely to develop DSA within the first 60 days posttransplantion; therefore, close monitoring is advised during this critical period.[30]

   4. Obtain blood type and crossmatch per protocol

      a. Blood products: (e.g., packed red blood cells, fresh frozen plasma, platelets) before, during, and after surgery are often required to correct coagulation abnormalities and replace intraoperative blood volume loss.

      b. Leukocyte-depleted blood is ordered in some centers.

         i. Leukocytes are removed by filtration of platelets and red blood cell concentrates that can lead to sensitization.

         ii. Giving leukopoor blood also reduces risk for cytomegalovirus (CMV) infection for patients with CMV-negative serologies.

      c. CMV-negative blood is ordered for CMV-negative patients.

         i. Giving CMV-positive blood (or an allograft from a CMV-seropositive donor) to a CMV-seronegative recipient increases the immunosuppressed recipient's risk of contracting CMV disease.

   5. Electrocardiogram: Particularly in patients who will have a repeat sternotomy; abnormal findings alert the anesthesiologist and surgeon to potential cardiac problems that may arise before cardiopulmonary bypass (CPB) is initiated.

B. Ensure that patient has nothing by mouth.

   1. Oral preoperative medications may be administered with a small sip of water.

C. Initiate telemetry monitoring, especially if patient's ICD has been deactivated.

   1. ICD is deactivated at some point prior to surgery because the electrocautery used during the procedure can cause the device to discharge unexpectedly.

D. Measure and record patient weight.

E. Measure and record vital signs per protocol.

F. Ensure that surgical informed consent document has been signed.

G. Start IV line.

H. Administer preoperative medications as directed or per protocol.

   1. Fresh frozen plasma or phytonadione (vitamin K) if patient has been on anticoagulant therapy

   2. Immunosuppressant(s)

   3. Antianxiety agent(s)

   4. Prophylactic antimicrobial therapy

TABLE 9-13 **Examples of Desensitization Therapies**

Therapy	Dose	Frequency
Plasmapheresis	1.5 volume exchanges	(A) 5 consecutive days
		(B) 5 times, every other day
		(C) 5 times, every other day every 2–3 wk
IVIG	(A) 2 g/kg IV divided over 2 d	(A) Every 2–4 wk
	(C) 0.1 mg/kg IV	(C) Every 2–4 wk
Rituximab	(A) 1 g IV	(A) Every week × 4
	(D) 500 mg	(D) Every 2 wk
Bortezomib	(A) 1.3 mg/m²/dose	(A) Twice-weekly for 2 wk (if rituximab fails)

(A) Cedars-Sinai Medical Center; (B) Stanford University; (C) University of Toronto; (D) University of Berlin.
Adapted from Kobashigawa J, Crespo-Leiro MG, Ensminger SM, et al. ISHLT consensus: report from a consensus on antibody-mediated rejection in heart transplantation. *J Heart Lung Transplant.* 2011;30:252–269; Velez M, Johnson MR. Management of allosensitized cardiac transplant candidates. *Transplant Rev.* 2009;23(4):235–247; Aggarwal A, Pyle J, Hamilton J, et al. Low-dose rituximab therapy for antibody-mediated rejection in a highly sensitized heart-transplant recipient. *Tex Heart Inst J.* 2012;39(6):901–905.

I.   Desensitization strategies
1. Plasmapheresis
   a. Mechanical removal of circulating antibodies may be used in highly sensitized patients to reduce the risk of allograft rejection preoperatively on the day of transplant (Table 9-13).[29–31]
   b. Plasmapheresis can also be done to desensitize (remove unacceptable antibodies) the patient while on the waiting list or prior to transplant to reduce antibodies and increase likelihood of finding a negative crossmatch. It can be combined with the administration of intravenous immunoglobulin (IVIG).[29]
2. Rituximab (Rituxan): A monoclonal antibody to CD20 that is used to desensitize patients prior to heart transplantation. Rituximab depletes B lymphocytes through complement-dependent cytotoxicity and can be used instead of, or in addition to, plasmapheresis.[31]
3. Long-term data regarding the use of pretransplant allosensitization with rituximab or plasmapheresis in the highly sensitized transplant recipient have shown an increase in antibody-mediated rejection (AMR) and posttransplant coronary artery vasculopathy (CAV) and a decrease in overall graft survival. Studies are small and more data and experience are needed with this complicated population of patients.[29]
4. Bortezomib (Velcade) is a 23S proteosome inhibitor used in the treatment of multiple myeloma. It may be used in conjunction with plasmapheresis and rituximab for desensitization.[32]

J.   Provide emotional support to patient and caregivers.
1. Give patient/family opportunity to ask questions or verbalize their concerns.

K.   Review immediate preoperative, intraoperative, and postoperative procedures with patient and family, such as
1. Approximate time surgery will begin and duration of surgery (typically 4 to 8 hours)
   a. Duration of surgery is typically longer if the recipient has had prior cardiac surgery, including implantation of a ventricular assist device.

2. Location of family waiting room
3. Provision of periodic updates by surgical team member
4. Location of the postanesthesia care unit (PACU) and/or ICU

L. Address cultural, religious, or psychosocial concerns such as spiritual care for the patient and/or caregiver(s).

M. Other: Have patient take antimicrobial shower per protocol.

N. If surgical procedure is canceled:

1. Make certain that ICD is turned back on.
2. Make certain that patient is adequately anticoagulated if anticoagulation had been reversed.
3. Provide emotional support to patient and family.
   a. Explain reason for cancelation of surgery.
   b. Given the long waiting times for donor hearts, patient and family are typically very distraught over this "missed opportunity" and often wonder if another donor heart will be found in time.
   c. Allow patient and family opportunity to express their emotions and disappointment.
   d. If needed, arrange consultation with mental health and/or spiritual care provider.

 IX. SURGICAL PROCEDURE

A. Placement of lines and catheters

1. Large-bore peripheral lines
2. Hemodynamic monitoring lines (e.g., pulmonary artery catheter, arterial line) that will facilitate intra- and postoperative monitoring of
   a. BP
   b. Pulmonary artery pressure
   c. PCWP (if ordered)
   d. Central venous pressure (CVP)
   e. Arterial blood gases (ABG)
   f. CO/cardiac index (CI)
3. Foley catheter to monitor urine output
4. Naso- or orogastric tube to decompress the stomach and remove secretions
5. Chest tubes

B. Initiation of CPB

C. Surgical techniques[33–35]

1. Median sternotomy
2. Biatrial (standard) technique[33,34]
   a. Cuffs of the recipient's native right and left atria are sutured to the donor right and left atria; donor aorta is sutured to recipient's aorta; donor pulmonary artery is sutured to recipient's pulmonary artery.
   b. The donor heart is denervated.
      i. With explanation of the donor heart, the sympathetic and parasympathetic nervous system fibers are severed (see "Denervation of the Cardiac Allograft").
      ii. The recipient's remaining *native* atrial tissue may still have electrical activity; however, these impulses do not cross the suture line.

    c. Disadvantages of biatrial technique are related to the large and anatomically abnormal atria created during the surgery and include the risk of
       i. Mitral and tricuspid valve regurgitation
       ii. Thrombus formation within the atria
       iii. Tachydysrhythmias
       iv. Persistent sinus node dysfunction requiring a permanent pacemaker
    d. Biatrial technique is shown in Figure 9-5. Anastomoses include left atrium, right atrium, pulmonary artery, and aorta.

3. Bicaval technique[35,36]
    a. More commonly used.
    b. Leaves recipient with more anatomically normal atria.
    c. Intact donor RA is preserved; anastomoses are at recipient's superior and inferior vena cava; left atrial cuff is reduced in size to a small area around the pulmonary veins.
    d. Advantages:
       i. Preserved sinoatrial (SA) node function
       ii. Decreased sinus node dysfunction
       iii. Decreased incidence of atrial dysrhythmias and mitral and tricuspid regurgitation.[34]
    e. Disadvantages: Longer surgical procedure prolongs ischemic time.
    f. Bicaval technique for orthotopic heart transplantation is shown in Figure 9-5.

4. Heterotopic transplantation is a procedure in which the donor heart is "piggybacked" onto the recipient's native heart.
    a. This procedure was first successfully performed in 1974.[37] During the 1970s, it was the primary method of heart transplantation due to the ability of the recipient's native heart to maintain cardiac function during acute rejection episodes.
    b. With the advent of cyclosporine and improved outcomes with orthotopic heart transplantation, use of the heterotopic technique subsequently waned.[38]
    c. More recently, heterotopic heart transplantation has increased in some centers owing to a number of factors, including
       i. Increased number of large (>80 kg) candidates with refractory pulmonary hypertension
       ii. Underuse of small donor hearts and marginal allografts
       iii. Small donor pool in some areas of the world
    d. Advantages of heterotopic transplantation include[38]
       i. More lenient size matching between recipient and potential donor
       ii. Ability of recipient's native heart to maintain hemodynamic stability during acute rejection episodes
       iii. Prevention of RV failure in recipients with severe pulmonary hypertension
    e. Disadvantages of heterotopic transplantation include[38]
       i. Continued pathology of native heart (e.g., ischemic disease, HF)
       ii. Difficulty in performing EMB
       iii. Persistent angina in recipients with ischemic cardiomyopathy
       iv. Need for anticoagulation in the setting of hypokinesis and clot formation
       v. Pulmonary complications associated with compression and subsequent atelectasis of the right lung by the heterotopically placed donor heart
    f. Example of a heterotopic heart transplant technique is shown in Figure 9-6.

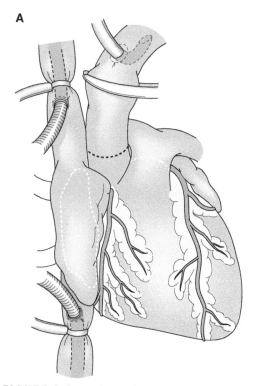

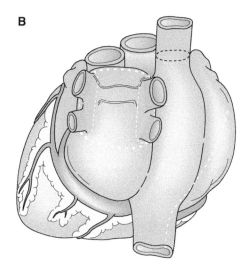

FIGURE 9-5 Native cardiectomy and donor graft preparation. **A.** Recipient pericardium after institution of cardiopulmonary bypass and ascending aortic occlusion with caval snares secured. The diseased native heart can then be safely excised by transecting the recipient aorta and pulmonary artery, and the atria can be divided as appropriate for intended implant technique. Shown is the right atrial incision for the traditional Lower/Shumway right atrial cuff. **B.** Posterior view of the explanted donor heart, indicating various incisions used for atrial cuff preparation. Donor atrial cuff incisions made in preparation for traditional Lower/Shumway biatrial implant are indicated by the *heavy gray dashed line*. The superior vena cava (SVC) is ligated or oversewn. Right and left pulmonary vein (*light gray dashed line*) and superior vena cava (*black dashed line*) incisions are indicated for the total atrioventricular implant technique. For the bicaval technique, the donor SVC and inferior vena cava (IVC) are retained as for the total atrioventricular technique (*black dashed line*), and the donor left atrial cuff trimmed as for the traditional biatrial approach (*heavy gray dashed line*). (Mulholland MW, Lillemoe KD, Doherty GM, et al. *Greenfield's Surgery: Scientific Principles and Practice.* 4th ed. Philadelphia, PA: Lippincott Williams & Wilkins; 2006.)

X. DENERVATION OF CARDIAC ALLOGRAFT[38]

A. In the normal heart, sympathetic and parasympathetic (vagal) chains affect the speed of electrical conduction, HR, and contractility.

B. Donor cardiectomy severs both sympathetic and parasympathetic nervous system connections. These connections are not restored when the donor heart is implanted. As a result, the transplanted heart is denervated; that is, it lacks sympathetic or parasympathetic innervation. This unique physiology has several effects:

1. Bradyarrhythmias may be observed in the immediate postoperative period; chronotropic support with isoproterenol (Isuprel) or pacing may be temporarily required.

2. Unique response to activity, exercise, and stressors such as hypovolemia, hypoxia, hemorrhage, and ischemia.

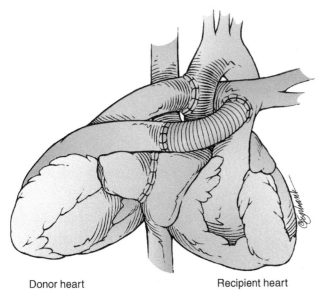

Donor heart   Recipient heart

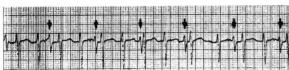

FIGURE 9-6 Heterotopic method of heart transplantation. The donor heart is anastomosed with a Dacron graft to the recipient's heart, resulting in this ECG tracing. Note the "extra" QRS at an independent rate. (From Smeltzer SC, Bare BG. *Brunner and Suddarth's Textbook of Medical-Surgical Nursing.* 10th ed. Philadelphia, PA: Lippincott Williams & Wilkins; 2004:775.)

   3. Heart transplant recipients have a higher than normal resting HR averaging 90 to 110 beats per minute (bpm).
   4. See Table 9-14 for a comparison of normal (innervated) and denervated heart.
   C. Major implications of cardiac denervation are as follows[39,40]:
      1. Response to vigorous physical activity and exercise
         a. Recipients require a longer warm-up period before exercise so that circulating catecholamines and increased venous return can increase HR.
            i.   Because the denervated heart's response to activity is slow, it is essential to have the patient do appropriate warm-up exercises (e.g., 5 to 10 minutes of leg pumping, ankle rotations) prior to engaging in activity (getting out of bed, ambulating). Failure to do so can result in orthostatic hypotension.

TABLE 9-14 Comparison of Normal and Denervated Heart

Factor	Normal Heart	Denervated Heart
Parasympathetic innervation	Resting HR 60–100 bpm due to inhibitory effect of parasympathetic stimulation	No parasympathetic stimulation Resting HR = 90–110 bpm[30]
Sympathetic innervation	Direct sympathetic stimulation that automatically increases CO with exercise	No direct sympathetic stimulation; other mechanisms increase CO with exercise:40 1. Early in exercise: ↑ venous return augments preload and ↑ CO 2. Later in exercise: inotropic and chronotropic effects of catecholamines released from noncardiac sites results in ↑ CO

bpm, beats per minute; CO, cardiac output; HR, heart rate.

   b. Similarly, recipients require a longer cooldown after exercise so that HR can gradually decrease as circulating catecholamines dissipate.

    i. Patients should not abruptly stop vigorous physical activity. Instead, they should gradually decrease their level of activity.

  2. The denervated heart does not respond well to stress that requires an abrupt increase in HR (e.g., hypoxia, hemorrhage, hypovolemia) in order to maintain or increase CO.

  3. The denervated heart will have an altered response to certain cardiac drugs. In particular, atropine is not useful in the setting of bradycardia, because atropine's mechanism of action is to block input from the parasympathetic nerves (see "Response of Denervated Cardiac Allograft to Medications").

   a. Isoproterenol (Isuprel) may be used to treat bradycardia because it directly stimulates cardiac adrenergic receptors (see "Hemodynamic Monitoring and Support").

   b. Theophylline (Theo-Dur) and terbutaline may also be considered.

   c. Terbutaline, dosed orally, may also be used for a period of time postoperatively to ensure adequate heart rate.

  4. The normal diurnal variation in blood pressure is eliminated.

  5. The transplanted heart lacks afferent innervation.[39] Although there is some evidence that partial reinnervation may develop over time,[39,40] most recipients with myocardial ischemia or infarction typically do not have angina, as there is no direct afferent sensory input.

   a. Clinical manifestations of ischemia in heart transplant recipients include the *sequelae* of ischemia or infarction such as shortness of breath, increased fatigue, decreased ability to perform usual activities, etc.

   b. However, it is important to teach recipients not to disregard angina, as angina can be a symptom of ischemia in some patients.

 XI. ROUTINE POSTOPERATIVE MONITORING AND MAINTENANCE: EVALUATE OBJECTIVE CRITERIA[41–49]

 A. Arrival in ICU

  1. Patient arrives in ICU sedated and intubated with

   a. Dressings in place over sternal incision, pacemaker/ICD removal site, MCS exit cannula removal site

    i. The surgical dressing is typically left in place for approximately 24 to 48 hours, unless bleeding from the surgical wound necessitates removal of the dressing.

   b. Mediastinal, pericardial, and, usually, pleural drains

    i. Mediastinal and pleural drains are typically placed to 20 cm of underwater seal suction[48]

   c. Atrial and ventricular temporary epicardial pacing wires (see "Telemetry and Epicardial Pacemaker")

  2. Goals of nursing care:

   a. Maintenance of graft function and hemodynamic stability

   b. Ensuring proper ventilation and oxygenation

   c. Maintenance (or recovery) of all organ system functions

   d. Prevention or early recognition of complications

  3. Patients are placed in protective isolation status per center protocol (see "Prevention of Infection").

B. Vital signs:
1. Systolic BP is typically maintained at 90 to 110 mm Hg.
2. HR is typically maintained at 100 to 120 bpm.

C. Hemodynamic monitoring and support
1. Hemodynamic monitoring includes
  a. BP via an arterial line
  b. Swan-Ganz catheter to monitor:
    i.   Pulmonary artery pressures
    ii. CVP
    iii. CO and CI
  c. Mixed venous oxygen saturation (SvO$_2$; normal: 60% to 80%)
  d. Pulse oximetry
2. Obtain specific guidelines from the physician regarding acceptable hemodynamic parameters; monitor hemodynamic profile and notify physician if patient deviates from acceptable parameters.
  a. Acceptable hemodynamic parameters differ from patient to patient and depend on a number of factors including
    i.   Preoperative conditions (e.g., pulmonary hypertension, renal insufficiency)
    ii. The intraoperative course
    iii. Preservation techniques
    iv. Ischemic time of the donor heart
  b. Due to the incidence of RV dysfunction in the transplanted heart, maintaining an RA pressure of 5 to 12 mm Hg is recommended.[42]
3. It is important to monitor, document, and report *trends*.
4. Normal hemodynamic parameters are shown in Table 9-15.[16,48,49]
5. The function of the cardiac allograft is influenced by donor selection, denervation, preceding cold ischemic time, intraoperative complications, and preexisting severity of patient illness.[42]
6. Contractility, systolic function, and HR may be impaired.
  a. Primary graft dysfunction can be seen within 24 hours posttransplant and should be considered in the setting of abnormal heart function.
  b. Certain IV medications may be required, depending upon the patient's hemodynamic state.
  c. The use of low-dose inotropic agents to promote hemodynamic stability is common and recommended in the early postoperative period (see Table 9-16).[49] These inotropic medications can be gradually weaned off as tolerated over 3 to 5 days.[41,42]
7. Response to certain medications may be altered due to the fact that the heart is denervated. See Table 9-17[49] for review of cardiac allograft response to medications.

D. Ventilator settings
1. Maintain ventilator settings per protocol.
2. Monitor blood gases.
  a. Normal adult blood gases (at sea level) are shown in Table 9-18.
  b. Blood gases are used to guide weaning from ventilator.
3. Weaning from mechanical ventilation typically begins 6 to 8 hours postoperatively when the patient
  a. Has recovered from anesthesia and is alert and awake
  b. Is hemodynamically stable and has no dysrhythmias or excessive bleeding

(*text continues on page 347*)

TABLE 9-15 **Normal Hemodynamic Parameters**

Parameter	Definition/ Description	Normal Range	Increased in	Decreased in
Cardiac output	Amount of blood ejected by the LV in 1 min	4–8 L/min	Sepsis	LV failure ↓ preload ↑ afterload ↓ contractility Dysrhythmias
Cardiac index	Cardiac output adjusted for body size; cardiac output divided by body surface area	2.5–4.0 L/min/m²	Sepsis	LV failure ↓ preload ↑ afterload ↓ contractility Dysrhythmias
Stroke volume	Amount of blood ejected by the LV in one contraction	60–130 mL/beat		HF
Stroke volume index	Stroke volume adjusted for body size; stroke volume divided by body surface area	36–48 mL/beat/m²		HF
Pulmonary artery pressures	PA systolic pressure: reflects pressure produced by RV	20–30 mm Hg	Hypertension Pulmonary hypertension	
	PA diastolic pressure: reflects LV end-diastolic pressure	5–10 mm Hg	Pulmonary emboli LV failure	
	PA mean	10–20 mm Hg	Volume overload Ischemia Mitral stenosis or regurgitation	
Pulmonary capillary wedge pressure	Reflects left atrial pressure	4–12 mm Hg	Fluid overload LV failure Ischemia Mitral stenosis Mitral regurgitation Cardiac tamponade Constrictive pericarditis	Hypovolemia Hypovolemic shock Septic shock Vasodilator therapy
Pulmonary vascular resistance	Measurement of flow resistance in the lung from pulmonary artery to left atrium	50–250 dynes/s/cm⁵ (0.625–3.12 Wood units)	Large pulmonary embolism Pulmonary hypertension Hypoxemia	Use of pulmonary vasodilators
Pulmonary vascular resistance index	Pulmonary vascular resistance divided by body surface area	80–240 dynes/s/cm⁵m²		

(continued)

TABLE 9-15 Normal Hemodynamic Parameters (*Continued*)

Parameter	Definition/ Description	Normal Range	Increased in	Decreased in
Central venous pressure or RA pressure	Reflects right atrial filling pressure and mean pressure of systemic veins	2–8 cm H_2O or 2–6 mm Hg	Pulmonary hypertension Pulmonary embolism Cardiac tamponade Cardiogenic shock Pulmonary stenosis Right-sided HF RV infarct	Hypovolemia (may be secondary to diuretics, blood loss, vomiting, etc.) Hypovolemic shock Vasodilation
RV pressure	Systolic	15–30 mm Hg	Pulmonary hypertension	Hypovolemia (may be secondary to diuretics, blood loss, vomiting, etc.)
	Diastolic	2–6 mm Hg	Left-sided failure LV ischemia LV infarct Pulmonary embolism Hypoxemia Mitral stenosis or regurgitation	Hypovolemic shock Vasodilation
Systemic vascular resistance	Vascular resistance across arterial and venous circuits	800–1,300 dynes/s/cm^5	Hypovolemia Hypothermia Vasoconstriction Cardiac tamponade	Vasodilator drugs Cardiogenic shock Septic shock
Systemic vascular resistance index	Systemic vascular resistance divided by body surface area	1,200–2,500 dynes/s/cm^{5}m^2		
SvO$_2$	Mixed venous oxygen saturation	60%–80%	Sepsis Anesthesia	Hypovolemia Hemorrhage Cardiac tamponade MI Dysrhythmias Tachycardia HF Pulmonary edema Anemia Fever Respiratory failure

HF, heart failure; LV, left ventricle; MI, myocardial infarction; PA, pulmonary artery; RA, right atrial.
From Heart Failure Society of America. *The Stages of Heart Failure—NYHA Classification*. Heart Failure Society of America; 2006; Hardin SE, Kaplow R. *Cardiac Surgery Essentials for Critical care Nursing*. Burlington, MA: Jones and Bartlett Publishers; 2010; Hollenberg SM. Vasoactive drugs in circulatory shock. *Am J Respir Crit Care Med*. 2011;183(7):847–855; Kittleson MM, Kobashigawa JA. Long-term care of the heart transplant recipient. *Curr Opin Organ Transplant*. 2014;19(5):515–524; Patel JK, Kittleson M, Kobashigawa JA. Cardiac allograft rejection. *Surgeon*. 2011;9(3):160–167.

TABLE 9-16 Properties of Intravenous Vasoactive Drugs Used after Heart Transplantation

Alpha to Beta Effects	Drug	Dose	Heart Rate	Contractility	Peripheral Vasoconstriction	Peripheral Vasodilation
Alpha	Phenylephrine (Neosynephrine)	20–200 µg/min	0	0	+++	0
	Norepinephrine (Levophed)	2–40 µg/kg/min	+	++	++++	0
	Dopamine	1–4 µg/kg/min	+	+	0	+
		4–20 µg/kg/min	++	++ or +++	++ or +++	0
	Epinephrine	1–20 µg/min	++++	++++	++++	+++
	Dobutamine	2–20 µg/kg/min	++	+++ or +++++	0	++
	Milrinone	0.375–0.75 µg/kg/min	+	+++	0	++
Beta	Isuprel	0.2–10 µg/min	++++	++++	0	+

From Hollenberg SM. Vasoactive drugs in circulatory shock. *Am J Respir Crit Care Med.* 2011;183(7):847–855.

TABLE 9-17 Response of Denervated Cardiac Allograft to Medications

Medication	Action	Response in Cardiac Allograft
Aminophylline FC: spasmolytic	↑ HR	Unchanged; not mediated by CNS
Atropine FC: parasympathetic blocking agent	↑ HR	No effect on AV conduction; does not ↑ ventricular HR in setting of bradycardia, sudden heart block, or asystole
Dobutamine FC: β₁-adrenergic agonist	Catecholamine ↑ contractility, SV and CO, coronary blood flow ↓ SVR	Unchanged inotropic and chronotropic effect; not mediated by CNS*
Dopamine FC: β₁- and α-adrenergic agonist	Vasopressor *High dose* (>10 mcg/kg/min): ↑ CO, ↑ peripheral vasoconstriction, and ↑ SVR *Low dose* (2.5 mcg/kg/min): may be used to ↑ renal blood flow, particularly in setting of cyclosporine-induced nephrotoxicity	↓ inotropic response*
Ephedrine FC: β-adrenergic agonist	↑ HR and contractility	↓ inotropic response
Epinephrine FC: β-adrenergic agonist	↑ SVR	Unchanged inotropic and chronotropic effect; not mediated by CNS*
Isoproterenol FC: β-adrenergic agonist	↑ HR (dose titrated upward until HR is typically 100–120 bpm); ↓ pulmonary vascular resistance; ↑ CO	Unchanged or ↑ inotropic effect or ↑ chronotropic effect
Norepinephrine FC: β-adrenergic agonist	↑ SVR	Unchanged inotropic and chronotropic effect; no reflex bradycardia with ↑ in BP
Milrinone FC: inotropic/vasodilator agent	Phosphodiesterase inhibitor Positive inotrope that ↑ contractility without ↑ HR Vasodilator properties ↓ preload and afterload by relaxing vascular smooth muscle	Unchanged; not mediated by CNS
Nitroglycerine FC: coronary vasodilator	Relaxes arteries and veins; ↓ preload and afterload	Unchanged; not mediated by CNS
Sodium nitroprusside FC: antihypertensive; vasodilator	Afterload reducer; improves LV function by dilating arteries; ↓ afterload; ↑ venous capacitance; ↓ preload; ↓ BP; ↑ CO; ↓ SVR; ↓ PCWP; ↑ SV with little ↑ in HR	Unchanged; not mediated by CNS
Terbutaline FC: selective β₂-agonist	Catecholamine ↑ HR	Unchanged; not mediated by CNS
Theophylline FC: spasmolytic	↑ HR	Unchanged; not mediated by CNS

*Due to denervation supersensitivity, there is an exaggerated response to most inotropes acting on beta receptors.
AV, atrioventricular; BP, blood pressure; CNS, central nervous system; CO, cardiac output; FC, functional class; HR, heart rate; PCWP, pulmonary capillary wedge pressure; SV, stroke volume; SVR, systemic vascular resistance.
From Hollenberg SM. Vasoactive drugs in circulatory shock. *Am J Respir Crit Care Med.* 2011;183(7):847–855.

TABLE 9-18 **Normal Adult Blood Gases**

Parameter	Arterial	Mixed Venous
pH	7.40 (7.35–7.45)	7.36 (7.31–7.41)
PCO_2	35–45 mm Hg	41–51 mm Hg
HCO_3	21–28 mEq/L	22–26 mEq/L
PO_2	80–100 mm Hg	35–40 mm Hg
SaO_2	95% or >	70%–75%
Base excess	+/– 2 mEq/L	–2 to +2

Note: This is a reference and may vary slightly depending on the lab.
Adapted from Malarkey L. *Nursing Guide to Laboratory and Diagnostic Tests.* Saunders; 2005:203.

    c. Is able to maintain adequate ventilation and oxygenation; can maintain airway and clear secretions

    d. Meets weaning criteria per protocol

4. Weaning may be delayed due to

    a. Pretransplant mechanical ventilation

    b. Preexisting pretransplant pulmonary complications

    c. Posttransplant complications such as

      i. Decreased metabolism of anesthetic agents and muscle relaxants secondary to hepatic dysfunction

      ii. Elevated PVR

      iii. Pleural effusions

5. Following extubation, maintain aggressive pulmonary toilet to decrease atelectasis and prevent risk of pneumonia through chest physiotherapy or equivalent hyperinflation therapy, turning, coughing, deep breathing, incentive spirometry, and early ambulation.

E. Neurologic status

1. Assess neurologic status upon admission to ICU and monitor closely throughout postoperative period. Depending on the patient's condition, elements of the neurologic assessment may include an evaluation of

    a. Level of consciousness: Spontaneous activity and responsiveness (e.g., with the Glasgow Coma Scale or similar tool)

      i. Alert, wakeful state

      ii. Lethargic state

      iii. Obtunded state

      iv. Stuporous state

      v. Deep coma

    b. Orientation to time, place, and person

    c. Motor function

      i. Involuntary movements

      ii. Motor response to stimuli

      iii. Strength testing

      iv. Muscle tone

    d. Reflexes

    e. Sensory function

    f. Coordination

F. Drainage output
    1. Monitor drainage from chest tube, naso- or orogastric tube, surgical drains, and incision.
    2. Report chest tube drainage that exceeds hospital protocol parameters (e.g., >100 mL/hr).
    3. Observe quality of chest tube drainage.
        a. Bright red blood can be indicative of active arterial bleeding.
        b. Old dark blood is usually not indicative of active bleeding.
    4. Assess patency of chest tubes; maintain patency per hospital protocol; inadequate chest tube drainage can lead to tamponade.
    5. Pericardial effusion can occur postoperatively and may be monitored by echocardiogram if the patient is stable. A soft surgical drainage catheter may be inserted in the posterior pericardial space when there is concern for hemodynamic compromise due to pericardial effusion.
        a. This catheter is connected to a drainage bulb.
        b. The drainage bulb is compressed to induce negative pressure.
        c. This drain may remain in place for 3 or 4 days following the removal of chest tubes.
        d. This drain is typically removed once the drainage is less than hospital protocol parameters (e.g., <40 mL/24 h).

G. Telemetry monitoring and epicardial pacemaker
    1. Cardiac dysrhythmias can occur immediately following heart transplantation due to ischemia, suture lines, or surgical trauma from manipulation of the heart. Development of dysrhythmias may also be an indication of rejection.[42,43]
    2. Bradycardia, a common dysrhythmia in cardiac allograft recipients, may occur in the early postoperative period and is often caused by SA node dysfunction.
    3. Dysrhythmias may be an indication of rejection or irritability secondary to ischemia and manipulation of the heart.[42-44]
    4. β-Adrenergic agonists and/or atrial or atrioventricular (AV) sequential pacing may be required to increase intrinsic HR.
    5. Preoperative administration of amiodarone (Cordarone) may blunt sinus node and/or AV node function.[44]
    6. Temporary epicardial pacemaker wires are routinely placed on the surface of the RA and ventricle.
        a. In early postoperative period, atrial pacing or AV sequential pacing may be required for relative bradycardia to maintain HR > 90 bpm.
        b. Often, pacing wires are left in place until after first EMB.

H. Fluid balance
    1. Measure and record weight daily.
    2. Measure and record intake and output per protocol.
    3. Fluid management
        a. Maintenance IV fluid administration may not be necessary during the first 24 to 48 hours due to
            i.   Extravascular fluid accumulation during CPB
            ii. IV fluids given with IV medications or to monitor CO
    4. Observe for clinical manifestations of hyper- or hypovolemia (see sections on Hypervolemia and Hypovolemia).

I. Pain management

1. Postoperative pain management is vital not only for the comfort of the patient but also to facilitate the patient's ability to participate in activities (e.g., coughing, turning, deep breathing, ambulation) that help to prevent atelectasis and pneumonia.

2. Review chart to determine if patient is allergic to any pain medication(s).

3. Assess for pain frequently; administer pain medications in a timely manner and document the effectiveness with a follow-up assessment.

4. While the patient is intubated, continuous morphine or fentanyl infusions may be used to control pain.

5. Following extubation and tolerance of oral intake, oral pain medications are administered (e.g., acetaminophen/oxycodone [Percocet]).

    a. Note: Nonsteroidal anti-inflammatory medications (NSAIDs) are avoided due to the increased potential for nephrotoxicity in the setting of calcineurin inhibitor immunosuppressive therapy.[45]

6. Pain control should be such that patient is able to ambulate at least two to three times per day.

7. Encourage patient to splint sternal incision with pillow while coughing and ambulating.

J. Laboratory test results

1. Baseline laboratory studies upon arrival in ICU typically include CBC count with differential, platelet count, serum electrolytes, creatinine, glucose, coagulation studies (fibrinogen, partial thromboplastin time, prothrombin time), and arterial blood gas.

2. Laboratory tests following transfer to the intermediate care unit typically include the following: CBC count with differential, platelet count, serum electrolytes, carbon dioxide, renal function panel, liver function panel, serum glucose, albumin, total protein, and prealbumin.

K. Immunosuppression trough blood levels (e.g., 12-hour cyclosporine or tacrolimus levels, mycophenolic acid levels).

1. It is extremely important to obtain accurate immunosuppression trough levels to enable the medical staff to titrate medications to goal and reduce the risk for renal toxicity.

L. Urinalysis and/or cultures (if infection is suspected)

1. Potential complications and associated laboratory test results are shown in Table 9-19.[14,41–43,49]

XII. MONITOR CARDIAC ALLOGRAFT GRAFT FUNCTION FOR POTENTIAL COMPLICATIONS: REJECTION

Over the past 40 years, cardiac allograft rejection has been classified in various ways. Recently, the results of several expert panel consensus conferences have been endorsed by the ISHLT to better understand the different mechanisms of rejection and to discuss optimal treatment modalities. Cardiac allograft rejection occurs when the recipient's immune system recognizes the transplanted organ as a foreign object and triggers a cascade of immune responses. Mediators of the immune system can lead to different forms of rejection in the heart transplant recipient and require differing treatment modalities.[43,49] Additionally, the patient's

TABLE 9-19 **Potential Complications and Associated Laboratory Test Results**

Complication	Associated Laboratory Test Results	Other Abnormal Findings	Comment/Potential Cause
Left ventricular failure	↑ serum creatinine ↑ blood urea nitrogen ↑ liver function tests ↑ BNP	↓ CO ↓ SV ↑ ventricular diastolic pressure ↓ EF ↓ tissue perfusion	See section on Ventricular Dysfunction below
Bleeding	↓ hemoglobin ↓ hematocrit ↓ red blood cells ↓ platelet count (↑ in acute hemorrhage) ↓ iron ↓ total iron binding capacity ↓ serum albumin ↑ total bilirubin ↓ total protein		Bleeding from anastomoses Effects of CPB Hepatomegaly secondary to HF (↓ ability of hepatocytes to produce coagulation factors) Splenomegaly (thrombocytopenia)
Infection	↑ white blood cell count ↑ sedimentation rate + C-reactive protein Positive cultures (serum, wound, sputum, stool, etc.)	**↑ neutrophils:** Acute infection Empyema Endocarditis Inflammation Pancreatitis Septicemia **↑ eosinophils:** Coccidioidomycosis Thrombophlebitis **↑ basophils:** Sinusitis **↑ lymphocytes:** Cytomegalovirus Endocarditis Hepatitis Mononucleosis Toxoplasmosis **↑ monocytes:** Epstein-Barr virus	Continuation of pretransplant infection Transmission of infection from allograft Surgical technique, iatrogenic sources Reactivation of viral infections Note: Corticosteroid therapy may blunt inflammatory response
Rejection	↑ BNP levels may indicate development of heart failure		Indications of dysfunction or failure of other organ systems may be indirect markers of decreased perfusion (e.g., ↑ serum creatinine level, ↑ liver function tests)

BNP, brain natriuretic peptide; CO, cardiac output; CPB, cardiopulmonary bypass; EF, ejection fraction; HF, heart failure; SV, stroke volume.

From Malarkey LM, McMorrow ME. *Nursing Guide to Laboratory and Diagnostic Tests.* Saunders; 2005; Gass AL, Emaminia A, Lanier G, et al. Cardiac transplantation in the new era. *Cardio Rev.* 2015;23(4):182–188; Davis MK, Hunt SA. State of the art: cardiac transplantation. *Trends Cardiovasc Med.* 2014;24(8):341–349; Kittleson MM. New issues in heart transplantation for heart failure. *Curr Treat Options Cardiovasc Med.* 2012;14(4):356–369; Hollenberg SM. Vasoactive drugs in circulatory shock. *Am J Respir Crit Care Med.* 2011;183(7):847–855.

clinical presentation directs the treatment administered. For the purposes of
this discussion, rejection is discussed on the basis of primary immune pathway
mediators: Cellular-mediated or antibody-mediated rejection. Types of cardiac
allograft rejection include hyperacute rejection, acute cellular rejection, acute
antibody-mediated rejection, and chronic rejection.[42,46,47,50-53]

A. Types of rejection
   1. Hyperacute cardiac allograft rejection[54]
      a. Description
         i. A catastrophic immune response that occurs within minutes to hours
            upon initiation of blood flow to the graft resulting in cardiogenic
            shock.
         ii. The process is thought to be caused by the recipient's circulating
            preformed cytotoxic antibodies to the donor graft.[54]
         iii. Most often occurs intraoperatively and patient has difficulty weaning
            from CPB due to profound organ hypoperfusion.
         iv. Patient will often require immediate MCS (e.g., extracorporeal
            membrane oxygenation [ECMO] for cardiopulmonary support [CPS]
            as well as continued intubation and IV inotropes).
      b. Primary mediators:
         i. The recipient's circulating, preexisting human leukocyte antigen (HLA)
            antibodies bind to antigens found on the endothelium of the donor
            heart and activate the complement pathway.
         ii. Complement activation initiates a cascade of subsequent events that
            lead to thrombosis and ultimately necrosis of the graft.
         iii. The heart dilates rapidly and turns dark red with damage to the
            capillary wall structure; hemorrhage and fibrillation ensue.[53]
      c. Risk factors for hyperacute rejection include
         i. Blood group mismatching
         ii. High levels of preformed antibodies to the donor cells
         iii. History of allosensitization prior to transplant associated with multiple
            blood transfusions, multiparity, pretransplant MCS support, and prior
            organ transplant[53-56]
      d. The prognosis is poor. Fortunately, the incidence of hyperacute rejection
         is rare (<1%) due to careful pretransplant screening of circulating
         antibodies in the recipient, prospective crossmatching of donor and
         recipient blood demonstrating compatibility, and careful ABO blood
         group matching.
      e. Report clinical manifestations of hyperacute rejection (similar to clinical
         manifestations of cardiogenic shock):
         i. Hypotension (systolic BP <80 mm Hg; mean arterial pressure [MAP]
            <60 mm Hg)
         ii. Decreased CO
         iii. Decreased CI (<2.0 L/min/m²)
         iv. Increased CVP
         v. Elevated PCWP (>18 mm Hg)
         vi. Elevated systemic vascular resistance (SVR)
         vii. Pulmonary congestion
         viii. Peripheral edema
         ix. Auscultation of S_3, S_4
      f. Retrospective crossmatch with recipient blood and donor cells (usually
         from the donor spleen) will be performed to determine cytotoxicity.

g. Treatment usually begins in the operating room (OR). Intraoperative biopsy is usually performed to confirm diagnosis. Treatment of hyperacute rejection may include most or all of the following[54,55]:
    i.   High-dose IV corticosteroids.
    ii. Plasmapheresis.
    iii. IVIG.
    iv. Cytolytic immunosuppressive therapy.
    v.   IV administration of immunosuppressive agents such as cyclosporine (Neoral), tacrolimus (Prograf), or mycophenolate mofetil (CellCept).
    vi. Initiation of IV inotropes and vasopressors.
    vii. MCS such as ECMO or other means of ventricular support is often required.
    viii. Intervene as ordered by physician; titration of inotropes; prepare patient for plasmapheresis or MCS.
h. Due to a high incidence of mortality in patients retransplanted for hyperacute rejection, this option is not viable. Aggressive treatment and stabilization is the appropriate plan.
i. In the setting of suspected hyperacute rejection, primary graft dysfunction (PGD) should also be considered (see "Primary Graft Dysfunction").
j. Collaborate with interdisciplinary team: Physicians (surgeon, cardiologist, intensivist), other providers (e.g., advanced practice registered nurses [APRN]), OR staff, transplant coordinator (for urgent relisting), social worker, and chaplain (for support for patient's family).

2. Acute cellular rejection (ACR)[53,56-58]
    a. Description:
        i.   ACR is a T-cell–mediated process.
        ii. ACR may have a subtle or gradual presentation but can lead to HF, dysrhythmias, or cardiogenic shock and requires treatment.
        iii. The diagnosis of ACR is confirmed by EMB.
    b. Primary mediators:
        i.   Characterized by infiltration of T lymphocytes and macrophages in the donor graft
        ii. In severe form, polymorphonuclear cell accumulation and myocyte necrosis
    c. T-cell response is the primary target for prevention and treatment via
        i.   Suppression of cytokine production (e.g., corticosteroids, calcineurin inhibitors such as cyclosporine (Neoral, Gengraf), or tacrolimus (Prograf, Astagraf XL)[57]
        ii. Prevention of clonal expansion of lymphocytes (e.g., immunosuppressive cell cycle inhibitors such as mycophenolate mofetil [CellCept, Myfortic])
        iii. Cytolytic therapy for treatment of severe ACR[46]

3. Acute Antibody-Mediated Rejection (AMR)[46,50-52]
    a. Description
        i.   Due to more advanced antibody screening methods, AMR is increasingly more recognized in heart transplant recipients. Although AMR was first described in 1987, diagnosis and treatment have been varied.
        ii. A consensus regarding the clinical significance and diagnosis of AMR was published in 2011.[55,56] The initial ground work from this consensus has led to a pathologic grading scale for AMR.
            • In the past, circulating donor-specific antibodies and cardiac dysfunction were required to reach diagnosis of AMR. Consensus

agreed that asymptomatic AMR, which occurs without cardiac dysfunction but is biopsy proven, is associated with greater mortality and greater development of cardiac allograft dysfunction.

- AMR may also be present in the absence of detectable circulating donor HLA antibodies as these antibodies may be adhered to the donor graft. The role of non-HLA antibodies in the development of AMR is also a potential consideration. Currently, no standard screening method exists to determine the presence of non-HLA antibodies.

    iii. AMR occurs in approximately 15% of heart transplant recipients.

    iv. The clinical presentation of AMR can vary. Some patients may be asymptomatic. Others may present with hemodynamic compromise and cardiogenic shock.

  b. Primary mediator

    i. Antibodies to activated endothelial cells may interact with the complement cascade resulting in macrophage infiltration and complement deposition leading to tissue injury.[42,43,50,53]

  c. Diagnosis of AMR

    i. Histologic and immunopathology changes noted on EMB

- Histologic changes on EMB include endothelial activation, accumulation of intravascular macrophages, capillary injury, thrombus, and myocyte necrosis.
- Immunoperoxidase or immunofluorescence stains of EMB positive for complement deposits such as C4d or as a marker for intravascular macrophages.[55,56]

  d. Circulating HLA antibodies to donor-specific antigens (DSA) may be present in recipient serum or concentrated in the donor graft (and therefore not detectable in the recipient's serum). Screening for DSA should be done routinely but the presence of these antibodies is not necessarily indicative of a diagnosis of AMR.[42] The presence of strong or complement-binding DSA may be cytotoxic and lead to AMR.[53-56]

  e. Risk factors for AMR include[56-58]

    i. Female gender

    ii. Preexisting PRA

    iii. Positive donor-specific crossmatch

    iv. Prior implantation of MCS

    v. CMV recipient seropositivity

    vi. Retransplantation

B. Signs and symptoms of acute rejection

1. Successful treatment of rejection depends on the early recognition of signs and symptoms.

  a. Prompt treatment may mean the difference between a successful recovery from a rejection episode and damage that leads to morbidity and mortality.

2. Because rejection is a natural process of the body's immune system, many of the signs and symptoms can mimic those of

  a. A generalized flu-like infection (e.g., malaise, nausea, vomiting, diarrhea)

  b. HF: Rejection in the cardiac transplant population involves irritation, damage, or destruction of cardiac myocytes that reduce the pumping ability of the heart—thus essentially causing HF. Many of the objective signs and symptoms of graft rejection can mimic those of HF.

BOX 9-2   Mnemonic for Signs and Symptoms of Rejection

R Rub (pericardial friction)*
E Electrocardiogram voltage decreased*
J Jugular venous distention*
E Edema (new onset, peripheral)*
C Cardiac dysrhythmias (atrial dysrhythmias; bradydysrhythmias)*
T Tiredness, fatigue
I Intolerance of exercise*
O Onset of low-grade fever
N New S_3 or S_4*

E Enlarged cardiac silhouette*
P Pulmonary crackles, wheezes*
I Increase in weight (particularly sudden weight gain of $\geq$1 lb/day)*
S Shortness of breath*
O Onset of hypotension*
D Disturbances in mood
E Echocardiogram findings: decreased systolic function, change in left ventricular mass and wall thickness, decreased in left ventricular chamber size*

*May indicate severe rejection.
Adapted from Cupples SA. Heart transplantation. In: Cupples SA, Ohler L, eds. *Transplantation Nursing Secrets*. Philadelphia, PA: Hanley & Belfus; 2003:85–105.

---

  c. The mnemonic "REJECTION EPISODE" may be useful for remembering the signs and symptoms of rejection (Box 9-2).

  d. Because of the potentially serious consequences of rejection, patients experiencing these signs and symptoms must be promptly evaluated by the transplant team.

  e. If rejection is suspected, an EMB is performed and treatment is initiated as soon as possible in order to control the rejection process, prevent further damage to the myocardium, and reverse the symptoms.

C. Diagnosis of acute rejection:

 1. Cardiac allograft rejection may present insidiously and symptoms may have latent development. Therefore, routine surveillance for rejection is standard practice.

 2. Laboratory markers exist for renal and liver transplant recipients but not for heart transplant recipients.

 3. Cardiac magnetic resonance imaging (MRI) is a promising noninvasive possibility for future detection of rejection but requires more investigation. MRI is currently not indicated for monitoring for rejection.

 4. The EMB remains the key diagnostic test for evaluating rejection in cardiac transplantation and is used commonly in heart transplant programs.[49,50,55]

  a. Most centers perform biopsies frequently in the early-phase posttransplant with biopsies becoming less frequent as time from transplant progresses.

  b. After 1 year posttransplant, biopsies are generally performed if the patient exhibits rejection symptoms. However, some centers may continue to perform surveillance biopsies at regular intervals.[58]

5. Risk factors for acute rejection include[56-62]
   a. Younger recipient age
   b. Female gender (donor or recipient)
   c. Higher number of HLA mismatches between the donor and recipient
   d. Black recipients
   e. Use of induction therapy
6. Biomarkers are emerging as viable options to monitor for rejection.
   a. A gene expression profile test, Allomap, was approved by the FDA in 2008 and is used for surveillance of acute cellular rejection. Studies concluded that this genetic test was noninferior to EMB in the determination of moderate or severe cellular rejection, and use of this test can minimize the potential risks associated with an invasive biopsy procedure.[58-60]
   b. Many programs use this blood test to evaluate for acute cellular rejection as indications allow.[59-62]
7. An immune cell functional assay, ImmuKnow, was approved by the FDA in 2002.
   a. This whole blood assay can be used to determine cell-mediated immunity in an immunosuppressed patient.
   b. Process:
      i. Lymphocytes are isolated and activated in vitro by plant phytohemagglutinin.
      ii. The activated lymphocytes are then lysed to measure adenosine triphosphate production (ATP). The level of ATP characterizes the immune state.[63]
      iii. An ATP level of <225 ng/mL indicates a low immune response.
      iv. At this time, studies have indicated the benefit of this bioassay in determining patients at risk for infection thereby allowing for the minimization of immunosuppression in such situations. There is contention among experts regarding the accuracy of this assay to predict rejection.[63]

D. EMB procedure

1. The biopsy procedure typically takes approximately 30 minutes and is generally done on an outpatient basis.
2. IV access for EMB is typically obtained via the right internal jugular (IJ) vein using local anesthetic. The right subclavian vein or femoral vein may be used as alternate access sites.[58]
3. With access achieved, the bioptome is advanced into the RV and small tissue samples are obtained under fluoroscopic or echo guidance. These samples are examined under the microscope and assigned a rejection grade (Figure 9-7).

E. EMB grading

1. AMR
   a. Prior (1992) guidelines for the histologic diagnosis of AMR included the following:
      i. Endothelial cell swelling
      ii. Immunoglobulin (IgM or IgG) deposition in perivascular spaces (with or without deposition of complement or fibrin)
      iii. Cellular infiltrates may be absent.
   b. The 2013 ISHLT working formulation for pathologic diagnosis of AMR is shown in Table 9-20.[55,56] Histologic and immunohistochemical criteria are used to equate severity of AMR.
   c. Treatment protocols for AMR are shown in Table 9-21.[53]

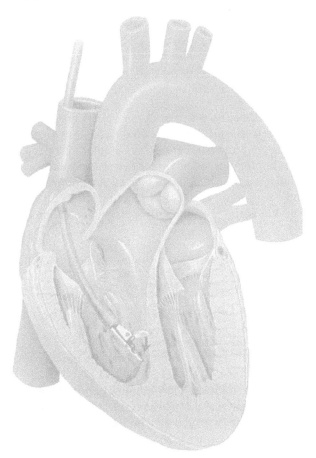

FIGURE 9-7 Positioning of bioptome for endomyocardial biopsy. (From Baughman KL. History and current techniques of endomyocardial biopsy. In: Baumgartner WA, Reitz B, Kasper E, Theodore J, eds. *Heart and Lung Transplantation.* 2nd ed. Philadelphia, PA: Saunders; 2002:267–281, Figure 25-4.)

TABLE 9-20 2013 ISHLT Working Formulation for Pathologic Diagnosis of Cardiac Antibody-Mediated Rejection

Grade	Definition	Substrates
pAMR 0	Negative for pathologic AMR	Histologic and immunopathologic findings are both negative
pAMR 1 (H+)	Histopathologic AMR alone	Histologic findings are present and immunopathologic findings are negative
pAMR 1 (I+)	Immunopathologic AMR alone	Histologic findings are negative and immunopathologic findings are positive (CD68+ and/or C4d+)
pAMR 2	Pathologic AMR	Both histologic and immunopathologic findings are present
pAMR 3	Severe pathologic AMR	Interstitial hemorrhage, capillary fragmentation, mixed inflammatory infiltrates, endothelial cell pyknosis, and/or karyorrhexis, marked edema, and immunopathologic findings are present. pAMR 3 cases are associated with severe hemodynamic dysfunction and poor clinical outcomes.

NB: Histologic changes include interstitial capillary injury and activated mononuclear cells, which are characterized by endothelial cell swelling and intravascular macrophage accumulation. Severe AMR is characterized by hemorrhage, neutrophilic or mixed inflammatory cell infiltrates, intravascular thrombus, and myocyte necrosis.
Szymanska S, Grajkowska W, Pronicki M. Pathologic diagnosis of antibody-mediated rejection in endomyocardial biopsy after heart transplantation based on renewed International Society for Heart and Lung Transplantation criteria. *Pol J Pathol.* 2014;65(3):176–181; adapted from Berry GJ, Angelini A, Burke MM, et al. The ISHLT working formulation for pathologic diagnosis of antibody-mediated rejection in heart transplantation: evolution and current status (2005–2011). *J Heart Lung Transplant.* 2011;30(6):601–611.

TABLE 9-21 Treatment Protocols for Antibody-Mediated Rejection (AMR)

Therapy	Dose	Frequency
Solu-Medrol	500 mg–1,000 mg IV × 3 d	(A) 500 mg × consecutive days (B) IV (C) IV (D) 1,000 mg IV × 3 d
Plasmapheresis	1.5 volume exchanges	(A) yes, no frequency reported (B) 5–6 cycles over 10–14 d (C) yes, no frequency reported (D) 7–10 cycles
IVIG		(A) 2 g/kg days 0 and 30 (B) used, no frequency reported (C) used, no frequency reported (D) used, no frequency reported
Rituximab	(A) 1 g IV (D) 500 mg	(A) 1 g on days 7 and 21 (D) × 4 wk
Antithymocyte globulin		(A) used on days 0 and 30 (D) used, no frequency reported

(A), Cedars-Sinai Medical Center; (B), Columbia Presbyterian Medical Center; (C), Cleveland Clinic; (D), Hospital University of Spain. Stewart S, Winters GL, Fishbein MC, et al. Revision of the 1990 working formulation for the standardization of nomenclature in the diagnosis of heart rejection. *J Heart Lung Transplant*. 2005;24:1710–1720; adapted from Kobashigawa J, Crespo-Leiro MG, Ensminger SM, et al. ISHLT Consensus: report from a consensus on antibody-mediated rejection in heart transplantation. *J Heart Lung Transplant*. 2011;30:252–269.

2. Cellular rejection
   a. Initial grading systems for acute cellular rejection were created in 1990. These systems were revised in 2005.
   b. Revised (2005) grading system: ISHLT Standardized Cardiac Biopsy Grading: Acute Cellular Rejection is shown in Table 9-22.[42]
   c. Diagnostic features/grading of ACR seen in Figure 9-8.

F. Postprocedure activity depends on the biopsy approach:
   1. IJ or subclavian vein approach: Patients may resume normal activities; maintaining an upright position decreases risk of venous oozing or bleeding.
   2. Femoral venous approach: Bed rest for 2 to 4 hours to facilitate venous plugging and endothelial repair.

G. Common (minor) side effects of the procedure are
   1. Pain or discomfort at the puncture site
      a. Pain may become more noticeable as the effect of the local anesthetic wears off.
      b. Pain is typically managed with acetaminophen or with prescription analgesics if needed.
   2. Small hematoma and bruising at the puncture site (typically resolves within 24 to 48 hours)

H. Complications of EMB include[57]
   1. RV perforation and pericardial tamponade (see section on Cardiac Tamponade below)
   2. Malignant ventricular dysrhythmias

TABLE 9-22 **International Society for Heart and Lung Transplantation Standardized Cardiac Biopsy Grading**

Grade	Description	Interpretation
0 R*	No acute rejection	No evidence of mononuclear inflammation or myocyte damage
Grade 1 R	Mild Low grade	Manifested in one of two ways: • Presence of perivascular and/or interstitial mononuclear cells • Up to one focus of mononuclear cells with myocyte damage
Grade 2 R	Moderate Intermediate grade	Two or more foci of infiltrate with associated myocyte damage Foci may be present in one or more biopsy fragment Areas of uninvolved myocardium are present between rejection foci Low-grade rejection (1 R) may be present in other biopsy fragments
Grade 3 R	Severe High grade	Diffuse inflammatory process that involves multiple biopsy fragments Majority of biopsy fragments are typically involved Involves multiple areas of myocyte damage Edema, interstitial hemorrhage, and vasculitis may or may not be present

*"R" denotes revised grade.
Adapted from Stewart S, Winters GL, Fishbein MC, et al. Revision of the 1990 working formulation for the standardization of nomenclature in the diagnosis of heart rejection. *J Heart Lung Transplant.* 2005;24:1710–1720; Davis MK, Hunt SA. State of the art: cardiac transplantation. *Trends Cardiovasc Med.* 2014;24(8):341–349.

3. Transient complete heart block
4. Pneumothorax
5. Carotid artery puncture
6. Supraventricular dysrhythmias
7. Nerve paresis (vocal cord paresis, temporary diaphragmatic weakness)
8. Venous hematoma

Cellular Rejection in Heart Transplant Biopsies

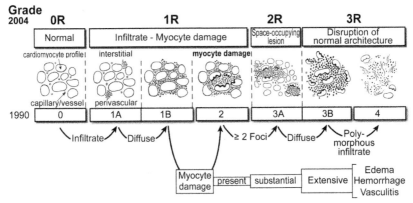

FIGURE 9-8 Grading of cellular rejection in heart transplant biopsies. The grading is illustrated from left to right, where the highest grade finding present determines the diagnosis. Comparison of original (1990) and revised grading (2004) schemes is schematically illustrated (see also e-Fig. 9.21). *Open circles* represent cardiomyocyte profiles; *small dots* represent vessels or inflammatory infiltrate. The main diagnostic feature of each grade is provided. The diagnostic features required for the 1990 grading are provided below the scheme. Based on Gassel AM, Hansmann ML, Radzun HJ, Weyand M. Human cardiac allograft rejection. Correlation of grading with expression of different monocyte/macrophage markers. *Am J Clin Pathol.* 1990;94(3):274–279; Stewart S, Winters GL, Fishbein MC, et al. Revision of the 1990 working formulation for the standardization of nomenclature in the diagnosis of heart rejection. *J Heart Lung Transplant.* 2005;24(11):1710–1720. Epub Jun 20, 2005. PMID:16297770; and Tan CD, Baldwin WM III, Rodriguez ER. Update on cardiac transplantation pathology. *Arch Pathol Lab Med.* 2007;131(8):1169–1191. Review. PMID:17683180.

I. Baseline (preprocedure) and postprocedure monitoring includes assessment of the following:

1. BP, HR, and rhythm
2. Respiratory rate and quality of respirations
   a. Increased respiratory rate or difficulty breathing may indicate cardiac tamponade, pneumothorax, or hemothorax and must be reported immediately.
3. Bruising or hematoma at puncture site
4. Bleeding from puncture site
   a. If bleeding occurs, apply pressure to the site for a minimum of 5 minutes (or longer as per protocol) and then apply an occlusive dressing.
5. In the event of cardiac tamponade (see "Cardiac Tamponade")
   a. Notify physician immediately.
   b. Administer oxygen as ordered.
   c. Obtain echocardiogram.
   d. Prepare patient for emergency pericardiocentesis or subxiphoid pericardial window.
   e. Obtain IV access for the administration of fluids.
6. PA and lateral chest radiograph or echocardiogram may be ordered by the physician post biopsy procedure as standard practice.

J. Patient education regarding the EMB procedure

1. Instruct patient to monitor the biopsy site and report the following:
   a. Severe pain at the site of the puncture wound
   b. Chest pain
   c. Shortness of breath
   d. Increased bruising, swelling, or bleeding at puncture site
2. Outpatients: Instruct patient to remove dressing after 12 to 24 hours unless bleeding or oozing continues.
3. Educate patient about potential interventions based on abnormal biopsy findings; for example:
   a. Increase in immunosuppression dose
   b. Prednisone "pulse" (e.g., prednisone 50 mg twice daily for 3 days; may be followed by prednisone taper)
   c. Administration of IV corticosteroids
   d. Hospitalization for administration of more potent antirejection agents

K. Postrejection follow-up

1. In the setting of rejection, EMB should be repeated approximately 1 to 2 weeks after treatment.
   a. Waiting approximately 2 weeks allows the edema and inflammation associated with myocyte damage to recede enough to allow for accurate grading of rejection.
2. Once rejection has been successfully treated, close monitoring of follow-up biopsy results, the immunosuppressive regimen, dose adjustments, and immunosuppressant levels must be continued in an attempt to prevent recurrent episodes of rejection.
3. Other factors that may have contributed to the episode of rejection should be assessed such as
   a. Tapering of corticosteroid therapy
   b. Change in immunosuppressant medications

          c. Patient nonadherence to immunosuppression regimen

          d. Rejection that occurs in the setting of infection due to up-regulation of the immune system to combat such infection

      4. Collaborate with interdisciplinary team.

          a. Rejection monitoring and treatment may require collaboration among the following interdisciplinary team members: physicians (surgeon, cardiologist, pathologist, intensivist), APRN, transplant pharmacist, immunologist, nurse practitioner, physician's assistant, and dietitian.

          b. Depending upon the immunosuppressant side effects that the patient may develop, collaboration with the following specialists may also be necessary: endocrinologist, neurologist, infectious disease physician, nephrologist, pulmonologist, gastroenterologist, ophthalmologist, hematologist, social worker, psychologist, or psychiatrist.

L. Other tests for rejection

    1. Gene expression profiling, Allomap, is a noninvasive test performed by a single laboratory using microarray technology to assess a gene expression profile with RNA isolated from peripheral blood mononuclear cells.

    2. An 11-gene expression signature associated with heart transplant rejection is evaluated to determine the absence of moderate or severe cellular rejection.

    3. The result is reported as a score between 0 and 40.

       a. Score of < 34 equates to a low likelihood of moderate or severe cellular rejection.

       b. A score of > 34 is suggestive of possible rejection warranting further confirmation of diagnosis by endomyocardial biopsy.

    4. In the proper clinical setting, Allomap testing may be used routinely and can reduce the number of biopsies and potential biopsy-related complications.

    5. Indications for use of Allomap are as follows[59–62]:

       a. Patients > 15 years of age.

       b. Patients >55 days posttransplant.[62]

       c. Corticosteroid dose >20 mg/day may artificially lower score.

       d. Use not established in patients receiving rejection therapy within 21 days.

       e. Use not established in patients receiving blood transfusion or hematopoietic growth factors within 30 days.

       f. Use not established in allosensitized patients at risk for antibody-mediated rejection. The test is not validated for AMR.

       g. Use not established in recipients >5 years posttransplant.

       h. Use in dual-organ recipients not validated.

M. Prevention of acute rejection

    1. Immunosuppression therapy is necessary to prevent allograft rejection and may be administered in several phases: as induction therapy in the early postoperative period, as a routine maintenance immunosuppressive regimen, or in the treatment of acute rejection.[51]

    2. Induction therapy provides intensive immunosuppression at the time of transplant when the risk of acute rejection is greatest. Currently, approximately 50% of all heart transplant programs use some form of induction therapy. However, there has not been a randomized trial supporting the use of routine induction therapy in all patients. Induction therapy may also be used for patients with significant renal dysfunction. Induction agents allow the delayed start of calcineurin inhibitor therapy, thereby limiting the nephrotoxic effects of these drugs.[45,46]

a. Generally used selectively in patients with increased risk of rejection such as recipients who are highly sensitized at the time of transplant or patients with renal insufficiency from prolonged HF.

b. Agents currently used include T-cell–depleting agents such as rabbit antithymocyte globulin (Thymoglobulin) or monoclonal IL-2 antibodies such as basiliximab (Simulect).

c. Although small randomized trials have shown decreased incidence of early rejection episodes with the use of induction therapy, long-term survival benefit over routine maintenance immunosuppression therapy has not been demonstrated.[45,46,52]

d. Induction therapy may be associated with increased infection risk.[52]

3. Routine Maintenance Immunosuppression Therapy[45,57,64]

a. Maintenance therapies are directed toward T-cell suppression.

b. Most commonly, a triple-drug combination regimen including calcineurin inhibitor, antimetabolite, and corticosteroid therapy is initiated at the time of transplant.

c. Calcineurin inhibitors(CNI) such as tacrolimus (Prograf, Astagraf XL) and cyclosporine (Sandimmune, Neoral, Gengraf) bind to intracellular proteins leading to suppression of T lymphocytes.

   i. CNIs

   - Some evidence suggests that tacrolimus may be associated with fewer acute rejection episodes but both agents are effective.
   - Additionally, tacrolimus may be associated with less hypertension and hyperlipidemia than cyclosporine; however, tacrolimus has been associated with an increased incidence of new-onset diabetes.[65-67]

   ii. Antimetabolite agents

   - Immunosuppressants such as mycophenolate mofetil (CellCept, Myfortic) and azathioprine (Imuran) block purine synthesis thereby inhibiting T- and B-lymphocyte proliferation.
   - Mycophenolate mofetil is generally the preferred antimetabolite used today. Studies have indicated fewer treated rejection episodes, less incidence of malignancy, less incidence of CAV, and increased survival with mycophenolate mofetil versus azathioprine.[51,57,64]

   iii. Corticosteroids

   - Anti-inflammatory, nonspecific panimmunosuppressive agents used in all three phases of immunosuppressive therapy.
   - Corticosteroids alter cytokine expression and leukocyte activity.
   - Long-term corticosteroid use is associated with many adverse effects.
   - Studies have demonstrated safety in slow withdrawal of corticosteroid therapy in patients.
   - For recipients at low risk for rejection, many programs withdraw steroid therapy completely by 1 year posttransplant. Patients are closely monitored for rejection during this withdrawal process by EMB or gene expression profile testing.[68]

d. Proliferation signal inhibitors (PSI), also known as mammalian target of rapamycin (mTOR) inhibitors, (sirolimus [Rapamune]or everolimus [Zortress]) are newer agents used in maintenance immunosuppression.

   i. Studies indicate lower incidence of CAV, CMV disease, and malignancy with these agents.

  ii. When used, sirolimus or everolimus will generally replace mycophenolate mofetil (CellCept, Myfortic) in the maintenance immunosuppression regimen.

  iii. Due to increased incidence of wound healing complications and infection, early postoperative use of proliferation signal inhibitors is often avoided.

  iv. Studies indicate that when everolimus (Zortress) is used, CNI doses may need to be lowered to minimize CNI nephrotoxicity, which is further potentiated by the use of PSI agents.[68-72]

 e. Pravastatin (Pravachol) therapy has been demonstrated in studies to have anti-inflammatory and immunomodulatory effects, particularly in suppression of T-cell responses.

  i. These immunomodulatory effects are independent of the cholesterol-lowering abilities of statin therapy.[73,74]

  ii. Use of statin therapy has been associated with a decreased incidence of acute rejection, CAV, and mortality.

  iii. Statin therapy is indicated for use post–heart transplant if tolerated.

  iv. Due to the potentiating effects of statin therapy when used in conjunction with calcineurin inhibitors, statin doses are much lower than in conventional populations in order to mitigate side effects such as myositis.[73,74]

N. Treatment of Acute Rejection

 1. In the event of acute rejection, more aggressive therapies will be required in addition to the maintenance immunosuppression mentioned above. These therapies will vary depending on the type or pathway of rejection as well as the clinical presentation of the recipient. See Table 9-23 for an overview.

 2. Treatment strategies are based on a number of factors including

  a. Histological grade of rejection

  b. Type of rejection (e.g., cellular vs. antibody mediated)

  c. Time elapsed since transplantation

  d. Effectiveness of previous rejection treatment strategies

  e. Patient's current hemodynamic status

  f. Patient's prior rejection pattern

  g. Patient's current immunosuppression regimen

  h. Patient's current comorbidities

 3. Treatment options for AMR (see Figure 9-9)[51,75]

  a. Initial therapies aimed at reducing the immune-mediated injury to the donor heart may include high-dose IV corticosteroids.

  b. In conjunction with IV steroid treatment, the following desensitization therapies are also used to remove circulating antibodies to the donor graft or decrease their reactivity (see Table 9-13):

   i. Plasmapheresis

   ii. IVIG

   iii. Anti–B-cell agents such as rituximab (Rituxan) may also be added to reduce the risk of recurrent AMR.

   iv. Bortezomib (Velcade)

   v. Cytolytic agents such as Thymoglobulin may also be considered.

  c. Treatment to maintain hemodynamic stability may include

   i. IV inotropic support or vasopressor therapy

   ii. Systemic anticoagulation may be used to reduce the risk of thrombosis in the cardiac allograft

   iii. MCS

TABLE 9-23 **Overiew of Types of Immunosuppressive Therapy**

Type of Therapy	Goal	Treatments

Desensitization therapy	Reduce or eradicate HLA antibodies pre- or posttransplant	• Plasmapheresis
		• Intravenous immunoglobulins (IVIG)
		• Interleukin-2 receptor antagonist
		  – Bortezomib (Velcade)
		• Monoclonal antibody
		  – Rituximab (Rituxan)

Induction therapy	Acute rejection prevention, delay calcineurin inhibitor use in patients with renal disease	Cytolytic therapy • Antithymocyte globulin
Maintenance therapy	Prevent rejection	Corticosteroids • Prednisone Calcineurin inhibitors • Tacrolimus (Prograf) • Cyclosporine (Gengraf, Neoral) Antimetabolites • Mycophenolate mofetil (CellCept) • Azathioprine (Imuran) Proliferation signal inhibitors • Sirolimus (Rapamune) • Everolimus (Zortress)

Rejection therapy	Treat acute rejection	• Pulse steroids IV or PO
		• Increase/change maintenance immune suppression
		• Consider mechanical support (IABP, VAD, TAH)
		Cytotoxic
		• Cytolytic therapy
		  – Antithymocyte globulin
		AMR
		• Plasmapheresis/IVIG
		• Interleukin-2 receptor antagonist
		  – Bortezomib (Velcade)
		• Monoclonal antibody
		  – Rituximab (Rituxan)
		• Photopheresis in severe recurrent cases

IABP, intra-aortic balloon pump; VAD, ventricular assist device; TAH, total artificial heart.

    d. Reassessment with EMB in 1 to 2 weeks including pathology and immunochemistry evaluation for resolution of AMR.
    e. Monitoring for presence of or increase in circulating DSA.
    f. Monitor for complement binding DSA.
    g. Adjustment of maintenance immunosuppression may be considered.
       i. Increased doses of current immunosuppression regimen
      ii. Addition of new immunosuppressive agents to the current regimen
     iii. Change to different agents

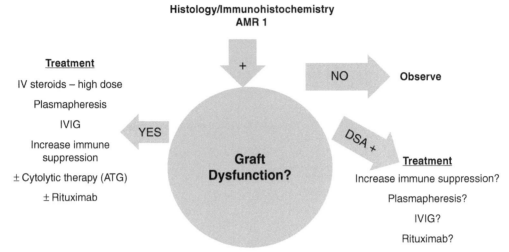

FIGURE 9-9 Treatment algorithm for antibody-mediated rejection. Periodic evaluations to include DSA titers, biopsy, histology, immunochemistry, allograft function, and intravascular ultrasound. AMR, antibody mediated rejection; IV, intravenous; ATG, antithymocyte globulin; IVIG, intravenous immune globulin. Adapted from Kobashigawa J, Crespo-Leiro MG, Ensminger SM, et al. ISHLT Consensus: Report from a consensus on antibody-mediated rejection in heart transplantation. *J Heart Lung Transplant*. 2011;30:252–269.

    h. Retransplantation is not an option in cases where heart function remains severely compromised as outcomes are not favorable in a situation of ongoing or recent rejection.

4. Treatment options for symptomatic ACR will depend on the biopsy grade of rejection (i.e., 2R or 3R) and the clinical presentation of the patient.[62,66,67]

    a. Treatment of symptomatic ACR starts with hospitalization of the patient to a cardiac monitoring unit. If hemodynamic compromise is present, admission to ICU will be necessary.

    b. Treatment will often include the following (Table 9-23)[42]

        i. Administration of high-dose IV corticosteroids is first-line therapy for symptomatic acute rejection regardless of ISHLT biopsy grade (e.g., 500 to 1,000 mg of methylprednisolone [Solu-Medrol] daily for 3 days).

        ii. In the presence of hemodynamic compromise, cytolytic immunosuppressive therapy with antithymocyte antibodies (Thymoglobulin) should be administered. Cytolytic therapy should also be administered 12 to 24 hours after high-dose IV corticosteroids if no signs of clinical improvement.

        iii. IV inotropes and vasopressor therapy may be needed for hemodynamic instability.

        iv. The use of MCS may also be required if cardiogenic shock ensues.

        v. Systemic anticoagulation may be used to reduce the risk of thrombosis in the cardiac allograft.

        vi. Reassessment with EMB should be performed 1 to 2 weeks after treatment.

        vii. Adjustment of maintenance immunosuppression may be needed such as
- Increased doses of current immunosuppression regimen
- Addition of new immunosuppressive agents to the current regimen
- Change to different agents

        viii. Monitoring response to treatment is usually done by serial echocardiograms.

      ix. AMR should be considered in the setting of ongoing hemodynamic compromise with low- or high-grade cellular rejection by biopsy.

5. Treatment of asymptomatic ACR
   a. Severe asymptomatic ACR (ISHLT Grade 3R) should be treated with high-dose IV corticosteroids.
   b. Treatment of moderate asymptomatic ACR (ISHLT Grade 2R)
      i. Moderate asymptomatic rejection may be treated with IV or increased oral corticosteroid therapy (e.g., 50 mg of prednisone twice daily for 3 days followed by a gradual wean back to baseline prednisone dose).
      ii. Reassessment with EMB should be performed 2 to 4 weeks after treatment.
      iii. Adjustment of maintenance immunosuppression may be needed in the setting of asymptomatic ACR such as
         - Increased doses of current immunosuppression regimen
         - Addition of new immunosuppressive agents to the current regimen
         - Change to different agents
   c. Asymptomatic mild cellular rejection (ISHLT grade 1R) does not require treatment in most cases.

6. Treatment of recurrent or resistant ACR:
   a. Cytolytic immunosuppressive therapy with antithymocyte antibodies (Thymoglobulin) should be considered
   b. Changes in maintenance immunosuppressive regimen may be necessary.
   c. Surveillance of cardiac allograft function by serial echocardiography is routinely done.
   d. Additional therapies that may be considered for recurrent or resistant cellular rejection include the following[55,56,75]:
      i. Addition of proliferation signal inhibitors such as sirolimus or everolimus to the maintenance antirejection regimen.
      ii. Photopheresis.
      iii. EMB specimens should be evaluated for the presence of AMR in the setting of resistant cellular rejection (see "Treatment of AMR").

7. Monitoring of rejection therapy
   a. The improvement or deterioration of the patient's hemodynamic parameters, clinical status, and follow-up test results (e.g., EMB, immunofluorescence stains, antibodies to DSA) are important indications of the effectiveness of antirejection therapy.
   b. Rejection therapy is administered cautiously and requires close monitoring for side effects including bone marrow suppression and opportunistic infections.
   c. Antimicrobial agents should be administered during periods of rejection therapy, for example, sulfamethoxazole/trimethoprim (Bactrim), clotrimazole (Mycelex), and valganciclovir (Valcyte).
   d. Potential side effects of major rejection therapies are shown in Table 9-24.

O. Chronic rejection: CAV[76–84]
   1. Description of CAV:
      a. A rapid and progressive form of coronary artery disease (CAD) that can develop early posttransplant and is characterized by endothelial injury leading to concentric diffuse intimal proliferation and eventual luminal stenosis, progressing to total occlusion of the smaller coronary arteries[78,79,83]
      b. Thought to be a form of chronic allograft rejection
      c. A major impediment to long-term survival following heart transplantation
      d. Remains the most common reason for retransplantation

(*text continues on page 368*)

TABLE 9-24 Side Effects of Major Rejection Therapies

Rejection Therapy	Potential Side Effects		Monitor
Corticosteroids	**Masking of infection** **Endocrine:** ↓ glucose tolerance Hyperglycemia Hypercholesterolemia Glycosuria ↑ insulin or sulfonylurea requirements Cushingoid appearance **Fluid and electrolyte balance:** Hypokalemia alkalosis Hypokalemia Hypocalcemia **CV:** Hypotension or hypertension Thromboembolism Thrombophlebitis Dysrhythmias ECG changes **Hematologic:** Leukocytosis **Dermatologic:** Impaired wound healing Thinning of skin Petechiae Ecchymoses Erythema Urticaria	**Ophthalmic:** Glaucoma Cataract formation Exophthalmos **GI:** Nausea, vomiting ↑ appetite (occasionally, anorexia) Diarrhea or constipation Abdominal distention Pancreatitis Gastric irritation Peptic ulcers **CNS:** Headache Vertigo Insomnia Restlessness Seizures Mood swings, personality changes	Blood glucose level Serum electrolytes Complete blood cell count with differential Impaired wound healing Cardiovascular status Gastrointestinal status Neurologic status Signs and symptoms of infection Patient's response to therapy
Antithymocyte globulin (Thymoglobulin)	Fever and chills Leukopenia Abdominal or other pain Headache	Thrombocytopenia Dyspnea Malaise Dermatologic reactions	Temperature Complete blood cell count Platelet count Respiratory status Patient's response to therapy
Basiliximab (Simulect)	Infection **Respiratory:** Pulmonary edema Dyspnea Wheezing Cough **CV:** Cardiac failure Chest pain Hypotension Hypertension Edema	**Electrolytes:** Hyperkalemia Hypokalemia Hypocalcemia Hypophosphatemia **Endocrine:** Hypercholesterolemia **GI:** GI bleeding Hepatotoxicity Nausea, vomiting Diarrhea	Temperature Complete blood cell count, differential Liver function Electrolytes Uric acid Symptoms of hepatotoxicity (dark urine, jaundice, itching, light-colored stools) Patient's response to therapy

TABLE 9-24 **Side Effects of Major Rejection Therapies (*Continued*)**

Rejection Therapy	Potential Side Effects		Monitor
	CNS:	Constipation	
	Pyrexia	Abdominal pain	
	Chills	Stomatitis	
	Tremors	Gingival hyperplasia	
	Headache	**Dermatologic:**	
	Weakness	Acne	
	Insomnia	**Other:**	
		Acidosis	
		Hyperuricemia	
Cyclophosphamide (Cytoxan)	Opportunistic infections	Hemorrhagic cystitis	Complete blood cell count, differential
	Leukopenia	Renal tubular necrosis	Platelet count
	Nausea, vomiting	Sterility (males and females)	Renal function
	Alopecia	Oligospermia	Hepatic function
	Urinary bladder fibrosis	Azoospermia	Urinalysis
			Patient's response to therapy
Rituximab (Rituxan)	**During infusion:**	**Respiratory:**	Complete blood cell count, differential
	Fever	Angioedema	Vital signs
	Chills	Bronchospasm	Respiratory status
	Rigor	Dyspnea	Cardiovascular status
	Nausea, vomiting	Cough	Neurologic status
	Urticaria	Rhinitis	Renal function
	Fatigue	Hypoxia	Patient's response to therapy
	Headache	Asthma	
	Pruritus	Sinusitis	
	Bronchospasm	Bronchitis	
	Hypotension	**Dermatologic:**	
	Angioedema	Pruritus	
	Dyspnea	Rash	
	Rhinitis	Urticaria	
	Flushing	Flushing	
	General:	**CNS:**	
	Asthenia	Headache	
	Arthralgia	Paresthesia, hyperesthesia	
	Pain	Anxiety, agitation	
	Malaise	Insomnia	
	CV:	**GI:**	
	Dysrhythmias	Abdominal pain	
	Hypotension or hypertension	Nausea, vomiting	
	Angina	Dyspepsia	
	Peripheral edema	Impaired taste	
	Hematologic:	Anorexia	
	Thrombocytopenia		
	Anemia		
	Neutropenia/leukopenia		
	Coagulation disorders		

(*continued*)

TABLE 9-24 **Side Effects of Major Rejection Therapies (*Continued*)**

Rejection Therapy	Potential Side Effects		Monitor
Plasmapheresis	Hypotension		Patient's response to therapy
Photopheresis	Fever	Hypotension	Serum electrolytes
	Myalgia	Infection	Complete blood cell count
	Nausea, vomiting		Patient's response to therapy
Total lymphoid irradiation	Leukopenia		Complete blood cell count
	Thrombocytopenia		Platelet count
			Clinical manifestations of infection
			Patient's response to therapy

CMV, cytomegalovirus; CNS, central nervous system; GI, gastrointestinal; GU, genitourinary; PTLD, posttransplant lymphoproliferative disease.

2. Prevalence of CAV[77]
   a. The cumulative prevalence of CAV in heart transplant survivors at 1 year posttransplant is 8% (follow-ups between January 1995 and June 2012).
   b. The cumulative prevalence of CAV in heart transplant survivors at 5 years posttransplant is 30% and 50% at 10 years posttransplant (follow-ups between January 1995 and June 2012).
3. Definition of CAV[78]
   a. A working formulation of a standardized nomenclature for CAV was commissioned by the ISHLT in 2010. The aim of this initiative was to standardize the definition and diagnosis of CAV. Several consensus points were reached. The points are as follows:
      i. Currently, a diagnosis of CAV is best reached with the use of coronary angiography and assessment of cardiac allograft function.
      ii. While use of intravascular ultrasound (IVUS) may detect an increase in intimal thickness and this increase can be a prognostic indicator for the future development of CAV, data regarding routine use of IVUS remain speculative.
      iii. Use of IVUS to evaluate change in intimal thickness within 1 year posttransplant is done by comparing 4- to 88-week and 1-year posttransplant IVUS results (Table 9-25).[62] Although an increase in intimal thickness of > 0.5 mm may be a prognostic indicator for the development of CAV, such use of IVUS is considered investigational.[79]
      iv. Use of noninvasive computed tomography (CT) angiography to assess for CAV is not validated. Sensitivity for branch vessel assessment in cardiac transplantation has not been determined. Additionally, the risks associated with iodinated contrast agents and radiation remain an issue.
      v. When defining CAV severity, use of EMB findings, immune-based markers, gene-based or protein-based biomarkers, microvascular function testing, or stress-based imaging has not been validated.
      vi. From the above consensus points, a nomenclature for the severity of CAV was established (Table 9-26).[78]
4. Characteristics of CAV:
   a. CAV is an unusual form of CAD that affects both epicardial and myocardial vessels. It differs from CAD as shown in Table 9-26.
   b. Traditional and nontraditional risk factors play a role in CAV (Table 9-27).[78,79]

TABLE 9-25 Basic Criteria for the Interpretation of Intravascular Ultrasound Measurements After Heart Transplantation

Timing of Intravascular Ultrasound	Intimal Thickness—Normal Findings	Abnormal Findings
Baseline measurements: 4–6 wk posttransplant	0.25–0.50 mm intimal thickness	Intimal lesions ≥0.5 mm suggest donor disease
1 y posttransplant	No change in intimal thickness	Any increase in intimal thickness >0.5 mm from baseline measurements is a prognostic indicator for accelerated coronary artery vasculopathy and coincides with adverse outcomes

Kobashigawa J, Patel J, Kittleson M, et al. Results of a randomized trial of allomap vs heart biopsy in the 1st year after heart transplant: early invasive monitoring attenuation through gene expression trial. *J Heart Lung Transplant.* 2013;32(4):S203; adapted from Costanzo MR, Dipchand A, Starling R, et al. The International Society of Heart and Lung Transplantation guidelines for the care of heart transplant recipients. *J Heart Lung Transplantation.* 2010;29(8):914–956.

TABLE 9-26 ISHLT-Recommended Nomenclature for Cardiac Allograft Vasculopathy

Coronary Artery Vasculopathy (CAV) Grade	Significance	Description
CAV_0	Not significant	No detectable lesion
CAV_1	Mild	Angiographic left main (LM) <50%, or primary artery with maximum lesion of <70%, or any branch with lesions <70% (including diffuse narrowing) without allograft dysfunction
CAV_2	Moderate	Angiographic LM <50%; or a single primary artery stenosis ≥70%, or isolated branch stenosis ≥70%, without allograft dysfunction
CAV_3	Severe	Angiographic LM ≥50%; or two primary arteries ≥70% stenosis or CAV1 or CAV2 with allograft dysfunction (EF ≤45% with presence of regional wall motion abnormalities) or evidence of restrictive physiology

Adapted from Mehra MR, Crespo-Leiro MG, Dipchand A, et al. International Society for Heart and Lung Transplantation working formulation of a standardized nomenclature for cardiac allograft vasculopathy-2010. *J Heart Lung Transplant.* 2010;29(7):717–727.

TABLE 9-27 Difference Between Natural Coronary Artery Disease (CAD) and Transplant Coronary Artery Vasculopathy (CAV)

Natural CAD	Transplant CAV
Asymmetrical lesions	Concentric intimal lesions
Involves focal lesions	Diffuse thickening of vascular wall affecting entire length of vessel (pruning)
Affects both large and small branches	Typically does not affect small branches
Internal elastic lamina disrupted	Internal elastic lamina intact
Does not affect intramyocardial vessels	Affects intramyocardial vessels
Calcification common	Calcification rare
Develops slowly over years	Develops rapidly (may develop over months)
Development of collaterals common	Development of collaterals rare
Symptomatic chest pain	Asymptomatic, no chest pain due to denervated heart
CAD may manifest as angina, MI, heart failure, arrhythmias, or sudden death	CAV manifests as MI, heart failure, arrhythmias, or sudden cardiac death

From Kobashigawa JA, Pauly DF, Starling RC, et al. Cardiac allograft vasculopathy by intravascular ultrasound in heart transplant patients: substudy from Everolimus versus mycophenolate mofetil randomized, multicentre trial. *JACC Heart Fail.* 2013;1(5):389–399; Mehra MR, Crespo-Leiro MG, Dipchand A, et al. International Society for Heart and Lung Transplantation working formulation of a standardized nomenclature for cardiac allograft vasculopathy *J Heart Lung Transplant.* 2010;29(7):717–727.

TABLE 9-28 Etiologic Factors in Development of CAV

Immunological Factors	Nonimmunological Factors
Human leukocyte antigen mismatching (cellular and humoral response) Presence of DSA—Classes I and II are associated with increased mortality and greater incidence of CAV Presence of non-HLA antibodies can be seen in chronic rejection	Donor characteristics: age (older donor), sex, smoking, HTN, ischemic time, preexisting CAD, explosive brain death (gunshot wound/trauma/fatal intracerebral bleed) Recipient characteristics: age, sex, obesity, hypertension, hyperlipidemia, diabetes mellitus, smoking, cytomegalovirus infection, oxidative injury, systemic inflammation, and CRP >3 mg/L
Suboptimal immunotherapy Long-term steroids or CNI use increases risk factors for CAV (HTN, hyperlipidemia, and CKD) Acute rejection (number and severity)	Immunosuppression—sirolimus and everolimus are shown to reduce progression of CAV by reducing growth factor–driven smooth muscle cell proliferation and reduce CMV infection rates and inhibit progression of existing CAV Donor organ procurement injury, prolonged ischemic time

Inflammation
Lymphocyte and macrophage activation Cytokine and chemokine release

Endothelial injury and dysfunction
Up-regulation of adhesion molecules Vascular smooth muscle cell proliferation and migration

Cardiac Allograft Vasculopathy
End result

From Colvin-Adams M, Agnihotri A. Cardiac allograft vasculopathy: current knowledge and future direction. *Clin Transplant.* 2011;25(2):175–184; Kobashigawa JA, Pauly DF, Starling RC, et al. Cardiac allograft vasculopathy by intravascular ultrasound in heart transplant patients: substudy from Everolimus versus mycophenolate mofetil randomized, multicentre trial. *JACC Heart Fail.* 2013;1(5):389–399; Mehra MR, Crespo-Leiro MG, Dipchand A, et al. International Society for Heart and Lung Transplantation working formulation of a standardized nomenclature for cardiac allograft vasculopathy *J Heart Lung Transplant.* 2010;29(7):717–727.

    5. Etiology of CAV
        a. Both immunological and nonimmunological processes are involved in the development of CAV.
        b. See Table 9-28 for etiology and pathogenesis of CAV.[76,79–83]
        c. Protective factors slowing progression of CAV are shown in Table 9-29.[83]
    6. Clinical manifestations of CAV
        a. Unlike classic CAD, angina is rarely associated with CAV because the allograft is denervated.

TABLE 9-29 Protective Factors Slowing Progression of CAV

Medications
Statins
Ace inhibitors
Sirolimus
Everolimus
Calcium channel blockers

Exercise
High-intensity exercise reduces progression of CAV

From Fishbein MC. Pathologic findings of cardiac dysfunction. In: Norman DJ, Turka LA, eds. *Primer on Transplantation.* 2nd ed. Mt. Laurel, NJ: American Society of Transplantation; 2016:370–374.

b. CAV may be a slow indolent process or a rapidly progressive process leading to allograft dysfunction and restrictive physiology. Signs of restrictive cardiac allograft physiology may include the following:
   i. Symptomatic HF
   ii. Right atrial pressure (RAP) >12 mm Hg
   iii. PCWP >25 mm Hg
   iv. CI < 2 L/min/m²
c. Other clinical manifestations may include
   i. Increasing fatigue
   ii. Exertional dyspnea or dyspnea at rest
   iii. Elevated LV filling pressures
   iv. Decreased LVEF by echocardiogram
   v. Clinical manifestations of allograft failure
      • Congestive HF
      • Dysrhythmias
      • Sudden death

7. Diagnosis of CAV
   a. CAV causes diffuse, concentric narrowing of arteries; focal stenoses are rare. Conventional coronary angiography may lack sensitivity to assess these diffuse lesions but remains the method of surveillance.
   b. From a multicenter study, IVUS has been shown to be an effective imaging modality by allowing early detection of risk for CAV.
   c. IVUS studies have indicated that an increase in intimal thickness of 0.5 mm or greater at 1 year posttransplant (compared with early posttransplant) denotes poor survival, but more investigation is needed.[79] Currently, routine use of IVUS has not been sanctioned by the ISHLT.
   d. IVUS permits
      i. Delineation of the actual lumen diameter
      ii. Assessment of vessel wall morphology
      iii. Quantification of the stenosis
   e. May be most helpful for negative predictor value at any time posttransplant rather than a routine surveillance tool for CAV.

8. Treatment of CAV
   a. Revascularization procedures such as percutaneous transluminal coronary angioplasty (PTCA) or coronary artery bypass graft surgery are limited treatment options because of the diffuse, concentric nature of CAV.[78,84]
   b. For those recipients with focal lesions in epicardial vessels, drug-eluting stents have shown some success with lower restenosis rates than conventional bare metal stents. Due to the high rate of restenosis post PTCA, re-evaluation by coronary angiography may be considered at 6 months postprocedure.[80]
   c. Surgical revascularization is rarely an option in CAV due to poor distal targets.
   d. Research has indicated some advantage in slowing the progression of CAV with the use of proliferation signal inhibitors such as everolimus (Zortress) and sirolimus.[70,71]
   e. Statin therapy has also been demonstrated to reduce the risk of CAV and improve survival.[72,73]
   f. Use of vitamin E and vitamin C as well as ACE inhibitors has also been shown to reduce the incidence of CAV.
   g. The only definitive treatment for severe CAV is retransplantation.

P. An at-a-glance summary of the key characteristics of the major types of rejection is shown in Table 9-30.[47,53–55,58,75,76,78,79]

(*text continues on page 374*)

TABLE 9-30 Key Characteristics of Major Types of Rejection

Type of Rejection	Hyperacute	Antibody Mediated (Humoral/Vascular)	Acute Cellular	Chronic Rejection (Coronary Artery Vasculopathy [CAV])
Timing	Within minutes to hours of reestablishment of circulation to allograft	1–12 mo posttransplant (but can occur later)	1–12 mo posttransplant (but can occur later)	The cumulative prevalence of CAV in heart transplant survivors at 1 y posttransplant is 8% (follow-ups between January 1995 and June 2012)
Occurrence	Rare ($\leq$ 1%)	Common Approximately 25% of recipients were diagnosed with rejection during the first posttransplant year (transplants performed between January 2004 and December 2010)*,† Number of treated rejection episodes during first posttransplant year was 14% (for transplants performed between January 2004 and December 2010)*,†		The cumulative prevalence of CAV in heart transplant survivors at 5 yr posttransplant is 30% and 50% at 10 y posttransplant (follow-ups between January 1995 and June 2012)
Primary mediators	Preformed circulating cytotoxic antibodies against donor antigens (ABO group antigens, major histocompatibility antigens, and endothelial antigens); complement	B cells	Leukocytes (T cells and macrophages) Cytokine activation (tumor necrosis factor, interleukin-2, gamma-interferon, alpha-interferon, interleukin-4)	Alloantibodies T-cell products Tissue growth factors
Pathophysiology	Antibody-antigen binding, activation of complement pathway, endothelial cell damage, platelet aggregation, vascular thrombosis, tissue infarction	Deposition of immunoglobulin (typically IgM) and complement components in capillary walls. HLA-DR expressed on endothelium following endothelial injury	Activation and proliferation of T lymphocytes; subsequent infiltration of lymphocytes and destruction of allograft tissue	
Diagnosis	Clinical manifestations	Immunofluorescence stains Donor-specific antibodies	Endomyocardial biopsy	Intravascular ultrasound (predictive value) Coronary angiography

Therapeutic options	Inotropic therapy Plasmapheresis Mechanical circulatory support Retransplantation	Plasmapheresis Photopheresis Total lymph node irradiation Corticosteroids Anti–B-cell agents such as cyclophosphamide Antithymocyte globulin	Immunosuppressive agents that (1) inhibit clonal expansion (e.g., azathioprine) and cytokine production (e.g., steroids, cyclosporine) and (2) deplete circulating T lymphocytes (monoclonal and polyclonal antilymphocyte antibodies)	Revascularization procedures are of limited utility due to the diffuse, concentric nature of CAV. Retransplantation is the only definitive treatment

*ISHLT Registry Data 2013.

†Based on type of immunosuppressant therapy.

From Costanzo MR, Dipchand A, Starling R, et al. The International Society of Heart and Lung Transplantation Guidelines for the care of heart transplant recipients. *J Heart Lung Transplant.* 2010;29(8):914–956; Stewart S, Winters GL, Fishbein MC, et al. Revision of the 1990 working formulation for the standardization of nomenclature in the diagnosis of heart rejection. *J Heart Lung Transplant.* 2005;24:1710–1720; Kaczorowski DJ, Datta J, Kamoun M, et al. Profound hyperacute cardiac allograft rejection rescue with biventricular mechanical circulatory support and plasmapheresis, intravenous immunoglobulin, and rituximab therapy. *J Cardiothorac Surg.* 2013;8:48; Berry GJ, Angelini A, Burke MM, et al. The ISHLT working formulation for pathologic diagnosis of antibody-mediated rejection in heart transplantation: evolution and current status (2005–2011). *J Heart Lung Transplant.* 2011;30(6):601–611; Patel JK, Kittleson M, Kobashigawa JA. Cardiac allograft rejection. *Surgeon.* 2011;9(3):160–167; Chih S, Tinckam KJ, Ross HJ. A survey of current practice for antibody-mediated rejection in heart transplantation. *Am J Transplant.* 2013;13(4):1069–1074; Colvin-Adams M, Agnihotri A. Cardiac allograft vasculopathy: current knowledge and future direction. *Clin Transplant.* 2011;25(2):175–184; Kobashigawa JA, Pauly DF, Starling RC, et al. Cardiac allograft vasculopathy by intravascular ultrasound in heart transplant patients: substudy from Everolimus versus mycophenolate mofetil randomized, multicentre trial. *JACC Heart Fail.* 2013;1(5):389–399; Mehra MR, Crespo-Leiro MG, Dipchand A, et al. International Society for Heart and Lung Transplantation working formulation of a standardized nomenclature for cardiac allograft vasculopathy *J Heart Lung Transplant.* 2010;29(7):717–727.

XIII. MONITOR PATIENT FOR POTENTIAL COMPLICATIONS: VENTRICULAR DYSFUNCTION/FAILURE

A. RV dysfunction/failure
1. RV failure is one of the leading causes of morbidity early in the posttransplant period.[84,85]
2. Etiology: RV failure can result from
    a. Loss of contractility in the allograft (may be associated with changes in the donor myocardium following brain death)
    b. Increased PVR in the recipient
        i.   Patients with HF often develop pulmonary hypertension as the disease progresses.
        ii. RV failure occurs when the donor RV fails due to the recipient's elevated PVR.
        iii. If a donor heart is transplanted into a recipient with severe pulmonary hypertension, the new RV is at high risk for failure as it may be unable to pump against the increased pressure found in the recipient's pulmonary vasculature.
        iv. Because the RV is a thin-walled chamber, it is compliant and able to accommodate increased amounts of blood volume; however, because the RV consists of only a thin wall of myocardium, it is unable to pump against a high-pressure system.
        v.   RV dysfunction can occur in the setting of a normal PVR.
    c. Ischemic injury; inadequate donor organ preservation
    d. Reperfusion injury
    e. Effects of CPB
    f. Donor-recipient size mismatch (considerably smaller donor heart implanted into larger recipient)
    g. Obstruction at site of pulmonary artery anastomosis
3. Report clinical manifestations of RV dysfunction/failure[75,83,85]:
    a. Hypotension.
    b. Tachycardia.
    c. S_3, S_4 gallop.
    d. Elevated CVP in the setting of decreased LV filling pressures and decreased CO.
    e. Increased RV diastolic pressure.
    f. Decreased CO: RV failure leads to RV dilation, ischemia, decreased contractility, decreased pulmonary blood flow, and shift of the interventricular septum toward the LV. These physiologic changes subsequently result in decreased LV filling and CO.
    g. Echocardiogram findings:
        i.   RV dilatation and hypokinesis
        ii. Shift of interventricular septum toward the LV
4. Intervene as ordered by physician[86,87]
    a. The goals of therapy are to
        i.   Optimize RV preload
        ii. Decrease RV afterload by decreasing PVR
        iii. Decrease pulmonary pressures via pharmacologic management
        iv. Decrease pulmonary vasoconstriction by ventilating with high inspiratory oxygen concentrations and/or increasing tidal volume
        v.   Maintain systemic BP and thus preserve coronary perfusion

b. RV dysfunction may begin in the OR with difficulty weaning from CPB. Potential interventions may include[47,86–88]

    i. Inotropic agents to augment RV function such as isoproterenol (Isuprel), milrinone (Primacor), enoximone (not approved in the United States), dobutamine, and epinephrine.

- In setting of normal or near normal PA pressures, administer/titrate inotropic agents as ordered to support RV contractility; adjust RV preload as needed.
- In setting of systemic hypotension, administer/titrate inotropic agents and optimize RV preload via volume resuscitation.

    ii. Systemic vasodilators with pulmonary vasodilating properties such as nitroglycerine, nesiritide (Natrecor), and sodium nitroprusside may be used in normotensive patients.

- In setting of elevated PA pressures and transpulmonary gradient, administer/titrate vasodilators as ordered.

    iii. Selective pulmonary vasodilators may be used to manage perioperative RV dysfunction such as prostaglandins (prostaglandin E1, prostaglandin I2, or inhaled iloprost), inhaled nitric oxide, and sildenafil (Revatio).

- Action: lowers PVR without affecting SVR
- Administered in setting of persistent, elevated PA pressure ($\geq$45 mm Hg) and severe RV dysfunction

    iv. In the event of ongoing hemodynamic instability despite increased pharmacotherapy, intra-aortic balloon pump (IABP) or other type of MCS may be considered. Temporary ventricular assist devices (VAD) provide RV, LV, and biventricular support but allow for explantation when the patient recovers.

    v. For persistent isolated RV failure, prepare patient for return to OR for implantation of an RV assist device.

- Prepare patient for return to OR if etiology is due to obstruction at site of pulmonary artery anastomosis (see Figure 9-9 for Treatment of Acute RV Dysfunction).

5. Follow-up monitoring: Monitor patient's response to therapy.

    a. Hemodynamic parameters: With effective interventions:

        i. CVP should decrease as RA filling pressure and mean pressure of systemic veins decrease.

        ii. CO should increase as RV contractility improves.

        iii. PVR should decrease with improvement in CO.

        iv. RV end-diastolic pressure should decrease as RV contractility improves.

    b. BP: With effective interventions, systemic hypotension should resolve as LV filling and CO improve.

6. Collaborate with interdisciplinary team: physicians (surgeon, cardiologist, pulmonologist, intensivist), APRN, critical care pharmacist, and OR staff; if patient's condition is critical, social worker and chaplain.

B. Left ventricular systolic dysfunction/failure[54,86,87]

1. Etiology of LV systolic dysfunction/failure

    a. Ischemic injury

    b. Reperfusion injury

    c. Damage to allograft due to trauma

    d. Poor preservation techniques

   e. Primary graft dysfunction
   f. Coronary artery vasculopathy
   g. Cellular or humoral rejection
2. Report clinical manifestations of LV systolic dysfunction/failure:
   a. ↓ CO
   b. ↓ CI (severe LV dysfunction: CI ≤ 2.0 L/min/m²)
   c. ↓ SV
   d. ↑ ventricular diastolic pressure
   e. ↓ EF (severe LV dysfunction: EF ≤ 30% or EF has decreased 25% from posttransplant baseline)
   f. Need for resumption or increased dose of inotropic therapy (severe LV dysfunction)
   g. ↓ tissue perfusion
   h. Renal failure (↑ serum creatinine, ↑ blood urea nitrogen)
   i. Liver failure (↑ bilirubin and liver enzymes)
   j. Evidence of HF: dyspnea, fatigue, orthopnea, and palpitations
3. Intervene as ordered by physician; potential interventions for LV systolic dysfunction/failure include
   a. Administration/titration of agents to augment CO without increasing SVR (e.g., milrinone [Primacor], low-dose dopamine, dobutamine)
   b. Administration/titration of isoproterenol (Isuprel) to increase HR
   c. Atrial pacing
   d. Volume correction to maintain PA diastolic pressure 15 to 20 mm Hg
   e. Preparation of patient for one of the following:
      i. IABP counterpulsation
      ii. ECMO
      iii. Implantation of MCS
4. Monitor patient's response to therapy; with effective interventions:
   a. Hemodynamic parameters
      i. CO, SV, and EF should increase as LV contractility improves.
      ii. LV diastolic pressure should decrease as LV contractility improves and volume status is optimized.
   b. Tissue perfusion should improve as CO increases.
   c. Renal function test results: Elevated blood urea nitrogen (BUN) and creatinine should decrease as CO improves and blood flow to the kidney increases.
   d. Liver function test results: Elevated bilirubin and liver enzymes should decrease as CO improves and blood flow to the liver increases.
5. Collaborate with interdisciplinary team: physicians (surgeon, cardiologist, intensivist), critical care pharmacist, APRN, and OR staff; if patient's condition is critical, social worker and chaplain.

C. Left ventricular diastolic dysfunction/failure[82]
   1. Etiology of LV diastolic dysfunction/failure:
      a. Ischemic injury
      b. Reperfusion injury
      c. Poor preservation techniques
   2. Report clinical manifestations of LV diastolic dysfunction/failure (ventricle becomes stiff)
      a. Elevated left atrial and left ventricular end-diastolic pressures as a consequence of poor LV compliance

b. Pulmonary congestion/edema secondary to elevated left atrial and left ventricular end-diastolic pressures

3. Intervene as ordered by physician: Potential interventions for LV diastolic dysfunction/failure include
   a. Administration/titration of IV nitroglycerine or nitroprusside (to decrease afterload)
   b. Administration of diuretics to decrease preload
   c. Restriction of IV fluids to decreased preload

4. Monitor patient's response to therapy; with effective interventions:
   a. Hemodynamic parameters
      i. LA pressures should decrease as afterload is decreased.
      ii. LV end-diastolic pressure should decrease as afterload is decreased.
   b. Oxygen saturation should improve as pulmonary congestion resolves.

5. Collaborate with interdisciplinary team: physicians (surgeon, cardiologist, intensivist, critical care pharmacist, APRN).

D. Primary Graft Dysfunction (PGD)[86,87]

1. Although PGD (also known as primary graft failure) is not a new process, a definition of PGD is newly emerging. In 2013, an ISHLT consensus conference was commissioned to better define the risk factors and severity of PGD.

2. PGD is a syndrome in which the cardiac allograft fails to meet the circulatory demands of the recipient in the immediate postoperative period thus leading to left, right, or biventricular failure and cardiogenic shock requiring supportive measures.

3. The incidence of PGD is unclear due to inconsistency in diagnosis.

4. A diagnosis of PGD should be entertained only when other forms of acute graft failure have been excluded such as rejection or cardiac tamponade.[86,87] (See Table 9-31.)

5. The etiology of PGD may include
   a. Donor brain death and its effects on the cardiac allograft
   b. Hypothermic ischemic injury
   c. Warm ischemic injury
   d. Reperfusion injury

6. Risk factors for PGD can be categorized by the following[86,87] (see Table 9-32):
   a. Donor risk factors
   b. Recipient risk factors
   c. Procedural risk factors

7. Clinical manifestation of PGD
   a. Echocardiographic evidence of right, left, or biventricular systolic dysfunction
   b. Cardiogenic shock occurring within 24 hrs posttransplantation
   c. Low systolic BP <90 mm Hg
   d. Decrease CO < 2 L/min/m^2
   e. CVP > 15 mm Hg or PCWP > 20 mm Hg despite optimal intracardiac filling pressure
   f. Use of multiple inotropic or vasopressor agents to support heart function

8. Treatment of PGD
   a. Management of cardiogenic shock symptoms.
   b. Inotropic or vasopressor therapy.
   c. Intervene as ordered by physician, titrate inotropes, and prepare patient for IABP or MCS (ECMO, LVAD).

TABLE 9-31 Definition of Primary Graft Dysfunction (PGD)

Ventricle Affected	Degree of PGD	Criteria for Diagnosis
PGD-left ventricle (PGD LV)	Mild PGD-LV	LVEF < 40% or hemodynamics with RAP > 15 mm Hg, PCWP >20 mm Hg, CI < 2.0 L/min, lasting ≥ 1 h requiring inotropes
	Moderate PGD-LV	Must have 1 criteria from both categories for diagnosis: Category I 1. LVEF < 40% 2. Hemodynamic compromise with RAP >15 mm Hg, PCWP > 20 mm Hg, CI < 2 L/min, hypotension = MAP < 70, lasting > 1 h Category II 1. High-dose inotropes 2. IABP use regardless of inotropes
	Severe PGD-LV	Left or biventricular mechanical support: any LVAD, BiVAD, or ECMO, not IABP
PGD-right ventricle (PGD-RV)	No severity score, either present or not	Must meet criteria from categories I and II or III alone for diagnosis: **Category I** 1. Hemodynamic compromise with RAP > 15 mm Hg, PCWP ≤ 15 mm Hg, CI < 2 L/min **Category II** 1. TPG < 15 mm Hg and/or PASP < 50 mm Hg **Category III** 1. Need for RVAD

LVEF, left ventricular ejection fraction; RAP, right atrial pressure; PCWP, pulmonary capillary wedge pressure; CI, cardiac index; MAP, mean arterial pressure; IABP, intra-aortic balloon pump; LVAD, left ventricular assist device; BiVAD, biventricular assist device; ECMO, extracorporeal membrane oxygenator; TPG, transpulmonary gradient; PASP, pulmonary artery systolic pressure; RVAD, right ventricular assist device. Iyer A, Kumarasinghe G, Hicks M, et al. Primary graft failure after heart transplantation. *J Transplant.* 2011;2011:175768; adapted from Kobashigawa J, Zuckermann A, Macdonald P, Leprince P, et al. Report from a consensus conference on primary graft dysfunction after cardiac transplantation. *J Heart Lung Transplant.* 2014;33(4):327–340.

TABLE 9-32 Risk Factors for Primary Graft Dysfunction

Donor Risk Factors	Recipient Risk Factors	Surgical/Procedural Risk Factors
• Age	• Age	• Donor-recipient sex mismatch
• Cause of death	• Weight	• Weight mismatch
• Trauma	• Mechanical support	• Ischemic time
• Cardiac dysfunction	• Congenital heart disease	• Experience of procurement team
• Inotropic support	• Multiple reoperations	• Transplant center volume
• Comorbidities	• LVAD explant	• Cardioplegic solution
– HTN, DM	• Comorbidities	• Blood transfusions required
• Cardiac arrest downtime	– Renal dysfunction, liver dysfunction, diabetes	• Elective vs. emergent transplant
• Substance abuse	• Ventilator dependence	
– Alcohol, cocaine, amphetamines	• Multiorgan transplant	
• Left ventricular hypertrophy	• Elevated PVR	
• Valvular disease	• Infection	
• Hormone therapy	• Retransplant	
• CAD/wall motion abnormalities on echo		
• Sepsis		
• Marginal donor use		
• Troponin trend		
• Hypernatremia		

Iyer A, Kumarasinghe G, Hicks M, et al. Primary graft failure after heart transplantation. *J Transplant.* 2011;2011:175768; adapted from Kobashigawa J, Zuckermann A, Macdonald P, Leprince P, et al. Report from a consensus conference on primary graft dysfunction after cardiac transplantation. *J Heart Lung Transplant.* 2014;33(4):327–340.

d. Urgent listing for retransplantation may be considered if no improvement in ventricular function.

e. Collaborate with interdisciplinary team: physicians (surgeon, cardiologist, intensivist), APRN, OR staff, transplant coordinator (for urgent relisting), social worker, and chaplain (for support to patient's family).

 XIV. MONITOR PATIENT FOR OTHER COMPLICATIONS

A. Bleeding

1. Potential etiology of bleeding:
   a. Preoperative liver dysfunction secondary to HF
   b. Hypothermia induced during surgery
   c. Administration of heparin during CPB
   d. CPB-associated platelet destruction and fibrinolysis
   e. Surgical site tissue trauma

2. Report clinical manifestations of bleeding:
   a. Excessive chest tube drainage (e.g., >100 mL/hour; check hospital protocol)
   b. Decreasing hematocrit and hemoglobin
   c. Tachycardia (HR >110 to 120 bpm)
   d. Low CO and CI (<3.0 L/min/m^2)
   e. Decreasing mixed venous saturation (SvO$_2$ < 65%)
   f. Hypotension (<90 mm Hg systolic)
   g. Increasing O$_2$ requirements
   h. Late signs of bleeding include hypotension and decreasing pulmonary artery and central venous pressures.[63]

3. Intervene as ordered; potential interventions for bleeding may include
   a. Administration of blood products (e.g., packed red blood cells, platelets, fresh frozen plasma)
      i. CMV is carried in the leukocytes that are in red blood cell and platelet transfusions; therefore
         • Platelets should be administered through a leukocyte filter
         • Packed red cells should be leukocyte-reduced if possible and infused via a leukocyte filter.
      ii. CMV-negative recipients should receive CMV-negative blood products.
   b. Administration of plasminogen inhibitors such as aminocaproic acid (Amicar) and factor VII as well as medications such as protamine, desmopressin (DDAVP), or aprotinin (Trasylol)
   c. If needed, preparation of patient for return to the OR for subxiphoid pericardial window or mediastinal reexploration

4. Follow-up monitoring:
   a. Continue to monitor hemoglobin, hematocrit, platelet count, prothrombin time, and partial thromboplastin time to assess the patient's response to therapy.
   b. Monitor patient for signs of cardiac tamponade.

5. Collaborate with interdisciplinary team: physicians (surgeon, cardiologist, intensivist), APRN, blood bank personnel, and OR staff (if needed).

B. Cardiac tamponade

1. Overview[88,89]
   a. Cardiac tamponade is a serious and life-threatening complication that occurs when the accumulation of blood and clots in the pericardial space

is so severe that it compresses the heart and impairs its ability to fill and/ or pump effectively, thereby severely diminishing the CO and causing massive hemodynamic compromise.

b. Can occur with as little as 150 mL of fluid in the pericardial space.

c. May occur suddenly or gradually over time.

d. Without immediate treatment, cardiac tamponade will ultimately lead to cardiac arrest and death.

2. Etiology of cardiac tamponade

a. Trauma (e.g., catheter or bioptome perforation, contusion during cardiopulmonary resuscitation [CPR])

b. Laceration during pericardiocentesis

c. Aortic dissection

d. MI with myocardial rupture

3. Report clinical manifestations of cardiac tamponade: Notify physician immediately as this is a life-threatening complication.

a. Patient's symptoms: shortness of breath, chest or arm pain, unexplained apprehension, or anxiety

b. Marked decrease in chest tube drainage (typically occurs suddenly)

c. Increased CVP or increased JVD on physical exam

d. Increased PCWP

e. Equalizing right- and left-sided heart pressures (RA mean, RV end-diastolic pressure, pulmonary artery (PA) diastolic pressure, PCWP) within 5 mm Hg

f. Decreased CO

g. Decreased CI

h. Hypotension (systolic pressure < 80 mm Hg or MAP < 60 mm Hg)

i. Narrowed pulse pressure

j. Pulsus paradoxus (drop of 10 to 15 mm Hg during inspiration; only valid in nonventilated patients)

k. Decreased MVO_2

l. Compensatory tachycardia (may subsequently progress to bradycardia)

m. Echocardiogram: presence of fluid in pericardial space

n. Chest radiograph: widened mediastinum

o. Distant or muffled heart sounds

p. Weak peripheral pulses

q. Decreased urinary output

r. Altered mental status

s. Inappropriately fluctuating mean arterial pressure

t. Diaphoresis

u. Low-voltage QRS or electrical alternans on electrocardiogram (ECG)

v. Hepatomegaly

w. Cyanosis or pallor[64]

x. Rapid assessment for cardiac tamponade includes this triad of physical findings: hypotension, distended neck veins, and muffled heart sounds

4. Intervene as ordered by physician; potential interventions for cardiac tamponade include

a. Administration of oxygen

b. Volume resuscitation to optimize filling pressures (care should be taken to prevent RV overload)

c. Inotropic support to improve CO

d. Preparation for bedside echocardiogram to confirm diagnosis

e. Preparation of patient for emergent pericardiocentesis

5. Monitor:
   a. Hemodynamic parameters
   b. Vital signs
   c. Oxygen saturation
   d. Patient's response to intervention(s); with effective therapy and improvement in heart's ability to fill and pump effectively:
      i. Patient's symptoms should improve (decreased shortness of breath, chest or arm pain, anxiety).
      ii. Elevated CVP and PCWP should decrease.
      iii. Right- and left-sided heart pressures should normalize.
      iv. CO and CI should increase.
      v. BP should increase.
      vi. Pulse pressure should widen.
      vii. Pulsus paradoxus should resolve.
      viii. MVO_2 should increase.
      ix. Weak peripheral pulses should become stronger.
      x. Chest tube drainage should normalize.
      xi. Urine output should increase.
6. Collaborate with interdisciplinary team: physicians (surgeon, cardiologist, intensivist, radiologist), APRN, echocardiographer, radiology technician, and cardiac catheterization laboratory or OR personnel (for pericardiocentesis).

C. Pericardial effusion[24,41]
   1. Etiology of pericardial effusion
      a. Transplant specific
         i. The recipient's native heart dilates as HF progresses and the pericardium stretches in order to accommodate the enlarging heart.
         ii. During transplantation, a normal-sized heart is placed into the space that was once occupied by an enlarged heart. The "unfilled" space is a potential site of fluid accumulation or effusion.
      b. General
         i. Infection
            - Viruses, for example, adenovirus, enterovirus, influenza, varicella virus
            - Bacteria, for example, streptococci, staphylococci, pneumococci, *Pseudomonas* species, *Mycobacterium tuberculosis*
            - Fungi, for example, *Histoplasma, Aspergillus, Candida*
         ii. Postcardiotomy syndrome
         iii. Chest trauma, for example, pacemaker insertion and fractured ribs secondary to CPR
         iv. Systemic disease, for example, severe hypothyroidism, uremia
   2. Report clinical manifestations of pericardial effusions promptly as large effusions can result in cardiac tamponade.
      a. Clinical manifestations can be subtle until the effusion becomes quite large and begins to cause hemodynamic compromise. At that point, the symptoms can be identical to that of tamponade (see "Cardiac Tamponade"). Pericardial effusions can also be seen on echocardiogram and by chest radiography (enlarging cardiac silhouette).
   3. Intervene as ordered by physician; potential interventions for pericardial effusions may include
      a. Withholding anticoagulants or substitution of heparin for other anticoagulants such as warfarin

  b. Check coagulation parameters
  c. Aspiration of pericardial fluid via pericardial catheter
  d. Pericardiocentesis
  e. Subxiphoid pericardiotomy
  f. Pericardial window
 4. Monitor:
  a. Hemodynamic parameters
  b. Vital signs
  c. Oxygen saturation
  d. Patient's response to intervention(s)
 5. Collaborate with interdisciplinary team: physicians (surgeon, cardiologist, intensivist), APRN, OR or cardiac catheterization lab staff if pericardial window, pericardiotomy, or pericardiocentesis is required).

D. Low cardiac output
 1. Potential etiology of low CO[43]
  a. ↓ HR
  b. Hypovolemia (due to bleeding, diuresis)
  c. Hemorrhage
  d. Fluid shift (third spacing)
  e. Elevated SVR (due to hypothermia, circulating catecholamines, hypovolemia)
  f. Graft failure (see sections on Left and Right Ventricular Dysfunction as well as PGD)
  g. Cardiac tamponade (see "Cardiac Tamponade")
  h. Dysrhythmias
  i. Rejection
 2. Report clinical manifestations associated with low CO.[42,89]
  a. Cardiovascular
   i. Hemodynamic changes: decreased BP; increased HR
   ii. Dysrhythmias
   iii. Decreased peripheral pulses
   iv. Jugular venous distention
   v. Cyanosis
   vi. Pallor
   vii. Cold, clammy skin
   viii. Slow capillary refill
  b. Renal
   i. ↑ serum creatinine level
   ii. ↑ BUN
   iii. Oliguria (typically <0.5 mL/kg/hr)
   iv. Anuria
  c. Respiratory
   i. Dyspnea
   ii. Crackles
   iii. Shortness of breath
   iv. Tachypnea
   v. Metabolic acidosis
  d. Neurologic
   i. Mental status changes (decreased mentation, confusion, agitation, etc.)
   ii. Loss of consciousness

3. Intervene as ordered by physician; depending on cause, potential interventions for low CO may include[56]
   a. Atrial or AV sequential pacing to achieve an adequate HR
   b. Volume infusion to increase PCWP to 15 to 20 mm Hg with SVR between 1,000 and 1,400 dynes/s/cm^5
   c. Blood products
   d. Vasopressors or vasodilators (depending on SVR)
   e. Increased dose of inotropes if CI is <2 L/min/m^2
   f. Agents to treat rejection
   g. IABP or other type of MCS for graft failure
4. Monitor response to intervention(s):
   a. Hemodynamic status: CO, PAWP, SVR, HR/rhythm, BP
   b. Perfusion status: skin temperature, capillary refill, presence of cyanosis or pallor
   c. Fluid status: intake and output; weight
   d. Respiratory status (pulse oximetry, breath sounds, respirations)
   e. Neurologic status
   f. Perfusion
5. Collaborate with interdisciplinary team: physicians (surgeon, cardiologist, neurologist, nephrologist, pulmonologist), APRN, social worker, chaplain (if patient's condition is critical).

E. Alterations in blood pressure
   1. Hypertension
      a. Hypertension is a fairly common complication after transplantation with a cumulative prevalence of 94% and 97% within 5 and 8 years posttransplant, respectively.[42,76]
      b. Pathophysiology
         i. Early postoperative period: Hypertension increases myocardial oxygen demand and increases the risk of postoperative bleeding.
         ii. Hypertension is a known risk factor for the development of CAV.
      c. Potential etiology of hypertension:
         i. Side effect of immunosuppressant medications (particularly corticosteroids and calcineurin inhibitor therapy)
         ii. Renal dysfunction
         iii. Pain
         iv. Anxiety
         v. Intracranial event (sedated and intubated patient)
      d. Report clinical manifestations of hypertension (note: hypertension may be asymptomatic)
         i. Headache
         ii. Visual disturbances
         iii. Nausea, vomiting
         iv. Seizures: Recipients who had been hypotensive prior to transplantation may be at risk for seizures posttransplant, even though they are normotensive or slightly hypertensive. Recipients who complain of a headache and have a systolic BP >140 mm Hg in the first weeks posttransplant require immediate antihypertensive therapy.
      e. Intervene as ordered by physician
         i. Early postoperative period:
            • Warming lights or blankets.

- IV antihypertensive agents (e.g., sodium nitroprusside, nitroglycerine) (see "Response of Denervated Cardiac Allograft to Medications").
- Sedation, analgesia.
- Optimize ventilation and oxygenation.

    ii. Long-term management:
- May require multidrug therapy consisting of a combination of calcium channel blockers, ACE inhibitors, alpha-2 adrenergic agonists, and ARBs.
- Persistent hypertension may require a change in immunosuppressant medications or management with multiple antihypertensive agents.

  f. Monitor
    i. BP
    ii. Hemodynamic parameters
    iii. Serum immunosuppressant levels
    iv. Renal function tests
    v. Patient's response to therapy
  g. Collaborate with interdisciplinary colleagues: physicians (surgeon, cardiologist, intensivist, nephrologist, etc.), APRN, and transplant pharmacist.

2. Hypotension
  a. Hypotension in the early postoperative phase decreases end-organ perfusion and places the recipient at risk of end-organ damage.
  b. Potential etiology of hypotension
    i. Decreased myocardial contractility due to
- Myocardial ischemia
- Allograft rejection
- Other causes such as acidosis

    ii. Cardiac tamponade
    iii. Dysrhythmias
    iv. ↓ SVR (due to sepsis, transfusion reaction, drug reaction, etc.)
    v. Pneumothorax
    vi. Pulmonary embolus
    vii. Bleeding
    viii. Hypovolemia (see section on Hypovolemia)
    ix. Excessive use of diuretics
    x. Impaired metabolism of antihypertensive medications
  c. Report clinical manifestations of hypotension (vary with etiology)
    i. Low BP (systolic pressure ≤80 to 90 mm Hg)
    ii. Light-headedness, dizziness
    iii. Weakness
    iv. Syncope
    v. Blurred vision
    vi. Mental status changes
  d. Intervene as ordered by physician; potential interventions depend on the etiology and severity of the hypotension and may include
    i. Placement of patient in Trendelenburg position
    ii. Administration of oxygen
    iii. IV fluid bolus
    iv. Administration of dopamine or increase in dopamine dose to obtain pressor effect (15 to 20 µg/kg/min)

        v. Administration of vasopressors such as norepinephrine and vasopressin may be required to maintain MAP > 65 mm Hg.[63]

        vi. Optimize preload, afterload, contractility (see "Response of Denervated Cardiac Allograft to Medications").

        vii. Treatment of primary cause.

   e. Monitor:

        i. BP

        ii. Hemodynamic parameters

        iii. Patient's mental status

        iv. Patient's response to therapy

   f. Collaborate with interdisciplinary team members: physicians (surgeon, cardiologist, intensivist), APRN, transplant pharmacist.

F. **Disturbances of cardiac rate and/or rhythm**

  1. Sinus node dysfunction[64,88]

   a. 25% to 50% of recipients have sinus node dysfunction.

   b. Etiology of sinus node dysfunction

        i. Surgical trauma to the SA node

        ii. Inadequate myocardial preservation

        iii. Cardiac denervation

        iv. Sinus node dysfunction in donor heart

        v. Ischemia

        vi. Sinoatrial nodal artery trauma

        vii. Perinodal atrial tissue injury

        viii. Pretransplant use of amiodarone

        ix. Sinus bradycardia (<70 to 80 bpm) has been linked to prolonged ischemic time, direct injury to the SA node, and preoperative use of amiodarone.[88]

        x. Junctional bradycardia

        xi. Bradycardia occurring early after surgery has minimal prognostic significance, but late-onset bradycardia could be an indication of allograft rejection or vasculopathy.[47]

   c. Report clinical manifestations of sinus node dysfunction.[86]

   d. Intervene as ordered by physician; potential interventions for sinus node dysfunction include

        i. Preparation of patient for pacing via epicardial wires that were placed during surgery

        ii. Administration/titration of isoproterenol (Isuprel) if pacing wires are nonfunctional

        iii. If bradycardia persists (>4 to 5 days), administration of aminophylline, theophylline (Theo-Dur), or terbutaline (Brethine) to increase HR

        iv. Preparation of patient for implantation of a temporary or permanent pacemaker (dual chamber) in the setting of persistent symptomatic bradycardia associated with decreased CO, persistent junctional escape rhythms, or persistent sinus bradycardia

   e. Monitor:

        i. ECG

        ii. HR

        iii. Patient's response to therapy

   f. Collaborate with interdisciplinary team: physicians (surgeon, cardiologist, intensivist, electrophysiologist), APRN, and electrophysiology lab staff (if pacemaker is required).

2. Atrial dysrhythmias
   a. Transient, asymptomatic atrial dysrhythmias are fairly common, occurring in approximately 25% of recipients while hospitalized.
   b. Etiology of atrial dysrhythmias
      i.   Rejection (particularly atrial fibrillation and flutter)
      ii. Electrolyte imbalances (hypokalemia and hypomagnesemia)
      iii. Preoperative use of amiodarone
      iv. Biatrial surgical technique (bicaval is most common technique used today)
   c. Report clinical manifestations of atrial dysrhythmias
      i.   Premature atrial complexes (most common type of atrial dysrhythmias)
      ii. Atrial flutter
      iii. Atrial tachycardia
      iv. Atrial fibrillation
   d. Intervene as ordered by physician; potential interventions for atrial dysrhythmias include
      i.   Administration of antirejection agents if dysrhythmias are due to rejection.
      ii. Atrial pacing (especially for atrial flutter).
      iii. Administration of electrolyte replacements where necessary; consider other possible causes of atrial dysrhythmias.
      iv. Administration of beta-blockers or calcium channel blockers with caution
      v.   *Note:* Digoxin is not used to treat atrial dysrhythmias because its effects are vagally mediated; therefore, it has no effect on the denervated SA or AV nodes[22]
      vi. Preparation of patient for cardioversion if atrial dysrhythmias do not respond to pharmacologic therapy or if they lead to hemodynamic instability
   e. Monitor:
      i.   ECG
      ii. HR and rhythm
      iii. Patient's response to therapy
   f. Collaborate with interdisciplinary team: physician (surgeon, cardiologist, electrophysiologist), APRN, and electrophysiology or cardiac catheterization lab staff (if cardioversion is required).
3. Ventricular dysrhythmias[88]
   a. Potential etiology of ventricular dysrhythmias:
      i.   Electrolyte imbalances (hypokalemia or hypomagnesemia)
      ii. Rejection
      iii. Increased sensitivity of the heart to catecholamines and inotropes
      iv. Reperfusion injury
      v.   Prolonged ischemic time
      vi. Manipulation of donor heart
   b. Report clinical manifestations of ventricular dysrhythmias:
      i.   Premature ventricular complexes
      ii. Ventricular tachycardia (rare)
      iii. Ventricular fibrillation (rare)
   c. Intervene as ordered by physician; potential interventions for ventricular dysrhythmias include
      i.   Administration of intravenous lidocaine or amiodarone

        ii.   Electrolyte replacement therapy

        iii. Advanced cardiac life support for malignant dysrhythmias

   d. Monitor:

        i.   ECG

        ii.   Serum electrolytes

        iii. Patient's response to intervention(s)

   e. Collaborate with interdisciplinary team: physicians (surgeon, cardiologist, intensivist, electrophysiologist), APRN, transplant pharmacist.

G. Fluid imbalance

  1. Hypovolemia: fluid volume deficit and loss of isotonic fluid and solutes from extracellular space[88]

   a. Potential etiology of hypovolemia:

        i.   Effects of CPB (movement of fluid into interstitial space; increased capillary permeability)

        ii.   Administration of diuretics during or after surgical procedure

        iii. Increase in intravascular space during rewarming

        iv. Excessive urine output

        v.   Excessive bleeding or drainage

        vi. Diabetes mellitus (DM)

        vii. Vomiting, diarrhea

        viii. GI tube drainage

        ix. Third space fluid shifts

   b. Report clinical manifestations of hypovolemia (Box 9-3).[17,90]

   c. Intervene as ordered by physician; potential interventions for hypovolemia include

        i.   Insuring that patient has a central line and/or two patent, large-bore IV lines available

        ii.   Administration of fluids to expand circulating volume and replace urine output with volume

             • Crystalloids (e.g., normal saline)

             • Colloids (e.g., albumin, Hespan)

             • Electrolyte solutions (e.g., PlasmaLyte)

        iii. Replacement of electrolytes

        iv. Oxygen therapy to enhance tissue perfusion

        v.   Administration of vasopressors

        vi. Meticulous skin care to prevent breakdown

   d. Monitor patient's response to interventions.

        i.   Vital signs at least hourly; more often if indicated

        ii.   Hemodynamic parameters (MAP, CVP, PCWP) to assess patient's response to therapy

        iii. Lab tests, for example:

             • Hematocrit: should decrease as hypovolemia is reversed.

             • Electrolytes: should normalize with the administration of electrolyte solution and as diarrhea, vomiting, excessive urine loss resolve.

             • BUN: should decrease as hypovolemia is reversed.

        iv. Intake and output (hourly or per protocol)

        v.   Weight (daily)

        vi. Mental status; changes in level of consciousness

        vii. Skin: color, turgor, temperature

        viii. Patient's response to sedatives and narcotic pain medications

---

BOX 9-3   Manifestations of Hypovolemia[17,90]

Hypotension or labile blood pressure
Tachypnea
↓ CI
↓ PAP/CVP
↑ HR; weak pulse
↓ urine output
↑ hematocrit
Increasing serum BUN/creatinine levels
↑ serum sodium levels
↑ urine specific gravity
Subnormal body temperature (unless there is a concurrent infectious process)
Poor skin turgor
Pallor
Dry skin and mucous membranes
Flat jugular veins
Weakness
Mental status changes (restlessness, anxiety, irritability, ↓ level of consciousness)
Exaggerated response (hypotension) to sedatives or narcotic pain medication
Weight loss
Thirst
Delayed capillary refill
Cool, pale skin over arms and legs
Negative intake and output balance (output > intake)
Postural hypotension (drop in systolic blood pressure >15 mm Hg or increase in heart rate >15 bpm when patient changes from supine to upright position)
Hypovolemic shock:
Low CVP (<5 to 10 cm H_2O)
Low PCWP (<6 to 12 mm Hg)
Low PAP (<10 to 20 mm Hg)
Low CO (< 4 to 8 L/min)
High SVR

BUN, blood urea nitrogen; CI, cardiac index; CVP, central venous pressure; HR, heart rate; PAP, pulmonary artery pressure; PCWP, pulmonary capillary wedge pressure; SVR, systemic vascular resistance.

---

ix. Clinical manifestations of volume overload and pulmonary edema (crackles, increased oxygen requirements) (see section on Hypervolemia).

e. Collaborate with interdisciplinary team: physicians (surgeon, cardiologist), APRN, dietitian, physical therapist, wound care nurse, ancillary nursing staff.

2. Hypervolemia: Excess of isotonic fluid (water and sodium) in extracellular (interstitial or intravascular) compartment[90]

a. Potential etiology of hypervolemia:

i. Fluid accumulation secondary to CPB

ii. Administration of IV fluids: Normal saline or lactated Ringer's solution; fluids used to administer medications or perform monitoring procedures (e.g., CO)

iii. Renal dysfunction

    iv.   Excessive oral fluid intake

    v.   High intake of dietary sodium

    vi.   Blood or plasma replacement

    vii.   Fluid or sodium retention secondary to HF, liver failure, nephrotic syndrome, corticosteroid therapy, low dietary protein intake

    viii.   Use of plasma proteins (e.g., albumin)

  b. Report clinical manifestations of hypervolemia (Box 9-4).[17,90]

  c. Intervene as ordered by physician; potential interventions for hypervolemia include

    i.   Administration of diuretics

    ii.   Restriction of fluid and sodium intake

    iii.   Administration of oxygen

    iv.   Good skin care to prevent breakdown of edematous areas

    v.   If pulmonary edema develops, administration of medications to dilate blood vessels (e.g., nitroglycerine, morphine), aggressive diuresis, and bilevel positive airway pressure (BiPAP)

    vi.   Hemodialysis

    vii.   Continuous renal replacement therapy for hemodynamically unstable patients

  d. Follow-up monitoring

    i.   Volume status and filling pressures (CVP, PCWP, and other hemodynamic parameters)

BOX 9-4   Manifestations of Hypervolemia[17,90]

↑ CVP

↑ PAP

↑ PCWP

Hypertension

Dependent edema (legs and feet when patient is standing; sacrum and buttocks when patient is lying down)

Anasarca (severe generalized edema)

Distended veins in neck and hands

Rapid, bounding pulse

S_3 gallop (in heart failure)

Pulmonary edema: crackles, shortness of breath, tachypnea, frequent frothy (pink) sputum, cough

Pulmonary congestion on chest radiograph

Dyspnea

Ascites

Weakness

Weight gain

Mental status changes

Intake exceeds output

Lab values:

↓ hematocrit (secondary to hemodilution)

↓ or normal serum sodium

↓ serum osmolality

↑ BNP

BUN, blood urea nitrogen; CO, cardiac output; CVP, central venous pressure; PAP, pulmonary artery pressure; PCWP, pulmonary capillary wedge pressure; BNP, B-type natriuretic peptide.

ii.   Respiratory rate and pattern
iii. Neck vein distention
iv.   Heart sounds
v.   Breath sounds (presence of crackles or rhonchi)
vi.   Arterial blood gases
vii. Weight (daily trends)
viii. Intake and output (hourly or per protocol)
ix.   Lab results: for example, with diuretic therapy
- Potassium may decrease.
- Hematocrit may increase.
x.   Clinical manifestations of hypovolemia (see section on Hypovolemia)
e. Collaborate with interdisciplinary team: physicians (surgeon, cardiologist nephrologist), APRN, transplant pharmacist, dietitian, physical therapist, ancillary nursing staff.

H. Electrolyte imbalance
1. Potential etiology:
a. Intra- and postoperative IV fluid administration
b. Renal dysfunction; decreased excretion of electrolytes
c. Inadequate intake or supplementation of electrolytes through IV solutions, diet, enteral feedings, total parenteral nutrition
d. Increased or decreased absorption of electrolytes in GI tract
e. Excessive loss of electrolytes through vomiting, diarrhea, gastric suctioning, severe diaphoresis, wound drainage
f. Excessive intake of electrolytes
g. Adverse effects of medications (e.g., antibiotics, diuretics, corticosteroids)
h. Infection
i. Rhabdomyolysis
j. Insulin deficiency
k. Acid-base imbalances
l. Lack of vitamins that promote absorption of electrolytes
m. Comorbidities (e.g., hypoalbuminemia, hyperparathyroidism)
2. Monitor:
a. Serum electrolytes
b. Associated lab tests
c. Patient's response to intervention(s)
3. Collaborate with interdisciplinary team: physicians (surgeon, cardiologist, intensivist, nephrologist, gastroenterologist, endocrinologist), APRN, dietitian, transplant pharmacist.

I. Disorders of glucose metabolism
1. Hyperglycemia (fasting blood glucose level ≥ 126 mg/dL or ≥ 6.9 μmol/L)
a. Potential etiology of hyperglycemia
i. Preexisting DM
- Insulin dependent
- Noninsulin dependent
ii. Side effects of medications such as corticosteroids and tacrolimus
b. Clinical manifestations of hyperglycemia (Table 9-33)
c. Intervene as ordered by physician:
i. Serum blood glucose monitoring
ii. Capillary blood glucose monitoring

TABLE 9-33 Manifestations of Hyperglycemia

Clinical Manifestation	Pathophysiology
Glycosuria	Amount of glucose molecules filtered by kidney exceeds amount of glucose that can be reabsorbed by renal tubules
Polyuria	Osmotic diuresis
Polydipsia	Intracellular dehydration as blood glucose levels ↑ and water is pulled out of cells, particularly those in thirst center
Polyphagia	In IDDM: cellular starvation and ↓ in carbohydrate, fat, and protein stores
Weight loss (particularly in IDDM)	Loss of fluid secondary to osmotic diuresis Loss of body tissue as body uses fat and protein stores for energy
Obesity (particularly in uncomplicated NIDDM)	Altered metabolism
Recurrent blurred vision	Exposure of lens and retina to hyperosmolar fluid
Weakness, fatigue	Lowered plasma volume
Paresthesias	Dysfunction of peripheral sensory nerves
Skin infections	Growth of yeast organisms

IDDM, insulin-dependent diabetes mellitus; NIDDM, non–insulin-dependent diabetes mellitus.

  iii. Administration of insulin (subcutaneous or IV insulin drip)
  iv. Oral hypoglycemic agents
  v. American Diabetic Association diet
  vi. Diabetes education for patient and family
 d. Monitor patient's response to interventions.
  i. Serum and capillary blood glucose level
  ii. Hemoglobin A_{1C}
  iii. Patient's and family's knowledge of diabetes
 e. Collaborate with interdisciplinary team: physicians (surgeon, cardiologist, intensivist, endocrinologist), APRN, dietitian, ancillary nursing staff, diabetes educator, home health care nurse.
2. Hypoglycemia (serum glucose level ≤50 mg/dL or ≤2.77 µmol/L)
 a. Potential etiology of hypoglycemia
  i. Insulin dose that exceeds patient's metabolic requirements
  ii. Oral hypoglycemic agents
  iii. Insufficient caloric intake
  iv. Strenuous activity or increased exercise that is not accompanied by appropriate increase in food intake or decrease in insulin dose
  v. Factors that potentiate the action of hypoglycemic medications:
   • Renal insufficiency
   • Medications (e.g., sulfonamides)
  vi. Weight loss
  vii. Decrease in corticosteroid dose
  viii. Comorbidities (e.g., liver disease)
 b. Report clinical manifestations of hypoglycemia (Table 9-34)
 c. Intervene as ordered by physician; potential interventions include
  i. Administration of oral or IV glucose
  ii. Discontinuation of IV insulin
  iii. Decrease in dose of insulin or oral hypoglycemic agent

TABLE 9-34 **Manifestations of Hypoglycemia**

Clinical Manifestation	Pathophysiology

Impaired cerebral function:
  Headache
  Slurred speech
  Motor dysfunction
  Impaired problem solving
  Feeling of vagueness
  Change in emotional behavior
  Convulsions
  Coma
	Results from ↓ availability of glucose for brain metabolism

Parasympathetic nervous system:
  Hunger
  Nausea
  Hypotension
  Bradycardia
	Compensatory changes due to activation of autonomic nervous system

Sympathetic nervous system:
  Anxiety, irritability
  Diaphoresis
  Cool, pale skin
  Tachycardia	

      d. Monitor

         i. Serum glucose level (keep between 80 and 110 mg/dL or 4.44 and 6.1 µmol/L)

         ii. Capillary glucose levels

         iii. Patient's mental status

         iv. Patient's response to intervention(s)

      e. Collaborate with interdisciplinary team: physicians (surgeon, cardiologist, endocrinologist), APRN, diabetes educator, dietitian, home health care nurse.

  J. Renal dysfunction

    1. Potential etiology of renal dysfunction:

      a. Preoperative factors: HF (cardiorenal syndrome), prolonged diuretic therapy, decreased perfusion[91]

      b. Intraoperative factors: abnormal renal perfusion with CPB

      c. Postoperative factors: low CO, nephrotoxic effects of immunosuppressive agents, particularly calcineurin inhibitors[43]

    2. Report clinical manifestations of renal dysfunction.

      a. Oliguria (typically <0.5 mL/kg/hr)

      b. Anuria

      c. Elevated serum creatinine level

    3. Intervene as ordered by physician; potential interventions for renal dysfunction include[41–44]

      a. Placement of Foley catheter to urimeter with gravity drainage.

      b. Administration of low-dose dopamine (2 to 3 µg/kg/min) to increase renal blood flow.

    c. Administration of medications to maintain MAP between 60 and 80 mm Hg (e.g., epinephrine, vasopressin, inotropes).

    d. Cautious volume administration if oliguria occurs early after transplantation (urine output < approximately 50 mL/h).

       i. Maintain CVP 5 to 12 mm Hg to ensure adequate hemodynamics without causing RV overload.

    e. Optimizing CO.

    f. Administration of loop diuretics by intermittent IV bolus or continuous IV infusion to prevent volume overload.

       i. If BUN and/or serum creatinine are elevated, it is important to maintain intravascular volume.

       ii. Colloid replacement is preferred in the first 24 h post–heart transplantation for optimal fluid management.

    g. Delaying initiation of calcineurin inhibitor therapy in setting of oliguria and rising serum creatinine level.

       i. If renal function fails to improve within 48 hours, or renal dysfunction was noted prior to transplant, other cytolytic therapy may be initiated (see induction therapy).

    h. Decreasing immunosuppressive dose.

    i. Changing immunosuppressive medications.

    j. Avoiding other nephrotoxic drugs, especially antibiotics.

    k. Hemodialysis should be considered early if recipient is anuric and oliguric or has a sharp increase in creatinine within 2 to 4 hrs postoperatively to allow for better volume management.

    l. In setting of ongoing elevated RAP > 20 mm Hg despite adequate pharmacologic therapy, ultrafiltration should be considered.

  4. Follow-up monitoring:

    a. Urine output per ICU protocol (e.g., hourly)

       i. As with other types of cardiac surgery patients, a urine output of at least 1 mL/kg/h is generally an indication of adequate CO, blood volume, and peripheral perfusion.

    b. Renal function (serum creatinine, BUN)

    c. Serum electrolytes

    d. Hemodynamic parameters

    e. Serum immunosuppressant levels

  5. Collaborate with interdisciplinary team members: physicians (surgeon, cardiologist, nephrologist), APRN, and critical care pharmacist.

K. Pleural effusions

  1. Potential etiology of pleural effusions[24]

    a. Postoperative bleeding into pleural space

    b. Increased hydrostatic pressure associated with a positive fluid balance

    c. Increased vascular permeability associated with certain infections such as pneumonia

    d. Decreased osmotic pressure associated with a low-protein state

    e. Increased intrapleural negative pressure associated with atelectasis

  2. Report clinical manifestations of pleural effusions.

    a. Patients with pleural effusions may not become symptomatic until the effusion becomes quite large.

    b. Clinical manifestations vary with the cause of the effusion and may be vague.

       i. Infection: fever and signs of inflammation

       ii. Shortness of breath due to decrease in lung volume on affected side

      iii.   Tachypnea

      iv.   Diminished breath sounds

      v.   Percussion: dullness or flatness

      vi.   Pleuritic pain (associated with inflammatory process)

      vii.   Visualization of effusion on chest radiograph (typically observed when there is an accumulation of 250 mL or more of fluid)

      viii.   Mediastinal shift toward contralateral side (with large, acute effusion)

3. Intervene as ordered by physician.

    a. Definitive therapy is directed to the cause of effusion.

    b. Potential interventions include

      i.   Preparation of patient for thoracentesis (for diagnostic and therapeutic purposes)

      ii.   Administration of antimicrobial agents if infection is the cause of the effusion

L. **Infection: General**

1. Immunosuppression places transplant recipients at risk for

    a. Nosocomial infections (particularly at surgical incisions and sites of vascular lines and percutaneous tubes)

    b. Emergence of latent endogenous infections

    c. Infections transmitted via allograft or blood products

    d. Opportunistic infections

    e. Community-acquired infections

2. Incidence of infection

    a. Non-CMV infections account for 13% of deaths in the first 30 days after heart transplantation. The incidence of fatal non-CMV infection increases to 33% within 2 to 12 months posttransplantation.

    b. Approximately 25% of patients have one or more major infections during the first 2 posttransplant months.

    c. Bacterial infections are the most frequently occurring type of infection during the transplant hospitalization; the peak risk is during first postoperative week.

    d. During the immediate postoperative period, the lung is the most common site of infection and the pulmonary infection is typically bacteria.

3. Prevention of infection

    a. Implement neutropenic protocol per physician's order.

      i.   For neutropenic patient, limit room traffic and place a visitor restriction sign on the door.

    b. Maintain protective isolation status per hospital policy.

      i.   Protocols differ widely among transplant centers.

      ii.   Most centers place patients in an ICU room that has been specially cleaned, observe strict hand-washing technique, and use gloves; some centers use complete reverse isolation.

      iii.   Proper hand-washing technique is the single most important and successful intervention aimed at decreasing the incidence of nosocomial infections.

    c. Administer appropriate blood products based on CMV serostatus as ordered by physician.

      i.   Leukocyte-poor blood products

      ii.   CMV-negative blood for CMV-negative recipient

    d. Strictly adhere to hospital protocol regarding care of indwelling lines and catheters, for example:

       i. Changing vascular access monitoring line dressings per protocol

       ii. Changing IV tubing, transducers, and flush solutions per protocol

       iii. Removing Foley catheter within 24 hours, if possible (per physician's order)

       iv. Discontinuing all drains, arterial lines, and large-caliber central venous lines within 3 to 4 days, if possible (per physician's order)

    e. Administer antimicrobial agents per protocol; examples of prophylactic antimicrobial agents include[46]

       i. Ganciclovir (Cytovene)/valganciclovir (Valcyte) for CMV-negative recipients who receive an allograft from a CMV-positive donor

       ii. Sulfamethoxazole/trimethoprim (Bactrim) for prophylaxis against Pneumocystis

       iii. Nystatin (Mycostatin) for prophylaxis against *Candida* infections

    f. Extubate as soon as possible (per physician's order).

    g. Maintain meticulous pulmonary toilet (frequent coughing, deep breathing, turning, chest physiotherapy).

    h. Facilitate mobility per physician's order.

       i. Get patient out of bed to chair on first postoperative day or as soon as possible.

       ii. Ambulate patient as soon as possible.

       iii. Increase ambulation as tolerated by patient.

    i. Instruct family members and other visitors in infection control techniques, particularly hand-washing.

  4. Recognize and report clinical manifestations of infection.[51,52]

    a. General (Box 9-5)

    b. Site specific (Table 9-35)

    c. It is important to note that the anti-inflammatory effects of steroid therapy may

       i. Blunt the patient's ability to produce pyrogens. As a consequence, the recipient's body temperature may be lower than would be expected.

         • Even small increases in body temperature should be noted and reported.

BOX 9-5   General Manifestations of Infection[50,51]

Fever (38°C/100.4°F)

Tachycardia

Tachypnea

Hypotension

↑ CO/CI

↓ SVR

↑ oxygen requirements

Chills

Leukocytosis

C-reactive protein (positive)

↑ sedimentation rate

CO, cardiac output; CI, cardiac index; SVR, systemic vascular resistance.

TABLE 9-35 **Site-Specific Manifestations of Infection**

Site	Example of Clinical Manifestations
Ear, nose, throat	Sinus drainage, rhinitis, cough, sneezing, ear ache, pruritus, fever, thrush, mouth sores, lesions, dental caries, swollen lymph glands
Respiratory tract	Cough, wheezing, change in color and quantity of sputum, shortness of breath
Gastrointestinal tract	Diarrhea, nausea, vomiting, abdominal pain, bleeding, loss of appetite
Urinary tract	Frequency, burning, urgency, dysuria, flank pain, cloudy urine, urine with foul odor
Skin	Purulent drainage from any surgical or line site; erythema; lesions, rash, pruritus, foot ulcers
Neurologic system	Mental status changes, neck pain, headache
Musculoskeletal system	Joint pain, muscle aches, fever

      ii. Mask symptoms of infection (e.g., urinary tract infections may be asymptomatic).

  5. Anticipate physician's order for cultures for evidence of infection—particularly in response to a fever; obtain samples and test results in a timely manner.

    a. A thorough fever workup (e.g., pan cultures [culture of blood, urine, sputum], urinalysis, CBC count with differential, etc.) should be initiated for temperature $\geq 38\,^{\circ}C$ ($\geq 100.4\,^{\circ}F$).

  6. Intervene as ordered by the physician; potential interventions include

    a. Administration of antimicrobial therapy

    b. Preparation of patient for additional diagnostic tests (e.g., chest radiograph, CT scan, bronchoscopy with bronchoalveolar lavage)

    c. Preparation of patient for surgical exploration/debridement (e.g., for mediastinitis)

  7. Monitor patient's response to therapy; depending on site and nature (local vs. systemic) of infection, with effective therapy:

    a. Test results should return to normal (e.g., CBC count, cultures, chest radiograph, CT scan).

    b. Hemodynamic parameters

      i. Elevated CO/CI should decrease.

      ii. Decreased SVR should increase.

    c. Vital signs, for example, body temperature should return to normal.

    d. Oxygen requirements; with effective therapy, oxygen requirements should decrease.

    e. Surgical incisions, drainage, and access lines: for example, drainage should decrease.

    f. Pain should decrease.

    g. Patient's mental status should improve.

  8. Collaborate with interdisciplinary team members: physicians (surgeon, cardiologist, infectious disease specialist), APRN, wound care nurse, transplant pharmacologist, and home health care nurse (e.g., if postdischarge IV antibiotics and wound monitoring are required).

  9. See chapter on Infectious Diseases for additional information.

M. Wound infection

  1. Types

    a. Suprasternal soft tissue infection

       i.   Treatment options: antibiotic therapy, wound care, drainage, and debridement

   b. Deep wound infection that causes mediastinitis

2. Mediastinitis[64]

   a. Incidence: <5%

   b. Etiology of mediastinitis:

       i.   Colonization of recipient

       ii. Less common: microbial colonization from donor

   c. Potential causative organisms

       i.   Most common: Gram-positive bacteria (*Staphylococcus aureus*, coagulase-negative *S. aureus*)

       ii. Gram-negative bacteria

       iii. Fungal pathogens: *Aspergillus fumigatus* and *Candida* spp.

   d. Report clinical manifestations of mediastinitis.

       i.   Purulent wound drainage

       ii. Mobile sternal fragments

       iii. Wound edge separation

       iv. Sternal pain or tenderness

       v. Fever

       vi. Leukocytosis

       vii. Erythema

       viii. Increasing wound drainage

   e. Treatment options (based on severity of infection)

       i.   Antimicrobial agents

       ii. Wound drainage

       iii. Surgical debridement

       iv. Tissue flap wound closure

   f. Monitor patient's response to therapy; with effective therapy:

       i.   Test results should normalize, for example:

          • White blood cell count should decrease.

          • Cultures should be negative.

       ii. Temperature should normalize.

       iii. At site of wound infection:

          • Drainage and redness should decrease.

          • Drainage should become less purulent.

          • Sternal mobility should decrease.

          • Wound edges should begin to approximate.

          • Pain or tenderness should decrease.

   g. Collaborate with interdisciplinary team members: physicians (surgeon, cardiologist, infectious disease specialist, plastic surgeon), APRN, wound care nurse, transplant pharmacologist, and home health care nurse (e.g., if postdischarge intravenous antibiotics and wound monitoring are required).

N. Impaired wound healing

1. Potential etiology of impaired wound healing:

   a. Corticosteroid therapy

       i.   Decreases collagen content in dermis; as a result, skin becomes thin and easily damaged and wound healing is impaired.

       ii. Increases risk of infection.

   b. Use of proliferation inhibitors (e.g., sirolimus [Rapamune])

      c. Poor nutritional status

      d. Poor blood glucose control

  2. Report clinical manifestations of impaired wound healing at any incisional or cannulation site.

      a. Purulent drainage and excessive drainage

      b. Wound edge separation

      c. Erythema

      d. Swelling

      e. Necrosis

      f. Dehiscence

  3. Intervene as ordered by physician; potential interventions for impaired wound healing may include

      a. Meticulous sterile wound care; dressing changes per protocol

      b. Enzymatic debridement

      c. Medications

         i. Antimicrobial therapy

        ii. Medications to improve blood glucose control

       iii. Changing immunosuppressant therapy (i.e., proliferation signal inhibitor therapy) is often avoided early posttransplant due to increased risk of wound infection.

      d. Dietary changes to enhance nutritional status

      e. Return to OR for surgical debridement

  4. Monitor patient's response to interventions.

      a. Incisions, IV access, and cannulation sites

         i. Drainage, wound edges, swelling, and erythema

      b. Serum glucose level

      c. Nutritional status (prealbumin, calorie counts)

  5. Collaborate with interdisciplinary team: physicians (surgeon, cardiologist, intensivist, plastic surgery specialist, infectious disease specialist, endocrinologist), APRN, wound care nurse, dietitian, physical therapist, and home health care nurse.

O. Neurologic complications

  1. Etiology of neurologic dysfunction

      a. Ischemic stroke

         i. The manipulation of the diseased native heart along with the cannulation, clamping, and unclamping of the aorta may dislodge material such as thrombus and atheromatous plaque that has the potential to embolize to the brain.[48]

      b. Cerebral emboli from dilated LV with thrombus

      c. Low CO with hypotension and watershed infarction

      d. Encephalopathy secondary to

         i. Operative or postoperative global hypoxic-ischemic insult (within first 48 hours)

        ii. Metabolic abnormalities (within first 48 hours)

       iii. Calcineurin inhibitor (cyclosporine or tacrolimus) toxicity (headache, depression, obtundation, cortical blindness)

       iv. High-dose steroids: psychosis

      e. Side effects of pre- and posttransplant medications (may be more pronounced in the setting of renal and/or hepatic dysfunction)

      f. Metabolic abnormalities

2. Clinical manifestations of neurologic complications (depend on etiology)
   a. Ischemic insult: hemiparesis, aphasia, visual deficits, severe delirium, and coma
   b. Medication side effects:
      i. β-Blockers: depression, confusion
      ii. Calcium channel blockers: headache, confusion, vertigo, tremor
      iii. Amiodarone: neuropathy, ataxia, tremor
      iv. Corticosteroid therapy: convulsions, vertigo, headache
      v. Calcineurin inhibitors: tremor, headache
   c. Encephalopathy: may range from mild confusion to coma
   d. Focal cerebral abnormalities: typically associated with embolic events
   e. Seizures: typically associated with drug toxicity (e.g., tacrolimus [Prograf, Astagraf XL])
3. Intervene as ordered by physician; potential interventions depend on etiology and may include
   a. Initiating seizure precautions—airway protection
   b. Optimizing CO
   c. Decreasing dose of immunosuppressant medications
   d. Changing immunosuppressant agents or other medications
   e. Correcting metabolic abnormalities
   f. Administering anticonvulsants
      i. It is important to note that certain anticonvulsants (e.g., phenytoin [Dilantin], phenobarbital, carbamazepine [Tegretol]) may increase the metabolism of calcineurin inhibitors (cyclosporine and tacrolimus); this may result in low serum levels of these immunosuppressants.
      ii. Monitor serum levels of calcineurin inhibitors carefully; dose of calcineurin inhibitor may have to be adjusted.
4. Monitor patient's response to therapy:
   a. Neurologic status
   b. Cognitive status
   c. Mood state
   d. Serum anticonvulsant levels (e.g., phenytoin [Dilantin] level)
5. Collaborate with interdisciplinary team members: physicians (surgeon, cardiologist, neurologist, neuropsychologist, psychologist), APRN, transplant pharmacist, physical therapist, occupational therapist.

P. Altered bowel function
   1. Constipation
      a. Potential etiology
         i. Effects of general anesthesia, especially the opioid component; the smooth muscles of the GI tract are often temporarily paralyzed and peristalsis may be impaired.[92]
         ii. Narcotic analgesics that may suppress peristalsis and lead to constipation or obstruction.
         iii. Reduced mobility: Inactivity slows progression of materials through the GI tract.
      b. Report clinical manifestations of constipation.
         i. Infrequent bowel movements
         ii. Difficult defecation
         iii. Passage of unduly hard and dry fecal material
         iv. Abdominal distention

      v. Abdominal pain or tenderness

      vi. Abnormal abdominal radiograph, ultrasound, or CT scan results

  c. Intervene as ordered by physician; potential interventions may include

      i. Increasing patient's level of activity (ambulation, scheduled exercise)

      ii. Administration of medications to relieve constipation (e.g., prokinetic agents, stool softeners, suppositories, laxatives)

         • Note: Aluminum-based laxatives may decrease absorption of medications in the gut.

      iii. Enemas

      iv. Nasogastric tube for decompression

      v. Increasing patient's intake of fluid and fiber

      vi. Changing type and/or frequency of pain medication

  d. Monitor:

      i. Bowel sounds (absent, hypoactive, hyperactive)

      ii. Abdominal pain, tenderness, distention

      iii. Patient's response to intervention(s):

         • Bowel movements (e.g., frequency, quantity).

         • Observe trend via stool charts.

  e. Collaborate with interdisciplinary team members: physicians (surgeon, cardiologist, intensivist, gastroenterologist), APRN, dietitian, physical therapist, ancillary nursing personnel

2. Diarrhea

  a. Potential etiology

      i. Medications that irritate the bowel and precipitate ulcerations, bleeding, and diarrhea

         • Mycophenolate mofetil (CellCept, Myfortic)

         • Antiplatelet agents

         • Antibiotics that alter the normal flora of the bowel and subsequently cause diarrhea

      ii. Opportunistic infections (e.g., CMV may cause gastritis or colitis)

      iii. Hospital-acquired infections such as *Clostridium difficile*

  b. Report clinical manifestations of diarrhea.

      i. Frequent passage of unformed, watery stool

      ii. Positive stool cultures

      iii. Weight loss

      iv. Abnormal test results (e.g., positive stool cultures, abnormal abdominal radiograph, ultrasound, or CT scan)

  c. Intervene as ordered by physician; potential interventions may include

      i. Altering medication time schedule (e.g., administering mycophenolate mofetil [CellCept] 500 mg three times daily instead of 750 mg twice daily)

      ii. Treatment of infection (e.g., metronidazole or oral vancomycin for *Clostridium difficile*)

      iii. Administration of binding agents for diarrhea caused by non–toxin secreting organisms (e.g., loperamide [Imodium])

  d. Monitor:

      i. Bowel sounds (absent, hypoactive, hyperactive)

      ii. Abdominal pain, tenderness, distention

      iii. Laboratory test values (e.g., electrolytes)

      iv.   Patient's response to intervention(s):
- Bowel movements (frequency, quantity, characteristics).
- Observe trend via stool charts.

    e. Collaborate with interdisciplinary team members: physicians (surgeon, cardiologist, intensivist, gastroenterologist), APRN, dietitian, physical therapist, ancillary nursing personnel.

Q. Altered nutrition

1. The patient's nutritional status at the time of transplantation may influence posttransplant nutrition.

    a. Heart transplant recipients are at risk for malnutrition due to pretransplant[93]:

       i.   Anorexia (secondary to gastric compression from ascites)

       ii.   GI symptoms (nausea, vomiting, diarrhea, constipation)

       iii.   Dysgeusia (impaired taste)

       iv.   Dysphagia

       v.   Hypermetabolism (increase in resting energy expenditure)

       vi.   Drug-nutrient interactions

       vii.   Malabsorption (secondary to engorgement of viscera with fluid)

       viii.   Poor nutrient delivery to tissues

       ix.   Early satiety

       x.   Restricted diets

       xi.   Impaired ability to prepare food

       xii.   Altered mental status

       xiii.   Cardiac cachexia[93]

2. The goal of pretransplant care is to optimize the candidate's weight and nutritional status.

3. Following transplantation, the energy expended by the body through the healing and recovery process is increased from basal levels and a greater amount of protein is required for tissue repair and regeneration.

4. Pretransplant heart failure dietary restrictions (e.g., sodium and fluid restrictions) are typically relaxed in the immediate postoperative period, thereby expanding the patient's food choices.

    a. For the long term, however, patients are encouraged to follow a heart-healthy (i.e., low-fat, low-salt, low-cholesterol) diet and maintain ideal body weight to prevent or reduce the severity of complications such as obesity, hypertension, DM, etc.

5. Nutrition remains an area that requires close monitoring as there is some evidence that cachexia and obesity increase the risk of poor posttransplant outcomes. In addition, obesity may increase the risk of other posttransplant complications.[89]

6. Report:

    a. Patient's baseline and current appetite

    b. Patient's baseline and current weight

    c. Low serum albumin level

       i.   Normal values: adults: 3.5 to 5.5 g/dL or 35 to 55 g/L

       ii.   Normal values: adults >60 years of age: 3.4 to 4.8 g/dL or 34 to 48 g/L

    d. Low prealbumin level

       i.   Normal values: 10 to 40 mg/dL or 100 to 400 mg/L

    e. Result of calorie counts

    f. Nausea, vomiting (may be associated with general anesthesia)

g. Diarrhea, constipation

h. Absent bowel sounds, increasing abdominal girth and tension, or reflux of feedings (may indicate hypomotility or the presence of a bowel obstruction or ileus)

7. Intervene as ordered by physician; potential interventions include

   a. Calorie counts to assess patients' ability to meet their nutritional needs

   b. Small, frequent feedings if patients continue to have early satiety

   c. Nutritional supplements

   d. Enteral feedings

      i. Confirm correct placement of feeding tube prior to initiating feeding.

      ii. Monitor for manifestations of aspiration: increased ventilator resistance, increased temperature, changes on chest radiograph, or the presence of tube feed in the secretions of intubated patients.

      iii. Early postoperative feeding must be initiated slowly due to the effects of general anesthetics on the motility of GI tract.

   e. Total parenteral nutrition (TPN) if the patient does not tolerate enteral feedings

      i. Monitor nutritional status, electrolyte and mineral levels, blood glucose level; triglycerides, liver function tests.

   f. Administration of medications to control nausea, vomiting, diarrhea

8. Monitor:

   a. Lab test results

      i. Serum albumin

      ii. Serum prealbumin

      iii. Electrolytes

      iv. Liver function tests

   b. Appetite

   c. Bowel sounds

   d. Activity level

   e. Patient's response to interventions:

      i. Weight gain or loss

      ii. Calories consumed

      iii. Presence or absence of nausea, vomiting, diarrhea, constipation

      iv. Tolerance of nutritional supplements, enteral feedings, or TPN

9. Collaborate with interdisciplinary team: physicians (surgeon, cardiologist, intensivist), APRN, dietitian, physiotherapists, social worker (for psychological etiology of altered nutrition), ancillary nursing personnel.

   a. Collaboration with the dietitian is of particular importance as this clinician can

      i. Conduct a pretransplant nutrition screening and assessment (history, physical assessment, analysis of laboratory test results)

      ii. Implement strategies to correct pretransplant malnutrition and/or optimize candidate's pretransplant weight, particularly with respect to requirements of calories, protein, vitamins, minerals, and electrolytes

      iii. Develop a plan of posttransplant nutritional support and monitor patient's progress (particularly if the recipient requires enteral or parenteral feedings)

      iv. Identify medication side effects that can interfere with posttransplant nutrition

      v. Provide continuity of care with respect to potential chronic posttransplant problems such as obesity, hyperlipidemia, DM, and hypertension

      vi. Serve as a resource regarding food safety issues

R. Altered mobility and/or self-care deficit

  1. Early mobility is an important factor in preventing postoperative complications and facilitating recovery.

  2. Potential etiology of altered mobility and/or self-care deficit:

    a. Pain or anticipatory pain

    b. Pre- or posttransplant deconditioning

    c. Altered mood state (e.g., depression, anxiety)

  3. Clinical manifestations:

    a. Inability or unwillingness to participate in self-care

    b. Inability or unwillingness to ambulate

  4. Interventions

    a. Administer adequate pain medication prior to self-care activities or ambulation.

      i. Assess effectiveness of pain medication before patient engages in self-care activities or ambulation.

    b. Establish mutual goals for self-care, ambulation, and exercise.

    c. Instruction in sternal precautions.

    d. Physical therapy.

      i. Establishment of mutual goals

      ii. Development of exercise program (in hospital and at home)

    e. Occupational therapy.

      i. Establishment of mutual goals

    f. Involve family in patient's care.

    g. Referral for home physical and/or occupational therapy, if needed.

    h. Referral to outpatient phase II cardiac rehabilitation program upon discharge.

    i. Referral for mental health services, if needed.

  5. Monitor

    a. Effectiveness of pain medication

    b. Patient's ability to perform self-care activities

    c. Patient's progress with physical and occupational therapy

  6. Collaborate with interdisciplinary colleagues: physicians (surgeon, cardiologist, intensivist), APRN, physical therapist, occupational therapist, home health care nurse mental health provider.

S. Noninfection complication topics discussed in Chapter 6 include

  1. Hyperlipidemia

  2. Metabolic syndrome

  3. Diabetes mellitus (DM)

  4. Obesity

  5. Malignancies

  6. Osteoporosis

  7. Gout

  8. Gingival hyperplasia

  9. Sexual dysfunction

  10. Neurocognitive impairment

REFERENCES

1. Arnold M. *The Merck Manual Professional Edition. Heart Failure Chapter;* 2013. Available at www.merckmedicus. com. Accessed on August 15, 2014. Content last modified October 2013.
2. Kailash S, Sunil A, Sirin Y, et al. Outpatient management of heart failure in the United States, 2006–2008. *Tex Heart Inst J.* 2014;41(3):253–261.
3. Garg A, Vignesh C, Singh V, et al. Acute right heart syndrome: rescue treatment with inhaled nitric oxide. *Indian J Crit Care Med.* 2014;18(1):40–42.
4. Jaski B. *The 4 Stages of Heart Failure.* Minneapolis, MN: Cardiotext Publishing; 2015:6–8, 21–31, 86–95, 103–110.
5. Kallikazaros I. Heart failure with preserved ejection fraction. *Hellenic J Cardiol.* 2014;55:265–266.
6. Komamura K. Review article. Similarities and differences between the pathogenesis and pathophysiology of diastolic and systolic heart failure. *Cardiol Res Pract.* 2013;2013:Article ID 824135.
7. Blair J, Huffman M, Shah S. Heart failure in North America. *Curr Cardiol Rev.* 2013;9:128–146.
8. Lindenfeld J, Albert NM, Boehmer JP, et al. Heart Failure Society of America (HFSA) 2010 Comprehensive Heart Failure Practice Guideline. *J Card Fail.* 2010;16(6):1–194.
9. McMurray JJ, Adamopoulos S, Anker SD, et al. European Society of Cardiology (ESC) Guidelines for the diagnosis and treatment of acute and chronic heart failure 2012. The Task Force for the Diagnosis and Treatment of Acute and Chronic Heart Failure 2012 of the European Society of Cardiology. Developed in collaboration with the Heart Failure Association (HFA) of the ESC. *Eur Heart J.* 2012;33:1787–1847.
10. Mehra MR, Kobashigawa J, Starling R, et al. Listing criteria for heart transplantation: International Society for Heart and Lung Transplantation Guidelines for the Care of Cardiac Transplant Candidates—2006. *J Heart Lung Transplant.* 2006;25:1024–1042.
11. Luo J, Huang R, et al. Value of STOP-BANG questionnaire in screening patients with obstructive sleep hypopnea syndrome in sleep disordered breathing clinic. *Chin Med J (Engl).* 2014;127(10):1843–1848.
12. Mehra R. Sleep apnea ABCs: airway, breathing, circulation. *Cleve Clin J Med.* 2014;81(8):479–489.
13. Beigel R, Cercek B, Siegel RJ, et al. Echo-Doppler hemodynamics: an important management tool for today's heart failure care. *Circulation.* 2015;131(11):1031–1034.
14. Malarkey LM, McMorrow ME. *Nursing Guide to Laboratory and Diagnostic Tests.* Philadelphia, PA: Saunders; 2005.
15. Hunt SA, Baker DW, Chin MH, et al. ACC/AHA Guidelines for the evaluation and management of chronic heart failure in the adult: executive summary. A report of the American College of Cardiology/American Heart Association Task Force on Practice Guidelines (Committee to revise the 1995 Guidelines for the Evaluation and Management of Heart Failure). *Circulation.* 2001:2996–3007.
16. Ammar KA, Jacobsen SJ, Mahoney DW, et al. Prevalence and prognostic significance of heart failure stages: application of the American College of Cardiology/American Heart Association heart failure staging criteria in the community. *Circulation.* 2007;115(12):1563–1570.
17. Hunt SA, Abraham WT, Chin MH, et al. *American College of Cardiology/American Heart Association 2005 Guideline Update for the Diagnosis and Management of Chronic Heart Failure in the Adult: A Report of the American College of Cardiology/American Heart Association Task Force on Practice Guidelines (Writing Committee to Update the 2001 Guidelines for the Evaluation and Management of Heart Failure);* 2005.
18. Starling R. Medical grand rounds advanced heart failure transplant, LVADs, and beyond. *Cleve Clin J Med.* 2013;80(1):33–40.
19. Fang KC, Ewald GA, Allen LA, et al. Advanced (stage d) heart failure: a statement from the heart failure society of America guidelines committee. *J Card Fail.* 2015;21(6):519–534.
20. Reed BN, Rodgers JE, Sueta, CA. Polypharmacy in heart failure: drugs to use and avoid. *Heart Fail Clin.* 2014;10(4):577–590.
21. Yancy CW, Jessup M, et al. 2013 ACCF/AHA Guideline for the Management of Heart Failure: a Report of the American College of Cardiology Foundation/American Association Task Force on Practice Guidelines. *J Am Coll Cardiol.* 2013;62(16):147–239.
22. Mancini GB, Howlett JG, Borer J, et al. Pharmacologic options for the management of systolic heart failure: examining underlying mechanisms. *Can J Cardiol.* 2015;31(10):1282–1292.
23. Barnard CN. Human cardiac transplantation: an evaluation of the first two operations performed at the Groote Schuur Hospital, Cape Town. *Am J Cardiol.* 1968;22:584–596.
24. Nguyen CT, Lee E, Luo H, et al. Echocardiographic guidance for diagnostic and therapeutic percutaneous procedures. *Cardiovasc Diagn Ther.* 2011;1(1):11–36.
25. Borel JF, Feurer C, Gubler HU, et al. Biological effects of cyclosporine A: a new antilymphocytic agent. *Agents Actions.* 1976;6:468–475.
26. Kahan BD. Forty years of publication of transplantation proceedings—the second decade: the cyclosporine revolution. *Transplant Proc.* 2009;41:1423–1437.
27. McCalmont V, Ohler L. Cardiac transplantation: candidate identification, evaluation, and management. *Crit Care Nurs Q.* 2008;31(3):216–229.

28. Lund LH, Edwards LB, Kucheryavaya AY, et al. The registry of the International Society for Heart and Lung Transplantation: thirty-first official adult heart transplant report—2014; focus theme: retransplantation. *J Heart Lung Transplant.* 2014;33(10):996–1008.

29. Velez M, Johnson MR. Management of allosensitized cardiac transplant candidates. *Transplant Rev.* 2009;23(4):235–247.

30. Kobashigawa J, Crespo-Leiro MG, Ensminger SM, et al. ISHLT Consensus: report from a consensus on antibody-mediated rejection in heart transplantation. *J Heart Lung Transplant.* 2011;30:252–269.

31. Aggarwal A, Pyle J, Hamilton J, et al. Low-dose rituximab therapy for antibody-mediated rejection in a highly sensitized heart-transplant recipient. *Tex Heart Inst J.* 2012;39(6):901–905.

32. Stegall MD, Gloor JM. Deciphering antibody-mediated rejection: new insights into mechanisms and treatment. *Curr Opin Organ Transplant.* 2010;15(1):8–10.

33. Lower RR, Stofer RC, Shumway NW. Homovital transplantation of the heart. *J Thorac Cardiovasc Surg.* 1961;41:196–204.

34. Miniati DN, Robbins RC. Techniques in orthotopic cardiac transplantation: a review. *Cardiol Rev.* 2001;9:131–136.

35. El Gamel A, Yonan NA, Grant S, et al. Orthotopic cardiac transplantation: a comparison of standard and bicaval Wythenshawe techniques. *J Thorac Cardiovasc Surg.* 1995;109:721–729.

36. Deleuze PH, Benvenuti C, Mazzucotelli JP, et al. Orthotopic cardiac transplantation with direct caval anastomosis: is it the optimal procedure? *J Thorac Cardiovasc Surg.* 1995;109:731–737.

37. Barnard CN, Losman JG. Left ventricular bypass. *S Afr Med J.* 1975;49:303–312.

38. Jahanyar J, Korener MM, Ghodsizad A, et al. Heterotopic heart transplantation: the United States experience. *Heart Surg Forum.* 2014;17(3):E132–E140.

39. Shah AB, Patel JK, Rafiei M, et al. The impact of mean first-year heart rate on outcomes after heart transplantation: does it make a difference? *Clin Transplant.* 2013;27(5):659–665.

40. Kittleson MM, Kobashigawa JA. Management of the ACC/AHA Stage D patient: cardiac transplantation. *Cardiol Clin.* 2014;32(1):95–112.

41. Gass AL, Emaminia A, Lanier G, et al. Cardiac transplantation in the new era. *Cardio Rev.* 2015;23(4):182–188.

42. Davis MK, Hunt SA. State of the art: cardiac transplantation. *Trends Cardiovasc Med.* 2014;24(8):341–349.

43. Kittleson MM. New issues in heart transplantation for heart failure. *Curr Treat Options Cardiovasc Med.* 2012;14(4):356–369.

44. Cotts WG, Oren RM. Function of the transplanted heart: unique physiology and therapeutic implications. *Am J Med Sci.* 1997;314:164–174.

45. Soderlund C, Radegran G. Immunosuppressive therapies after heart transplantation—the balance between under- and over-immunosuppression. *Transplant Rev (Orlando).* 2015;29(3):181–189.

46. Ansari D, Lund LH, Stehlik J. Induction with anti-thymocyte globulin in heart transplantation is associated with better long-term survival compared with basiliximab. *J Heart Lung Transplant.* 2015. pii: S1053-2498(15)01204–01208.

47. Costanzo MR, Dipchand A, Starling R, et al. The International Society of Heart and Lung Transplantation Guidelines for the care of heart transplant recipients. *J Heart Lung Transplant.* 2010;29(8):914–956.

48. Hardin SE, Kaplow R. *Cardiac Surgery Essentials for Critical care Nursing.* Burlington, MA: Jones and Bartlett Publishers; 2010.

49. Hollenberg SM. Vasoactive drugs in circulatory shock. *Am J Respir Crit Care Med.* 2011;183(7):847–855.

50. Mandras SA, Crespo MD, Patel HM. Innovative application of immunologic principles in heart transplantation. *Ochsner J.* 2010;10:231–235.

51. Chang DH, Kobashigawa JA. Cardiac allograft immune activation: current perspectives. *Transpl Res Risk Manag.* 2014;7:13–22.

52. Ansari D, Lund LH, Stehlik J. Induction with anti-thymocyte globulin in heart transplantation is associated with better long-term survival compared with basiliximab. *J Heart Lung Transplant.* 2015;34(10):1283–1291.

53. Stewart S, Winters GL, Fishbein MC, et al. Revision of the 1990 working formulation for the standardization of nomenclature in the diagnosis of heart rejection. *J Heart Lung Transplant.* 2005;24:1710–1720.

54. Kaczorowski DJ, Datta J, Kamoun M, et al. Profound hyperacute cardiac allograft rejection rescue with biventricular mechanical circulatory support and plasmapheresis, intravenous immunoglobulin, and rituximab therapy. *J Cardiothorac Surg.* 2013;8:48.

55. Berry GJ, Angelini A, Burke MM, et al. The ISHLT working formulation for pathologic diagnosis of antibody-mediated rejection in heart transplantation: evolution and current status (2005–2011). *J Heart Lung Transplant.* 2011;30(6):601–611.

56. Szymanska S, Grajkowska W, Pronicki M. Pathologic diagnosis of antibody-mediated rejection in endomyocardial biopsy after heart transplantation based on renewed International Society for Heart and Lung Transplantation criteria. *Pol J Pathol.* 2014;65(3):176–181.

57. Kittleson MM, Kobashigawa JA. Long-term care of the heart transplant recipient. *Curr Opin Organ Transplant.* 2014;19(5):515–524.

58. Patel JK, Kittleson M, Kobashigawa JA. Cardiac allograft rejection. *Surgeon.* 2011;9(3):160–167.

59. Wu YL, Ye Q, Ho C. Cellular and functional imaging of cardiac transplant rejection. *Curr Cardiovasc Imaging Rep.* 2011;4(1):50–62.

60. Pham MX, Deng MC, Kfoury AG, et al. Molecular testing for long-term rejection surveillance in heart transplant recipients: design of the Invasive Monitoring Attenuation Through Gene Expression (IMAGE) trial. *J Heart Lung Transplant.* 2007;26(8):808–814.

61. Pham MX, Teuteberg JJ, Kfoury AG, et al. Gene-expression profiling for rejection surveillance after cardiac transplantation. *N Engl J Med.* 2010;362(20):1890–1900.

62. Kobashigawa J, Patel J, Kittleson M, et al. Results of a randomized trial of allomap vs heart biopsy in the 1st year after heart transplant: early invasive monitoring attenuation through gene expression trial. *J Heart Lung Transplant.* 2013;32(4):S203.

63. Kobashigawa JA, Kiyosaki KK, Patel JK, et al. Benefit of immune monitoring in heart transplant patients using ATP production in activated lymphocytes. *J Heart Lung Transplant.* 2010;29(5):504–508.

64. Soderlund C, Radegran G. Immunosuppressive therapies after heart transplantation—the balance between under- and over-immunosuppression. *Transplant Rev.* 2015;29(3):181–189.

65. Kobashigawa JA, Miller LW, Russell SD, et al. Tacrolimus with mycophenolate mofetil (MMF) or sirolimus vs. cyclosporine with MMF in cardiac transplant patients: 1-year report. *Am J Transplant.* 2006;6(6):1377–1386.

66. Eisen HJ, Kobashigawa J, Keogh A, et al. Three-year results of a randomized, double-blind, controlled trial of mycophenolate mofetil versus azathioprine in cardiac transplant recipients. *J Heart Lung Transplant.* 2005;24(5):517–525.

67. Eisen HJ, Kobashigawa JA, Starling RC, et al. Everolimus versus mycophenolate mofetil in heart transplantation: a randomized, multicenter trial. *Am J Transplant.* 2013;3(5):1203–1216.

68. Baraldo M, Gregoraci G, Livi U. Steroid-free and steroid withdrawal protocols in heart transplantation: the review of literature. *Transpl Int.* 2014;27(6):515–529.

69. Kobashigawa J, Ross H, Bara C, et al. Everolimus is associated with a reduced incidence of cytomegalovirus infection following de novo cardiac transplantation. *Transpl Infect Dis.* 2013;5(2):150–162.

70. Eisen HJ, Kobashigawa J, Starling RC, et al. Everolimus versus mycophenolate mofetil in heart transplantation: a randomized, multicenter trial. *Am J Transplant.* 2013;13(5):1203–1216.

71. Guethoff S, Stroeh K, Grinninger C, et al. De novo sirolimus with low-dose tacrolimus versus full dose tacrolimus with mycophenolate mofetil after heart transplantation—8 year results. *J Heart Lung Transplant.* 2015;34(5):634–642.

72. Alberú J, Pascoe MD, Campistol JM, et al. Lower malignancy rates in renal allograft recipients converted to sirolimus-based, calcineurin inhibitor-free immunotherapy: 24-month results from the CONVERT trial. *Transplantation.* 2011;92(3):303–310.

73. Kobashigawa JA, Moriguchi JD, Laks H, et al. Ten-year follow-up of a randomized trial of pravastatin in heart transplant patients. *J Heart Lung Transplant.* 2005;24(11):1736–1740.

74. Kittleson MM, Kobashigawa JA. Statins in heart transplantation. *Clin Transpl.* 2013:135–143.

75. Chih S, Tinckam KJ, Ross HJ. A survey of current practice for antibody-mediated rejection in heart transplantation. *Am J Transplant.* 2013;13(4):1069–1074.

76. Colvin-Adams M, Agnihotri A. Cardiac allograft vasculopathy: current knowledge and future direction. *Clin Transplant.* 2011;25(2):175–184.

77. Lund LH, Edwards LB, Kucheryavaya AY, et al. The Registry of the International Society for Heart and Lung Transplantation: Thirtieth Official Adult Heart Transplant Report—2013; focus theme: age. *J Heart Lung Transplant.* 2013;32(10):951–964.

78. Mehra MR, Crespo-Leiro MG, Dipchand A, et al. International Society for Heart and Lung Transplantation working formulation of a standardized nomenclature for cardiac allograft vasculopathy—2010. *J Heart Lung Transplant.* 2010;29(7):717–727.

79. Kobashigawa JA, Pauly DF, Starling RC, et al. Cardiac allograft vasculopathy by intravascular ultrasound in heart transplant patients: substudy from Everolimus versus mycophenolate mofetil randomized, multicentre trial. *JACC Heart Fail.* 2013;1(5):389–399.

80. Nascimento BR, Gomes TO, Borges JC, et al. Primary angioplasty for cardiac allograft vasculopathy presenting as ST-Elevation acute myocardial infarction during endomyocardial biopsy. *Case Rep Transplant.* 2013;2013;Article ID 606481.

81. Beygui F, Varnous S, Montalescot G, et al. Long-term outcome after bare-metal or drug-eluting stenting for allograft coronary artery disease. *J Heart Lung Transplant.* 2010;29(3):316–322.

82. Tremmel JA, Ng MK, Ikeno F, et al. Comparison of drug-eluting versus bare metal stents in cardiac allograft vasculopathy. *Am J Cardiol.* 2011;108(5):665–668.

83. Fishbein MC. Pathologic findings of cardiac dysfunction. In: Norman DJ, Turka LA, eds. *Primer on Transplantation.* 2nd ed. Mt. Laurel, NJ: American Society of Transplantation; 2016:370–374.

84. Seki A, Fishbein MC. Predicting the development of cardiac allograft vasculopathy. *Cardiovasc Pathol.* 2014;23:253–260.

85. Mastouri R, Batres Y, Lenet A, et al. Frequency, time course, and possible causes of right ventricular systolic dysfunction after cardiac transplantation: a single center experience. *Echocardiography.* 2013;30(1):9–16.

86. Iyer A, Kumarasinghe G, Hicks M, et al. Primary graft failure after heart transplantation. *J Transplant.* 2011;2011:175768.

87. Kobashigawa J, Zuckermann A, Macdonald P, et al. Report from a consensus conference on primary graft dysfunction after cardiac transplantation. *J Heart Lung Transplant.* 2014;33(4):327–340.

88. Iyer V, Garan AR, Mancini D, et al. Ablation of ventricular tachycardia originating from the papillary muscle of the left ventricle early after heart transplantation. *Circ Heart Fail.* 2014;7(1):223–224.

89. Pinney SP, Mancini DM. Myocarditis and specific cardiomyopathies—Endocrine disease and alcohol. In: Fuster V, O'Rourke RA, et al., eds. *Hurst's The Heart.* 13th ed., Vol. 2. New York: McGraw-Hill; 2011:1949–2674.

90. Prenner G, Wasler A, Fahreleinter-Pammer A, et al. The role of serum albumin in the prediction of malnutrition in patients at least five yr after heart transplantation. *Clin Transplant.* 2014;28(6):737–742.

91. Cruz D. Cardiorenal syndrome in critical care: the acute cardiorenal and renocardiac syndromes. *Adv Chronic Kidney Dis.* 2013;20 (1):56–66.

92. Mythen MG. Postoperative gastrointestinal tract dysfunction. *Anesth Analg.* 2005;100:196–204.

93. Grady KL, Naftel D, Pamboukian SV, et al. Post-operative obesity and cachexia are risk factors for morbidity and mortality after heart transplant: multi-institutional study of postoperative weight change. *J Heart Lung Transplant.* 2005;24:1424–1430.

SELF-ASSESSMENT QUESTIONS

1. A 65-year-old male transplant candidate is admitted to the hospital for decompensated heart failure. His signs and symptoms would likely include:
   a. serum creatinine > 2.0 mg/dL, serum sodium < 130, heart rate > 100 bpm, and systolic blood pressure < 100 mm Hg.
   b. serum creatinine > 2.0 mg/dL, serum sodium > 145, and decreasing brain natriuretic peptide level.
   c. heart rate < 60 bpm, systolic blood pressure < 80 mm Hg, and decreasing brain natriuretic peptide level.
   d. increasing peripheral edema, decreasing abdominal fullness, and increased responsiveness to diuretics.

2. Absolute contraindications to heart transplantation would be:
   1. history of carcinoma within the last year.
   2. history of active alcohol abuse.
   3. recent pulmonary infarction.
   4. history of poor compliance with drug regimens.
   a. 1 and 3.
   b. 1 and 4.
   c. 2 and 4.
   d. 3 and 4.
   e. all of the above.

3. Ventricular tachycardia after giving diuretics in the heart failure patient is most likely due to:
   a. hypercalcemia and/or hypophosphatemia.
   b. hypokalemia and/or hypomagnesemia.
   c. hyperkalemia and/or hypermagnesemia.
   d. hypophosphatemia and/or hypernatremia.

4. Heart failure medical treatment may include all of the following except:
   1. sodium restriction.
   2. immune suppression.
   3. inotropic drips.
   4. daily weights.
   5. fluid restriction.
   a. all of the following except # 1.
   b. all of the following except # 2.
   c. all of the following except # 3.
   d. all of the following except # 4.
   e. includes all of the above.

5. Which respiratory disorder is a risk factor that can worsen heart failure?
   a. Asthma
   b. COPD
   c. Sleep apnea
   d. Pneumonia

6. A 32-year-old male transplanted 3 months ago is admitted from a clinic with new-onset fatigue, shortness of breath, and palpitations. 12-lead EKG shows aflutter with HR 142, and clinical exam reveals S3 gallop. Likely diagnosis is:
   a. cardiac allograft vasculopathy.
   b. renal failure.
   c. cardiac tamponade.
   d. rejection.

7. A 52-year-old female is admitted to ICU post heart transplant. Within 24 hours, the patient develops bradycardia with HR down to 52 beats per minute. Anticipate orders for one or more of the following:
   1. AV sequential pacing via temporary epicardial pacing wires
   2. Chest x-ray
   3. Endomyocardial biopsy
   4. Initiation of isoproterenol (Isuprel)
   a. 1 and 3
   b. 2 and 4
   c. 1 and 4
   d. 3 and 4

8. Right ventricular failure is common post heart transplant. Risk factors include:
   a. ischemic injury or inadequate donor organ preservation.
   b. pulmonary hypertension in the recipient due to prolonged heart failure.
   c. smaller donor heart transplanted into larger recipient.
   d. all of the above.

9. Cardiac allograft vasculopathy is considered a chronic rejection process. Treatment may include:
   1. drug-eluting stent to occluded vessels.
   2. change in immunosuppressive therapy.
   3. management of restrictive heart physiology.
   4. retransplantation.
   a. 1 and 3.
   b. 2 and 3.
   c. 1 and 2.
   d. All of the above.

10. A 58-year-old woman received heart transplant 12 hrs ago and is recovering in ICU. Lab work shows acute rise in serum creatinine from 1.1 initially postoperatively to now 2.4. Expect orders for the following:
    1. Induction therapy to delay the initiation of calcineurin inhibitors
    2. Fluid replacement
    3. Initiation of renal dose dopamine at 2 to 3 mcg/kg/min
    4. Increase in corticosteroid dose
    a. 1, 2, and 4
    b. 1, 2, and 3
    c. 2, 3, and 4
    d. All of the above

11. You are caring for a 55-year-old female heart transplant recipient who had severe liver dysfunction prior to transplantation. On postoperative day 2, you assume care of this patient at 7 AM and you observe the following trends that occurred on the night shift: decreasing hemoglobin and hematocrit, decreasing cardiac output and cardiac index, increasing chest tube output, and increasing oxygen requirements. During your first assessment, you note the following: cardiac index 2.8 L/min/m^2, systolic pressure 88 mm Hg, HR 140 bpm, and chest tube output 200 mL/hour. You notify the physician and anticipate orders for:
    1. antirejection therapy.
    2. blood products.
    3. protamine.
    4. stripping of chest tubes.
    5. increased immunosuppression.
    6. preparation of patient for return to OR.
    a. 1, 2, and 3.
    b. 1, 4, and 5.
    c. 2, 3, and 6.
    d. 2, 3, and 4.

12. A 56-year-old male transplant recipient develops metabolic acidosis secondary to hyperkalemia. His symptoms of hyperkalemia would likely include:
    a. skeletal muscle weakness, irregular pulse, and inverted T waves on ECG.
    b. increased deep tendon reflexes, nausea, and vomiting.
    c. constipation, small muscle hypoactivity, and irregular pulse.
    d. skeletal muscle weakness, tall peaked T waves on ECG, nausea, and vomiting.

13. Immediately following heart transplantation, the nurse notices the following vital signs:

Time	Urine Output	CVP	Blood Pressure	Heart Rate
11 AM	200 mL/h	12 mm Hg	150/100	110 bpm
12 noon	150 mL/h	10 mm Hg	140/98	90 bpm
1 PM	100 mL/h	8 mm Hg	128/78	88 bpm
2 PM	25 mL/h	4 mm Hg	98/70	100 bpm

The nurse should anticipate an order for:
    a. a diuretic.
    b. an IV fluid bolus.
    c. a vasodilator.
    d. a pacemaker.

14. A 56-year-old male transplant candidate is admitted to the hospital for worsening heart failure. His signs and symptoms would likely include:
    a. rising serum creatinine level, decreasing serum sodium level, and increasing brain natriuretic peptide level.
    b. rising serum creatinine level, increasing serum sodium level, and decreasing brain natriuretic peptide level.
    c. heart rate > 85 bpm, systolic blood pressure < 80 mm Hg, and decreasing brain natriuretic peptide level.
    d. increasing peripheral edema, decreasing abdominal fullness, and increased responsiveness to diuretics.

15. You are caring for a 44-year-old male heart transplant recipient in the step-down unit who suddenly becomes bradycardic. You should anticipate an order for:
    a. atropine.
    b. isoproterenol.
    c. nitroprusside.
    d. digoxin.

16. The clinical manifestations of rejection are likely to include:
    1. hypertension.
    2. fever >101°F.
    3. hypotension.
    4. atrial dysrhythmias.
    a. 1 and 2.
    b. 3 and 4.
    c. 2 and 4.
    d. 1 and 4.

17. Your patient is 5 days post–heart transplantation and has just had his first endomyocardial biopsy. When he returns to the step-down unit, you notice the following vital signs:

Time	CVP	Blood Pressure	Heart Rate	Urine Output
11 AM	6 mm Hg	110/90	110 bpm	200 cc/h
12 noon	8 mm Hg	100/86	90 bpm	150 cc/h
1 PM	12 mm Hg	90/84	72 bpm	100 cc/h
2 PM	15 mm Hg	80/62	68 bpm	25 cc/h

You suspect that the patient has:
    a. rejection.
    b. acute renal failure.
    c. cardiac tamponade.
    d. sepsis.

18. Clinical manifestations of infection in a heart transplant recipient may include:
    1. fever ($\geq$ 38°C/100.4°F).
    2. negative C-reactive protein.
    3. leukocytosis.
    4. elevated sedimentation rate.
    a. 1, 2, and 3.
    b. 1, 2, and 4.
    c. 2, 3, and 4.
    d. 1, 3, and 4.

19. Premature atrial or ventricular contractions in a heart transplant recipient are most often due to:
    a. hypokalemia and/or hypomagnesemia.
    b. hypercalcemia and/or hypophosphatemia.
    c. hyponatremia and/or hyperphosphatemia.
    d. hypophosphatemia and/or hypernatremia.

20. As a result of denervation of the donor heart, heart transplant recipients are likely to:
    1. have a higher resting heart rate.
    2. have a lower resting heart rate.
    3. experience angina.
    4. have an altered response to certain cardiac drugs.
    5. have an altered diurnal variation in blood pressure.
    a. 2, 3, and 5.
    b. 1, 3, and 5.
    c. 1, 4, and 5.
    d. 2, 4, and 5.

21. In your discharge teaching, you would tell patients to report which of the following signs and/or symptoms that might indicate complications after an endomyocardial biopsy?
    1. Severe pain at site of puncture wound
    2. Nausea or vomiting
    3. Shortness of breath
    4. Chest or arm pain
    a. 1, 2, and 4
    b. 2, 3, and 4
    c. 1, 2, and 3
    d. 1, 3, and 4

22. Coronary artery vasculopathy is thought to be a form of:
    a. chronic graft rejection.
    b. hyperacute rejection.
    c. acute humoral rejection.
    d. acute cellular rejection.

23. In a heart transplant recipient, the clinical manifestations of a myocardial infarction *typically* may include:
    1. fatigue.
    2. dyspnea.
    3. angina.
    4. dysrhythmias.
    a. 1, 2, and 3.
    b. 1, 2, and 4.
    c. 2, 3, and 4.
    d. 1, 3, and 4.

Correct Answers:
1.a 2.e 3.b 4.b 5.c 6.d 7.c 8.d 9.d 10.b 11.c 12.d 13.b 14.a 15.b
16.b 17.c 18.d 19.a 20.c 21.d 22.a 23.b

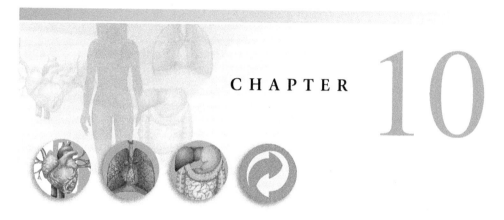

CHAPTER 10

Mechanical Circulatory Support

Suzanne R. Chillcott, RN, BSN

Leslie Hazard, RN, MS, ANP-BC, CNS

 ## I. INTRODUCTION

A. Scope of the problem

1. Heart failure is a global health problem with a US and worldwide prevalence of 5.8 million and 23 million, respectively.[1]

2. The annual number of reported heart transplant procedures worldwide peaked at nearly 5,000 in 1993 and declined steadily until 2004. More recently, the annual number of heart transplants seems to be increasing slightly. However, the demand for donor hearts greatly exceeds the supply.[2]

3. Given that heart transplantation is available to relatively few patients due to the shortage of suitable organ donors, it is not surprising that the need for mechanical circulatory support (MCS) is increasing.

B. Overview

1. Heart failure results in low cardiac output (CO) and leads to inadequate blood pressure and subsequent reduced blood flow to vital organs including the brain, kidneys, heart, and lungs.

2. Mechanical circulatory support (MCS) consists of the implantation of a pump to supplement or replace the blood flow generated by the native heart.

3. MCS can be used to provide temporary or long-term (durable) support. This chapter will focus on pumps that are used to provide long-term support, particularly left ventricular assist devices (LVADs).

C. LVADs

1. The LVAD is a pump that supplements or replaces the function of the damaged left ventricle. LVADs are increasingly used for mechanical support for patients with severe systolic heart failure (HF).

2. Purpose of LVAD support:

   a. Long-term (durable) LVADs can be implanted as a bridge to transplantation (BTT) or destination therapy (DT).

b. Long-term LVADs have also been implanted as bridge to recovery of the native heart, but this use is not currently recognized as a treatment option by the Food and Drug Administration (FDA) or the Centers for Medicare and Medicaid (CMS).

3. BTT: LVADs are implanted in listed patients when it is determined that they may not survive until a suitable donor is identified.

   a. While patients are on the heart transplant waiting list, the LVAD:
      i. Preserves end-organ function by maintaining perfusion
      ii. Minimizes the risk of clinical deterioration from heart failure, which might adversely affect their transplant candidacy
      iii. Reduces their risk of death
   b. Recent International Society for Heart Transplantation Registry data indicate that in 2012:
      i. Approximately 35% of adult heart transplant recipients were bridged to transplant with LVADs[2]
      ii. Approximately 23% of pediatric recipients were bridged to transplantation with a ventricular assist device or total artificial heart.[3]

4. DT: LVADs have also effectively supported patients who are ineligible for transplantation.[4]

   a. CMS guidelines for patient selection for DT include patients who are not transplant candidates and meet the following conditions:
      i. Failed optimal medical management for at least 45 of the last 60 days, are intra-aortic balloon pump (IABP) dependent for 7 days, or are continuously inotrope dependent for 14 days
      ii. Left ventricular ejection fraction (LVEF) <25%
      iii. Peak oxygen consumption (VO$_2$ max) < or = 14 mL/kg/min (unless patient is dependent on an IABP or inotropes or is physically unable to perform this test)
      iv. New York Heart Association (NYHA) functional class IV[5]
   b. MCS as DT represents a major proportion of all implants in the United States[6]:
      i. The proportion of implants for DT increased from 14% in 2006–2007 to 41.6% in 2011–2013.
      ii. Conversely, the proportion of patients on the heart transplant waiting list at time of implantation decreased from 42.4% (2006–2007) to 21.7% (2011–2013).

II. TYPES OF MCS DEVICES

A. MCS devices can be categorized according to the type of flow, duration of support, anatomic positioning of the pump, and ventricle(s) supported.

B. Type of flow:
   1. Pulsatile: these pumps generate a pulse of blood similar to native cardiac function (Thoratec paracorporeal ventricular assist device, Berlin Heart, SynCardia Total Artificial Heart [TAH]).
   2. Continuous flow: these pumps deliver blood as a continuous jet of laminar blood flow. Both axial and centrifugal flow pumps are classified as "continuous" (HeartMate II, HeartWare).
      a. It should be noted that some of the new continuous flow pumps have a slightly pulsatile feature (not enough to generate a palpable pulse but may provide better washing of the pump and left ventricle).

C. Duration of support:
1. Short-term devices: those devices that can be used to support a patient for a few hours to days, such as
    a. IABP
    b. Continuous flow devices that can be used for right- or left-sided support such as Tandemheart, Impella, or CentriMag
    c. Extracorporeal membrane oxygenation (ECMO), which provides
        i. Support for both right- and left-sided cardiac function and oxygenation (venoarterial)
        ii. Pulmonary support alone (venovenous)
2. Long-term or durable devices: those that can be used to support a patient for years and enable the patient to be discharged to home while on support.
    a. These types of devices can be used as either BTT or DT
    b. Currently approved continuous flow devices include the HeartMate II (axial flow) or HeartWare HVAD (centrifugal flow)[6]
    c. Future preference may favor continuous flow with a slight pulsatile component. Pulsatility, smaller components, and implantable controllers with transcutaneous energy transfer (which eliminates the need for a percutaneous driveline) are all in clinical trials or development at this time.

D. Anatomic positioning of pump:
1. Internal (intracorporeal) versus external (paracorporeal) positioning

E. Ventricle(s) supported:
1. An LVAD supports the left ventricle.
    a. LVADs are the most common type of devices used for long-term support.
    b. Examples:
        i. Long-term support: HeartMate II, HeartWare HVAD, Thoratec paracorporeal ventricular assist device, or Berlin Heart
        ii. Short-term support: IABP, Impella, Tandem Heart, CentriMag, Maquet, or Medtronic VADs
2. A right ventricular assist device (RVAD) supports the right ventricle; examples include the
    a. HeartWare HVAD (off-label use)
    b. Thoratec paracorporeal ventricular assist device
    c. Berlin Heart
    d. Short-term devices:
        i. CentriMag
        ii. Maquet VAD
        iii. Medtronic VAD
3. A biventricular assist device (BiVAD) supports both ventricles; examples include
    a. Thoratec paracorporeal ventricular assist device
    b. Berlin Heart
    c. Short-term support devices:
        i. Bilateral CentriMag
        ii. Maquet VAD
        iii. Medtronic VAD

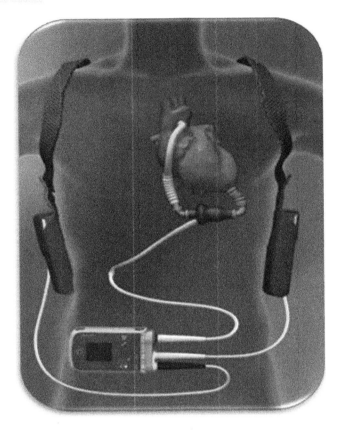

FIGURE 10-1   HeartMate II LVAD with Pocket Controller. (Picture provided by Thoratec Inc.)

4. Total artificial heart (TAH): both ventricles are removed and replaced with the device.
    a. Example: SynCardia TAH with freedom driver, which allows for discharge to home as BTT patients.
5. See Figure 10-1: HeartMate II
6. See Figure 10-2: HeartWare HVAD

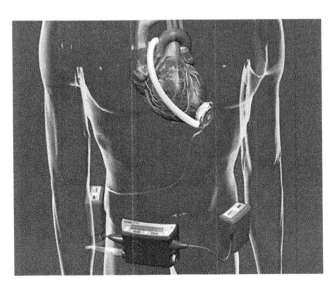

FIGURE 10-2   HeartWare HVAD. (Picture provided by HeartWare Inc.)

III. SURVIVAL RATES[6]

A. Interagency Registry for Mechanically Assisted Circulatory Support (INTERMACS) data indicate a 1-year actuarial survival rate of 80% and a 2-year actuarial survival rate of 70% following implantation of a continuous flow device (LVADs, BiVADs)

B. 1-year survival is highest for continuous flow LVADs (81%) followed in decreasing order by pulsatile flow LVADs (65%), total artificial heart (59%), continuous flow BiVADs (57%), and pulsatile flow BiVADs (45%)

IV. PHYSIOLOGIC BENEFITS OF MCS

A. LVADs assist the failing heart by
  1. Decreasing myocardial workload through reduction of left ventricular preload and myocardial oxygen consumption
  2. Augmenting systemic circulation maintaining adequate and consistent cardiac output (CO), which in turn improves organ perfusion
  3. Decreasing venous pressure

B. RVADs assist the failing heart by
  1. Unloading the right ventricle
  2. Augmenting pulmonary circulation
  3. Improving preload to left ventricle

V. PREIMPLANT PHASE: PATIENT SELECTION

A. An interdisciplinary team identifies patients who could benefit from transplantation or LVAD implantation as BTT or DT.
  1. This team typically includes interdisciplinary clinicians from the following services: cardiology, cardiovascular surgery, MCS coordinators, heart transplant coordinators, social service, nutrition, and palliative care, and optimally includes representatives from physical therapy, rehabilitation services, the finance department, pharmacy, infectious disease, endocrinology, and others involved in the care of these complex patients.[7]

B. Decisions regarding MCS are typically based on
  1. Clinical parameters (ability to meet eligibility criteria for cardiac transplantation or CMS guidelines for coverage noted above).
  2. International Society for Heart and Lung Transplantation (ISHLT) Guidelines for mechanical circulatory support (Table 10-1)[8]:
     a. See Table 10-2 for ISHLT classes of recommendations and levels of evidence.[9]
  3. Cardiac risk scores such as the ones listed below may be used to assist the team with selection and presenting patients with possibly a more accurate assessment of their survival and outcome should they proceed with LVAD:
     a. Seattle Heart Failure Score[10,11]: estimates mean life expectancy at 1, 2, and 5 years. The score is derived from the following variables:
        i. Continuous variables: age, LVEF, New York Heart Association class, blood pressure, weight-adjusted diuretic dose, lymphocyte count, hemoglobin, serum sodium, total cholesterol, uric acid
        ii. Categorical variables: sex, ischemic cardiomyopathy, QRS interval >120 ms, implantable cardioverter defibrillator (ICD)/cardiac

TABLE 10-1 International Society for Heart and Lung Transplantation Guidelines for Mechanical Circulatory Support (MCS): Recommendations for Evaluation, Clinical Classification, and Risk Stratification

	Recommendation	Class	Level of Evidence
Evaluation process	Assess patient for any reversible causes of heart failure.	I	A
	Assess patient for potential transplant candidacy.	I	A
Clinical classification	Assess patient's New York Heart Association functional class.	I	C
	Determine patient's Interagency Registry for Mechanically Assisted Support profile.	I	C
Risk stratification	Long-term MCS for patients in acute cardiogenic shock: reserve for patients: • With ventricular function that is unrecoverable or unlikely to recover without long-term MCS • Who are so ill that they cannot: – Maintain normal hemodynamics and organ function with temporary MCS. – Be weaned from temporary mechanical circulatory device or inotropic support. • Who have the capacity for recovery of end-organ function and quality of life: • Without irreversible end-organ damage	IIa	C
	Patients who are dependent on inotropic support: consider for MCS due to high mortality associated with medical management.	IIa	B
	Patients with end-stage systolic failure who are not in two previous risk stratification categories: monitor at regular intervals to reassess: • Level of risk • Need for MCS • Potential timing of MCS	IIa	C
	Patients at high risk for 1-year mortality: refer for advanced therapy such as: • Heart transplantation • MCS as bridge to transplantation • MCS as destination therapy	IIa	C

From Feldman D, Pamboukian SV, Teuteberg JJ, et al. The 2013 International Society for Heart and Lung Transplantation Guidelines for mechanical circulatory support: executive summary. *J Heart Lung Transplant.* 2013;32(2):157–187.

resynchronization therapy, and use of certain medications (β-blockers, angiotensin-converting enzyme inhibitors, angiotensin receptor blockers, potassium-sparing diuretics, statins, and allopurinol)

b. Heart Failure Survival Score: used to predict death, urgent heart transplantation (UNOS status 1), and ventricular assist device (VAD) implantation. The score is derived from the following variables[11,12]:
   i. Continuous variables: LVEF, resting heart rate (HR), mean blood pressure, peak oxygen consumption, and serum sodium
   ii. Categorical variables: ischemic cardiomyopathy and QRS interval > 120 ms

TABLE 10-2 International Society for Heart and Lung Transplantation Classes of Recommendations and Levels of Evidence

Class	Definition	Level of Evidence	Definition
1	Evidence and/or general agreement that a given treatment or procedure is beneficial, useful, and effective	A	Data derived from multiple randomized clinical trials or meta-analyses
2a	Conflicting evidence and/or divergence of opinion about the usefulness or efficacy of the treatment or procedure	B	Data derived from a single randomized clinical trial or large nonrandomized studies
2b	Weight of evidence or opinion is in favor of usefulness or efficacy.	C	Consensus of opinion of the experts and/or small studies, retrospective studies, registries
2c	Usefulness/efficacy is less well established by evidence/opinion.		
3	Evidence or general agreement that the treatment or procedure is not useful or effective and in some cases may be harmful.		

From International Society for Heart and Lung Transplantation Standards and Guidelines Document Development Protocol. Available at http://www.ishlt.org/ContentDocuments/ISHLT_Standards_and_Guidelines_Development_Protocol.pdf. Accessed June 27, 2015.

4. A psychosocial assessment (e.g., with the Stanford Integrated Psychosocial Assessment for Transplant [SIPAT] tool).[13]
5. It should be noted that individual centers use, score, and weigh these tools differently.

C. Decisions regarding patient selection and timing of LVAD implantation for DT are often guided by data from:
   1. The Randomized Evaluation of Mechanical Assistance for the Treatment of Congestive Heart Failure (REMATCH) trial[14]
   2. The Heart Mate II Trial[15]
   3. INTERMACS Registry[16]

D. Patients undergo a rigorous interdisciplinary evaluation of cardiovascular, noncardiovascular, and psychosocial factors that could influence postoperative outcomes.[8]

E. See Table 10-3 for the ISHLT Guidelines for MCS: Contraindications and Recommendations

 VI. INFORMED CONSENT PROCESS[8,17,18]

A. As part of the informed consent process, topics discussed with the patient/family include, but are not limited to, the following:
   1. Patient's and family's goals and expectations
   2. Patient's prognosis
   3. Progression of heart failure if LVAD is not implanted
   4. Risk/benefits of MCS implantation
   5. Impact (if any) on patient's eligibility for heart transplantation
   6. Transplant status post implant (if applicable)
   7. Potential perioperative and postoperative complications; impact of complications on potential eligibility for heart transplantation
   8. Survival rate post implant

TABLE 10-3 International Society for Heart and Lung Transplantation Guidelines for Mechanical Circulatory Support (MCS): Contraindications and Recommendations

	Contraindications	Class	Level of Evidence
Absolute in setting of:	Acute valvular infectious endocarditis with active bacteremia	III	C
	Active infection of an implantable cardioverter defibrillator or pacemaker with bacteremia	III	C
	Patient's inability to: • Operate the pump and/or respond to device alarms • Notify the MCS team of signs or symptoms of device malfunction or other health care problems	III	C
	Unsafe living environment for patient	III	C
	Demonstrated nonadherence with medical recommendations on several occasions	III	C
	Active substance abuse (including alcohol)	III	C
	Permanent dialysis	III	C
Relative in setting of:	Diabetes-related proliferative retinopathy, or severe nephropathy, vasculopathy, or peripheral neuropathy	IIb	C
	Very poor glycemic control	IIb	C
	Peripheral vascular disease (depends on extent and severity)	IIa	C
	Lack of sufficient social support	IIa	C
	Limited coping skills	IIa	C
	Significant caregiver burden or lack of any caregiver	IIb	C
MCS not recommended in setting of:	Irreversible multiorgan failure	III	C
	Neuromuscular disease that severely compromises the patient's ability to use and care for the device, ambulate, and exercise	III	C
	Active malignancy with a life expectancy of <2 y	III	C
	Active pregnancy	III	C
	Active psychiatric illness that impairs a patient's ability to care for the device or that requires long-term institutionalization.	III	C
Other	Patients with confirmed cirrhosis or increased Model for End-Stage Liver Disease score are poor candidates for MCS.	III	B

From Feldman D, Pamboukian SV, Teuteberg JJ, et al. The 2013 International Society for Heart and Lung Transplantation Guidelines for mechanical circulatory support: executive summary. *J Heart Lung Transplant*. 2013;32(2):157–187; International Society for Heart and Lung Transplantation Standards and Guidelines Document Development Protocol. Available at http://www.ishlt.org/ContentDocuments/ISHLT_Standards_and_Guidelines_Development_Protocol.pdf. Accessed June 27, 2015.

9. Necessary social support, including caregiver responsibilities and burden
10. Postoperative recovery, including pain management
11. Postimplant restrictions
12. Medications while MCS is in place
13. Device-specific instructions
14. Long-term care implications
15. Potential for survival following serious complications
16. Endpoints for and alternatives to MCS therapy
17. Advance directives

18. Insurance coverage and financial impact to the patient and family
19. Impact of noncompliance
20. Impact on Quality of Life, including limits imposed by the LVAD (such as no underwater activities)

B. Assessment of the patient's current quality of life can assist the patient in the decision-making process.

C. Although seemingly counterintuitive, an interdisciplinary palliative care consult at this time may be useful for[19]:
1. Providing emotional support for the patient and family
2. Documenting patient's and family's goals for implant
3. Developing a plan for potential complications
4. Advance care planning regarding end-of-life care and withdrawal of VAD support in alignment with the patient's advance directives

D. It is beneficial for both patients and their caregivers to meet with current LVAD patients and their caregivers to get a better understanding of what it is like to live with an LVAD.

E. Given the interplay of complex clinical, psychosocial, and ethical issues associated with VAD implantation, Petrucci and colleagues[20] proposed a triphase model for the informed consent process (Table 10-4). The timing and duration of each phase depends on the clinical status of the patient and is tailored to the patient's and family's needs.

TABLE 10-4 Triphase Model for Ventricular Assist Device Patient/Family Education and Informed Consent Process

Phase*	Topic	Description
Phase 1: initial information	Surgical intervention	Reason for VAD implantation
		Implications of elective vs. urgent VAD implantation
		Anticipated time of VAD implantation
		Specific devices available at institution
		Potential for device failure
		Potential need for device replacement
		Potential complications
	Device technology	Current device technology
		Risks, benefits, possible outcomes
		Potential need for additional surgical procedures
		VAD as "rescue" device rather than "cure" for heart failure
		Morbidity, mortality rates
	Expected recovery	Anticipated length of hospitalization
		Recovery trajectory
	Potential modification of care plan	Plan of care may change depending on physical, hemodynamic, or neurologic needs.
		Potential for change from "bridge to transplantation" to "destination therapy"
		Potential unexpected events: technical failure, pump replacement, withdrawal of device

(continued)

TABLE 10-4 **Triphase Model for Ventricular Assist Device Patient/Family Education and Informed Consent Process (*Continued*)**

Phase*	Topic	Description
Phase II: preimplant information	Care planning	Psychological and social aspects of "life with a VAD"
		Preparation of advance directives, living will, or health care power of attorney
	Appointing a decision-maker	Potential need for assessment of patient's mental capacity (e.g., neurologic and/or psychiatric evaluations)
		Appointment of family spokesperson to facilitate communication between interdisciplinary team and patient's family/friends
	Religious or cultural preferences	Patient's preferences in the event of withdrawal of VAD support
	Conflict resolution	Potential for ethics consultation in the event of unresolvable conflicts between family expectations and patient's clinical status and prognosis
Phase III: VAD-specific end-of-life care	Plan for palliative care	Potential postimplant end-of-life scenarios (e.g., device failure)
		Patient's preferences regarding potential aggressive management, palliative, or comfort care
		Definition and discussion of do not resuscitate/do not intubate orders
		Palliative care in home, hospital, hospice, other facility
	Plan for withdrawal of VAD support	Development of acceptable device withdrawal process for patient and family

*Timing and duration of each phase depends on the clinical status of the patient and is tailored to the patient's and family's needs.
From Petrucci RJ, Benish LA, Carrow BL, et al. Ethical considerations for ventricular assist device support: a 10-point model. *ASAIO J.* 2011;57(4):268–273.

E. With the increasing use of LVADs, numerous LVAD-related Internet, print, and multimedia educational resources materials are now available to patients and families.

1. A recent review of these materials indicated that many of these materials were suboptimal because they frequently[21]:
   a. Were biased toward proceeding with LVAD implantation
   b. Emphasized the benefits of LVADs but provided limited information on the risks, operative procedure, postimplant lifestyle, instructions for caregivers, or alternative therapies (e.g., palliative care)
   c. Cited outdated statistics
   d. Failed to explain the difference between DT and BTT
   e. Had a reading comprehension level > the eighth grade
   f. Failed to meet International Patient Decision Aid Standards
2. Clinicians should caution patients and family members about these shortcomings and encourage them to discuss their questions/concerns with members of the interdisciplinary MCS team.

VII. PREOPERATIVE EVALUATION AND PATIENT OPTIMIZATION

A. Renal function[8]

1. Assess and monitor renal function.
2. Patients with renal dysfunction, volume overload, and/or poor output:
   a. Optimize hemodynamic status (consider inotropic support).
   b. Aggressive diuresis or mechanical volume removal.
3. Following optimization of hemodynamic status, assess and monitor:
   a. Serum creatinine
   b. Blood urea nitrogen
   c. 24-hour urine for creatinine clearance and protein

B. Hepatic function

1. Screen for cirrhosis with ultrasound of the liver in the setting of:
   a. History of liver disease
   b. Abnormal liver function tests
   c. Chronic right heart failure
   d. Fontan physiology
2. Suspected cirrhosis[8]:
   a. Radiologic and tissue confirmation
   b. Hepatology consult
3. Abnormal liver function and hemodynamic decompensation:
   a. Aggressive therapy to restore hepatic blood flow and decrease hepatic congestion
4. In setting of elevated international normalized ratio (INR), which is not due to warfarin administration[8]:
   a. Consider treatment prior to MCS implantation.
   b. Optimize nutrition and right-side intracardiac filling pressures.
5. Note: Antiplatelet therapy is typically held for 4 to 7 days prior to LVAD implantation; INR should be normalized to minimize risk of bleeding.
6. Preoperative abnormal coagulation is common due to hepatic dysfunction.[22]

C. Pulmonary function[8]

1. Obtain chest radiograph and arterial blood gas.

D. Right ventricular function

1. Assessment with:
   a. Echocardiogram
   b. Invasive determination of intracardiac filling pressures
2. Management of right ventricular (RV) dysfunction
   a. Hospitalization for aggressive therapeutic options:
      i.   Diuresis
      ii. Ultrafiltration
      iii. Inotropic support
      iv. Pulmonary/RV afterload reduction
      v.   IABP
      vi. Short-term temporary MCS

E. Thoracic anatomy[8]

1. Computed tomography (CT) imaging or magnetic resonance imaging (MRI):
   a. Prior to MCS implantation
   b. In setting of prior surgery or suspected thoracic anomalies

F. Nutritional status
1. Malnutrition is common in patients with end-stage HF.[22]
    a. Approximately half of all patients with advanced HF experience weight loss
    b. Cardiac cachexia[23]:
        i.   Progressive wasting with concomitant inflammatory response
        ii. Body mass index (BMI) <24, weight loss of at least 5 kg over 6 months, and current weight <85% of ideal body weight
    c. Sequelae of malnutrition include[22,23] the following:
        i.   Compromised immune function
        ii.   Poor wound healing
        iii. Skeletal muscle atrophy that negatively impacts potential for postoperative recovery
        iv.   Prolonged hospitalization
        v.   Increased morbidity and mortality
2. Malnutrition may be due to a number of medical and psychological factors including[23] the following:
    a. Anorexia
    b. Early satiety
    c. Nausea subsequent to delayed gastric emptying
    d. Chronic, low-grade, systemic inflammation
    e. Excess production of gastric acid associated with emotional and physical stressors
    f. Decreased tolerance of food or medications
    g. Poor eating habits
3. A registered dietician, pharmacist, and physician with expertise in nutrition are key members of the interdisciplinary MCS team.[24]
4. Potential assessment tools[23]
    a. Physical examination
    b. Handgrip assessment
    c. Anthropometric assessment: BMI (may be misleading due to fluid retention)
    d. Diet and weight history
    e. Biochemical assessment: serum albumin and prealbumin; C-reactive protein[8]:
        i. Note: results may be influenced by many factors.[23]
5. Nutritional support[8]:
    a. Consider nutritional support for patients with malnutrition.[8]
    b. Potential nutritional support options:
        i.   Oral nutritional supplements
        ii.   Enteral nutrition
        iii. Parenteral nutrition
6. In the setting of severe malnutrition, consider delaying MCS implantation and optimizing nutritional status if the patient's clinical status permits.[8]
7. See Table 10-5 Nutrition Recommendations for VAD Patients.[23,25,26]

G. Infection[8]
1. Infection risk: prior to MCS implantation:
    a. Remove all unnecessary lines and catheters.
    b. Dental assessment and remedial treatment, time, and patient's clinical status permitting.
    c. Nasal swab to screen for methicillin-resistant *Staphylococcus aureus*; if results are positive, administer topical antibiotic treatment.
2. Active infection: administer appropriate antibiotic therapy per infectious disease specialist.

TABLE 10-5 **Nutritional Recommendations for Ventricular Assist Device Patients**

Parameter	Normal Weight	Obesity
Energy requirements	30–35 kcal/kg OR Resting metabolic rate + 15%–25% minimal, physical activity; additional 10% for hypermetabolism	Recommendation: metabolic cart to determine resting energy expenditure by measuring oxygen consumption and carbon dioxide production. Average: 21 kcal/kg actual weight
Protein requirements	1–1.5 g/kg	1.5–2.0 g/kg of ideal body weight
Sodium	2 g sodium	
Fluid	1.5–2.0 L	
Diet—oral	Small, frequent meals Encourage protein intake to meet metabolic demand.	
Enteral nutrition	Consider in following setting: severely ill patients who cannot start on oral diet within 24–48 h of ICU admission; hemodynamically unstable patients, particularly malnourished patients and/or those on vasopressors Consider placement of feeding tube into small intestine Hypo-osmolar, fiber-free formula, concentrated (i.e., 1.5 kcal/mL) In setting of enteral intolerance or ischemic bowel: initial rate = 10–20 mL/h	
Supplements	B vitamin: supplement in setting of poor oral intake or known deficiency Vitamin D: supplement in setting of known deficiency Zinc: supplement in setting of known deficiency	

Adapted from Montgomery TD, Cohen AE, Garnick J, et al. Nutrition assessment, care, and considerations of ventricular assist device patients. *Nutr Clin Pract.* 2012;27(2):352–362; Anderegg BA, Worrall C, Barbour E, et al. Comparison of resting energy prediction methods with measured resting energy expenditure in obese, hospitalized adults. *J Parenter Enteral Nutr.* 2009;33(2):168–175; Glynn CC, Greene GW, Winkler MF, et al. Predictive versus measured energy expenditure using limits-of-agreement analysis in hospitalized, obese patients. *J Parenter Enteral Nutr.* 1999;23(3):147–154.

 VIII. IMMEDIATE PREOPERATIVE PERIOD

A.   Patient/family education includes, but is not limited to
  1. Anticipated duration of surgery
  2. Periodic updates for family during surgery
  3. Transfer of patient from operating room (OR) to postanesthesia care unit (PACU) or intensive care unit (ICU)
  4. Plan of care following implant
  5. Plan for discharge education and training on use of LVAD

B.   Antibiotic prophylaxis:
  1. Preoperative antibiotics:
    a. Broad-spectrum gram-positive or gram-negative coverage as indicated[8]
  2. Routine prophylaxis[8]:
    a. Should include at least one dose prior to surgery (given within 60 minutes of first incision).
    b. Levels should remain within the therapeutic range throughout course of administration.
    c. Usual duration of coverage: 24 to 48 hours.[8,27]
  3. Whole-body skin prep to cleanse skin should be done the night before and morning of surgery.

C.   New Swan Ganz and arterial pressure lines are placed in the OR just prior to start of surgery to facilitate continuous monitoring.[8]

IX. SURGICAL PHASE

A. The surgical procedure, performed under general anesthesia, typically takes 6 to 8 hours, depending on
   1. The ventricle(s) supported (e.g., LVAD vs. BiVAD)
   2. History of prior sternotomy, prior coronary artery bypass graft surgery
   3. Preexisting comorbidities (e.g., coagulopathies)

B. OR personnel typically provide periodic updates to family members during the procedure.

C. The most common surgical approach is a mediastinal incision, but other methods have been used in certain circumstances.

D. Concurrent procedures are frequently performed as part of the primary LVAD implant surgery.
   1. These frequently include mitral or tricuspid valve replacement or repair as well as aortic valve repair or closure.[28]

E. Driveline site infection prevention starts in the OR by ensuring that the driveline is secured in a fixed location before the patient is transported from the OR.

F. A VAD-trained coordinator or other personnel responsible for the VAD should be in the OR during procedure for pump prep, monitoring and troubleshooting.[7]

X. POSTOPERATIVE PHASE: ICU

A. Arrival in the ICU
   1. Patient transferred to the ICU after surgery, intubated with
      a. Dressings in place over sternal incision and around driveline site
         i. The surgical dressings are typically left in place for 24 to 48 hours, unless bleeding from surgical wound necessitates removal.
         ii. Driveline dressings are changed by LVAD-trained personnel.
      b. Mediastinal, pericardial, and pleural drains
      c. Epicardial pacing wires
   2. Baseline laboratory studies upon arrival to the ICU typically include
      a. Complete blood cell (CBC) count
      b. Complete metabolic panel (CMP)
      c. Arterial blood gases (ABGs)
      d. Coagulation studies

B. Blood pressure (BP) monitoring
   1. Patients with nonpulsatile LVADs typically do not have a wide pulse pressure, which makes BP pressure measurement difficult.
   2. Typical mean arterial pressure (MAP) goal: 65 to 100 until right heart function is stabilized.
      a. It should be noted that the centrifugal flow pumps (such as the HeartWare HVAD) are more sensitive to delta p than axial flow devices.
         i. Delta p is the difference of pressure across the pump (preload pump pressure to afterload pressure the pump is pumping against). For this reason, tighter control of the MAP may be beneficial in patients with

centrifugal pumps, allowing them to have higher blood flow than if the delta p was higher.

b. The speed at which the pump is spinning determines if the BP is pulsatile with a systolic and diastolic pressure or laminar with just a mean arterial pressure. With current pump technology, any pulsatility is supplied by the native heart. Higher pump speeds, however, generally attenuate pulsatility by reducing LV volume available for ejection during systole.

c. Typically, current preference is to allow some pulsatility. Therefore, the LVAD speed is generally set to allow for this. However, the systolic pressure will be lower and the diastolic pressure higher than would be expected in patients without an LVAD.[8]

3. MAP is determined with direct arterial line measurement.

4. With a continuous flow VAD: once the arterial line has been removed, Doppler BP readings are correlated with automatic cuff pressure readings at least once per shift.

C. HR monitoring

1. Goal: typically normal sinus rhythm, 80 to 110 beats per minute

a. Keeping the HR on the higher end of this range may enhance right-sided heart function and output

D. Hemodynamic monitoring

1. Includes the following:

a. BP via an arterial line and, following removal of the arterial line, blood pressure via Doppler reading.

i. Note: pulsatile pumps will generate a normal BP reading, and continuous flow pumps will generate a lower systolic BP and a higher diastolic BP with normal MAP.

b. Pulmonary artery pressure (PAP) should be within normal limits.

c. Central venous pressure (CVP) should be within normal limits.

d. CO should provide a cardiac index (CI) >2.2.

e. Mixed venous oxygen saturation (SvO_2): maintain >70.

f. Oxygen saturation (pulse oximetry): maintain >92%.

g. Direct left atrial pressure (LAP) monitoring can simplify postoperative management and is used by some institutions.

i. Maintaining the LAP within normal limits helps with setting the speed of the pump; higher LAP allows for speed increases; lower LAP indicates that the pump may need to be slowed.

2. Obtain specific guidelines from the physician regarding acceptable hemodynamic parameters, monitor trends, and notify physician of any deviations.

3. NOTE: invasive lines including peripherally inserted central catheters, CVP, right atrial pressure, or PAP lines are contraindicated in patients with a TAH.

E. LVAD monitoring

1. The LVAD measures or calculates revolutions per minute (RPM), blood flow through the pump, power, and, in the case of HeartMate II, the pulsatility index (PI).

a. RPM and power are direct measurements.

b. Blood flow through the pump (flow) and PI are calculated values based on power and RPM.

2. Power is a direct measurement of the amount of energy needed to spin the rotor and is displayed as watts.
   a. Power can be affected by a variety of variables chief of which is the pump set speed.
   b. An increase in pump speed results in an increase in pump power.
   c. Note: a significant increase in power may indicate thrombosis formation on the rotor.
3. RPM:
   a. Pump speed is a direct measurement of the rotation rate of the rotor, which is the one variable that the clinician sets. Typical speed ranges vary according to the type of pump and are available from the manufacturer. Changes in speed more than 100 above or below the set speed should be addressed (could indicate a problem with the pump).
   b. RPM are adjusted to optimize flow. However, optimizing preload and afterload to the pump will have a greater impact on flow than RPM changes.
   c. Typically, a ramp (or sometimes referred to as a speed) echocardiogram is used to set RPM; during this study:
      i.   Pump speed is decreased to provide a low level of support.
      ii. Then the pump speed is increased over brief time intervals.
      iii. An echocardiogram displays the left heart volume, septal position, and valve function as LVAD speed is increased.[29]
      iv. A clinician familiar with the LVAD and ramp procedure adjusts the speed.
4. Flow is an approximation of the blood flow through the LVAD and is calculated from pump speed and power. Some VADs also take hematocrit into account when calculating flow. The flow rate should be sufficient to provide adequate CI for the patient.
5. PI is the magnitude of change in flow through the VAD during cardiac cycle associated with HR and contractility over a 15-second interval.
   a. Low PI may indicate a decrease in native right ventricular contractility or circulating blood volume.[28]
   b. NOTE: PI is only available with the HeartMate II LVAD.
   c. With the HeartWare HVAD, the waveform is the analogous parameter to PI.
6. Obtain specific guidelines from the physician regarding acceptable VAD parameters, monitor trends, and notify physician of any deviations.

F. Telemetry monitoring[30]

1. Ventricular dysrhythmias are common postoperatively and can impact LVAD flow by decreasing right-sided cardiac output resulting in less preload to the pump.[30]
   a. Average incidence, 33%; range, 22% to 53%
   b. Highest rates observed in the early postimplant period, particularly in the first 2 weeks. However, the absence of these dysrhythmias in the early postimplant period does not preclude their development later on.
2. Incessant ventricular dysrhythmias can precipitate hemodynamic compromise.[8]
3. Risk factors for ventricular dysrhythmias[30]:
   a. History of preimplant ventricular dysrhythmias (may double the risk of postimplant ventricular arrhythmias)
   b. Other potential risk factors:
      i.   Early increase in QT interval
      ii. Electrolyte imbalances
      iii. Preimplant history of atrial fibrillation

4. Potential etiology of ventricular dysrhythmias:
   a. Intracavitary suction events that obstruct the inflow cannula:
      i. Changes in venous return, high pump speed, or an increase in pulmonary resistance can cause negative pressure at the inflow cannula and precipitate a "suction event."
      ii. The "suction event" can draw the septum or left ventricular free wall closer to the inflow cannula and thereby precipitate the mechanical stimulation of the ventricular dysrhythmia.
   b. Myocardial fibrosis:
      i. Can increase susceptibility to dysrhythmias by changing myocyte excitability, decreasing conduction, and increasing ectopic activity
5. ISHLT guidelines for the management of ventricular tachycardia (VT)[8]:
   a. Identification and correction of electrolyte abnormalities or drug toxicities
   b. Cardioversion in the setting of poor device flows or hemodynamic compromise
   c. Antiarrhythmic agents for chronic VT:
      i. Beta-blockers
      ii. Amiodarone
   d. VT refractory to medical therapy: catheter ablation by an electrophysiologist with expertise in treating MCS patients
6. See section on "Dysrhythmias" below for additional information.

G. Respiratory function
1. Ventilator monitoring:
   a. Maintain ventilator settings per protocol.
   b. ISHLT ventilation parameters[8]:
      i.   Mode: assist/control
      ii. Rate: 10 to 12 breaths/min
      iii. Tidal volume: 6 to 8 mL/kg
      iv. Positive end-expiratory pressure: 5 cm H_2O
2. Blood gas monitoring:
   a. Pulse oximetry can be unreliable due to the variability of pulsatility with continuous flow pumps and the software within the pulse oximetry machinery.
   b. Therefore, it is important to confirm pulse oximetry values with arterial blood gas (ABG) analysis and observe pulse oximetry waveform for reliability.
3. Nitric oxide or other inhaled pulmonary vasodilators may be administered through the endotracheal tube to dilate the pulmonary vasculature and thus improve right ventricular function.
4. Ventilator weaning typically begins 8 to 10 hours after surgery when the patient
   a. Is off inhaled nitric oxide
   b. Has recovered from anesthesia and is alert and awake
   c. Is able to maintain adequate ventilation and oxygenation
   d. Meets weaning protocol parameters
5. Daily chest radiographs are obtained to monitor for respiratory infections or fluid collections.
6. Aggressive pulmonary toileting is continued post extubation to decrease the risk of pneumonia.

H. Fluid balance
  1. Measure and record daily weights:
     a. Note: a weight gain of more than 2 pounds in 24 hours could indicate fluid retention.
  2. Measure and record intake and output per protocol.[7]

I. Anticoagulation
  1. Generally, within a few days of surgery, both warfarin (Coumadin) and aspirin will be started to prevent thrombus formation within the LVAD.
  2. The anticoagulation regimen is specific to the patient, postoperative day, type of device, and institution.
     a. See Table 10-6 for ISHLT anticoagulation guidelines.[8]

J. Driveline site care
  1. Each institution has its own protocol for driveline site care with the goal of preventing infection.
  2. Driveline site infection remains the most prevalent adverse event for patients and has a direct impact on quality as well as length of life.
  3. Driveline site care is generally preformed using sterile technique initially.
     a. Some institutions will continue with sterile technique for the entire time the device is implanted.
     b. Other institutions use a sterile technique while the patient is hospitalized and change to a clean technique once the patient is discharged to home.

TABLE 10-6 International Society for Heart and Lung Transplantation Guidelines for Postoperative Anticoagulation Management

Time	HeartMate II Or Implantable Centrifugal Pump		Pulsatile MCS Device	
ICU admission—24 h	Consider acetylsalicylic acid		No action	
Postoperative day 1–2	If no evidence of bleeding: start IV heparin or other anticoagulation	Target PTT: 40–60 s		
Postoperative day 2			If no evidence of bleeding: start IV heparin or other anticoagulation	Target PTT: 40–60 s
Postoperative day 2–3	Continue heparin After removal of chest tubes, start warfarin and aspirin (81–325 mg/d)	Target PTT: 60–80 s Target INR: 2.0–3.0		
Postoperative day 3			Continue heparin After removal of chest tubes, start warfarin and aspirin (81–325 mg/d)	Target PTT: 60–80 s Target INR: 2.5–3.5

IV, intravenous; PTT, partial thromboplastin time; INR, international normalized ratio.
Adapted from Feldman D, Pamboukian SV, Teuteberg JJ, et al. The 2013 International Society for Heart and Lung Transplantation Guidelines for mechanical circulatory support: executive summary. *J Heart Lung Transplant.* 2013;32(2):157–187.

    4. Most institutions require the use of some type of dressing and device to secure the driveline during the entire time of the MCS is implanted.

      a. Trauma to the driveline site is directly related to development of an infection at the site.

      b. For this reason, some type of driveline securement device is generally used to prevent the driveline from being tugged or pulled out of position.

      c. Devices used to secure the driveline may include a modified abdominal binder, a driveline stabilization device, an adhesive dressing or a combination of these items.

    5. Observe site for signs of infection: redness, swelling, and exudate.

K. ISHLT Guidelines for Removal of Invasive Lines, Catheters, and Drains[8]:

    1. Pulmonary artery catheter: typically discontinued in 24 to 48 hours:

      a. Do not remove if the patient has severe right heart failure and is receiving high doses of inotropic agents.

    2. Arterial line: typically discontinued in 48 to 72 hours:

      a. Do not remove if the patient is receiving vasoactive medications.

    3. Central venous line: keep in place until no longer needed:

      a. Do not remove if the patient is receiving vasoactive medications.

    4. Chest tubes: typically removed at 48 hours or when chest tube drainage is < 100 mL in the preceding 6 hours

    5. Pocket drain: typically removed at 72 hours or when drainage is < 100 mL in the preceding 8 hours

L. Nutritional status[8]

    1. Goal: postoperative day 1: oral feeding

    2. Nutritional consult post implant and ongoing follow-up to monitor patient's progress and ensure that nutritional status is optimized

    3. If patient is not able to meet nutritional goals with oral feeding:

      a. Begin enteral feeding via a feeding tube.

      b. Parenteral nutrition: start only if enteral nutrition is not possible.

M. Mobility goal[8]

    1. Goal: postoperative day 1: up in chair

N. Other therapies

    1. Physical and occupational therapy should be started as soon as the patient is able to participate.

    2. Speech therapy is frequently consulted to assess the patient's swallowing ability and cognitive functioning.

      a. In some centers, speech therapists assist with LVAD education.

O. Discharge from ICU goal: postoperative day 3 to 5[8]

XI. POSTOPERATIVE PHASE: COMPLICATIONS

A. Infection

    1. Infections may be patient related or VAD related; infection-related complications remain a major limitation of LVAD therapy[31,32]

    2. ISHLT guidelines for evaluation of suspected infection[8]:

      a. All patients:

        i. CBC

        ii. Chest radiograph

iii. Blood cultures—at least:
- Three sets over 24 hours
- One culture from indwelling central venous catheters

b. Suspected cannula or driveline infection:
  i. Gram stain
  ii. Potassium hydroxide (KOH) test
  iii. Bacterial and fungal cultures

c. Aspirate from potential source of infection.

d. Radiographic studies as indicated.

e. Consider sedimentation rate or serial C-reactive protein levels.

3. Patient-related infections:
   a. Potential etiology:
      i. Organisms (bacterial or fungal) in blood, sputum, urine, or stool
      ii. Invasive lines
      iii. Surgical incisions
      iv. Prolonged intubation, immobilization, or hospitalization
      v. Reoperation
      vi. Poor nutritional status
   b. Potential manifestations:
      i. Increased temperature, HR, white blood cell count
      ii. Decreased BP, systemic vascular resistance (SVR)
   c. Potential considerations/interventions:
      i. Organism-specific antimicrobial therapy
      ii. Infectious disease consult
      iii. Removal of invasive lines and catheters if possible
      iv. Aggressive pulmonary toilet; extubate if possible
      v. Pharmacologic agents to increase BP and SVR
      vi. Fluid resuscitation as applicable
      vii. Small bowel feeding tube as applicable to maximize nutritional status
      viii. Mobilize patient as tolerated
      ix. Aggressive and appropriate VAD equipment cleaning protocols
   d. Monitor:
      i. Lab test results, particularly CBC count and differential
      ii. Wound site(s) for redness, swelling, exudate
      iii. Temperature (pan culture for temperature > 38.3 °C or >101 °F)
      iv. SVR, BP
      v. Nutritional status

4. VAD-related infections:
   a. Potential etiology[32]:
      i. The presence of a driveline that connects the device to an external control unit and power source through an open skin incision can lead to high rates of VAD-related infections.
      ii. Organisms (bacterial or fungal) in blood, sputum, urine, or stool:
         - Potential pathogens: span the entire spectrum of organisms.
         - Most common pathogens: gram-positive organisms (*Staphylococcus aureus* and coagulase-negative *Staphylococcus*).
         - Fungal infections, particularly *Candida* species, are associated with a high risk of mortality.
         - Antimicrobial-resistant organisms are common due to the prolonged hospitalizations and widespread use of broad-spectrum antimicrobial agents in this patient population.

  b. Classification: can involve any part of the LVAD[32]
   i. Driveline site:
- Can be localized or widespread, including infection of the bloodstream, endocarditis, and sepsis
- Can occur soon after implantation or later
- The most typical bacteria causing driveline infections are *Staphylococcus aureus* and *Pseudomonas aeruginosa*
- Frequently the source of other VAD-related infections

   ii. Pump pocket:
- Onset may be insidious.
- May lead to systemic manifestations and dissemination.

   iii. Pump:
- The inner portion of the device itself becomes infected.
- Can be caused by infection in other parts of the device or urinary or pulmonary infections.

  c. Potential manifestations:
   i. Elevated temperature, HR, white blood cell count
   ii. Decreased BP, decreased SVR

  d. Potential considerations/interventions:
   i. Infectious disease consult
   ii. Organism-specific antimicrobial therapy
   iii. Strict, sterile dressing changes using antiseptic solution (not creams) and occlusive dressing (on daily basis or more frequently if needed)
   iv. Antibiotic irrigation of exit site including driveline tunnel if applicable
   v. Surgical intervention with debridement and wound vac[33]
   vi. Replace VAD

  e. Monitor:
   i. Amount and characteristics of exudate on dressings
   ii. CBC with differential
   iii. Wound site(s) for redness, swelling, exudate
   iv. Temperature (pan culture for temperature > 38.3°C or >101°F)
   v. SVR, BP
   vi. Nutritional status

B. Bleeding
 1. Patient related:
  a. Potential etiology:
   i. Coagulopathy related to
- Liver dysfunction
- Preoperative anticoagulant therapy

   ii. Platelet dysfunction related to
- Prolonged cardiopulmonary bypass (CPB) time
- Preoperative antiplatelet therapy

   iii. Postoperative hemolysis
   iv. Clotting factor deficiency
   v. Hypothermia
   vi. History of cardiac surgery causing scar tissue, which is more prone to bleeding

b. Potential manifestations:
   i.   Chest tube drainage > 200 mL/hour within the first 12 hours postoperatively
   ii. Hypotension
   iii. Decreased hemoglobin, hematocrit
   iv. Sinus tachycardia
   v.   Hemodynamic parameters:
        • Decreased CVP
        • Decreased left atrial pressure
   vi. Signs/symptoms of tamponade:
        • Sudden decrease in chest tube drainage
        • Increased right atrial pressure/CVP
        • Hypotension; narrow pulse pressure
        • Sinus tachycardia
        • Decreased oxygen saturation
        • Diminished or absent peripheral pulses
        • Cyanosis
        • Decreased urine output
        • Widening cardiac silhouette on chest radiograph

c. Potential considerations/interventions:
   i.   Administration of blood products:
         • For transplant candidates: blood products should be leukocyte depleted and cytomegalovirus negative; may increase patient's panel reactive antibody (PRA) level.
         • Blood products may precipitate right-sided HF.
   ii.   Maintain slightly elevated filling pressures
   iii. Volume resuscitation
   iv.   Inotropic therapy
   v.   Pharmacologic agents (e.g., protamine)
   vi.   Discontinuing, decreasing, delaying, and/or reversing anticoagulant therapy
   vii. Increase positive end-expiratory pressure
   viii. Warming blanket for hypothermia
   ix.   Transesophageal echocardiogram (TEE) to diagnose or confirm tamponade
   x.   Reoperation to
         • Identify source of bleeding
         • Stabilize bleeding site
         • Evacuate hematomas

d. Monitor:
   i.   CBC, coagulation profiles.
   ii. Chest tube drainage.
   iii. Vital signs and hemodynamic parameters (particularly BP, HR, CVP, and left atrial pressure).
   iv. Volume status.
   v.   Signs/symptoms of right-sided HF.
   vi. Transplant candidates: recheck PRA.
   vii. For patients undergoing reoperation: observe for signs and symptoms of infection.

2. VAD related:
   a. Potential etiology:
      i.   Cannulation with bleeding at cannulation site
      ii. Fibrinolysis
   b. Potential manifestations:
      i.   Decreased VAD flows
      ii. Incomplete VAD filling
      iii. Decreased VAD stroke volume with pulsatile VAD
      iv. Tamponade:
         • Decreased VAD flows
         • Incomplete VAD filling
         • Decreased VAD stroke volume
   c. Potential considerations/interventions:
      i.   Reoperation to:
         • Identify source of bleeding
         • Stabilize bleeding site
         • Evacuate hematomas
   d. Monitor:
      i.   VAD parameters (flow rate, filling, stroke volume).
      ii. For patients undergoing reoperation: observe for signs or symptoms of infection.

C. Gastrointestinal (GI) bleeding
   1. Etiology:
      a. Patients with LVADs have frequent GI bleeding, especially from arteriovenous malformations that can occur throughout the GI tract, thought to be possibly related to the low pulse pressures associated with continuous flow pumps.[34]
   2. Source of bleeding:
      a. Bleeding can occur anywhere in the GI tract.
         i.   Esophagus
         ii. Stomach
         iii. Small intestine
         iv. Colon/rectum
      b. Often, it is difficult to determine the site of the bleeding.
      c. Published reports indicate that bleeding tends to occur more often in the upper GI tract.
   3. Manifestations:
      a. Decreased hemoglobin and hematocrit
      b. Blood in emesis or stool
   4. Diagnosis:
      a. Diagnosis of GI bleeding should include upper and lower endoscopy.
      b. If the suspected source of the bleeding is the small bowel, video capsule endoscopy may be warranted.
      c. Tagged red blood cell scan or angiography for persistent bleeding and negative endoscopic studies.[8]
   5. Potential considerations/interventions[8]:
      a. Gastroenterology consult for comanagement of patient.
      b. Anticoagulation therapy typically stopped during GI bleeding episode and may or may not be restarted depending on the patient and institution protocol.

   c. ISHLT guidelines for management of anticoagulation and antiplatelet therapy[8]:
     i. Patient presents with clinically significant bleeding:
- Hold anticoagulation and antiplatelet therapy.
- In absence of pump dysfunction, continue to hold anticoagulation and antiplatelet therapy until significant bleed resolves.
- Reverse anticoagulation if INR is elevated.
- Monitor patient, pump, and device parameters.

     ii. Recurrent GI bleeding:
- Gastroenterology consult with repeat endoscopic studies.
- If source of bleeding cannot be identified or cannot be treated, consider the severity of the bleeding and type of pump:
  - Reevaluate the use, type, and dose of antiplatelet therapy.
  - Reevaluate target INR and whether or not to continue warfarin therapy.
  - Monitor patient and device parameters.
- If recurrent bleeding is due to arteriovenous malformations and patient is on a continuous flow pump: consider reducing pump speed.

   d. Replace blood or blood products as needed.

6. Monitor:
   a. Labs (e.g., hemoglobin, hematocrit, INR, etc.)
   b. Pallor, feeling of fatigue
   c. BP
   d. Shortness of breath
   e. Patient, pump parameters

D. Dysrhythmias
  1. Patient related:
   a. Potential etiology:
     i. Myocardial ischemia or infarction
     ii. Drug toxicity
     iii. Hypoxia
     iv. Electrolyte imbalance
     v. Invasive monitoring lines
     vi. Underlying disease
   b. Potential manifestations:
     i. Hypotension
     ii. Decreased pump flow
     iii. Shortness of breath
     iv. Deterioration in mental status
     v. Thrombus formation in native heart
     vi. Pulmonary edema
     vii. Change in exercise tolerance
   c. Potential considerations/interventions:
     i. Determine clinical/hemodynamic effect of dysrhythmia.
     ii. Correct any electrolyte imbalance(s).
     iii. Remove invasive cardiac monitoring lines.
     iv. Wean inotropic support as soon as possible.
     v. Antiarrhythmic pharmacologic agents.

          vi. Electrical cardioversion.

          vii. Anticoagulation therapy.

     d. Monitor:

          i.   Electrocardiogram

          ii. Serum electrolytes; effectiveness of electrolyte replacement therapy

          iii. Oxygen saturation

2. VAD related:

     a. Potential etiology:

          i.   Irritability of native ventricle due to stimulation by inflow cannula

     b. Potential manifestations:

          i.   Decreased VAD flows

     c. Potential considerations/interventions:

          i.   Assess VAD performance.

          ii. Cardioversion, depending upon

            • Type of VAD

            • Type of dysrhythmia

          iii. Patients on LVAD with refractory dysrhythmia may require implantation of RVAD.

     d. Monitor:

          i.   Electrocardiogram

          ii. VAD flows

          iii. Patient's response to interventions

3. ISHLT guidelines for the management of atrial fibrillation and flutter[8]:

     a. Cardioversion in setting of rapid ventricular rates and compromised device function.

     b. In the setting of atrial fibrillation that does not compromise device function: follow current American College of Cardiology/American Heart Association guidelines.

4. ISHLT guidelines regarding implantable cardioverter defibrillators (ICD)[8]:

     a. Patients who had an ICD before implantation: reactivate ICD post implant.

     b. Consider ICD placement for patients without a prior ICD.

     c. Consider inactivation of the ICD for patients on optimal medical therapy and biventricular support who have

          i.   Persistent VT or ventricular fibrillation

          ii. Frequent sustained runs of VT

5. LVAD patients typically tolerate dysrhythmias.[35] However, defibrillation or cardioversion may be required, particularly in the setting of hemodynamic compromise. It is safe to defibrillate or cardiovert the patient with an LVAD if indicated. Follow hospital protocol.

6. Chest compressions, when needed, have produced successful outcomes and should be performed with care due to risk of dislodging the device.[35]

E. Hemolysis

1. Patient related:

     a. Potential etiology:

          i.   Effects of CPB

          ii. Blood transfusions

          iii. Liver failure

          iv. Coagulopathies

     b. Potential manifestations:

          i.   Decreased hemoglobin, hematocrit.

      ii.   Hematuria; tea-colored urine.

      iii. Plasma free hemoglobin value >15 mg/dL with or without clinical signs of deterioration.[36,37]

      iv. Increased lactate dehydrogenase (LDH) >100 or three times the baseline value or the upper limit of normal.

      v.   A Ramp echocardiogram can be used in conjunction with LDH levels.

  c. Potential considerations/interventions:

      i.   Judicious administration of blood products

  d. Monitor:

      i.   Vital signs

      ii.   Labs: CBC, liver function tests, and LDH

      iii. Coagulation profile

      iv. Plasma-free hemoglobin

      v.   Resolution of hematuria

2. VAD related:

  a. Potential etiology:

      i.   Passage of blood through foreign surface of the VAD

      ii.   Device thrombosis (early warning sign)

  b. Potential manifestations:

      i.   Decreased VAD flow

      ii.   Decreased VAD inflow or stroke volume (pulsatile VADs)

      iii. Incomplete filling of pump (pulsatile VADs)

  c. Potential considerations/interventions:

      i.   TEE to determine:

         • Position of VAD cannulae

         • Integrity of VAD valve (pulsatile VADs)

      ii.   Maximize filling of VAD pump to minimize trauma to blood cells (with pulsatile VADs)

  d. Monitor:

      i.   VAD function

F. Thromboembolism

1. Overview:

  a. Postimplant anticoagulation strategies require a balance between providing adequate anticoagulation to prevent complications such as hemolysis or thrombosis while preventing bleeding (e.g., gastrointestinal bleeding or neurological events).[36]

  b. These strategies are further complicated by the hematologic effects of continuous flow VADs.

  c. Potential sequelae of device thrombosis include neurological events (transient ischemic attacks, cerebral embolism, ischemic or hemorrhagic stroke) hemodynamic compromise, and death.[36]

2. Patient-related thromboembolism:

  a. Potential etiology:

      i.   Inadequate coagulation

  b. Potential manifestations: signs and symptoms of:

      i.   Organ or peripheral arterial occlusion

      ii.   Transient ischemic attack or cerebrovascular accident (e.g., mental status changes, neurologic deficits, seizures)

      iii. Abnormal computed tomography scan, electroencephalogram, ultrasound

    c. Potential considerations/interventions:
       i. Obtain coagulation profile.
       ii. Maintain adequate device-specific anticoagulation.
       iii. Maintain adequate blood pressure.
       iv. TEE to determine presence of native heart thrombus.
    d. Monitor:
       i. Coagulation profiles
       ii. Patient for resolution of presenting signs/symptoms

3. VAD-related thromboembolism:
    a. Potential location of thrombus:
       i. LVAD thrombosis is evidenced by the development of a blood clot in one of the components of the LVAD, including the inflow cannula, outflow cannula, or the rotor.
       ii. Pump thrombus is defined as recurrent, consistent pump controller power spikes, echocardiographic demonstration of thrombus, or pump failure.
    b. Potential etiology:
       i. Incomplete VAD ejection
       ii. Kinking or obstruction of cannulae
       iii. Low VAD flows
       iv. Low VAD stroke volume (with pulsatile VAD)
    c. Potential manifestations:
       i. Obstruction of inflow or outflow valves, which leads to decreased filling or emptying of VAD (pulsatile VADs).
       ii. Failure of the left ventricular end-diastolic diameter to decrease in response to increasing LVAD speed.
       iii. The echocardiogram is typically checked to measure left ventricular end-systolic and end-diastolic diameter, mitral regurgitation, aortic insufficiency, inflow cannula velocity, and right ventricular function.
          • The echocardiogram can show a dilated ventricle, severe mitral regurgitation, and frequency of aortic valve opening.
    d. Potential considerations/interventions:
       i. Check for kinking of cannulae or pneumatic cables.
       ii. Confirm and maintain adequate VAD ejection and flow.
       iii. Determine presence and location of thrombus with:
          • TEE
          • A left ventriculogram
       iv. Hospitalization advised if pump thrombus suspected.
       v. Patients may be started on heparin infusion therapy unless contraindicated.
       vi. Patients experiencing HF symptoms may require diuresis and inotropic support.
       vii. Severe pump thrombosis that does not respond to therapy may necessitate pump exchange and is favored over the use of lytic therapies.
    e. Monitor:
       i. VAD flows
       ii. Coagulation profiles
       iii. Fluid status in patients requiring diuresis
       iv. Daily hematologic markers and echocardiogram for signs of improvement

G. Right-sided HF
  1. Patient related:
     a. Potential etiology:
        i. Preoperative risk factors for right HF (e.g., pulmonary edema, increased need for inotropic support).
        ii. Bleeding: multiple blood transfusions can precipitate volume overload and increased pulmonary vascular resistance (PVR), which in turn can cause right-sided HF.
        iii. Pulmonary hypertension.
        iv. Pulmonary infarct.
        v. Right ventricular infarct or septal defects.
        vi. Dysrhythmias.
     b. Potential manifestations
        i. Increased right atrial pressure ± decreased left atrial pressure
        ii. Increased PVR
        iii. Decreased SaO$_2$
        iv. Liver congestion; jaundice
        v. Peripheral edema
        vi. Atrial dysrhythmias
        vii. On TEE: dilated right ventricle, acute tricuspid regurgitation, inadequate filling of left atrium and left ventricle; septal shift to the left ventricle
     c. Potential considerations/interventions:
        i. Inotropic agents (milrinone [Primacor]; dobutamine)
        ii. Pulmonary vasodilators; nitric oxide
        iii. Fluid management to avoid overloading right ventricle
        iv. Judicious use of blood products (if required)
        v. Hyperventilation (patients with increased PVR)
        vi. TEE to evaluate native heart
        vii. Reduce VAD speed to allow septum to move to midline
        viii. Implantation of RVAD (Note: progressive decline of right ventricle should initially respond to medical management but may ultimately require off-label use of RVAD.)
     d. Monitor:
        i. Fluid status
        ii. Hemodynamic parameters
        iii. Patient's response to treatment
        iv. LVAD flow
  2. VAD related:
     a. Potential etiology:
        i. Physiological implications associated with unloading the left ventricle
     b. Potential manifestations:
        i. Decreased LVAD flow, PI, waveforms (continuous flow VADs)
        ii. Decreased LVAD filling (pulsatile VADs)
        iii. Decreased LVAD stroke volume (pulsatile VADs)
        iv. Decreased LVAD outflow
     c. Potential considerations/interventions:
        i. Consider TEE to evaluate function of native heart and VAD.
        ii. Implant RVAD.
        iii. Adjust VAD parameters to maximize forward flow.

      d. Monitor:
         i. VAD flows
         ii. Patient's response to therapeutic interventions
   3. RV dysfunction following LVAD implantation[8]:
      a. Potential late manifestation
      b. Clinical presentation:
         i. Signs/symptoms of right-sided HF
         ii. Decrease in flow and pulsatility
      c. Workup:
         i. Right heart catheterization
         ii. Echocardiogram
      d. Potential treatment option: inotropic support

H. Aortic Insufficiency (AI)
   1. Acquired AI can be complication of long-term VAD support.
      a. Noted in 25% to 50% of patients at 1 year post implantation of a continuous flow LVAD[38]
   2. Severity of AI often progresses in patients with preimplant AI.[39]
   3. Potential etiology[38]:
      a. Degeneration of the aortic valve
      b. Dilatation of the aortic sinus
      c. Increased transvalvular gradients with high pulsitile LVAD support
      d. Results in flow loop from aorta through aortic valve and back to LV
   4. Diagnosis: thoracic echocardiogram
   5. Potential manifestation:
      a. Signs and symptoms of HF[38]:
         i. Left-sided HF symptoms associated with elevated left ventricular end-diastolic pressures
         ii. Right-sided HF symptoms secondary to left-sided HF and reactive pulmonary hypertension
      b. Signs and symptoms of end-organ malperfusion[39]:
         i. Severe AI can compromise LVAD output and lead to decreased end-organ perfusion.
   6. Potential considerations/interventions[38]:
      a. Lesser degrees of AI can be managed medically.
      b. Patients with clinical HF and significant AI:
         i. Diuretic therapy to maintain euvolemia:
            • Monitor patient for hypovolemia, orthostatic hypotension, and device alarms.
         ii. Patient with refractory dyspnea: continuous flow LVAD pump speed optimization:
            • Performed under right heart catheterization guidance
         iii. Severe AI refractory to medical management: surgical correction

I. Device malfunction
   1. Patient related:
      a. Potential etiology:
         i. Patient mismanagement of VAD
      b. Potential manifestations:
         i. Decompensating hemodynamic parameters
         ii. Decreased level of consciousness
         iii. Mental status changes
         iv. Cool, clammy extremities, cyanosis

c. Potential considerations/interventions:
   i. Volume resuscitation.
   ii. Inotropic and/or chronotropic support.
   iii. Reinforce patient/family education on VAD operation, alarms, activation of EMS, etc.
d. Monitor
   i. Patient's response to therapeutic interventions
   ii. Patient's/family's understanding of VAD operation

2. VAD related:
   a. Potential etiology:
      i. Motor failure of corporeal VAD
      ii. Kink or air leak in pneumatic cables (pulsatile VAD)
      iii. Fractured wires in driveline cables
      iv. Console or controller malfunction
      v. Power source malfunction
   b. Potential manifestations:
      i. Audible or visual VAD alarms
      ii. Absence of audible or visual indicators of pump function
      iii. Severely low to no VAD filling (stroke volume) or emptying (flow or output)
   c. Potential considerations/interventions:
      i. Manually pump to avoid blood stasis and clotting (pulsatile VAD).
      ii. Systemic anticoagulation.
      iii. Check all connections; correct any obstructions.
      iv. Replace any defective equipment (e.g., consoles, controllers, cables, power source, etc.).
      v. Access backup equipment.
      vi. Exchange pump if necessary and patient is sufficiently stable to undergo surgery (noting potential for increased risk of mortality associated with exchange of corporeal pumps).
   d. Monitor:
      i. Patient's response to VAD interventions
      ii. VAD parameters

 XII. POSTOPERATIVE PHASE—TRANSFER FROM ICU

A. Transfer protocols are hospital specific.

B. In some cases, the patients remain in the same unit from OR to discharge home, while in other institutions, the patients will be transferred from a higher to lower level of nursing care as they recover, moving from the ICU to telemetry floor and then possibly to the rehabilitation unit prior to discharge.

C. Staff caring for the LVAD patient must have had initial LVAD training as well as ongoing competency evaluation.

D. The organization provides training to the staff in accordance with the interaction they have with the patient.[7]
   1. Awareness training is specific to the center and may vary in complexity from general awareness of the program to more detailed instruction regarding the types of VADs used and simplified emergency procedures.

XIII. DISCHARGE PREPARATION

A. Education for patients and family members/caregivers includes detailed information regarding self-care maintenance, self-care monitoring, and self-care management (Table 10-7).

B. In addition, patients are given information regarding:

1. Standard postcardiac sternotomy instructions:
   a. No lifting >10 lb for the first 6 weeks following surgery
   b. No driving for 6 weeks
   c. Incisional care

TABLE 10-7 Self-Care Education After Left Ventricular Assist Device Implantation

Domain	Definition	Examples

Self-care maintenance	"Behaviors to improve well-being, preserve health or maintain physical and emotional stability"[41 (p. 196)]	**Maintenance of LVAD**
		Operation of LVAD system:
		• System maintenance
		• Adequate power source
		Percutaneous lead care:
		• Immobilization of lead
		• Wound surveillance and management
		Lifestyle:
		• Hygiene and personal care
		• Adherence with medication taking
		• Adaptation of physical activity:
		  – Physical exercise
		  – Restriction from certain activities
		  – Sexual activity (e.g., performance enhancing agents; birth control)
		• Nutrition
		• Smoking abstinence/cessation
		• Sleep and rest
		• Optimization of caregiver well-being

Self-care monitoring	"Process of routine, vigilant body monitoring, surveillance, or 'body listening'"[41 (p. 196)]	**Monitoring**
		• LVAD device/system:
		  – Checking wires, controllers, batteries
		  – Recognition of pump malfunction
		• Visual inspection of percutaneous lead + exit site
		• Signs and symptoms:
		  – Heart failure
		  – Volume status
		  – Blood pressure
		• Side effects + complications:
		  – Infection
		  – Bleeding
		  – Neurological events
		• Psychological distress
		• Caregiver burden

(continued)

TABLE 10-7 **Self-Care Education After Left Ventricular Assist Device Implantation (*Continued*)**

Domain	Definition	Examples

Self-care management	"Evaluation of changes in physical and emotional signs and symptoms to determine if action is needed"[41 (pp. 196–197)]	**Management**
		• LVAD alarm recognition and response; emergency response skills
		• Emergency identification card with device information
		• Emergency on-call algorithm for notification of LVAD team
		• Adaptation of percutaneous lead and wound management
		• Adjustment of medications, diet, rest
		• Exercise guidelines and precautions
		• Patient and caregiver coping:
		  – Adjustment of self-concept, self-image
		  – Coping skills

Adapted from Kato N, Jaarsma T, Ben Gal T. Learning self-care after left ventricular assist device implantation. *Curr Heart Fail Rep.* 2014;11:290–298, Ref.[40]; Riegel B, Jaarsma T, Stromberg A. A middle-range theory of self-care of chronic illness. *ANS Adv Nurs Sci.* 2012;35(3):194–204, Ref.[41]

2. Showering:
   a. Patients are advised to avoid showering until the skin is well approximated around the driveline.
   b. Patients are provided with a shower kit and taught how to protect equipment as well as driveline site while showering.
3. Medications: see Table 10-8.
4. Follow-up appointments.

C. The MCS coordinator will be primarily responsible for this education, but all staff members must assist in the education process as it takes repetition for patients and caregivers to become familiar with the equipment and be able to safely manage their VAD equipment at home.

D. Community outreach:
   1. Notification of life safety personnel:
      a. Prior to discharge, the patient's home electric power provider must be notified of the potential need for emergency power.
      b. The local emergency medical system (EMS) should be notified of the patient's discharge:
         i. Regional EMS training is provided by the implanting hospital in conjunction with the EMS education department and the device manufacturer's training clinicians.
   2. Notification of patient's local health care providers and emergency department.
   3. Patients and their caregivers are frequently asked to visit their local fire station to ensure that the local responders are aware that they live in the area and know how to contact the implanting facility's MCS coordinators for further questions.[7]

TABLE 10-8 **Common Medications Postimplantation of a Left Ventricular Assist Device: Indications and Rationale**

Medication	Indication	Rational
Antiplatelet therapy		
H$_2$ antagonist (e.g., ranitidine)	Prevent gastric reflux	Gastrointestinal distress, potentiated by abdominal placement of the pump, can compromise nutritional status.
Prokinetic (e.g., metoclopramide [Reglan])	Stimulates muscles of gastrointestinal tract; promotes upper gastric motility	Premature satiation, due to abdominal placement of pump, can compromise nutritional status.
Antihypertensive agents	Prevent hypertension	In certain pumps, hypertension can compromise pump output.
Diuretics	Prevent fluid overload	Third spacing of fluid secondary to end-stage heart failure may require pharmacologic support initially as immediate postoperative extra- and intravascular volumes equilibrate.
Antimicrobial therapy	Prevent or treat infection	Both the device and the patient are susceptible to infection that may result in life-threatening sepsis.

E. Home environment: safety requirements[8]:
1. Supply of electricity; development of emergency plan if home electricity becomes unavailable. This should be evaluated preoperatively and is part of the evaluation for candidacy.
2. Use of grounded outlets
3. Avoidance of extension cords or outlets controlled by a switch
4. Working telephone. This should be evaluated preoperatively and is part of the evaluation for candidacy.
5. Placement of VAD equipment in a manner that minimizes risk of falls and permits caregivers to hear alarms
6. Other equipment as needed (e.g., shower chair, portable commode)

F. A discharge checklist is useful in ensuring that all predischarge preparations have been completed; for example:
1. Patient/caregiver completed and passed training on VAD operation and care of exit site.
2. Discharge teaching; demonstrations and return demonstrations.
3. Predischarge echocardiogram.
4. Completion of "day passes," or "field trips" either remaining within hospital grounds or leaving the hospital (if applicable and dependent on insurance company acceptance).
5. Supplies for VAD home use ordered and delivered (including supplies for dressing changes).
6. Patient provided with hospital emergency contact names/numbers.
7. Medical identification bracelet (if applicable).
8. Follow-up appointment date; equipment to bring to appointment.

XIV. FOLLOW-UP CLINIC APPOINTMENTS[8]

A.   Patients are followed by an interdisciplinary team that includes cardiovascular surgeons, advanced heart failure cardiologists, specialized MCS coordinators, and consultants with additional expertise as required.

B.   Frequency of outpatient clinic visits is determined by the patient's clinical status.

C.   Tests are scheduled on a routine basis to evaluate, assess, and screen patients:
1. Evaluate end-organ function.
2. Reassess any device-related issues.
3. Identify or monitor any patient- or device-related complications.

D.   Clinic visit:
1. Patient assessment:
a. Clinical:
i.   Vital signs
ii. Driveline exit site
b. Psychosocial:
i.   Patient/caregiver adjustment to discharge status
ii. Problems encountered
2. VAD assessment:
a. Integrity and performance of device, including VAD parameters
b. VAD history interrogation to detect unreported malfunctions
c. Position and immobilization of driveline
3. VAD equipment and supplies needed
4. Education:
a. Patient/caregiver recall of device operation, alarms, etc.
b. Reinforcement of need for ongoing gender- and age-specific health care screening tests, vaccinations, and dental care

XV. LVAD PATIENTS AT HOME

A.   Most patients with LVADs are able to live at home. Many return to work and resume their previous activities.

B.   Long-term activity restrictions for LVAD patients include
1. Underwater activities or those with risk of submersion
2. Contact sports (to prevent trauma to the driveline site and damage to the LVAD equipment)
3. MRIs

C.   Pregnancy is contraindicated during the course of MCS implantation.

D.   Many patients with LVADs travel for work or pleasure. The MCS team should provide the patient with
1. A travel letter directed to Transportation Security Administration agents describing the equipment implanted and what must remain with the patient in the cabin of an aircraft
2. A list of local contacts for emergency assistance as close as possible to where the patient will be staying

XVI. PERIOPERATIVE MANAGEMENT OF LVAD PATIENTS UNDERGOING NONCARDIAC SURGERY

A. The care of the LVAD patient intraoperatively can be challenging.

   1. Ideally, these patients should be cared for at an institution that is familiar with dealing with the complexities of the LVAD.[42]

   2. For noncardiac procedures near the area of the device itself, a cardiovascular surgeon should be in the OR or immediately available.[8]

B. The MCS team should be notified when an MCS patient requires noncardiac surgery.[8]

   1. The MCS team can provide information regarding anticoagulation or antiplatelet therapy (Table 10-9), LVAD settings, duration of implantation, and any complications associated with the LVAD.

C. All LVAD patients should be accompanied by an experienced clinician who is familiar with the device management and alerts.[7,8]

D. Patient monitoring[8]:

   1. MCS parameters should be continuously monitored by MSC nurses or perfusionists.

   2. Minor procedures: blood pressure monitoring with Doppler.

   3. Procedures with risk of hemodynamic instability:

      a. Arterial catheter for blood pressure monitoring

      b. Central venous catheter for monitoring CVP or administering medications

TABLE 10-9 International Society for Heart and Lung Transplantation: Recommendations for Management of Mechanical Circulatory Support Patients Undergoing Noncardiac Procedures: Anticoagulation and Antiplatelet Therapy

Type of Procedure	Recommendation	Class	Level of Evidence
Nonemergency	May continue warfarin and antiplatelet therapy if procedure-associated risk of bleeding is low	I	C
	If therapy must be stopped: hold for appropriate length of time based on operative procedure and risk of bleeding	1	C
	Consider use of heparin or heparin alternative while patient is not receiving warfarin.	1	C
Emergency	May need to rapidly reverse warfarin (fresh frozen plasma, prothrombin protein concentrate)	1	B
	Vitamin K: give with caution; slow onset of action		
Following surgical procedure	When postoperative risk of bleeding is considered acceptable, resume warfarin and antiplatelet therapy.	1	B
	May bridge patient with heparin or heparin alternative until INR reaches target	1	B

INR, international normalized ratio.
From Feldman D, Pamboukian SV, Teuteberg JJ, et al. The 2013 International Society for Heart and Lung Transplantation Guidelines for mechanical circulatory support: executive summary. *J Heart Lung Transplant.* 2013;32(2):157–187.

XVII. PALLIATIVE CARE, END-OF-LIFE CARE, AND DEACTIVATION OF DEVICE

A. It is important to discuss end-of-life issues with patient and caregivers prior to implant and readdress this issue when major events occur.

1. This open discussion should address the patient's concept of end of life (e.g., what "end of life" would look like to the patient).[43]

2. Informed consent should include the completion of advance directives prior to implant, particularly when the LVAD is implanted for DT.

B. In the United States[44]:

1. Patients have the right to refuse or request the withdrawal of unwanted life-sustaining treatments (e.g., mechanical ventilation, hemodialysis, artificial hydration, and nutrition).

2. Clinicians can ethically and legally comply with such requests.

3. Physicians are not obliged to provide treatments that they believe are futile.[45]

C. Many experts agree that if a patient is informed of and understands the alternatives to and consequences of withdrawing support, clinicians should honor such requests or transfer the patient's care to another clinician who is willing to honor the patient's request.[46]

D. An ethics consult is useful in addressing concerns raised by the patient, family, or members of the health care team.

E. The palliative care team can optimize end-of-life care by assisting with clinical decision-making, symptom management, and the provision of psychological, psychosocial, and spiritual care for the patient and family[47]

F. If a patient requests end-of-life care, the patient and family members should be advised of[44]

1. Potential symptoms the patient may experience

2. Appropriate treatment to palliate symptoms (e.g., opioids for dyspnea)

3. The availability of spiritual care

G. The LVAD pump should be disconnected from power once the patient requests withdrawal of support, is declared brain dead, or has stopped breathing. Disconnecting the LVAD is withdrawal of life-sustaining support and should be done per hospital policy.

H. Steps to disconnecting the LVAD pump:

1. Confirm do not resuscitate (DNR)/do not intubate (DNI) status.

2. The process of disconnecting the LVAD should be clearly outlined and understood by those who are participating.

3. If the patient is receiving other forms of life-sustaining treatments including an implantable defibrillator, dialysis, tube feedings, vasopressors, and mechanical ventilation, these should be discontinued before or at time of disconnecting the LVAD.

4. Survival after disconnecting the LVAD can range from minutes to a few days.

5. As with any patient during the withdrawal of life support, staff must be prepared to treat labored breathing, agitation, and/or other signs of discomfort.[44]

REFERENCES

1. Chen-Scarabelli C, Saravolatz L, Hirsh B, et al. Dilemmas in end-stage heart failure. *J Geriatr Cardiol.* 2015;12:57–65.
2. Lund LH, Edwards LB, Kucheryavaya AY, et al. The Registry of the International Society for Heart and Lung Transplantation—2014; Focus Theme: Retransplantation. *J Heart Lung Transplant.* 2014;33(10):1009–1024.
3. Dipchand AI, Edwards LB, Kucheryavaya AY, et al. The Registry of the International Society for Heart and Lung Transplantation: Seventeenth Official Pediatric Heart Transplantation Report—2014; Focus Theme: Retransplantation. *J Heart Lung Transplant.* 2014;33(10):985–995.
4. Adamson R, Stahovich M, Chillcott S, et al. Clinical strategies and outcomes in ventricular assist device. *J Am Coll Cardiol.* 2011;57(25):2487–2495.
5. The Centers for Medicare and Medicaid. *MLN Matters.* Available at http://www.cms.gov/Outreach-and-Education/Medicare-Learning-Network-MLN/MLNMattersArticles/downloads/MM7220.pdf. Accessed June 25, 2015.
6. Kirklin JK, Naftel DC, Pagani FD, et al. Sixth INTERMACS annual report: a 10,000-patient database. *J Heart Lung Transplant.* 2014;33:555–564.
7. The Joint Commission. Modified: ventricular assist device destination therapy requirements. *Jt Comm Perspect.* 2014;34(2):6–7. Available at http://www.jointcommission.org/assets/1/18/Ventricular_Assist_Device_Destination_Therapy_Requirements.pdf. Accessed June 26, 2015.
8. Feldman D, Pamboukian SV, Teuteberg JJ, et al. The 2013 International Society for Heart and Lung Transplantation Guidelines for mechanical circulatory support: executive summary. *J Heart Lung Transplant.* 2013;32(2):157–187.
9. International Society for Heart and Lung Transplantation Standards and Guidelines Document Development Protocol. Available at http://www.ishlt.org/ContentDocuments/ISHLT_Standards_and_Guidelines_Development_Protocol.pdf. Accessed June 27, 2015.
10. Levy WC, Mozaffarian D, Linker DT, et al. The Seattle heart failure model: prediction of survival in heart failure. *Circulation.* 2006;113(11):1424–1433.
11. Alba AC, Agoritsas T, Jankowski M, et al. Risk prediction models for mortality in ambulatory patients with heart failure. *Circ Heart Fail.* 2013;6:881–889.
12. Aaronson KD, Schwartz JS, Chen TM, et al. Development and prospective validation of a clinical index to predict survival in ambulatory patients referred for cardiac transplant evaluation. *Circulation.* 1997;95:2660–2667.
13. Maldonado JR, Dubois HC, David EE, et al. The Stanford Integrated Psychosocial Assessment for Transplantation (SIPAT): a new tool for the psychosocial evaluation of pre-transplant candidates. *Psychosomatics.* 2012;53(2):123–132.
14. Rose EA, Gelijns AC, Moscowitz AJ, et al. Long-term use of a left ventricular assist device for end-stage heart failure. *N Engl J Med.* 2001:345(20):1435–1443.
15. Miller LW, Pagani FD, Russell SD, et al. Use of a continuous-flow device in patients awaiting heart transplantation. *N Engl J Med.* 1997;357:885–896.
16. The Interagency Registry for Mechanically Assisted Circulatory Support. Available at http://www.uab.edu/medicine/intermacs. Accessed June 26, 2015.
17. McLean S, Dhonnchu TN, Mahon N, et al. Left ventricular assist device withdrawal: an ethical decision. *BMJ Support Palliat Care.* 2014;4:193–195.
18. Edlund JE, Edlund AE, Carey MG. Patient understanding of potential risk and benefit with informed consent in a left ventricular assist device population: a pilot study. *J Cardiovasc Nurs.* 2015;30(5):435–439.
19. McGonigal P. Improving end-of-life care for ventricular assist device (VAD) patients: paradox or protocol? *Omega.* 2013;67(1–2):161–166.
20. Petrucci RJ, Benish LA, Carrow BL, et al. Ethical considerations for ventricular assist device support: a 10-point model. *ASAIO J.* 2011;57(4):268–273.
21. Iacovetto MC, Matlock DD, McIlvennan CK, et al. Educational resources for patients considering a left ventricular assist device: a cross-sectional review of Internet, print, and multimedia materials. *Circ Cardiovasc Qual Outcomes.* 2014;7:905–911.
22. Khazanie P, Rogers JG. Patient selection for ventricular assist devices. *Congest Heart Fail.* 2011;17(5):227–234.
23. Montgomery TD, Cohen AE, Garnick J, et al. Nutrition assessment, care, and considerations of ventricular assist device patients. *Nutr Clin Pract.* 2012;27(2):352–362.
24. Holdy K, Dembitsky W, Eaton LL, et al. Nutrition assessment and management of left ventricular assist device. *J Heart Lung Transplant.* 2005;24(10):1690–1696.
25. Anderegg BA, Worrall C, Barbour E, et al. Comparison of resting energy prediction methods with measured resting energy expenditure in obese, hospitalized adults. *J Parenter Enteral Nutr.* 2009;33(2):168–175.
26. Glynn CC, Greene GW, Winkler MF, et al. Predictive versus measured energy expenditure using limits-of-agreement analysis in hospitalized, obese patients. *J Parenter Enteral Nutr.* 1999;23(3):147–154.

27. Walker PC, DePestel DD, Miles NA, et al. Surgical infection prophylaxis for left ventricular assist device implantation. *J Card Surg.* 2011;26(4):440–443.

28. Slaughter MS, Pagani FD, Rogers JC, et al. Clinical management of continuous-flow left ventricular assist devices in advanced heart failure. *J Heart Lung Transplant.* 2010;29:S1–S39.

29. Estep JD, Stainback RF, Little SH, et al. The role of echocardiography and other imaging modalities in patients with left ventricular assist devices. *JACC Cardiovasc Imaging.* 2010;3:1049–1064.

30. Pedrotty DM, Rame JE, Margulies, KB. Management of ventricular arrhythmias in patients with ventricular assist devices. *Curr Opin Cardiol.* 2013;28(3):360–368.

31. Topkara VK, Kondareddy S, Malik F, et al. Infectious complications in patients with left ventricular assist device: etiology and outcomes in the continuous-flow era. *Ann Thorac Surg.* 2010;90:1270–1277.

32. Califano S, Pagani FD, Malani PN. Left ventricular assist device-associated infections. *Infect Dis Clin North Am.* 2012;26:77–87.

33. Stahovich M, Baradarian S, Chillcott S, et al. Management of LVAD driveline site using the vacuum-assisted closure (VAC) device. *ASAIO J.* 2005;51(2):22A.

34. Islam S, Cevik C, Madonna R, et al. Left ventricular assist devices and gastrointestinal bleeding: a narrative review of case reports and case series. *Clin Cardiol.* 2013;36(4):190–200.

35. Shinar Z, Bellezzo J, Stahovich M, et al. Chest compressions may be safe in arresting patients with left ventricular assist devices (LVADs). *Resuscitation.* 2014;82(5):702–704.

36. Whitson BA, Eckman P, Kamdar F, et al. Hemolysis, pump thrombus, and neurologic events in continuous-flow left ventricular assist device recipients. *Ann Thorac Surg.* 2014;97:2097–2103.

37. Bartoli CR, Ghotra AS, Pachika AR, et al. Hematologic markers better predict left ventricular assist device thrombosis than echocardiographic or pump parameters. *Thorac Cardiovasc Surg.* 2014;62(5):414–418.

38. Cowger J, Rao V, Massey T, et al. Comprehensive review and suggested strategies for the detection and management of aortic insufficiency in patients with a continuous-flow left ventricular assist device. *J Heart Lung Transplant.* 2015;34(2):149–157.

39. Cowger J, Pagani FD, Haft JW, et al. The development of aortic insufficiency in LVAD supported patients. *Circ Heart Fail.* 2010;3(6):668–674.

40. Kato N, Jaarsma T, Ben Gal T. Learning self-care after left ventricular assist device implantation. *Curr Heart Fail Rep.* 2014;11:290–298.

41. Riegel B, Jaarsma T, Stromberg A. A middle-range theory of self-care of chronic illness. *ANS Adv Nurs Sci.* 2012;35(3):194–204.

42. Slininger KA, Haddadin AS, Mangi AA. Perioperative management of patients with left ventricular assist devices undergoing noncardiac surgery. *J Cardiothorac Vas Anesth.* 2013;27(4):752–759.

43. Brush S, Budge D, Alharethi R, et al. End-of-life decision making and implementation in recipients of a destination left ventricular assist device. *J Heart Lung Transplant.* 2010;29:1337–1341.

44. Mueller PS, Swetz KM, Freeman MR. Ethical analysis of withdrawing ventricular assist device support. *Mayo Clin Proc.* 2010;85(9):791–797.

45. Beauchamp TL, Childress JF. *Principles of Biomedical Ethics.* 7th ed. New York: Oxford University Press; 2013.

46. Swetz KM, Cook KE, Ottenberg AL, et al. Clinicians' attitudes regarding withdrawal of left ventricular assist devices in patients approaching the end of life. *Eur J Heart Fail.* 2013;15:1262–1266.

47. Ben Gal T, Jaarsma T. Self-care and communication issues at the end of life of recipients of a left ventricular assist device as destination therapy. *Curr Opin Support Palliat Care.* 2013;7:29–35.

SELF-ASSESSMENT QUESTIONS

1. Patient and caregiver education related to implantation of a left ventricular assist device (LVAD) implant begins with the first interaction with a nurse. The patient and caregiver need to learn about living with an LVAD early in the evaluation phase to help them:
   a. make informed decisions.
   b. understand the plan of care should they receive a LVAD.
   c. understand what will be required of them should they be implanted with a long-term LVAD.
   d. All of the above.

2. Prior to discharge, patients and their caregiver(s) should have an understanding of:
   a. caring for their driveline exit site.
   b. proper management and changing of power source.
   c. appropriate response to any and all possible alarms.
   d. whom to call for assistance in an emergency.
   e. all of the above.

3. Which of the following are Food and Drug Administration-approved reasons for implanting durable LVADs?
   1. Bridge to cardiac transplantation
   2. Destination therapy
   3. Bridge to cardiac recovery
   a. 1 and 2 only
   b. 1 and 3 only
   c. 2 and 3 only
   d. All of the above

4. An interdisciplinary team is used to identify patients that could benefit from implantation of a LVAD. This team typically includes the clinicians from the following services:
   1. Cardiology
   2. Cardiovascular surgery
   3. Social services
   4. Palliative care
   a. 1, 2, and 3 only
   b. 1, 2, and 4 only
   c. 2, 3, and 4 only
   d. All of the above

5. Following implantation of a long-term LVAD, antibiotic prophylaxis is typically provided for a duration of:
   a. 6 hours
   b. 24 to 48 hours
   c. 2 weeks
   d. 2 months

6. Blood flow through a LVAD is affected by:
   1. speed at which the pump is set.
   2. preload volume to the pump.
   3. afterload pressure against the pump.
   a. 1 and 2 only
   b. 2 and 3 only
   c. 1 and 3 only
   d. All of the above

7. Postoperative complications related to the LVAD may include which of the following?
   1. Infection
   2. Bleeding
   3. Dysrhythmias
   4. Hemolysis
   5. Thromboembolism
   a. 1, 3, and 4 only
   b. 2, 4, and 5 only
   c. 3, 4, and 5 only
   d. All of the above

8. Follow-up care following discharge from the hospital may include:
   1. local EMS notification.
   2. clinic visits to asses clinical and psychosocial aspects of LVAD acceptance.
   3. integrity and performance of the LVAD.
   4. travel letter when the patient wishes to travel.
   a. 1, 2, and 3 only
   b. 1, 3, and 4 only
   c. 2, 3, and 4 only
   d. All of the above

9. Which of the following should be recorded at least daily for all VAD patients?
   a. Daily weights
   b. Hematocrit
   c. Potassium level
   d. All of the above

10. Which of the following LVAD parameters is set by the clinician?
    1. Revolutions per minute
    2. Flow
    3. Pulsatility index
    a. 1 only
    b. 1 and 3 only
    c. 2 and 3 only
    d. All of the above

Correct Answers:
1.d   2.c   3.a   4.d   5.b   6.d   7.d   8.d   9.a   10.a

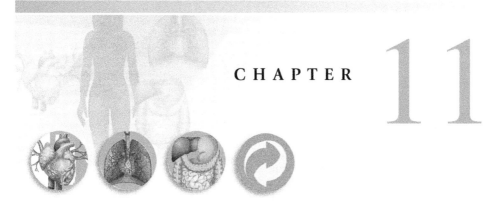

CHAPTER 11

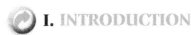

Lung and Heart-Lung Transplantation

Kevin C. Carney, MSN, CRNP, CCTC

J. Eric Hobson, MSN, CRNP

Vicki McCalmont, RN, MS, ANP-BC, CNS, CCTC

I. INTRODUCTION

A. Lung transplantation has evolved into a treatment option for patients with end-stage pulmonary disease.

1. It has been over 50 years since the first human lung transplant was performed by Hardy and colleagues at the University of Mississippi in 1963.[1]

   a. The donor died from a myocardial infarction and the donation after cardiac death (DCD) lungs were transplanted into the recipient who succumbed 18 days later of renal failure. Similar to the experiences of other solid organ transplant pioneers, dismal outcomes resulted in slow progress.[2,3]

   b. It took another 20 years before the Stanford group performed the first successful heart-lung transplant in 1981.[4]

   c. Subsequently in 1983, the Toronto Lung Transplant Group reported the first successful single-lung transplant.[5]

   d. In 1993, the University of Wisconsin team reported the first successful lung transplant using a DCD lung.[6]

   e. These noteworthy events led to a series of clinical advances in the area of lung transplantation, including improved selection criteria, implementation of the lung allocation score (LAS), refined surgical techniques, advancements in immunosuppression, and avoidance of steroids immediately postoperatively.[7-11]

2. Three decades later, lung transplantation has become an established treatment of choice for selected patients with a variety of end-stage lung diseases, leading to increased survival and improvement in quality of life.

   a. Remarkable progress continues to evolve with improved understanding of transplant immunology, microbiology, and pathology. Surgeons continue to explore opportunities to improve techniques such as the omentopexy, bronchial wrap, or telescoping or end-to-end anastomosis, which result in fewer airway-related complications.[12]

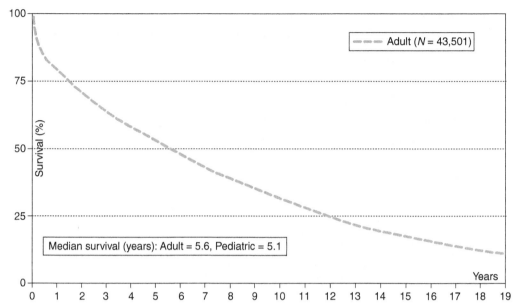

FIGURE 11-1 Adult lung transplant survival (Transplants: January 1990–June 2012). These survivals are estimates as some patients were lost to follow-up. (Data retrieved from ISHLT registry. Yusen RD, Edwards LB, Kucheryavaya AY, et al. The registry of the international society for heart and lung transplantation: thirty-first adult lung and heart–lung transplant report—2014; focus theme: retransplantation. *J Heart Lung Transplant.* 2014;33(10):1009–1024.)

    b. For adults, recent unadjusted survival rates are 80% and 53% at 1 and 5 years, respectively. Median survival is 5.6 years (Figure 11-1).[13]

    c. Despite these improvements in short- and intermediate-term survival, long-term survival of lung transplant recipients is less than that of other solid organ transplant recipients. Survival is limited by the prevalence of chronic allograft rejection, known as bronchiolitis obliterans syndrome (BOS), and by the worldwide shortage of donor organs, which leads to mortality rates on the waiting list of approximately 8% to 10%.[13,14]

II. INDICATIONS AND CONTRAINDICATIONS FOR LUNG TRANSPLANT

    A. Indications for lung transplantation[15–17]

      1. Patients with chronic, end-stage lung disease and who meet all of the following criteria should be considered for lung transplantation per 2014 International Society for Heart and Lung Transplant (ISHLT) consensus guidelines.[15]

        a. High (>50%) risk of death from lung disease within 2 years if lung transplant is not performed.

        b. High (>80%) likelihood of surviving at least 90 days after lung transplantation.

        c. High (>80%) likelihood of 5-year posttransplant survival from a general medical perspective, provided that there is adequate graft function.

      2. Diseases currently accepted as indications for lung transplantation (single or bilateral) or a combined heart and lung transplant (HLT) are listed in Table 11-1.[13,15]

TABLE 11-1 Diseases Treated by Lung Transplantation

Diagnosis	SLT (N = 15,321)	BLT (N = 26,579)	HLT (N = 3,255)
COPD/emphysema	6,594 (43.0%)	7,078 (26.6%)	141 (4.3%)
Idiopathic pulmonary fibrosis	5,354 (34.9%)	4,825 (18.2%)	121 (3.7%)
Cystic fibrosis	234 (1.5%)	6,628 (24.9%)	459 (13.9%)
Alpha-1	771 (5.0%)	1,572 (5.9%)	62 (1.9%)
Idiopathic pulmonary arterial hypertension	92 (0.6%)	1,158 (4.4%)	907 (27.4%)
Pulmonary fibrosis, others	677 (4.4%)	970 (3.6%)	121 (3.7%)
Bronchiectasis	62 (0.4%)	1,069 (4.0%)	30 (0.9%)
Sarcoidosis	280 (1.8%)	776 (2.9%)	54 (1.6%)
Retransplant: obliterative bronchiolitis	312 (2.0%)	379 (1.4%)	24 (0.7%)
Connective tissue disease	177 (1.2%)	409 (1.5%)	n/a
Obliterative bronchiolitis (not retransplant)	105 (0.7%)	351 (1.3%)	25 (0.8%)
LAM disease	138 (0.9%)	302 (1.1%)	n/a
Retransplant: not obliterative bronchiolitis	205 (1.3%)	227 (0.9%)	32 (1%)
Congenital heart disease	58 (0.4%)	291 (1.1%)	1,178 (35.5%)
Cancer	7 (0.0%)	29 (0.1%)	n/a
Others	255 (1.7%)	515 (1.9%)	101 (3%)

Data collected from ISHLT registry: 1995–2013.
Adapted from Yusen RD, Edwards LB, Kucheryavaya AY, et al. The registry of the international society for heart and lung transplantation: thirty-first adult lung and heart–lung transplant report—2014; focus theme: retransplantation. *J Heart Lung Transplant.* 2014;33(10):1009–1024.

    a. The most common indications for lung transplantation are[13–15]
       i. Chronic obstructive pulmonary disease (COPD); approximately 33% of patients
      ii. Idiopathic pulmonary fibrosis (IPF); approximately 24% of patients
     iii. Cystic fibrosis (CF); approximately 16% of patients[13]
    b. The number of combined HLTs continues to decline.[13]
       i. The highest number of HLTs was approximately 170 cases in 1994 and 1995, out of a total of approximately 1,200 lung and heart-lung transplant procedures worldwide.
      ii. Since 1999, the number of HLTs has declined overall; however, since 2003, the number appears to have stabilized between 62 and 94 procedures per year.
     iii. As of 2012, only 75 HLTs out of a total of approximately 3,000 lung and heart-lung transplant procedures were performed worldwide.
     iv. Congenital heart disease (CHD), pulmonary arterial hypertension (PAH), and CF remain the most common indications (see Table 11-1).
  3. Contraindications to lung transplantation:
    a. In 2014, selection criteria were updated by the ISHLT to standardize the selection process and to provide evidence-based guidelines.[15]
    b. See Tables 11-2 and 11-3[15,16] for detailed criteria concerning medical conditions that may have an impact on transplant selection eligibility for and contraindications to lung transplantation.

TABLE 11-2 Medical Conditions Impacting Lung Transplantation Eligibility

- Colonization of respiratory tract with fungi or atypical mycobacterium
- Requirement of mechanical ventilation
- Previous thoracotomy, sternotomy, pneumonectomy, or extensive pleural scarring
- Active infection/sepsis
- Active or recent malignancy/cancer
- Substance abuse or addiction
- Cigarette smoking within 4–6 mo of activation on the waiting list
- Irreversible left heart failure
- Severe osteoporosis (e.g., symptomatic compression fractures)
- Severe musculoskeletal disease
- Malnutrition: <70% or >130% of ideal body weight
- Psychosocial problems that place patient at high risk of poor outcome
- Severe, untreated psychiatric disease

Data from Weill D, Benden C, Corris P, et al. A consensus document for the selection of lung transplant candidates: 2014 an update from the pulmonary transplantation council of the International Society for Heart and Lung Transplantation. *J Heart Lung Transplant.* 2015;34(1):1–15; Kreider M, Hadjiliadis D, Kotloff RM. Candidate selection, timing of listing, and choice of procedure for lung transplantation. *Clin Chest Med.* 2011;32(2):199–211.

c. Despite these selection criteria, controversies persist regarding[11,15–18]:

   i.   Upper age limits for lung or heart-lung transplantation

   ii.   Selection of patients colonized or infected with antibiotic-resistant organisms

   iii.   Selection of patients with a history of nonadherence or with limitations due to physical conditions

   iv.   Lack of reliable social support

TABLE 11-3 Absolute Contraindications to Lung Transplantation

- Malignant disease—patients should be tumor-free for at least 5 y prior to consideration for transplantation. A 2-year disease-free interval may be reasonable for localized, nonmelanoma skin cancer that has been appropriately treated.
- Irreversible end-stage organ disease in another organ (other than in the setting of a combined organ transplant)
- Atherosclerotic disease with end-organ ischemia that is not able to be revascularized.
- Acute medical instability (e.g., sepsis, myocardial infarction, and liver failure)
- Bleeding diathesis that cannot be corrected
- Chronic infection with resistant microbes that are poorly controlled prior to transplant
- Active tuberculosis infection
- Significant spinal or chest wall deformity that may limit allograft expansion
- Class II or III obesity: body mass index > 35 kg/m^2
- Current, prior, repeated, or prolonged nonadherence to medical regimen that would increase the risk of posttransplant nonadherence
- Psychiatric or psychologic conditions that preclude ability to cooperate with the interdisciplinary transplant team or adhere to the therapeutic regimen
- Lack of an adequate and dependable social support system
- Functional status that is severely limited and not amenable to rehabilitation
- Alcohol, tobacco, or other illicit substance abuse or dependence
  - Note: Long-term participation in therapy and periodic blood and urine testing should be required before transplantation is considered.

TABLE 11-3 Absolute Contraindications to Lung Transplantation (*Continued*)

Relative Contraindications to Lung Transplantation[15]

- Age > 65
- Class I obesity (body mass index 30.0–34.9 kg/m²)
- Malnutrition that is progressive or severe
- Osteoporosis that is severe and/or symptomatic
- Prior extensive lung resection surgery
- Mechanical ventilation, extracorporeal life support
- Chronic infection with resistant microbes that are poorly controlled prior to transplant
- Hepatitis B or C virus infection
  - Consider transplantation* for stable patients on appropriate therapy if there are no clinical, radiological, or biochemical evidence of cirrhosis or portal hypertension.
- Human immunodeficiency virus (HIV)
  - Consider transplantation* for patients who are compliant with antiretroviral therapy in the setting of controlled disease, undetectable HIV-RNA
- Other infections* (e.g., multidrug-resistant mycobacterium abscesses); infections caused by certain types of organisms (e.g., *Burkholderia* species)
- Atherosclerotic disease that would increase the patient's risk for posttransplant end-organ disease
- Note: Treatment for other diseases that have not yet caused end-organ damage should be optimized before transplantation (e.g., diabetes mellitus)

*In transplant centers with expertise in this condition.
Data from Weill D, Benden C, Corris P, et al. A consensus document for the selection of lung transplant candidates: 2014 an update from the pulmonary transplantation council of the International Society for Heart and Lung Transplantation. *J Heart Lung Transplant.* 2015;34(1):1–15.; Kreider M, Hadjiliadis D, Kotloff RM. Candidate selection, timing of listing, and choice of procedure for lung transplantation. *Clin Chest Med.* 2011;32(2):199–211.

 III. PATIENT REFERRAL AND EVALUATION OF POTENTIAL CANDIDATES

A. Patients are typically referred to the lung transplant program by their local pulmonologist or primary care physician.
  1. Medical information is sent to the transplant center for review.
  2. The patient is then scheduled for a clinic visit to determine
     a. Whether the patient does indeed have end-stage disease
     b. If the patient has any conditions that may preclude lung transplantation
  3. Timing of the referral is one of the most important aspects in lung transplantation.
     a. Referrals that are late in the disease process may result in the patient being too sick for transplantation.
     b. Careful consideration of the natural history and prognosis of the underlying primary disease is crucial in this decision process.[16,19]
     c. Measures of quality of life with and without transplant must be weighed.[11,20,21]
     d. Attention should be given to
        i. The patient's age at time of referral
        ii. Associated consequences of the lung disease on other organ systems
        iii. Current physical condition

e. Waiting time on the list for donor lungs or combined heart-lungs must be factored into the decision regarding the timing of referral.
   i. Per 2012 Organ Procurement and Transplantation Network (OPTN) data, 12.7% of patients waiting had an LAS of 50% to 100%, and 65% of patients were transplanted within 1 year of listing.[22] Data accessed on October 1, 15 from www.optn.transplant.hrsa.gov/.
   ii. Per Scientific Registry of Transplant Recipients (SRTR) data, 2014 waitlist mortality was 13.3%.[23]
f. Referring a patient late in the disease process state or at an older age may prevent the patient from being listed for transplantation. Older adults have difficulty enduring prolonged wait times, and this may lead to an increased waitlist mortality or removal from the list due to a deterioration in health if they become "too sick to transplant." Blood type and HLA reactivity may also lead to prolonged wait times and higher waitlist mortalities.[16]
g. Patient referrals can also come from another transplant center when dual listing is advantageous to the patient. The United Network for Organ Sharing (UNOS) mandates that patients are informed of the right to be dual listed, as this may provide more opportunities for organ offers and expedite transplantation. Potential dual listing may be recommended for patients with
   i. Elevated HLA antibodies
   ii. Worsening disease progression
   iii. Uncommon size
   iv. Adequate health care insurance
      • Prior approval from insurance company is typically required.

IV. TRANSPLANT EVALUATION

A. Patients referred for lung transplantation undergo a thorough evaluation, which includes a medical history and physical and consultations with specialists and interdisciplinary team members (social workers, dieticians, pharmacists, etc.; lab and diagnostic testing). This evaluation process is detailed in Table 11-4.[15-17]
   1. Tests are tailored to the patient's specific lung disease.
   2. The purpose of this evaluation is to
      a. Ensure that the individual meets medical and psychosocial eligibility criteria for transplantation
      b. Minimize the risk associated with the transplant surgery
   3. The evaluation is typically done as an outpatient and takes 3 to 5 days to complete. It consists of
      a. Objective measures of end-stage organ failure
         i. Series of assessments, tests, and procedures (see Tables 11-4 and 11-5)[15-17]
      b. Psychosocial assessment, including, but not limited to
         i. Cognitive functioning
         ii. Psychiatric disorders
         iii. Substance abuse
         iv. Social support[24,25]
      c. Informed consent is obtained from the patient to proceed with the evaluation after comprehensive patient education is provided regarding the nature and rationale for all tests, procedures, and consults. Refer to the Patient Education chapter for additional information.

TABLE 11-4 Evaluation Protocol for Lung Transplantation

General
- Vital signs
- Height, weight, body mass index
- Functional level

Lab tests/blood chemistries
- Liver function tests (bilirubin, aspartate aminotransferase; alanine transaminase, and alkaline phosphatase)
- Blood urea nitrogen, creatinine, and estimated glomerular filtration rate
- Calcium
- Phosphorus
- Magnesium
- Serum electrolytes
- Fasting lipid profile
- Stool for heme (×3), or recent colonoscopy
- Prostate-specific antigen (males)*
- Beta-hCG (females)

Hematology and coagulation profile
- Complete blood cell count with differential and platelet count
- Prothrombin time (or international normalized ratio) and partial thromboplastin time

Urine tests
- Urinalysis
- 24-Hour urine for creatinine clearance
- 24-Hour urine for protein if diabetic or if urinalysis positive for protein*

Scans
- Ventilation-perfusion scan (V-Q scan)*
- Computed tomography scan with high resolution to chest

Radiology and ultrasound
- Mammography*
- Sinus films*
- Chest radiograph
- Abdominal ultrasound study (liver, pancreas, gallbladder, and kidney evaluation)
- Carotid ultrasound*

Consultations and evaluations
- Complete history and physical examination
- Respiratory therapist
- Pulmonologist
- Cardiologist*
- Transplant coordinator
- Surgeon
- Infectious disease specialist
- Dietician
- Social worker
- Psychiatric evaluation*
- Neuropsychiatric evaluation (neurocognitive evaluation)*
- Dental evaluation

(continued)

TABLE 11-4 **Evaluation Protocol for Lung Transplantation (*Continued*)**

Pulmonary
- Pulmonary function testing with arterial blood gases
- Six-minute walk (at most centers)
- Cardiopulmonary exercise test (CPET)* optional test
  - Measure as oxygen uptake and abbreviated as VO_2
  - $VO_2 \leq 8.3$ mL/kg/min is associated with increased mortality risk

Cardiovascular
- Electrocardiogram
- Two-dimensional echocardiogram with Doppler study
- Right heart catheterization with detailed hemodynamic evaluation
- Left heart catheterization with coronary angiography*

Immunology
- ABO blood type and antibody screen
- Panel-reactive antibody screen
- Human leukocyte antigen typing (if listed for transplantation)

Digestion and gastrointestinal
- Barium swallow or esophagram
- pH probe testing and manometry
- Gastric emptying study

Infectious disease screening Serologies for:
- Hepatitis virus A, B, and C
- Herpes simplex virus
- Human immunodeficiency virus
- Cytomegalovirus (CMV)
- Toxoplasmosis
- Varicella virus
- Rubella
- Epstein-Barr virus
- Venereal disease research laboratory
- Lyme titers*
- Histoplasmosis

Cultures
- Throat swab for viral cultures (CMV, adenovirus, and herpes simplex virus)*
- Urine culture and sensitivity*
- Sputum for bacterial, fungal, and mycobacterial cultures*

Skin test
- Purified protein derivative skin test with controls (i.e., mumps, dermatophytin, histoplasmosis, and coccidioidomycosis) or QuantiFERON Gold, a blood test to screen for exposure to tuberculosis

Vaccinations
- Hepatitis A and B series
- Pneumovax every 5 y
- Influenza vaccine each fall
- Consider shingles vaccine and measles, mumps, and rubella for age-appropriate, *nonimmunocompromised* candidates.

*Only performed if appropriate or indicated.
From Weill D, Benden C, Corris P, et al. A consensus document for the selection of lung transplant candidates: 2014 an update from the pulmonary transplantation council of the International Society for Heart and Lung Transplantation. *J Heart Lung Transplant.* 2015;34(1):1–15; Kreider M, Hadjiliadis D, Kotloff RM. Candidate selection, timing of listing, and choice of procedure for lung transplantation. *Clin Chest Med.* 2011;32(2):199–211; Dudley KA, El-Chemaly S. Cardiopulmonary exercise testing in lung transplantation: a review. *Pulm Med.* 2012;2012:237852.

TABLE 11-5 Objective Measures of Deteriorating Medical Condition, Guidelines for Selection

Primary Disease	Clinical Criteria
COPD/emphysema	BODE index of 7–10 or at least 1 of the following: • History of hospitalization for lung exacerbation associated with hypercapnia (pCO_2 > 50 mm Hg) • pO_2 < 50 mm Hg (rest) • Pulmonary hypertension or cor pulmonale or both despite O_2 therapy • FEV1 <25% and either DLCO <20% or homogeneous distribution of emphysema without reversibility
Cystic fibrosis	• FEV1 < 30 % predicted • pCO_2 > 50 mm Hg • pO_2 < 50 mm Hg (rest) • Rapid decline in FEV1, particularly if female (*list urgently*) • Increased antibiotic resistance and/or incomplete recovery from exacerbations. • Frequent hospitalization, use of noninvasive ventilation • Recurring hemoptysis • Pneumothoraces, loss of body weight • Pulmonary hypertension
Pulmonary fibrosis	Histologic or radiologic evidence of usual interstitial pneumonia • FVC < 60%–80% predicted or ≥ 10% decrease in FVC during 6-month follow-up • DLCO < 40% predicted • PAPm > 25 mm Hg • ANY O_2 requirement. • Honeycombing on high-resolution CT scan (fibrosis score > 2) • Symptomatic, progressive disease with failure to maintain lung function despite steroids and good medical therapy
Pulmonary hypertension	• NYHA class III or IV despite combination medical therapy including prostanoids. • Low or declining 6 MWT (350 m) • Right arterial pressure > 15 mm Hg • Pulmonary arterial pressure > 50 mm Hg • Cardiac index < 2 L/min/m² • Uncontrolled syncope, hemoptysis, pericardial effusions, or progressive right heart failure • Right arterial pressure >15 mm Hg
Sarcoidosis	• NYHA functional class III or IV and any of the following: • Hypoxemia at rest • Pulmonary hypertension • Elevated right atrial pressure > 15 mm Hg
Lymphangioleiomyomatosis (LAM)	• VO_2 max < 50% predicted (severe impairment in exercise and lung function) • Hypoxemia at rest

*Special circumstances.
BODE index, **b**ody mass index, airflow **o**bstruction, **d**yspnea, **e**xercise. Scores range from 0 to 10 and provide mortality risks based on data entered. CT, computed tomography; FEV1, forced expiratory volume in 1 second; MWT, minute walk test; pCO_2, carbon dioxide tension; PAPm, pulmonary arterial pressure by mean; VC, vital capacity; DLCO, diffusing capacity of carbon monoxide; oxygen, O_2; NYHA, New York Heart Association.
Adapted from Hook J, Lederer D. Selecting lung transplant candidates: where do current guideline fall short? *Expert Rev Respir Med.* 2012;6(1):51–61; Weill D, Benden C, Corris P, et al. A consensus document for the selection of lung transplant candidates: 2014 an update from the pulmonary transplantation council of the International Society for Heart and Lung Transplantation. *J Heart Lung Transplant.* 2015;34(1):1–15; Kreider M, Hadjiliadis D, Kotloff RM. Candidate selection, timing of listing, and choice of procedure for lung transplantation. *Clin Chest Med.* 2011;32(2):199–211.

d. If the patient is acutely ill, an expedited inpatient evaluation can be done. This type of evaluation has limitations as it does not
   i. Provide the most accurate assessment of the patient's functional status, compliance, and social support
   ii. Allow for a demonstration of commitment by the patient and his/her support system
4. The evaluation process can be a very stressful time for the patient and family.
   a. Many patients experience feelings of anxiety, ambivalence, and hopelessness during this process.
   b. The needs of the patient should be addressed by providing educational and emotional support to the patient and family.[24-26]
   c. Members of the patient's support system are evaluated for their willingness and ability to provide care for the patient long term, as caregiver burden can become problematic with prolonged illness.[25-27]
   d. Please see chapters on the Evaluation of Transplant Patients and Psychosocial Issues in Transplantation for additional information.

V. LISTING PATIENTS FOR LUNG TRANSPLANTATION

A. Patients considered for transplant are presented to the interdisciplinary transplant selection committee after the evaluation process is complete. All information is compiled prior to the meeting and formally presented for discussion by the team. Members of the transplant team requested to participate in the transplant evaluation and selection meeting include
   1. Pulmonologists
   2. Cardiothoracic surgeons
   3. Cardiologists, for patients who may require combined HLT
   4. Respiratory, speech, and physical therapists
   5. Dietitians
   6. Nurse coordinators
   7. Social workers
   8. Psychiatrists or psychologists
   9. Pharmacists
   10. Ethicists
   11. Research staff
   12. Financial counselor/coordinator

B. After a comprehensive discussion, the transplant selection team may
   1. Determine that the patient meets disease-specific criteria for lung transplantation (see Table 11-5).[11,14-16]
      a. If candidate meets medical criteria to be placed on the transplant waiting list, the timing of listing must be determined.
         i. Is the patient ready to list?
         ii. Is the patient above the functional threshold for listing, in which case the patient is monitored for disease progression and functional decline (Figure 11-2) as indicated by
            • Decline in FVC ≥10% during 6 months of follow-up
            • Decline in D_{LCO} ≥15% during 6 months of follow-up
            • Desaturation to <88% or walking <250 m on 6-minute walk test over a 6-month follow-up period

Whole-lung function

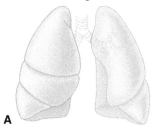

$\left\{\begin{array}{ll}\text{ABG (Fio}_2 = 0.21) & \text{Paco}_2 > 46 \text{ mm Hg} \\ & \text{Pao}_2 < 60 \text{ mm Hg} \\ \text{FVC} & < 50\% \text{ or } 1.5 \text{ mL/kg} \\ \text{FEV}_1 & < 50\% \\ \text{VC} & < 2 \text{ L} \\ \text{MVV} & < 50\% \text{ or } < 50 \text{ L/min} \\ \text{Lung Volume} & \text{RV/TLC} > 50\% \\ \text{DLco} & < 50\% \end{array}\right.$

A

Split-lung function

1. Split-lung spirometry with DLT
2. Regional lung radiospirometry
   Regional perfusion (^{133}Xe, ^{131}I-MAA)
   Regional ventilation ^{133}Xe

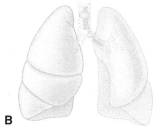

$\left\{\begin{array}{l}\text{Predicted postresection FEV}_1 < 800 \text{ mL} \\[1em] \text{Blood flow to the resected lung} > 70\% \end{array}\right.$

B

FIGURE 11-2   The order of tests to determine the cardiopulmonary status of the patient and the extent of lung resection that would be tolerated. **A.** The whole-lung function test is a basic screening test. **B.** The split-lung function tests are regional tests to determine the involvement of the diseased lung to be removed. ABG, arterial blood gas; FVC, forced vital capacity; FEV1, forced expiratory volume in 1 second; VC, vital capacity; MVV, maximum voluntary ventilation; RV/TLC, residual volume/total lung capacity; DLT, double-lumen tube. DLCO, diffusing capacity for carbon monoxide. (Adapted from Neustein SM, Cohen E. Preoperative evaluation of thoracic surgical patients. In: Cohen E, ed. *The Practice of Thoracic Anesthesia.* Philadelphia, PA: JB Lippincott; 1995:187, with permission.)

- Pulmonary hypertension on right heart catheterization
- Acute hospitalization for respiratory failure, pneumothorax, or disease exacerbation[28,29]

2. Decide that the patient does not meet medical or psychosocial transplant eligibility criteria at this time and determine whether or not
   a. The issue can be corrected or resolved over time, with recognition of current medical status and if feasible and realistic
   b. The patient should consider alternative centers for listing if the contraindications are center specific and not universal
   c. The patient should be reassessed after current medical and/or psychosocial concerns are resolved and reconsidered for listing
3. If all viable treatment options are exhausted and a decision is made to offer transplant listing to the patient, the patient must then decide if he/she wants to be placed on the waiting list for a donor organ.

C. Candidates for lung transplantation are listed on a national computerized waiting list maintained by UNOS, a private, nonprofit organization contracted by the US Department of Health and Human Services to allocate organs according to OPTN policies.[15]

1. Listing information is outlined in Table 11-6 per UNOS guidelines.

TABLE 11-6 UNOS Listing Information

Listing information consists of

1. Social security number
2. Organ—heart-lung or lung
3. Age group—adult or pediatric
4. Patient name
5. Locality
6. Date of birth
7. Race
8. Diagnosis and blood group
9. Height and weight
10. Forced expiratory volume in 1 sec (FEV1) and forced vital capacity (FVC)
11. Right heart catheterization pressures
12. 6-Minute walk test distance
13. Acceptable smoking history for a donor >20 pack years
14. Acceptable donor serologies (human immunodeficiency virus, hepatitis B virus, and hepatitis C virus)
15. Acceptable donor height range and age range
16. A maximum distance the organ recovery team is willing to travel
17. Whether a donor-specific crossmatch will be needed at the time of transplant

Adapted in part from United Network of Organ Sharing (UNOS). Available at https://www.unos.org/wp-content/uploads/unos/Lung_Professional.pdf?b2d5de. Accessed October 12, 2015 and personal experience.

2. The patient's LAS is calculated using a series of data factors that determine the probability of a patient surviving the next year without a transplant (urgent need) and the projected survival with a transplant (long-term benefit).[15,28-30]
    a. Data for clinical variables are entered into the LAS calculator and the LAS score is calculated (see Table 11-7).[15,28-30]
    b. The LAS ranges from 0 to 100 with a higher score suggestive of a higher severity of illness/increased urgency for transplantation and a higher probability of success following transplant.
        i. The LAS is used to prioritize patients on the lung transplant waiting list.
        ii. The score is typically provided to the patient at the time of official listing notification.
3. Candidates are typically required to reside or establish temporary residency within a 2-hour distance to the transplant center (by ground or air transportation).
    a. When distance precludes arrival at the transplant center via ground transportation within the 2-hour time limit, some transplant centers assist patients and families with alternate air transportation arrangements when a donor organ becomes available. Such arrangements
        i. Afford patients the opportunity to wait for their transplant in their own home, which is an important consideration in areas of the country where there are few lung transplant programs (e.g., rural communities). This allows patients to remain close to family and friends for support.
        ii. Attempt to maintain equity of organ allocation and distribution
    b. Other centers will allow for long-distance travel by notifying patients of organ offers earlier in the process and thus for car travel at the time of donor organ offers.
        i. Patients are notified that there is a risk that the organ offer may not be accepted as additional clinical information regarding the donor is obtained while the patient is en route.

TABLE 11-7 Lung Allocation Score (LAS)

Lung Allocation Score Data

- Diagnosis
- Date of birth
- Height
- Weight
- Forced vital capacity
- Supplemental oxygen—(amount of FiO_2 in liters or %):
  - At rest
  - At night
  - With exercise
  - Not needed
- Need for mechanical ventilation and type
- Arterial blood gases (need pCO_2's—current, highest, and lowest)
- 6-Minute walk (feet)/functional status
- Serum creatinine
- Right heart catheterization pressures (right atrial pressure, pulmonary artery pressures, and cardiac index)
- Presence or absence of diabetes mellitus (with/without Insulin use)

From Weill D, Benden C, Corris P, et al. A consensus document for the selection of lung transplant candidates: 2014 an update from the pulmonary transplantation council of the International Society for Heart and Lung Transplantation. *J Heart Lung Transplant.* 2015;34(1):1–15; Smits JM, Nossent GD, Vries ED, et al. Evaluation of the lung allocation score in highly urgent and urgent lung transplant candidates in Eurotransplant. *J Heart Lung Transplant.* 2011;30(1):22–28; Braun AT, Dasenbrook EC, Shah AS, et al. Impact of lung allocation score on survival in cystic fibrosis lung transplant recipients. *J Heart Lung Transplant.* 2015;34(11):1436–1441. doi: 10.1016/j.healun.2015.05.020; Organ Procurement and Transplantation Network. Policy 10: Allocation of Lungs, 134–150. Available at http://optn.transplant.hrsa.gov/ContentDocuments/OPTN_Policies. Accessed September 29, 2015.

VI. MANAGEMENT OF PATIENTS AWAITING LUNG TRANSPLANTATION

A.   During the waiting period, the health status of the lung transplant candidate is monitored regularly. This monitoring differs from center to center.

   1. Stable patients are typically followed in an outpatient clinic every 8 to 12 weeks.

      a. To maintain a current LAS, certain variables including functional status, diabetic status, assisted ventilation, and oxygen requirements are updated as frequently as every 2 weeks for patients with a LAS > 50 and at least every 6 months when the LAS <50.[14,28–30]

   2. Other variables including pulmonary function tests, 6-minute walk, and serum creatinine are updated at least every 6 months.[15,28–30]

   3. It is important to impress upon the patient and family that the transplant team must be notified of any hospitalizations, deterioration in pulmonary or general health status, and change in insurance or contact information and must keep all scheduled appointments.

   4. Many transplant centers require patients to participate in cardiopulmonary rehabilitation two to three times a week while they are on the waiting list.

VII. INDICATORS OF DETERIORATION

A. Subjective complaints may include the following:
1. Symptoms of increased anxiety and depression.
2. Fear of dying.
3. Increased shortness of breath.
4. Decreased exercise tolerance.
5. Increased dependence on others.
6. Complaints of weight loss despite increase caloric intake.
7. Early satiety or decreased appetite.
8. These factors are multidimensional influences and may be interrelated.

B. Objective findings may include the following[11,15]:
1. Weight loss.
2. Decline in pulmonary function measurements ($\downarrow$ forced vital capacity [FVC] or $\downarrow$ diffusing capacity of the lung for carbon monoxide [D_{LCO}]).
3. Pulmonary hypertension (elevated right heart pressures).
4. Decline of walk distance on a 6-minute walk test (6 MWT).
5. Increasing supplemental O_2 requirements at rest and/or with exertion:
   a. 6 MWT O_2 requirements may be increased.
6. Respiratory support requirements (continuous positive airway pressure [CPAP], bilevel positive airway pressure [BIPAP], mechanical ventilation).
7. Increased work of breathing.
8. Hospitalization for respiratory distress indicates higher urgency for transplant.

VIII. EDUCATION FOR THE LUNG TRANSPLANT PATIENT ACROSS THE TRANSPLANT CONTINUUM

A. Patient and family/caregiver education is an essential component of solid organ transplantation patient care and aids in managing expectations and optimizing adherence.
1. Education begins at the time the patient is referred for transplant evaluation and continues throughout the transplant continuum.

B. Pretransplant education for critically ill patients and their families requires special attention.
1. Given poor oxygenation and high levels of anxiety and overstimulation, patients may have less ability to concentrate and learn.
2. Small amounts of information shared at each interaction with repetition and gradual expansion of concepts optimizes retention.

C. Topics that should be covered while the patient is in the pretransplant phase of care could include, but are not limited to, the following:
1. The evaluation process:
   a. Expected time line from beginning of evaluation to completion (scheduling testing and consultations, follow-up appointments, review of results, and recommendations from the selection team)
   b. Evaluation tests (see Table 11-4)[15-17]:
      i. These vary from transplant program to transplant program.
   c. Consultation with interdisciplinary team members

  i. Note: the Centers for Medicare and Medicaid (CMS) requires the following:
- All patients must be evaluated using an interdisciplinary team approach.
- Notes from each discipline must be documented in the patient record for CMS review.
- If the patient does not have a need for a specific interdisciplinary team assessment, this must be documented in lieu of the consult note.
- Interdisciplinary team assessments from a social worker, dietician, and pharmacist must occur prior to listing, immediately after transplantation, and prior to discharge.

  ii. In addition to patient education, discipline-specific consults may include the following assessments:
- Social worker:
  - Emotional status and coping skill
  - Support system and resources
  - Existing stressors and prior mental health support
  - History of adherence to medical regimen
  - See chapter on Psychosocial Issues in Transplantation for additional information
- Dietician:
  - Body habitus
  - Nutritional status
  - Bone health indicators and osteoporosis status
- Pharmacist:
  - Current medications and tolerance
  - Medication allergies
  - Potential problems with posttransplant immunosuppression regimen
- Financial coordinator:
  - Current health care insurance, including medication benefits
  - Disability status
- Transplant coordinator:
  - Overall patient and family awareness of health status and disease state
  - Current status of routine health screening (e.g., mammography, prostate-specific antigen tests, dental examinations)

2. Waiting for a transplant
   a. Self-care
   b. Follow-up care with the transplant center; periodic labs and other tests
   c. Exercise program
   d. Nutrition and weight management:
      i. Cachectic patients may require nutritional supplements to achieve a body mass index (BMI) > 18.
      ii. Obese patients may be required to lose weight to achieve a BMI < 30.
   e. Support groups
   f. Communication with the transplant center reporting:
      i. Admission to other hospitals during the waiting period
      ii. Deterioration of condition and change in O_2 requirement
      iii. Signs and symptoms of infection
      iv. Change of insurance, address, or phone number

3. Optimal donor:
   a. Donor evaluation, matching, and selection[31]
4. Immediate preoperative period:
   a. When the donor offer comes[31-33]:
      i.   Offer reviewed by surgeon and accepted if
           * The donor/recipient are ABO compatible
           * The size of the donor is appropriate for the size of the patient
           * The donor organ is deemed suitable for transplant
      ii. Patient notification of donor offer and admission to hospital:
           * Appropriate hospital entry to use
      iii. Estimated time line of events; potential for delays
   b. Testing on admission:
      i.   Lab work
      ii. Chest radiograph (CXR)
      iii. Electrocardiogram (ECG)
      iv. Preoperative shower/scrub preparation
   c. Placement of lines and catheters
   d. Holding area
   e. Family waiting area
5. Surgical procedure[34,35]:
   a. Consent
   b. Completion of central lines and arterial line placement
   c. Initiation of anesthesia
   d. Type of incision
   e. Duration of surgical procedure
   f. Updating family during surgical procedure
   g. Transfer from the operating room directly to the intensive care unit (ICU). Postanesthesia management and recovery occur in the critical care unit, rather than in a postanesthesia care unit (PACU). Anesthesia is nearby if needed.
6. Immediate postoperative course:
   a. Length of stay in the ICU and intermediate care unit
   b. Lines, tubes, and devices insertion, maintenance, and removal
   c. Ventilator and ventilator weaning protocol
   d. Bronchoscopy for airway inspection and culture collection
   e. Supplemental O_2
   f. Pain management
   g. Medications:
      i.   Tolerance and safety for oral administration of medications
      ii. Weaning of intravenous (IV) inotropic and vasopressor support
      iii. Weaning of inhaled medications
      iv. Immune suppression:
           * In addition, antifungal medications interact with immunosuppression and complicate management.
             ◦ Precautions vary from center to center and even provider to provider.
   h. Postoperative routines:
      i.   Frequent vital sign/hemodynamic assessments
      ii. Diet progression
      iii. Ambulation (progressive increase in activity and physical therapy)
      iv. Use of incentive spirometer
      v.   Wound care and dressing changes
   i. Visitation by family and significant others

7. Long-term follow-up care posttransplantation:
   a. Adherence with the medical regimen.
   b. Posttransplant clinic appointments.
   c. Strategies to prevent infections, for example:
      i. Wearing a mask for a specified time after surgery (per transplant program protocol). May include use when the patient is
         * Exposed to crowds during the first 3 months following transplant
         * Around sick people during the cold/flu season
         * Returning to the hospital or physician's office where exposure to sick people is possible
      ii. Good hand hygiene.
      iii. Patients should not accompany others to physician office appointments.
      iv. Patients should not visit other patients in the hospital within 3 months posttransplant.
      v. Patients should avoid crowded times at restaurants, movie theaters, banks, grocery stores, shopping malls, and indoor sporting events.
      vi. Limit hand contact with contaminated surfaces such as handrails, doorknobs, and countertops.
      vii. Proper food preparation and food handling and preparation surface maintenance and cleaning.
      viii. Pet care:
         * Patients should not have contact with domestic birds (risk for psittacosis, histoplasmosis, and other diseases).
         * Patients should not have contact with cat litter boxes due to risk of toxoplasmosis exposure.
         * Obtaining a new pet is typically discouraged during the first year posttransplant.
      ix. Home construction or gardening can be hazardous due to risk of dust/spore inhalation.
      x. Dust inhaled related to these activities may often contain mold spores and can lead to fungal infections, which are difficult to treat.
   d. Some are more conservative and instruct patients to avoid all of the above activities at all costs, while others allow patients to participate, but instruct patients to use protective masks of varying quality.
      i. Wearing masks will reduce, but not completely eliminate, the risk.
      ii. In general, programs typically advise recipients to avoid the following activities:
         * Pulling up carpets
         * Repairing or replacing walls/ceilings
         * Gardening and yard work involving digging, fertilizing, and leaf raking
   e. Daily use of a home spirometry device to monitor the lung function.
   f. Immunosuppressants and other medications:
      i. Purpose
      ii. Adherence regarding timing, exact dosing, and intervals
      iii. Potential side effects

    iv. Potential drug interactions:
        • Prescription drugs
        • Over-the-counter medications
    v. Food/drug interactions such as those with grapefruit and/or grapefruit juice
    vi. Supplements and herbal remedies (avoid Echinacea, probiotics, and other remedies that are contraindicated posttransplant)
    vii. Monitoring medication supply, availability, and trough levels
    g. Management of symptom distress:
        i. When to call the transplant center or coordinator on call
        ii. Quality of life and realistic expectations
    h. Posttransplant health care costs:
        i. Coverage of health care costs for the posttransplant treatment and potentially expensive immunosuppressant medications can be one of the greatest concerns for patients and health care professionals.
        ii. Without prescription drug, transplant recipients face a significant financial challenge.
        iii. Patients should be referred to a social worker, pharmacist, and/or transplant financial coordinator who can
            • Identify potential financial resources.
            • Help the patient apply for pharmacy assistance programs or grants or engage in fundraising to defray future costs.
            • Patients should not share medications with one another as this is illegal.
    i. Returning to work after lung transplantation should be encouraged.
        i. The social worker may assist patients and families with return to work issues, including, but not limited to
            • Insurance coverage concerns
            • Potential loss of Medicare or other public insurance benefits

D. See chapter on Education for the Transplant Patient for additional information.

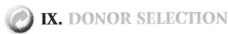 IX. DONOR SELECTION

A. Successful lung transplantation is dependent on optimal donor selection.[30-32]

B. Guidelines for the identification and management of potential lung donors have been established by UNOS.

C. Characteristics of optimal lung donor[31-33]:
    1. Usually younger than 55 years of age.
    2. Chest radiograph: clear:
        a. Ventilator recruitment maneuvers may clear areas of atelectasis.
    3. Arterial blood gas (ABG) with normal gas exchange and PaO_2 > 300 mm Hg on 100% FiO_2, 5 cm positive end-expiratory pressure (PEEP) for 5 minutes (Figure 11-3).
    4. No previous thoracic surgery, pulmonary contusions, or chest trauma.
    5. No evidence of aspiration.

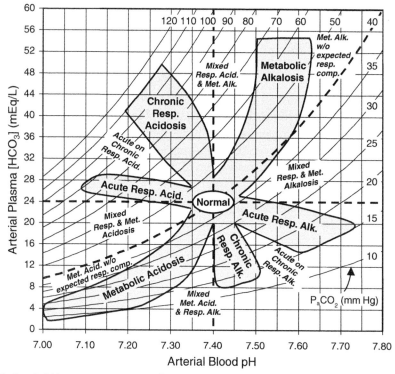

FIGURE 11-3 Acid-base nomogram NB. If ABG not available, can use VBG, but note that pH ~0.04 ↓, PaCO$_2$ ~8 mm Hg ↑, and HCO$_3$ ~2 mEq ↑. (Adapted from Brenner BM, ed. *Brenner & Rector's The Kidney.* 8th ed. Philadelphia, PA: Elsevier; 2007; Ferri F, ed. *Practical Guide to The Care of the Medical Patient.* 7th ed. Philadelphia, PA: Elsevier; 2007.)

6. Bronchoscopy should demonstrate clear airways:
   a. Free of purulent or aspirated material.
   b. Cultures should be negative, no lung infection.
7. Tobacco history < 20 pack/years.
8. Absence of any transmittable diseases.
9. If considering DCD lungs, follow above criteria and use direct visualization of lungs in the operating room.
10. Some programs will consider extended criteria lung donors (ECLD). These donors may be above age 55 and have an abnormal CXR or infiltrate, smoking history >20 pack/years, positive sputum cultures, and heavy secretions upon bronchoscopy.

D. Donor and recipient size match is also an important factor considered during the selection process.

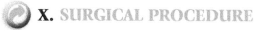 **X. SURGICAL PROCEDURE**

A. Several types of lung procedures are utilized[33,34]:
   1. Single-lung transplantation (SLT), either left or right
   2. Bilateral sequential lung transplant
   3. Double-lung en bloc
   4. Heart-lung transplantation
   5. Living donor lobar transplant

B. Determining the type of surgery depends on
1. Underlying disease
2. Recipient age
3. Recipient anatomy
4. Surgeon's preference (to some degree)

C. Patients who are candidates for deceased donor lung transplantation may be considered for living donor lobar transplantation at select transplant centers.
1. Procedure requires two living donors.
2. Each donates a lower lobe of a lung to the recipient.
3. This procedure is usually reserved for pediatric patients.

D. Surgical incision[34,35]:
1. Clamshell approach (standard and modified) (see Figure 11-4)
2. Standard median sternotomy incision
3. Standard thoracotomy incision
4. Minimally invasive thoracotomy incisions

E. Single-lung transplant[34,35]:
1. A standard posterolateral or anterolateral thoracotomy incision is used.
2. Mechanical ventilation is given to the contralateral lung, and the lung to be excised is deflated and removed. During removal, the surgeon is careful to protect the phrenic and vagus nerves and if on the left side will protect

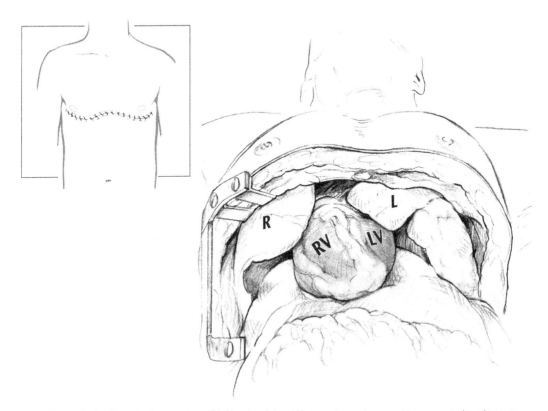

FIGURE 11-4 Clamshell extension of left anterolateral thoracotomy. In urgent/emergent situations, a clamshell incision, formed by extending a left anterolateral thoracotomy incision, transversely across the sternum, provides access but only suboptimal exposure of intrathoracic and mediastinal structures except the right ventricle and atrium. R, right lung; RV, right ventricle; LV, left ventricle; L, left lung.

the laryngeal nerve. Once the native lung is removed, the donor graft can be implanted. Three anastomoses are made in a posterior to anterior anastomosis sequence: (1) bronchus, (2) pulmonary artery, and (3) pulmonary veins and left atrium.

    a. The bronchial anastomosis has historically been the most vulnerable site for complications as the bronchial blood supply is disrupted during transplantation.

    b. A variety of bronchial anastomosis and revascularization techniques have been developed over the years. Discuss potential options with patient.

F. Bilateral lung transplant[33,34]:

    1. Can be performed using the "clamshell" approach (Figure 11-4) or a median sternotomy.

    2. Patient may be placed on cardiopulmonary bypass (CPB).

    3. After the chest is opened, both lungs are mobilized for removal.

        a. The native lung with the worst function is removed first and transplanted while the native lung remains ventilated.

        b. Once the first graft is completed, the second native lung is deflated, removed, and transplanted, while the new transplanted lung is ventilated.

        c. After completion of both grafts, chest tubes are placed in the pleural space and the chest is closed.

XI. IMMUNOSUPPRESSION[36–39]

A. The goal of immunosuppressive therapy is to prevent rejection of the allograft[36]:

    1. Immune suppression typically begins on the day of surgery.

    2. Example: preoperative dose of mycophenolate mofetil (CellCept) and an intraoperative dose of methylprednisolone (Solu-Medrol)

B. Optimal management of immunosuppressive therapy involves[36,38]

    1. Maintaining immunosuppressant drug levels within a therapeutic range

    2. Balancing immune suppression while minimizing the risk of infection, rejection, or cancer

    3. Preventing or minimizing side effects of immunosuppressive agents

    4. Preventing or minimizing complications associated with immunosuppressive agents

C. The immunosuppressive regimen for lung transplant patients is individualized and varies from center to center.

    1. Recent ISHLT data indicate that approximately 60% of adult patients who underwent heart and lung transplantation between 2001 and 2013 received some type of induction therapy.[13]

        a. Maintenance therapy consists of a triple drug regimen.[36–39]

            i. Calcineurin inhibitor (tacrolimus [Prograf] or cyclosporine [Neoral; Gengraf]):

              • Most centers use tacrolimus as the primary calcineurin inhibitor agent.[13]

              • Data suggest a potential role of calcineurin inhibitors in retarding the development of BOS.[38] See section on BOS below.

            ii. Corticosteroids: prednisone (Rayos).

            iii. Antimetabolites: mycophenolate mofetil (CellCept), mycophenolic acid (Myfortic), or azathioprine (Imuran).

    iv. mTOR inhibitors: sirolimus (Rapamune) or everolimus (Zortress).

    v. See chapter on Transplant Pharmacology for additional information on immunosuppressive drug therapies.

XII. IMMEDIATE POSTOPERATIVE CARE

A. Monitoring and maintenance of the lung transplant recipient begin as transport is completed from the operating room (OR) to the ICU.

B. Communication and collaboration between intraoperative and postoperative teams are essential to ensure a seamless transition.

C. Arrival in ICU[40–44]: patients typically arrive in the ICU with the following in place:

1. Airway is secured. Ventilator is often in use, though some single-lung transplant recipients may arrive in the ICU on mask O_2 support if extubated in the operating room.

2. Initiate bedside ECG monitoring.

3. Arterial line calibrated and pressures verified with a manual cuff reading.

4. Pulmonary artery (PA) catheter (Swan-Ganz) calibrated and measurements collected (Figure 11-5):

    a. Right atrial (RA) pressures or central venous pressure (CVP)

    b. Pulmonary artery pressures (PAP)

    c. Pulmonary capillary wedge pressure (PCWP), *not measured posttransplant*

    d. Cardiac output (CO) and cardiac index (CI)

    e. Mixed venous oxygen (SvO_2)

5. Pulse oximetry

6. Wounds dressings:

    a. Posterior-lateral thoracotomy or minimally invasive thoracotomy incisions are typical in SLT procedures.

Variable	Calculation	Normal values
Cardiac index (CI)	CO/BSA	2.5–4.0 l/min/m^2
Stroke volume (SV)	CO/HR	60–90 mL/beat
Stroke index (SI)	SV/BSA	40–60 mL/beat/m^2
Mean arterial pressure (MAP)	Diastolic blood pressure plus one-third pulse pressure	80–120 mm Hg
Systemic vascular resistance (SVR)	MAP-CVP/COX80	1200–1500 dynes/cm/sec^{-5}
Pulmonary vascular resistance (PVR)	PAP-PWP/COX80	100–300 dynes/cm/sec^{-5}
Right ventricular stroke work index (RVSWI)	0.0136 (PAP-CVP)/SI	5–9 g-m/beat/m^2
Left ventricular stroke work index (LVSWI)	0.136 (MAP-PWP)/SI	45–60 g-m/beat/m^2

CVP = central venous pressure; BSA = body surface area; CO = cardiac output; PAP = mean pulmonary artery pressure; PWP = pulmonary wedge pressure; MAP = mean arterial pressure; g-m = gram meter.

FIGURE 11-5   Hemodynamic variables: calculations and normal values.

      b. Transverse "clamshell," thoracosternotomy, or traditional midsternal sternotomy are typical incisions for bilateral lung transplant (BLT) or HLT procedures.

    7. Chest tubes and mediastinal tubes:

      a. Unilateral in SLT patients on the side of the transplant.

      b. Bilateral tubes in BLT recipients or if a patient develops a perioperative pneumothorax in the contralateral side from transplant.

      c. These tubes are typically placed to a pleuravac at –20 cm H_2O wall suction.

    8. Epicardial pacing wires in the HLT recipient

    9. Urinary catheter

  10. Naso- or orogastric tube to decompress stomach and remove secretions

  11. Compression stocking to legs[41]

  D. Role of the nurse during this phase of recovery is[40-45]

    1. Ensure physiologic stability:

      a. Obtain and document baseline measurements.

        i. Vital signs:

- Vital signs fluctuate due to a physiological response to thoracic surgery and immunosuppressive therapy during the initial postoperative period.
- Core body temperature will gradually increase with rewarming but might remain slightly hypothermic (96°F to 97°F) due to corticosteroid therapy.
- During the early postoperative period, a decrease in blood pressure is typically a response to vasodilatation secondary to rewarming.
  - Regulation of blood pressure is generally achieved by vasopressor administration and judicious use of colloid fluids if necessary.[42,44]
- Heart rate will vary according to
  - Fluid volume status and IV infusions running
  - Vasopressor and inotropic therapy
  - Hypothermia
  - Pain
  - Cardiac dysrhythmias (which are common); potential etiology
  - Irritation of the pericardium subsequent to intrusion into the pericardial space or electrolyte imbalances related to CPB and diuretic-induced fluid shifts
  - Suture line on the right atrium
- Respirations should remain within standard normal limits (normal respiratory rate [RR] 12 to 20) as ventilatory support is weaned.
- Oxygen saturation should remain within 90% to 100%.

    2. Monitor telemetry:

      a. Cardiac dysrhythmias are fairly common after surgery, most often including

        i. Tachycardia may develop initially as a response to

- Fluid loss
- Bleeding
- Nebulizers
- Corticosteroids
- Pain
- Catecholamine release with stress response to surgery
- Diuretic therapy (preoperative)

      ii. Atrial flutter or fibrillation:
- One study reported 34% of lung transplant recipients experiencing postoperative atrial fibrillation or flutter.[46]
- Atrial flutter may be due to circus electrical movement related to inflammation near pulmonary vein and atrial cuff suture lines.[43]
- Initial management of atrial dysrhythmias includes
  - ○ Rate-controlling drugs such as diltiazem (Cardizem), metoprolol (Lopressor), or amiodarone (Cordarone).[44]
  - ○ Chronic anticoagulation therapy might be necessary should sinus rhythm not be restored.[41,42,44]

     iii. Supraventricular tachycardia (SVT):
- Dysrhythmias may be associated with electrolyte imbalances post surgery.

3. Hemodynamic monitoring:
   a. Hemodynamic instability:
      i. Hemodynamic status is closely monitored via a PA catheter and peripheral arterial catheter.
      ii. Most patients will have a normalizing pulmonary artery pressures with healthy lungs and improved cardiac output due to the decrease in pulmonary hypertension.[41,43]
   b. Maintaining normal hemodynamic parameters is essential in order to[41,43,45]
      i.   Protect anastomosis sites
      ii. Prevent pulmonary edema in the early postoperative period
      iii. Normal systolic PAP: 15 to 25 mm Hg
      iv. Normal diastolic PAP: 8 to 15 mm Hg
      v.   An easy way to remember PA pressures is to think of a *"quarter on top of a dime"* 25/10.
      vi. Due to en bloc and sequential anastomosis techniques of lung transplantation, PAWP is not typically measured because an increase in arterial pressure during balloon inflation may precipitate rupture of the pulmonary artery anastomosis.[35,40]
      vii. CI (normal 2.0 to 4.0 L/min) and mixed venous oxygen saturation (SvO$_2$ normal range is 60% to 80%) trends should be followed to ensure adequate tissue perfusion and oxygenation to end organs.
   c. PA pressures are maintained by[39,44]
      i.   Diuretic administration.
      ii. Inhaled nitric oxide therapy.
      iii. Nebulized epoprostenol (Flolan).
      iv. If fluid administration is necessary, judicious administration of colloid fluids are preferred over crystalloid due to increased capillary permeability common in transplanted lung tissue.
      - Measurement of PAWP is typically an institution-specific practice based on patient population within each unit. Consult your unit nursing policy.
      - If measured, maintain PAWP at low normal level (normal 6 to 12 mm Hg).

4. Monitor fluid and electrolyte balance[40,42,44]:
   a. Fluid volume status is critically important in the early postoperative phase. The optimal volume replacement in the transplant patient is unknown. Most programs will give fluids to achieve a goal blood pressure and CVP set by the surgeon.

b. Some degree of pulmonary edema in the newly transplant lung is common due to increased vascular permeability and severed lymphatic drainage.

c. Most programs keep PA pressures and CVP on the lower side to optimize oxygenation and minimize pulmonary edema.

d. See Table 11-8 for a review of hypervolemia and hypovolemia following lung transplant.

e. For hyper- and hypovolemia, monitor patient's response to treatment.
   i. Vital signs; respiratory rate and pattern
   ii. Hemodynamic parameters
   iii. Heart sounds; breath sounds
   iv. Weight
   v. Intake and output
   vi. Mental status
   vii. Skin: color, turgor, temperature
   viii. Lab tests—for example:
   ix. With reversal of hypovolemia, hematocrit should decrease:
   - Electrolytes should normalize with administration of electrolyte solution and as diarrhea, vomiting, and excessive urine output resolve; BUN should decrease.
   - With reversal of hypervolemia, hematocrit should increase. (Note: serum potassium level may decrease with diuretic therapy.)
   - Monitor electrolytes that may contribute to cardiac dysrhythmias:
     ○ Potassium
     ○ Magnesium

5. Monitor patient for alterations in blood pressure:
   a. Hypotension:
      i. Potential etiologies:
      - Intravascular volume depletion
      - Blood loss from surgical site
      - Rewarming and vasodilation
      - Acute myocardial injury
      - Autopositive end-expiratory pressure (PEEP)
      - Tension pneumothorax (in setting of airway anastomotic leak)
      - Pneumopericardium, pericardial effusion, or cardiac tamponade
      ii. Clinical manifestations:
      - Low blood pressure (<80/50)
      - Light-headedness, dizziness
      - Weakness
      - Syncope
      - Blurred vision
      - Mental status changes
      iii. Potential interventions:
      - Administration of O_2
      - IV fluid bolus
      - Consider holding diuretics
      - Medications:
        ○ Dopamine
        ○ Vasopressin
        ○ Epinephrine
        ○ Neo-Synephrine

TABLE 11-8 Hypervolemia Versus Hypovolemia Posttransplant

Hypervolemia	Hypovolemia
Fluid volume excess predisposes transplant recipients to pulmonary and peripheral edema, which can precipitate PGD.	Fluid volume depletion predisposes transplant recipients to hypotension.
Potential etiology	**Potential etiology**
• Fluid accumulation secondary to cardiopulmonary bypass, corticosteroid therapy, or heart, liver, or renal failure • Administrative of IV fluids or blood products • Excessive dietary intake of fluids or sodium • Physiological or systemic responses to therapy should be included in the baseline assessment of the patient and throughout their care continuum.[30]	• Effects of CPB lead to movement of fluid into interstitial space and increased capillary permeability. This can occur more prevalently in the lung transplant patient as they have interrupted lymphatic drainage and hemodynamic changes from surgery, thus increasing the risk of PGD • Increase in intravascular space during rewarming • Third space fluid shifts • Administration of diuretics • Excessive urine output, bleeding, or drainage • Diabetes mellitus • Vomiting, diarrhea
Clinical Manifestations	**Clinical Manifestations**
• Hemodynamic parameters: increase in CVP and PA pressures • Hypertension • Ventricular gallop (S_3 sound) • Rapid, bounding pulse • Jugular venous distention (JVD) • Pulmonary edema (e.g., rales, shortness of breath, tachypnea, cough, and crackles) • Pulmonary congestion on chest radiograph • Generalized edema or ascites • Weight gain • Positive fluid balance using strict I&O • Mental status changes • Potential treatment options • Administration of diuretics • Restriction of fluid and sodium intake • Administration of oxygen • Meticulous skin care to prevent breakdown of edematous areas • Lab values: decreased hematocrit (secondary to hemodilution, decreased or normal serum sodium, and decreased serum osmolality)	• Hemodynamic parameters: ↓ CI, ↓ CVP, ↓ PAP • Increased heart rate; weak pulse • Hypotension; postural hypotension • Tachypnea • Decreased urine output • Integument: poor skin turgor, pallor, and dry skin • Dry mucous membranes • Thick respiratory secretions • Delayed capillary refill • Flat jugular veins • Mental status changes: restlessness, anxiety, irritability, decreased level of consciousness • Lab values: increased hematocrit, urine specific gravity, serum BUN, creatinine, and sodium levels **Hypovolemic shock**: ↓CVP, ↓ PAP, ↓CO, ↑SVR • Potential treatment options • Administration of IV fluids to expand circulating volume and replace urine output with crystalloids • Electrolyte replacement • O_2 administration to enhance tissue perfusion • Vasopressors • Meticulous skin care to prevent breakdown

PGD, primary graft dysfunction; CVP, central venous pressure; I&O, intake and output; CPB, cardiopulmonary bypass; CI, cardiac index; PAP, pulmonary artery pressures; CO, cardiac output; SVR, systemic vascular resistance.
From Rang HP, Ritter JM, Flower RJ, et al. *Rang & Dale's Pharmacolog*. 8th ed. Philadelphia, PA: Elsevier; 2015; Floreth T, Bhorade SM. Current trends in immunosuppression for lung transplantation. *Semin Respir Crit Care Med*. 2010;31(2):172–178.

- Monitor patient's response to treatment:
  - ○ Blood pressure
  - ○ Hemodynamic parameters
  - ○ Patient's mental status
  b. Hypertension:
  i. Potential etiology:
  - Immunosuppressants, particularly corticosteroids and calcineurin inhibitors
  - Preexisting essential hypertension
  - Renal dysfunction
  - Stress
  ii. Potential clinical manifestations (note that hypertension may be asymptomatic):
  - High blood pressure >140
  - Headache
  - Visual disturbances
  - Nausea, vomiting
  - Chest pain
  - Dyspnea
  - Palpitations
  iii. Potential interventions[40,42,44]:
  - Vasopressor therapy is titrated to maintain mean arterial pressure.
    - ○ Normal (70 to 105) and adequate end-organ perfusion until hemodynamic stability is achieved.
  - Optimization of ventilation and oxygenation.
  - Antihypertensive agents—Note: Use caution with calcium channel blockers because they can potentiate calcineurin inhibitors, which can result in increased circulating immunosuppressant drug levels.
  iv. Monitor patient's response to therapy:
  - Blood pressure
  - Hemodynamic parameters
  - Serum immunosuppressant levels
  v. Patient education: patients should be instructed to:
  - Monitor and record blood pressure at home
  - Notify transplant team if blood pressure exceeds stipulated parameters
  - Report symptoms of worsening hypertension, headache, nausea and vomiting, chest pain, dyspnea, and palpitations
6. Monitor patient for disorders of glucose metabolism[42,44]:
  a. Hyperglycemia:
  i. Potential etiology:
  - Preexisting diabetes mellitus (DM)
  - Stress response
  - Side effects of corticosteroid therapy and calcineurin inhibitors
  b. Note: Hyperglycemia frequently resolves as steroids are tapered to a daily maintenance dose.
  i. Potential clinical manifestations:
  - Glycosuria
  - Polyuria

- Polydipsia
- Polyphagia
- Weight loss (particularly in insulin-dependent DM)
- Obesity (particularly in non–insulin-dependent DM)
- Recurrent blurred visions
- Weakness, fatigue
- Paresthesias
- Skin infections

ii. Potential interventions:
- Blood glucose monitoring: glucose levels are checked regularly in the early postoperative phase when corticosteroid dosages are higher or whenever the corticosteroid dosage is increased to treat rejection.
- Administration of insulin or oral hypoglycemic agents.
- American Diabetic Association diet.

iii. Monitor patient's response to treatment:
- Blood glucose level
- Hemoglobin A$_{1c}$ level
- Resolution of clinical manifestations

c. Hypoglycemia:
i. Potential etiology:
- Patient's metabolic requirements.
- Insufficient caloric intake.
- Dose of insulin or oral hypoglycemic agents exceeds the patient's metabolic needs.
- Strenuous activity or increase in exercise that is not accompanied by appropriate increase in food intake or decrease in dose of insulin or oral hypoglycemic agents.
- Factors that potentiate the action of hypoglycemic agents, such as renal insufficiency or certain medications (e.g., sulfonamides).
- Decrease in corticosteroid dose.

ii. Potential parasympathetic nervous system manifestations:
- Hunger
- Nausea
- Hypotension
- Bradycardia

iii. Potential sympathetic nervous system manifestations:
- Anxiety
- Irritability
- Diaphoresis
- Cool, pale skin
- Tachycardia

iv. Potential interventions:
- Administration of oral or IV glucose
- Discontinuation of IV insulin
- Decrease in dose of IV insulin or oral hypoglycemic agent

v. Monitor patient's response to therapy:
- Serum glucose level
- Patient's mental status
- Resolution of clinical manifestations

vi. Patient education should include
- Explanation of the goal of glucose control: prevention of long-term end-organ damage and peripheral circulatory and microvascular complications resulting from poorly controlled DM.
- Instructions on when and how to test, monitor, track, treat, and report glucose levels.
- Clinical manifestations of hyperglycemia (3 Ps, polyuria, polydipsia, and polyphagia):
  ○ Insulin resistance or inadequately treated DM causes hyperglycemia, which causes an osmotic diuresis creating polyuria (increased urination), dehydration, followed by polydipsia (increased thirst), and occasionally polyphagia (increased hunger).
  ○ Unexplained weight loss may be related to a ketoacidotic state.
- Clinical manifestations of hypoglycemia: cool and clammy skin, diaphoresis, fatigue, and confusion.
- Collaborate with social workers, case managers, dietitians, pharmacists, and physicians to ensure that patients and families have access to educational materials, diabetes educators, monitoring supplies, equipment, and medications.

7. Monitor patient for alterations in bowel functioning:
a. Potential etiology[47,48]:
   i. Gastroparesis may occur due to a vagus nerve injury from surgical manipulation of the posterior mediastinum at the time of transplant.
   ii. Colonic perforation due to glucocorticoid therapy.
   iii. Ischemic bowel may occur due to hypotension or hypoperfusion.
   iv. Infection (e.g., cytomegalovirus [CMV] colitis, *Clostridium difficile*).
   v. Distal intestinal obstruction syndrome (DIOS):
   - DIOS causes abdominal pain due a sticky mass of fecal matter and mucosa obstructing the small intestines.
   - More common in patients with pancreatic insufficiency due to lack of enzymes to break down fecal fat, this can lead to increased stool viscosity and risk for inflammation or obstruction.
   vi. Malabsorptive gastrointestinal (GI) complications may stem from primary disease processes.[48,49]
   - CF proteins can be found on epithelial cells in the lungs, intestines, pancreas, and biliary system where they regulate chloride and fluid secretion. With diffuse disease, these extrapulmonary complications become more evident.
   - Patients who undergo transplantation for CF are especially at risk for small bowel obstructions.
     ○ Early postoperative dehydration, anesthesia, and delayed ambulation slow gastric motility.[47,48]
     ○ Thick secretions may occlude the GI lumen at the level of the terminal ileum, thus placing the patient at risk for meconium ileus.
     ○ Risk for DIOS.
   - CF patients: bowel prophylaxis for this patient population should include[47]
     ○ Advancement to a high-fiber, low-fat diet
     ○ Increased oral fluid intake
     ○ Regular stool softeners

b. Potential clinical manifestations:
   i.   Abdominal distention and pain
   ii. Absence of bowel sounds
   iii. Abdominal rigidity or guarding
   iv. Abnormal frequency and consistency of bowel movements
   v.   Early satiety, reflux, and vomiting
   vi. Fever
   vii. Patient monitoring (see Table 11-9):
c. Potential treatment options:
   i.   Diarrhea or constipation (see Table 11-9):
8. Gastroesophageal reflux disease (GERD)[47-50]:
   a. Gastroesophageal reflux disease (GERD) is a motility disorder caused by reflux of gastric contents into the esophagus. GERD commonly occurs before or after transplant. Causes of GERD may be due to[47,48]
      i.   Delayed gastric emptying.
      ii. Cough or percussive therapy.
      iii. Lung pathology from microaspirations causing reflexive bronchoconstriction from irritated esophageal mucosa.
      iv. Some medications can lower esophageal sphincter tone and lead to GERD. These medications may include, but not be limited to, steroids, bronchodilators, calcium channel blockers, beta-blockers, alpha-adrenergics, opioid analgesics, theophylline (Theodur), anticholinergics, and antibiotics.
      v.   Other foods and substances that can also lower esophageal sphincter tone are chocolate, peppermint, yellow onions, coffee, tobacco, and alcohol.
      vi. After transplant, 50% of CF patients report GERD.[47]
      vii. GERD has been implicated as a causative or additive factor leading to BOS due to the microaspiration of gastric contents. In addition, the normal defense mechanisms preventing reflux are impaired in the allograft.[50-52]
   b. Symptoms of GERD:
      i.   Heartburn or dyspepsia due to the acid irritating the esophagus
      ii. Noncardiac chest pain
      iii. Hoarseness
      iv. Cough
      v.   Asthma
      vi. Unexplained weight loss
   c. Treatments may include[47]
      i.   Histamine-2 (H$_2$) antagonists such as famotidine (Pepcid)
      ii. Proton pump inhibitors (PPI) such as omeprazole (Prilosec) or pantoprazole (Protonix):
           • Medications to stimulate gastric motility, such as metoclopramide (Reglan): Note: Administer with caution due to risk of neurotoxicity and cardiac dysrhythmias.
   d. Following transplant, GERD may occur due to esophageal dysmotility, an altered foregut motility, which delays gastric emptying after lung transplant surgery; this may be attributed to vagal nerve injury, ischemia, and local scarring related to surgery.[48]

TABLE 11-9 Posttransplant Diarrhea and Constipation: Etiology, Clinical Manifestations, Interventions, and Monitoring

	Diarrhea	Constipation
Potential etiology	• Medications that irritate bowel and precipitate ulcerations, bleeding, diarrhea (e.g., mycophenolate mofetil [CellCept], antiplatelet agents, magnesium supplements, and antibiotics that alter normal bowel flora) • Opportunistic infections (e.g., cytomegalovirus gastritis or colitis) • Hospital-acquired infections (e.g., *Clostridium difficile*)	• Effects of general anesthesia • Narcotic analgesics • Reduced mobility
Potential clinical manifestations	• Frequent passage of unformed, watery stool • Positive stool cultures • Weight loss • Abnormal abdominal radiograph, ultrasound, or computed tomography test results	• Infrequent bowel movements • Difficult defecation • Passage of unduly hard, dry fecal material • Abdominal distention • Abdominal pain, tenderness • Abnormal abdominal radiograph, ultrasound, or computed tomography scan results
Potential interventions	• Altering medication time schedule • Treatment of infection • Administration of binding agents for diarrhea caused by nontoxin secreting organisms • Note: infectious causes must be ruled out prior to administering medications to decrease gastric and intestinal motility.	• Increase patient's level of activity as tolerated (ambulation, exercise) • Increase patient's intake of fluid and fiber as tolerated • Medications to relieve constipation (prokinetic agents, stool softeners, suppositories, and laxatives). Note: aluminum-based laxatives may decrease absorption of medications from the gut. • Enemas • Nasogastric tube for decompression • Changing type and/or frequency of pain medication
Patient monitoring	• Bowel sounds (absent, hypoactive, and hyperactive) • Abdominal pain, tenderness, and distention • Lab test results (e.g., electrolytes) • Patient's response to interventions: • Frequency, consistency, and quantity of bowel movements (observe trend via stool chart)	• Bowel sounds (absent, hypoactive, and hyperactive) • Abdominal pain, tenderness, and distention • Patient's response to interventions: • Frequency, consistency, quantity of bowel movements (observe trend via stool chart)

Chronic rejection, OB (grade C), is described as present (C1) or absent (C0), without reference to presence of inflammatory activity.

   i.   CF patients have a six- to eightfold higher rate of esophageal acid and reflux than the normal population.[47]

  ii.   Typical symptoms of GERD are not seen following transplant and in some cases are found when the patient presents with BOS.[45]

 iii.   Prevention strategies may include assessing patients posttransplant for GERD using pH testing on and off H_2 or PPI drug therapy, gastric emptying study, and esophageal manometry to measure lower esophageal sphincter tone.[45]

    iv. In severe cases of GERD, a fundoplication is used as treatment post transplant.

9. Monitor patient for alterations in nutrition:

    a. During the pretransplant period, efforts focused on optimizing the transplant candidate's nutritional status because:

        i. Deconditioning and cachexia prior to transplantation can impede rehabilitation efforts after surgery.

        ii. Intercostal muscle wasting can lead to difficulty weaning from mechanical ventilation and poor pulmonary toileting postoperatively.

    b. Potential etiology of altered nutrition:

        i. Patients with end-stage heart disease are at risk for malnutrition due to:

- Anorexia (secondary to gastric compression from ascites)
- GI symptoms (nausea, vomiting, diarrhea, constipation)
- Dysgeusia (impaired taste)
- Dysphagia
- Hypermetabolism (increase in resting energy requirements)
- Drug-nutrient interactions
- Malabsorption (secondary to engorgement of viscera with fluid)
- Poor nutrient delivery to tissues
- Early satiety
- Restricted diet
- Impaired ability to prepare food
- Altered mental status

        ii. Potential etiology: CF patients:

- Malabsorptive disease processes
- Gastroparesis

    c. Potential clinical manifestations:

        i. Abnormal weight

        ii. Abnormal lab values (e.g., serum albumin, prealbumin, electrolytes)

        iii. Insufficient caloric intake

        iv. Impaired wound healing

    d. Potential interventions:

        i. Calorie counts to assess patient's ability to meet nutritional needs

        ii. Small, frequent feedings for patients with early satiety

        iii. Nutritional supplements

        iv. Enteral feedings as indicated

        v. Total parenteral nutrition (TPN) as indicated

        vi. Administration of medications to control nausea, vomiting, diarrhea

    e. Monitor patient's response to treatment:

        i. Lab results (e.g., serum albumin, serum prealbumin, electrolytes, liver function tests)

        ii. Calories consumed

        iii. Appetite

        iv. Bowel sounds

        v. Activity level

        vi. Weight

        vii. Resolution of nausea, vomiting, diarrhea, constipation

        viii. Tolerance of nutritional supplements, enteral feedings, or TPN

    f. Following transplant assess speech and swallow for oropharyngeal dysphagia (OPD).[50]
        i. In one study, OPD was found in over 50% of lung transplant recipients and reported as a common problem following thoracic surgical procedures.[50]
        ii. OPD can be assessed with a bedside swallow, fiberoptic endoscopic evaluation of swallowing (FEES), or modified barium swallow.
        iii. OPD presents an aspiration risk that can lead to infection or rejection (BOS) if left untreated.
        iv. Enteral nutrition is needed until effective swallowing returns and OPD resolves.
        v. Vocal cord paralysis can occur during surgery and may require treatment with speech therapy or an ear, nose, and throat (ENT) specialist.
    g. Collaborate with patient/family and interdisciplinary team: physicians (surgeon, cardiologist, pulmonologist, intensivist), nursing personnel, dietician, physiotherapists, social worker, or mental health provider (for psychological etiology of altered nutrition).

10. Monitor patient for altered mobility and self-care deficit:
    a. One of the major goals of lung and heart-lung transplantation is to restore adequate oxygenation to vital organs.
    b. Early mobility is an important factor in preventing postoperative complications.
    c. Potential etiology of altered mobility and/or self-care deficit:
        i. Pain or anticipation of pain
        ii. Altered mood state (e.g., depression and anxiety)
        iii. Deconditioning
    d. Potential clinical manifestations:
        i. Inability or unwillingness to participate in self-care
        ii. Inability or unwillingness to ambulate
    e. Potential interventions:
        i. Administer pain mediation prior to ambulation and self-care activities:
          • Assess effectiveness of pain medication before patient ambulates or engages in self-care activities.
        ii. Establish mutual goals for self-care, ambulation, exercise, physical therapy, and occupational therapy.
        iii. Teach the patient to monitor and record activity levels and progress:
          • Note: Decreases in activity tolerance may indicate allograft rejection.
        iv. Instruct the patient on sternal precautions.
        v. Involve family or other members of the patient's support system.
        vi. Obtain consultations as indicated (e.g., mental health services).
        vii. Provide encouragement, reassurance, and support.
        viii. Provide comprehensive discharge planning:
          • Home physical and/or occupational therapy
          • Outpatient cardiac rehabilitation for HLT recipients or pulmonary rehabilitation for SLT or BLT
          • Ambulatory assistive devices as indicated
          • Supplemental O_2 as indicated
    f. Monitor the patient's response to interventions:
        i. Effectiveness of pain medications

   ii. Patient's ability to ambulate and perform self-care activities

   iii. Patient's ability to participate in physical and occupational therapy

   iv. Patient's progress toward mutually established goals

  g. Collaborate with patient/family and interdisciplinary team members: physicians (surgeon, cardiologist, pulmonologist, intensivist), physical therapist, occupational therapist, mental health provider, and home health care nurse.

11. Ensure adequate pain management:

  a. Adequate pain management[52]:

   i. Facilitates earlier ambulation, physical therapy, and rehabilitation

   ii. Maximizes ventilation and decreases risk of atelectasis

  b. A multimodal approach to pain control and optimization includes the use of

   i. Epidural catheters and patient-controlled analgesia (PCA).[53]

   ii. A gradual transition to oral medications for pain management.

   iii. Alternative strategies such as Reiki therapy or healing touch.

   iv. Use of neuropathic agents such as like gabapentin (Neurontin) and pregabalin (Lyrica) is gaining acceptance.

    • Note: Nonsteroidal anti-inflammatory drugs should be avoided due to the synergistic nephrotoxic effects when combining with immunosuppressant drugs or antibiotics.[39]

12. Prevent infections[42,51,52]:

  a. Ensure strict hand hygiene for all caregivers and visitors.

  b. Maintain appropriate protective isolation.

  c. Maintain methicillin-resistant *Staphylococcus aureus* (MRSA) precautions, if indicated.

  d. Maintain vancomycin-resistant enterococcus (VRE) precautions, if indicated.

  e. Administer antimicrobial agents as ordered.

  f. Provide meticulous surgical site care:

   i. Daily care of surgical wounds and invasive line sites is especially important in the postoperative care phase:

    • Immunosuppressive therapy increases the risk of infections.

    • Infection prevention strategies may include the following:

     ◌ Invasive lines are assessed daily and removed as soon as possible to prevent catheter-borne infections and reduce the risk of thrombus.

     ◌ Surgical wounds are assessed in the early postoperative period in order to detect the early signs of any infectious process. Any signs of infection should be reported immediately to the transplant team.

    • Bacterial infections are typically the most common infection in the transplant recipient within the first posttransplant month.[51]

   ii. Most health care organizations have established protocols especially developed for transplant recipients and other types of immunocompromised patients.

13. Monitor and report lab results and trends:

  a. Monitor liver and renal function tests for complications of immunosuppressive therapy such as hepatotoxicity or acute renal insufficiency.

  b. Monitor daily complete blood counts (CBC) with differential to assess for medication-induced bone marrow depression (neutropenia) and infection.

  c. Monitor trough immunosuppression levels to determine if levels are within the prescribed therapeutic range.

14. Assess neurologic status[54]:
   a. Neurologic assessment is important in order to
      i. Determine arousal from anesthesia
      ii. Assess patient's level of comfort
      iii. Identify deleterious sequelae of high serum immunosuppressant drug levels:
         • Calcineurin inhibitors such as cyclosporine (Neoral; Gengraf) and tacrolimus (Prograf) have been associated with encephalopathy and vasculitis when serum drug levels become toxic.[38,54]
   b. Posterior reversible encephalopathy syndrome (PRES)[54]:
      i. PRES is a cliniconeuroradiologic entity characterized by typical neurologic symptoms with characteristic cerebral image alterations.
      ii. It has been reported in solid organ transplantation recipients, especially related to the use of calcineurin inhibitors.
      iii. The true incidence of PRES in lung transplantation is unknown and probably underreported in the literature.
      iv. The intensity and severity of clinical manifestations of PRES vary in different patients.
      v. Symptoms may range from confusion, somnolence, and lethargy to deep coma and eventually death.
      vi. Image findings also vary in severity, and thorough familiarity with imaging and clinical criteria is crucial to the diagnosis of this syndrome.
      vii. The combination of suggestive clinical manifestations and radiologic criteria establishes the diagnosis of PRES.[54]
      viii. The most common abnormality on neuroimaging is edema involving the white matter in the posterior portions of the cerebral hemispheres, especially bilaterally in the parieto-occipital regions. However, edema has also been described in the frontal lobes, temporal, basal ganglia, or cerebellum and brainstem in the posterior fossa and cortical gray matter.[54]
      ix. These abnormalities subsequently manifest as seizure activity, visual disturbances, headaches, confusion, or neuropathies.[54]

 XIII. MONITOR FOR POSTOPERATIVE COMPLICATIONS

A. There are three types of rejection:
   1. Hyperacute:
      a. Acute antibody-mediated rejection (AMR):
         i. An antibody-mediated process, which can develop immediately post implantation or within hours of transplant
      b. Primary graft dysfunction (PGD):
         i. Occurs within the first 72 hours following transplant thought to be due to an ischemic or reperfusion injury
   2. Acute:
      a. Most commonly seen during the first year following transplant:
         i. May be cellular or antibody mediated
   3. Chronic:
      a. Bronchiolitis obliterans syndrome (BOS)
      b. Chronic lung allograft dysfunction (CLAD)

4. All types of "rejection" listed above will be discussed in detail later in this chapter and in Tables 11-10[55,56] and 11-11.[56-59]

B. Surgical complications[47,58-64]:
   1. Inadequate bronchial anastomosis:
      a. Along with PGD, inadequate bronchial anastomosis remains a major cause of morbidity during the early postoperative period following lung transplantation.[56,60,61]
      b. Bronchial dehiscence and stenosis are the two major airway complications.
      c. Tracheal stenosis:
         i. Typically occurs concurrently with acute allograft rejection
         ii. Clinical manifestations include
            * Stridor
            * Cough
            * Shortness of breath
            * Palpable tracheal rumble on examination
            * Intermittent hypoxemia resolved by expectoration of secretions
         iii. Diagnosis: urgent bronchoscopy and/or chest CT is done to determine presence of stenosis and/or dehiscence diagnoses.[56,58,61]
         iv. Treatment typically includes
            * High-dose corticosteroids
            * Balloon dilatations of stenotic area
            * Bronchial stenting[64]
   2. Airway dehiscence:
      a. Improvements in organ preservation and surgical anastomosis techniques have decreased the incidence of dehiscence.
         i. Treatment includes
            * Balloon dilatation of the stenotic area and bronchial stenting
            * Reduction in immunosuppression, particularly high-dose corticosteroids (to promote healing)[58-63]

C. Pleural complications:
   1. Pneumothorax:
      a. Resolution of pneumothorax typically occurs within 1 to 2 days postoperatively (may be longer in some patients).
      b. The patient arrives in the ICU with two thoracostomy drains that are placed in the anterior and posterior pleura during surgery.
      c. A small but persistent air leak may occur due to undersized donor lungs.[49]
         i. The patient should be assessed at least each shift for the presence of subcutaneous air and addressed expeditiously[40,42]:
            * Assessment of subcutaneous air (crepitus) involves palpation of skin in the area of suspected air leak, but can be noted more remotely depending on the path the air has taken to escape.
            * Exam findings of popping of small air bubbles beneath the surface of the skin and dysphonia, which is observed as changes in the sound of the patient's voice becoming raspier or a nasal congestion sound despite not having a cold.

    d. Reexpansion of the transplanted lung is evaluated with daily chest radiographs.
       i. Following re-expansion, the chest tube suction system is generally weaned from −20 mm H_2O suction to water seal.
         • Chest tubes placed to water seal allow serous and sanguineous drainage to occur by gravity.
       ii. Chest tube drains are removed sequentially:
         • Fluid typically drains from anterior to posterior in the supine position.
         • The anterior tube is typically discontinued first.
         • The posterior tube is typically removed after there is no further evidence of persistent pneumothorax, air leak, or drainage.
    e. Following removal of the chest tube, the patient is assessed for a pneumothorax.
       i. Assess breath sounds for symmetry.
       ii. Assess patient for any signs and symptoms of respiratory distress.
       iii. Observe for sudden chest pain, shortness of breath, tachycardia, tachypnea, cough, cyanosis, or fatigue.
2. Chylothorax[47,48,50,65]:
    a. Occurs more commonly in pediatric transplant recipients
    b. Appears as a milky white discharge of lipid-rich lymphatic drainage in pleural fluid
    c. May occur in adults in the setting of
       i. Trauma to or manipulation of the thoracic duct occurs during surgery
       ii. Polycystic lung disease
       iii. Women with lymphangioleiomyomatosis (LAM)
    d. Clinical manifestations:
       i. Dyspnea
       ii. Cough
       iii. Hemoptysis
       iv. Chest and abdominal pain
       v. Unexplained weight loss
       vi. Effusions in pleural and abdominal cavities (frequent)
       vii. Pneumothorax (in certain cases)
    e. Definitive diagnostic testing includes pleural fluid analysis for triglycerides and cholesterol levels.[47,48,50]
       i. A rapidly reaccumulating chylothorax should be reported and treated, as this may inhibit lung expansion and oxygenation.
    f. Chest tube drains remain in place until the chylous drainage resolves.
    g. Standard treatment options include the following:
       i. Restriction of dietary fat.
       ii. Hyperalimentation therapy and transthoracic duct ligation may be required but should be initiated with caution due to infection concerns.[62,64]
3. Pleural effusions and/or pulmonary edema[63,65]:
    a. Varying degrees of pulmonary edema are commonly seen immediately after transplant.
    b. Pleural effusions are commonly observed during the first 2 weeks posttransplant.

      i. Early etiology:
- Interrupted bronchial lymphatic drainage
- Low serum albumin related to poor nutrition prior to transplantation

      ii. Late etiology:
- Infection
- Rejection

c. Diagnosis:
- i. Pulmonary edema can be diagnosed using PA pressure monitoring and CXR.
- ii. Early postoperative pleural effusions do not require any evaluation.
- iii. Late occurring pleural effusion are concerning for possible rejection or infection (empyema), a diagnosis of rejection is typically made by transbronchial biopsy (TBB), and bronchoscopy with bronchoalveolar lavage (BAL) or thoracentesis may be used to evaluate the pleural fluid (cell count, cytology, and culture) for infection.[64-66]

d. Treatment strategies are determined when diagnosis is confirmed.[66,67]
- i. Pulmonary edema and pleural effusions often respond to diuretic therapy and restoration of protein stores.
- ii. Keep PA pressures and CVP low to minimize pulmonary edema.
- iii. Occasionally, pleural effusions require therapeutic thoracentesis to drain accumulated fluid in order to prevent complications, which prevent lung expansion such as
  - Trapped lung
  - Pleural thickening

4. Impaired wound healing:
- a. May result from poor nutritional status prior to transplantation, general deconditioning, or immunosuppression.
- b. Meticulous assessment and care of surgical sites is essential to prevent and manage infections.
- c. All incisions should be assessed daily to monitor for
  - i. Dehiscence
  - ii. Erythema
  - iii. Edema
  - iv. Tissue necrosis
  - v. Amount and type of drainage
- d. Antibiotics may be administered for a specific time period or until chest tubes have been removed.
  - i. Typical classes of antibiotics administered during the perioperative period include
    - Cephalosporins
    - Glycopeptides
    - Fluoroquinolones
    - Nitroimidazoles

XIV. POSTTRANSPLANT MONITORING AND FOLLOW-UP

Lung and heart-lung transplant recipients are closely monitored to optimize medical therapy and reduce risks associated with infection and rejection. This monitoring includes, but is not limited to, bronchoscopies, biopsies, lab tests, chest radiographs, clinical examinations, and consultations. Patients are given transplant program-specific protocols to facilitate scheduling of follow-up clinic visits, tests, and procedures. Communication between the interdisciplinary transplant team and the patient is key to promoting patient understanding of and adherence to the posttransplant regimen.

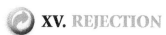 XV. REJECTION

A. Types of rejection (listed in order of possible occurrence):
1. Hyperacute rejection:
   a. An antibody-mediated process that can develop immediately post implantation or within hours of transplant.[56]
   b. Routine screening for preformed or panel-reactive antibodies (PRA) prior to transplantation has made hyperacute rejection a relatively uncommon occurrence.
   c. May present as acute O_2 desaturation[60]:
      i. O_2 saturation <90% if previously it had been well above this range
      ii. O_2 saturation that acutely falls more than 5% from baseline and requires additional supplemental O_2 titration to bring O_2 saturation back above 90% or to prior baseline level
      iii. Tissue hypoxia evidenced by perioral cyanosis, blue coloration to the fingers or toes
      iv. Noticeable radiographic changes suggesting infiltrates, consolidation, effusions, or pulmonary edema
2. Primary graft dysfunction (PGD)[56,60,61]:
   a. Formerly known as "reperfusion injury" or "implantation response"[61]
   b. Occurs within the first 72 hours following transplant[60]
   c. Major cause of early morbidity and mortality in lung transplant recipients
   d. Comparable to acute respiratory distress syndrome (ARDS)
   e. Possible causes related to[60,61]:
      i. Increased capillary permeability of transplanted lung tissue
      ii. Interrupted lymphatic drainage related to surgical procedure and CPB
      iii. Edema subsequent to prolonged ischemic time
      iv. Overall change in compliance and vascular resistance in donor and recipient
      v. Unrecognized fluid overload and suboptimal fluid management with volume resuscitation efforts
      vi. HLA mismatch ≥3 loci, which places higher risk for rejection[68,69]
   f. Potential warning signs/symptoms for graft dysfunction that should be reported promptly:
      i. General malaise
      ii. Increased work of breathing
      iii. Activity intolerance
      iv. Frequent O_2 desaturation (hypoxemia) with increasing supplementation requirements
      v. Pulmonary edema or diffuse opacities on chest radiograph
   g. Treatment options for PGD are similar to those for ARDS:
      i. Generally, patients require high FiO_2 support (70% to 100%).
      ii. Use of lower tidal volumes (TV) 100 to 300 mL (6 mL/kg) or low-stretch ventilator modes seem to have a lung-protective benefit.[61]
      iii. Positive pressure ventilation of 6 to 8 cm H_2O, along with the lower TV, recruits more alveoli and reduces ARDS risk.[62]

    h. Aggressive diuresis.

    i. For extubated patients:

        i. Recovery is typically quite slow.

        ii. Generally, 40% to 60% NRB O_2 mask as patients progress in the recovery.

        iii. Aggressive pulmonary toileting to prevent further complications and reduce requirement for reintubation.

        iv. Patients may exhibit persistent PGD refractory to the interventions listed above. In this instance

- Venovenous extracorporeal membranous oxygenation (VV-ECMO) may provide temporary support and allow the lung to rest.
- Long-term efficacy of ambulatory VV-ECMO is gaining acceptance but is not widely available in all centers.[61]

3. Acute rejection:

    a. Two types of acute rejection[69-71]:

        i. Cellular rejection:

- T-cell–mediated perivascular or bronchiolar mononuclear inflammation affects over 50% of lung transplant recipients within the first year.[71]

        ii. Antibody-mediated (humoral) rejection (AMR)[56]:

- AMR after lung transplantation remains unclassified and there is no consensus on its definition, diagnosis, histopathology, grading, or immunologic testing.[55]
  - There is no worldwide consensus regarding its significance and treatment.
- Etiology:
  - Immune-mediated response to the foreign transplanted organ.
  - When the recipient has positive serum anti-HLA antibodies to the donor, a humoral reaction occurs, and complement is deposited in alveolar tissue that can lead to fibrosis and scarring via stimulation of epithelial cells within the airway.
  - These humoral immune responses are also implicated in the pathogenesis of OB.
- This ISHLT consensus group[55] could not create a formal recommendation for evaluating and treating patients with AMR They did agree that AMR is an emerging problem, and if the recipient presents with allograft dysfunction and AMR is suspected, then a formal evaluation should occur.
  - Immunopathologically, blood is sent to the HLA lab to assess for the presence of donor-specific antibodies (DSA).[56,70]
  - Presence of donor antibodies can lead to complement activation and rapid graft loss.
  - Testing is done using the HLA antibody screening test used for serologic typing of the donor and recipient. If the DSA is positive in the recipient, the recipient may be at risk for rejection. Similar to "viral loads," the higher the DSA, the higher risk for antibody-mediated rejection.
  - Transbronchial biopsies are assessed for histologic evidence of capillary injury, and if present, then immunohistochemistry could be performed using special staining: C3d, C4d, CD31, and CD68.

- The use of C4d staining in particular may allow the humoral response to a lung graft to be interpreted along the lines of the NIH recommendations and may vary by interpreter.
b. Facts:
   i. Most lung transplant recipients will experience at least one acute rejection episode during the first year post transplant.[70]
   ii. The risk of rejection is highest in the first few months post transplant and decreases over time.
   iii. Acute rejection is a risk factor for bronchiolitis obliterans syndrome (BOS).
   iv. Current emphasis is placed on the prevention, early diagnosis, and complete eradication of acute rejection episodes to assure optimal short- and long-term outcomes.
c. Risk factors for acute rejection include
   i. Recipient PRA >10%
   ii. HLA mismatching (the more HLA mismatches between the donor and recipient, the higher the risk for rejection; increased risk if with class II HLA loci [DR] mismatch)[68,71]
   iii. Immunosuppressant drug levels that are not in therapeutic range
   iv. Nonadherence to immunosuppressive regimen
   v. Age: younger recipients (18 to 34) had higher incidence of rejection
   vi. Vitamin D deficiency[72]
   vii. Cytomegalovirus (CMV) mismatch (donor positive/recipient negative)
   viii. Donor issues (younger donor age, death by blunt trauma to head, and nonblack race)
d. Early acute rejection[70] is often nonspecific and may include one or more of the following clinical findings:
   i. Low-grade fever
   ii. Nonspecific respiratory symptoms
   iii. Flu-like syndrome
   iv. Hypoxemia
   v. Dyspnea
   vi. Tachypnea
   vii. Cough
   viii. Fatigue
   ix. Decreased exercise tolerance
   x. Pulmonary infiltrates
   xi. Pleural effusions
   xii. Chest pressure, new pain, or tenderness in the lung
   xiii. Notify provider immediately of these symptoms and anticipate prompt intervention.
      - Note: The symptoms of rejection may be similar to those of infection; therefore, it may be difficult to differentiate between infection and rejection.
e. Diagnosis is made by
   i. Clinical presentation
   ii. Objective findings on chest radiograph
   iii. Pulmonary function tests
   iv. Bronchoscopy

TABLE 11-10 **Grading Lung Rejection**

Type of Rejection	Grade	Severity	Appearance
Acute cellular rejection grading is based on perivascular and interstitial mononuclear infiltrates			
	0	None	Normal lung parenchyma
	1	Minimal	Inconspicuous small mononuclear perivascular infiltrates
	2	Mild	More frequent, more obvious, perivascular infiltrates, and eosinophils may be present
	3	Moderate	Dense perivascular infiltrates, extending into interstitial space, may see endothelialitis, eosinophils, and neutrophils
	4	Severe	Diffuse perivascular, interstitial, and airspace infiltrates with lung injury. Neutrophils may be present.
Airway inflammation graded looking at small airway inflammation, lymphocytic bronchiolitis			
	B0	None	No evidence of bronchiolar inflammation
	B1R	Low grade	Infrequent, scattered, or single-layer mononuclear cells in bronchiolar submucosa
	B2R	High grade	Larger infiltrates of larger and activated lymphocytes in bronchiolar submucosa. May involve eosinophils and plasmacytoid cells
	BX	Ungradable	No bronchiolar tissue available to grade
Chronic airway rejection/obliterative bronchiolitis			Chronic rejection, OB (grade C), is described as present (C1) or absent (C0), without reference to presence of inflammatory activity.
	C0	Absent	No evidence of BOS
	C1	Present	Describes intraluminal airway obliteration with fibrous connective tissue
Chronic vascular rejection/or accelerated graft vascular sclerosis	Ungraded		
		Findings	Fibrointimal thickening of arteries and poorly cellular hyaline sclerosis of veins. May be seen if an older donor is used.
			Usually requires open lung biopsy for definitive diagnosis.

From Stewart S, Fishbein MC, Snell GI, et al. Revision of the 1996 working formulation for the standardization of nomenclature in the diagnosis of lung rejection. *J Heart Lung Transplant.* 2007;26(12):1229–1242; Hechem R. Antibody-mediated lung transplant rejection. *Curr Respir Care Rep.* 2012;1(3):157–161.

  v. Surveillance transbronchial biopsies[55,66,73]:
    ● Note: Some patients may be asymptomatic and diagnosis of rejection may be based upon routine biopsy.
  f. Grading of acute rejection (see Table 11-10).[55,56,70]
  g. Treatment is based on the severity and type of rejection and clinical findings.
    i. Acute rejection is typically usually treated with
     ● High-dose corticosteroids
     ● Optimizing maintenance immunosuppression
     ● Replacing one immunosuppressive agent with another agent (considered in certain settings)

- T-cell–depleting agent: rabbit antithymocyte globulin (rATG) to thymoglobumin
- Antibody-mediated rejection may include the above strategies (1 to 4), plus:
  - Plasmapheresis
  - IVIG
  - Rituximab (Rituxan)
  - Bortezomib (Velcade)

ii. Follow-up:
- Office visits per protocol and dependent on severity of rejection.
- More severe rejection will require frequent return visits for medical care and surveillance biopsies.
- Transbronchial biopsy in 4 weeks with transplant labs to allow for treatment response.

4. Chronic rejection: bronchiolitis obliterans with or without BOS
   a. Overview:
   i. Bronchiolitis obliterans (BO) is the predominant feature of chronic rejection and is seen pathologically as dense fibrous scar tissue affecting the small airways.
   ii. Alloimmune and nonalloimmune factors have been shown to produce the fibroproliferative airway response seen in patients with OB.[72]
   - The final common pathway is the release of proinflammatory cytokines and growth factors that cause fibrous scarring and airway obliteration.[59,74,75]
   iii. The term "BOS" is also used to describe *chronic* rejection in lung transplant recipients.[76,77]
   - A delayed allograft dysfunction associated with a persistent decline in FEV1 that is not due to other known, potentially reversible causes of decreases in lung function.
   - Potential etiology: inflammation, destruction, and fibrosis of small airways.
   - BOS can lead to OB.
   iv. Note: the terms "BOS," "bronchiolitis obliterans" (BO), and "obliterative bronchiolitis" (OB) are used interchangeably; however, BO/OB refers to the histologic findings on biopsy, and BOS refers to the declining allograft lung function and is graded using spirometry.
   v. Facts:
   - Approximately 48% of recipients develop BO or BOS by 5 years after lung transplant and 76% after 10 years.[13]
   - Recurrent acute rejection has been associated with the development of BOS.[76,77]
   - Compared with chronic rejection in other transplanted organs, chronic rejection is a particularly pervasive problem in lung transplantation.
   - BOS is the most significant obstacle to long-term, morbidity-free survival and occurs typically after the first year of transplant.
   - BOS equally affects single-lung, double-lung, and heart-lung transplant recipients.

- No difference in incidence of BOS has been observed when recipients were stratified by age or diagnosis at time of transplant.[13]

b. Risk factors for BOS include[74,76,77]
  i. HLA mismatching
  ii. Elevated panel-reactive antibodies
  iii. CMV mismatch (donor CMV seropositive; recipient CMV seronegative)
  iv. PGD, severity correlates to development of BO
  v. Acute cellular or antibody-mediated rejection, particularly frequent episodes during the first year
  vi. Late-onset acute rejection after the first year
  vii. Inadequate immunosuppression
  viii. Viral infection
  ix. Bacterial infections
  x. GERD
  xi. Lymphocytic bronchiolitis
  xii. Community-acquired respiratory virus infection—symptomatic
  xiii. Colonization and infection of lung with *Pseudomonas aeruginosa* or *Aspergillus*
  xiv. Organizing pneumonia
  xv. Autoimmune sensitization to collagen V
  xvi. Neutrophilia on bronchiolar lavage differential

c. Clinical manifestations of BOS:
  i. Progressive shortness of breath; possible hypoxemia
  ii. Nonproductive cough
  iii. Symptoms resembling upper respiratory infection (URI)
  iv. Decreased exercise tolerance
  v. Airflow limitation
  vi. Progressive and persistent decline in the FEV1 to values <80% of posttransplantation baseline.
  vii. Changes on chest computed tomography (CT) scan (inspiratory and expiratory views) that suggest air trapping

d. Measuring rejection:
  i. Formulated in 1990 and last revised in 2007, the grading schema for pulmonary allograft rejection was developed by leading lung transplant specialists.[75]
  ii. Lung biopsy specimens are graded for acute rejection (grades A0 to A4), airway inflammation (grades B0 to B4), and bronchiolitis obliterans (C0 absent and C1 present) described in Table 11-10.[55,56,70]

e. ISHLT BOS stages:
  i. The ISHLT classified severity of BOS in stages based on a comparison of the patient's current FEV1 with his/her best posttransplant FEV1.[76,77]
  ii. This FEV1 decline should be demonstrated in two measurements at least 3 weeks apart.
    - Stage 0: FEV1 is >90% of baseline and FEF (25% to 75%) >75% of baseline.
    - Stage 0–p: FEV1 is 81% to 90% of baseline and/or FEF (25% to 75%) ≤75% of baseline.
    - Stage 1: FEV1 equals 66% to 80% of baseline.
    - Stage 2: FEV1 equals 51% to 65% of baseline.
    - Stage 3: FEV1 is ≤50% of baseline.

        iii. BOS does not necessarily require histologic confirmation.

        iv. HRCT is used to evaluate abnormalities seen on routine x-ray or abnormal pulmonary function tests (as seen above in the BOS grading).

   f. Potential strategies to prevent BOS may include

        i. Aggressive prophylaxis and management of acute rejection and CMV infection[77]

        ii. Individualization of treatment based on current immunosuppressive regimen and severity of disease and symptoms

        iii. Close monitoring of pulmonary function and early intervention

           • Decreased pulmonary function associated with chronic rejection is generally irreversible.

   g. Potential treatment options for BOS[77]:

        i. Optimization of immunosuppression regimen by

           • Adding the macrolide antibiotic azithromycin (Zithromax), which is typically dosed three times weekly.

              ○ Note: Perform a baseline EKG and monitor QT interval and increase risk of torsades ventricular tachycardia.[39]

           • Consider changing azathioprine (Imuran) to mycophenolate mofetil (CellCept).

           • Consider converting cyclosporine (Gengraf/Neoral) to tacrolimus (Prograf).

           • Consider a short course of high-dose corticosteroid therapy.

           • Consider additional agents such as sirolimus (Rapamune).

           • Other drug therapies such as antithymocyte globulin and thymoglobulin may be given, but the risk of infection is significant.

           • Consider trial of azathioprine (Imuran), particularly for patients with bronchoalveolar lavage (BAL) neutrophilia.

        ii. Recent evidence suggests that some patients with BOS may respond to azithromycin with >10% improvement in their FEV1.[76]

           • Consider antireflux surgery (fundoplication of the gastroesophageal junction) for select patients with a declining FEV1 and histologic evidence of gastroesophageal reflux aspiration on bronchoscopy biopsy specimens or a positive impedance study with symptomatic reflux.[59]

        iii. Consider referral for retransplantation.

 5. Chronic lung allograft dysfunction (CLAD):

   a. The term CLAD was first introduced in 2010 to cover all forms of graft dysfunction.[66,67]

   b. Definition of CLAD[57–59]:

        i. A restrictive allograft syndrome (RAS) that exhibits restrictive functional changes with fibrotic processes in peripheral lung tissue rather than the classical radiologic or pathologic findings of the small airway obliteration and obstructive findings seen in BOS.

        ii. A progressive form of chronic rejection that may be irreversible.

        iii. A complicated heterogeneous spectrum of disease that is not fully classified or understood at this time.

        iv. See Table 11-11 for further CLAD definitions and emerging phenotypes.[58–61]

   c. Measuring CLAD[58–61]:

        i. A baseline FEV1 (as defined by ISHLT) is the average of the two best measurements obtained at least 3 weeks apart.

TABLE 11-11 CLAD: Emerging Phenotypes and Key Features

Key Features	CLAD	CLAD: Emerging Phenotypes		
		Classic BOS	ARAD	RAS
Pulmonary function	• Full PFT testing done • Suspect CLAD if ≥10% decline in FEV1 and/or FVC from stable baseline function	• Obstructive • FEV1 decline ≥20% upon two measurements at least 3 wk apart • Graded on FEV1 decline	• Obstructive • FEV1 ≤80% of stable baseline value	• Restrictive • Persistent decline in VC and TLC and FEV1 decreased ≥20% from baseline posttransplant
HRCT imaging	• Used to assess phenotypes	• Air trapping usually present • No/minimal infiltrates—± bronchiectasis	• Changes of constrictive bronchiolitis ("tree-in-bud" peribronchiolar infiltrates often present)—± air trapping	• Upper lobe dominant fibrosis • Infiltrates (ground-glass opacities, interstitial, or honeycombing) usually present • Bronchiectasis air trapping
Histopathology	• BAL with total and differential cell counts	• OB (difficult to diagnose via transbronchial biopsy)	• Cellular bronchiolitis	• Diffuse alveolar damage • Extensive parenchymal/pleural fibroelastosis • w/wo scattered alveolar damage and OB lesions
Clinical findings	• A persistent decline in lung function in comparison to the best postoperative FEV1 • Efforts to determine the underlying cause should be made.	• Typically progressive but may stabilize • Recipients may have coexistent chronic bacterial infection. • May evolve to RAS	• High likelihood of significant response to azithromycin • They no longer meet criteria for persistent BOS if they have azithromycin-responsive BOS/allograft dysfunction.	• Tends to be relentlessly progressive • May start as/coincide with BOS
Miscellaneous	• CLAD encompasses all forms of chronic lung dysfunction.	• Usually responds poorly to pharmacologic therapies including azithromycin therapy • Nonresponders may be characterized as fibrotic OB.	• BAL neutrophilia (e.g., ≥15% on differential cell count) • May correlate with response to azithromycin therapy but is not necessary for a response • May require long-term azithromycin treatment	• Correlates with the presence of early DAD post transplant

BAL, bronchoalveolar lavage; BOS, bronchiolitis obliterans syndrome; CLAD, chronic lung allograft dysfunction; DAD, diffuse alveolar damage; ARAD, azithromycin-responsive allograft dysfunction; OB, obliterative bronchiolitis; RAS, restrictive allograft syndrome.
From Hechem R. Antibody-mediated lung transplant rejection. *Curr Respir Care Rep.* 2012;1(3):157–161; Sato M, Waddell T, Wagnetz D, et al. Restrictive allograft (RAS): a novel form of chronic lung allograft dysfunction. *J Heart Lung Transplant.* 2011;30(7):735–742; Saito T, Horie M, Sato M, et al. Low-dose computed tomography volumetry for subtyping chronic lung allograft dysfunction (CLAD). *J Heart Lung Transplant.* 2016;35(1):59–66. doi: 10.1016/j.healun.2015.07.005; Verleden S, Todd J, Sato M, et al. Impact of CLAD phenotype on survival after lung transplantation: a multicenter study. *Am J Transplant.* 2015;15(8):2223–2230.

      ii. The baseline TLC measurement is taken at the time of the best FEV1 measurements.

      iii. CLAD is defined as an irreversible decline in FEV1 ≥ of baseline.

      iv. CLAD is formally diagnosed when a functional decline persists despite appropriate treatment for infection, acute rejection, or both.

         • RAS is described as CLAD with an irreversible decline in TLC >10% of baseline.

      v. Persistent parenchymal infiltrates and (sub)pleural thickening on chest CT scan.[68]

    d. Clinical manifestations of CLAD:

      i. All symptoms are noted in prior rejection and BOS with a persistent decline.

    e. Treatment:

      i. All treatments are aimed at improving pulmonary function.

      ii. Recent evidence suggests that some patients with BOS phenotype CLAD may respond to azithromycin with >10% improvement in their FEV1 but complete recovery is unlikely.[66]

         • Azithromycin nonresponders do not have the BOS phenotype.[70]

      iii. Intensified immune suppression.

      iv. Retransplant.

  6. Future research:

    a. Further CLAD definitions, phenotyping, and treatment strategies

    b. New emerging posttransplant disorders, such as "acute lung allograft dysfunction" (ALAD), which may be due to acute rejection, infection, pulmonary embolism, etc. and is potentially reversible depending on the etiology and treatment options

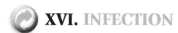 XVI. INFECTION

A. Overview:

  1. Infection is one of the major complications of immunosuppression therapy after transplantation.[38]

  2. The lung is the most common site of infection in all organ solid transplant recipients.

  3. The risk of infection is highest during the first months after transplantation and decreases subsequently thereafter.

B. Timing of infections:

  1. Bacterial and fungal infections comprise the majority of infections that occur in the transplanted lung in the first months after transplant.[49,51]

  2. Viral infections are most prevalent during the second to third posttransplant months.[51]

  3. Use of the procalcitonin (PCT) level is a promising biomarker for the assessment of early bacterial infections.[78]

    a. PCT levels did not elevate during viral episodes or rejections.

C. Prevention of infection:

  1. Broad-spectrum antibiotics are routinely used perioperatively to prevent infection.

  2. Additional antibiotics are used accordingly if the donor's cultures were positive.

   a. Antifungal medications are used if the *Candida* or *Aspergillus* are isolated in the recipient's early sputum cultures

D. Respiratory infections:

  1. Respiratory infections are the leading cause of morbidity after lung transplantation.[51]

  2. The transplanted lung is particularly susceptible due to the impairment of both mucociliary clearance and the cough reflex due to potential nerve damage from surgery.[50]

E. CMV infections:

  1. CMV infection is the most common and debilitating viral infection after lung transplantation.

  2. CMV can be a primary or secondary infection.

   a. Primary infections occur when an allograft from a CMV-seropositive donor is implanted into a CMV-seronegative recipient.

   b. Secondary infections develop as a result of reactivation of the disease in the recipient who has been exposed to CMV in the past (recipient is CMV sero-seropositive prior to transplantation).

  3. CMV infections can develop in the blood, lungs, GI tract, and retina.

  4. Most lung transplant programs have an aggressive posttransplant CMV prophylactic protocol, which may include ganciclovir (Cytovene), valganciclovir (Valcyte), or intravenous immunoglobulin (IVIG).

  5. See Infectious Diseases chapter for additional information and routine solid organ prophylaxis strategies.

XVII. OUTCOMES AND QUALITY OF LIFE

A. Although lung transplantation is an accepted therapy for select patients with end-stage pulmonary disease, certain patients may experience complications that make long-term survival suboptimal.

  1. 2014 ISHLT data indicate the following[13]:

   a. Primary lung transplantation: adults who underwent transplantation between 1990 and 2012 and 5-year survival rates of 82% and 53.6%, respectively:

    i. Approximately 48% and 76% of recipients developed BO or BOS at 5 and 10 years posttransplant, respectively.13

    ii. Younger (18 to 34 years) and female each had higher survival rates than older (>34 years) and male recipients.

   b. Primary heart-lung transplantation: adults who underwent primary heart-lung transplantation between 1982 and 2012:

    i. 1- and 5-year survival rates of 63% and 45%, respectively.

B. Although there is an extensive body of quality of life (QOL) research in other transplant cohorts, additional QOL research is needed in the lung transplant population.[79]

  1. This section will highlight select lung transplant QOL studies that have been done to date.

   a. In an early study, Lanuza and colleagues[80] examined functional status among 10 lung transplant patients before and 3 months after transplantation.

    i. Following transplantation, patients reported improvement in physical strength, current health, and QOL.

  ii. However, as reported in other studies, there was no significant pre- to posttransplant improvement in psychological functioning.

  iii. Ninety percent of patients reported satisfaction with their decision to undergo transplantation.

  iv. Patients who had developed BOS grade ≥1 had significantly poorer QOL than did those with a BOS = 0.6.

 b. Looking at different lung transplant populations, Yazdani and colleagues[20] compared patients with rheumatoid arthritis-associated interstitial lung disease (RA-ILD; n = 10), idiopathic pulmonary fibrosis (IPF; n = 53), and scleroderma-associated interstitial lung disease (SSc-ILD; n = 17) who underwent lung transplantation.

  i. There were no significant differences among the three groups with respect to survival at 1, 2, or 5 years post transplant.

  ii. The RA-ILD and IPF patients had marked improvement in pre- to posttransplant QOL.

  iii. Lung transplantation should be considered for end-stage RA-ILD patients as it appears to confer significant QOL benefits, particularly with regard to respiratory symptoms

 c. In their 2013 systematic review of 73 studies published between 1983 and 2011, Singer and colleagues[20] noted that adult lung transplantation is associated with substantial and sustained improvements in health-related quality of life (HRQOL), particularly in the domains of physical health and functioning.

  i. The greatest improvement is seen between 6 and 12 months post transplant, after which time HRQOL was negatively affected by BOS and comorbidities.

  ii. Posttransplant HRQOL does not decline to pretransplant levels.

  iii. Physical rehabilitation may augment the early improvements in HRQOL, whereas BOS and psychological conditions have a negative impact.

 d. In their 2014 retrospective study, Cohen and colleagues[27] examined cognitive function, mental health, and HRQOL in 42 lung transplant recipients. Mild and moderate cognitive impairment was noted in 67% and 5% of the recipients, respectively. Additionally, these investigators noted that

  i. Prolonged allograft ischemic time was independently associated with worse posttransplant cognitive impairment (perhaps due to ischemia-reperfusion injury, oxidative stress, and neuroinflammation).

  ii. Posttransplant HRQOL was higher than pretransplant HRQOL.

  iii. Approximately 20% of recipients continued to experience moderate to severe anxiety following transplantation.

  iv. Functional improvement at the conclusion of posttransplant physical rehabilitation was independently associated with improved cognitive function.

 e. In summary, most studies found patient physical QOL significantly improved from before to after transplantation, but psychological health did not demonstrate similar improvement.

 f. Future research regarding the psychosocial outcomes of lung and heart-lung transplantation should

  i. Focus less on descriptive studies and more on prospective clinical trials designed to

- Identify the risk factors and clinical sequelae of transplant recipients' psychosocial status
- Test the efficacy and effectiveness of psychosocial interventions
ii. Focus on long-term outcomes (>5 years posttransplant)
iii. Include appropriately sized samples to ensure adequate statistical power
iv. Include samples that are truly representative of the cardiothoracic transplant population[20,79]
v. Validate the psychometric performance of HRQOL instruments in the lung transplant population
vi. Employ qualitative methods to characterize disease-specific QOL constructs
vii. Include both generic and pulmonary-specific QOL tools to capture both changes in allograft function and the effects of transplant-specific comorbidities and side effects of posttransplant treatment modalities

XVIII. LUNG TRANSPLANTATION SUMMARY

A. Lung transplantation is an alternative therapy for select patients with end-stage pulmonary disease.
1. Long-term survival is limited by the development of BOS.
2. However, patient's perceptions of global QOL improve pre- to posttransplant; these perceptions either remain stable or further improve over time.[79]

B. The future of lung transplantation will be defined by
1. New immunosuppressive therapies to prevent long-term complications
2. Further refinement of selection criteria
3. Increasing the availability of donor organs
4. Ex vivo lung perfusion (EVLP)
a. This technology creates effective prolonged cold preservation with the use of the Perfadex solution, which is a colloid-containing preservation fluid and has played a significant pioneering role in the development of this procedure; the effective preservation time for lungs has been extended from about 4 hours before the introduction of Perfadex to well beyond 25 hours today. This major advance has revolutionized access to suitably matched donor lungs where transcontinental transport times have previously restricted utilization, in effect significantly expanding the very restricted donor pool.

XIX. HEART-LUNG TRANSPLANTATION

A. The first successful HLT was performed in 1981 by Shumway and Reitz at Stanford University on a patient with primary pulmonary hypertension (PPH).[4]
1. The patient survived 5 years following this combined heart and double-lung transplant surgery.
2. The total number of adult procedures has stabilized since 2003 and ranges from 62 to 94 per year due to the donor organ shortage. In 2012, only 75 HLT were reported to the ISHLT worldwide.[36]

B. Indications:
1. Idiopathic pulmonary arterial hypertension (IPAH):
a. End-stage pulmonary hypertension with right ventricular failure on inotropic support

2. CHD complicated by Eisenmenger syndrome
3. CF with decompensated right heart failure
4. Hypertrophic cardiomyopathy and chronic pulmonary obstructive disease

C. Evaluation:
1. Evaluation for HLT combines individual organ tests, procedures, and consults and, when completed, is presented to the transplant selection committee for listing consideration.

D. Listing:
1. Patient demographic and clinical information are entered into the UNOS database.
2. HLT recipients are listed on both the heart and lung transplant lists.
3. Both the heart transplant and lung transplant data are entered, and a status is given for the heart and a LAS is generated for the lung.

E. Organ allocation:
1. Considerable debate exists on a fair and equitable system for allocating heart-lung organs.

F. Per UNOS policy 6.5.E (allocation of heart-lungs), there are two match runs for HLT:
1. Candidates: a combined heart-lung match list run and a lung-alone match list run.
2. If the candidate is allocated a heart, the lung from the same deceased donor must be allocated to the HLT candidate.
3. If the candidate is offered a lung, the heart from the same donor is only allocated with the lung if no suitable 1A heart candidate is eligible to receive the heart.

G. Surgical procedure:
1. Cardiac anesthesia provides airway support:
   a. The requirement for a single- or dual-lumen ETT depends on the type of procedure.
   b. The ventilation of the lung during the lung transplant surgery is the same as described during the lung transplant procedure.
2. Invasive lines, tubes, and catheters are placed.
3. Skin prep is completed.
4. The chest is opened using a median sternotomy.
5. Donor heart and lungs are examined and deemed suitable for transplant.
6. ABO verification is rechecked prior to implant.
7. Surgeon cross clamps the aorta and places the patient on CPB.
8. For HLT, cardiectomy of the diseased heart is done by cutting the proximal ascending aorta, inferior and superior vena cava, or right atrial cuff and vena cava for single-lung transplant (SLT); following removal of the heart, the lung(s) is removed by resecting the trachea for bilateral lung transplants (BLT) or left/right mainstem bronchus for an SLT (Figure 11-6).[81]
9. The heart-lung bloc is readied for implant. The surgeon starts with the tracheal anastomosis (the lower end of the recipient trachea to the upper end of the donor trachea). Followed by the anastomosis of the donor and recipient aorta and remaining right atrial cuff or blood vessels. Upon completion, the cross clamp is removed and the heart-lung are reperfused and assessed for leaks/bleeding. The ETT is deliberately placed above the tracheal

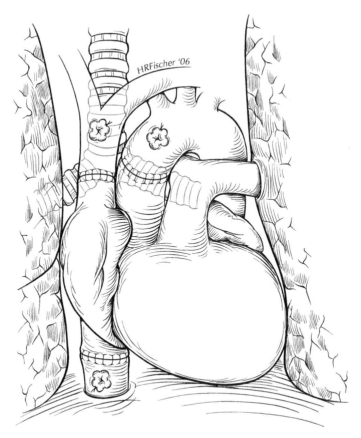

FIGURE 11-6   The completed implantation of the heart-lung transplant. The tracheal anastomosis lies in the space between the superior vena cava and posterior to the ascending aorta. Angled chest drains are placed bilaterally and a straight drain in the anterior mediastinum. The chest closure is routine.

anastomosis site and confirmed by fiberoptic bronchoscope to assess correct position. Low tidal volume ventilation is started (4 to 6 mL/kg) to promote tracheal healing.

10. See chapter on Heart Transplantation for additional information.

H. Advantages of HLT include[81]

1. Improved perfusion

a. Following HLT, the donor trachea and lungs receive blood from the right bronchial artery, whereas in lung transplantation alone, there is no bronchial blood supply.

b. HLT minimizes ventilation and perfusion defects by removing all diseased tissue.

REFERENCES

1. Hardy JD, Webb WR, Dalton ML, et al. Lung homotransplantation in man. *JAMA.* 1963;186:1065–1074.
2. Nelems JM, Rebuck AS, Cooper JD. Human lung transplantation. *Chest.* 1980;78:569–573.
3. Kamholz SL, Veith FL, Mollenkopf FP, et al. Single lung transplantation with cyclosporine immunosuppression. *J Thorac Cardiovasc Surg.* 1983;86:537–542.
4. Reitz BA, Wallwork JL, Hunt SA, et al. Heart–lung transplantation: successful therapy for patients with pulmonary vascular disease. *N Engl J Med.* 1982;306:557–564.

5. Toronto Lung Transplantation Group. Unilateral lung transplantation for pulmonary fibrosis. *N Engl J Med.* 1986;314:1140–1145.

6. Wigfield CH, Love RB. Donation after cardiac death lung transplantation outcomes. *Curr Opin Organ Transplant.* 2011;16(5):462–468.

7. Cooper JD, Pearson FG, Patterson GA, et al. Technique of successful lung transplantation in humans. *J Thorac Cardiovasc Surg.* 1987;93(2):173–181.

8. Morgan WE, Lima O, Goldberg M, et al. Improved bronchial healing in canine left lung reimplantation using omental pedicle wrap. *J Thorac Cardiovasc Surg.* 1983;85:134–139.

9. Lima O, Cooper JD, Peters WJ, et al. Effect of methylprednisolone and azathioprine on bronchial healing following lung autotransplantation. *J Thorac Cardiovasc Surg.* 1981;82:211–215.

10. American Society for Transplant Physicians, Thoracic Society, European Respiratory Society, International Society for Heart and Lung Transplantation. International guidelines for the selection of lung transplant candidates. *Am J Respir Crit Care Med.* 1998;58:335–339.

11. Hook J, Lederer D. Selecting lung transplant candidates: where do current guideline fall short? *Expert Rev Respir Med.* 2012;6(1):51–61.

12. Inci I, Walter W. Managing surgical complications. In: Vigneswaran WT, Garrity ER Jr, eds. *Lung Transplantation.* London: Informa Healthcare; 2010:249–265.

13. Yusen RD, Edwards LB, Kucheryavaya AY, et al. The registry of the international society for heart and lung transplantation: thirty-first adult lung and heart–lung transplant report—2014; focus theme: retransplantation. *J Heart Lung Transplant.* 2014;33(10):1009–1024

14. Valapour M, Skeans MA, Heubner BM, et al. OPTN/SRTR 2013 annual data report: lung. *Am J Transplant.* 2015;15(suppl 2):1–28.

15. Weill D, Benden C, Corris P, et al. A consensus document for the selection of lung transplant candidates: 2014 an update from the pulmonary transplantation council of the International Society for Heart and Lung Transplantation. *J Heart Lung Transplant.* 2015;34(1):1–15.

16. Kreider M, Hadjiliadis D, Kotloff RM. Candidate selection, timing of listing, and choice of procedure for lung transplantation. *Clin Chest Med.* 2011;32(2):199–211.

17. Dudley KA, El-Chemaly S. Cardiopulmonary exercise testing in lung transplantation: a review. *Pulm Med.* 2012;2012:237852.

18. Shah P, Orens J. Guidelines for the selection of lung transplant candidates. *Curr Opin Organ Transplant.* 2012;17(5):3467–3473.

19. Shoham S, Shah PD. Impact of multidrug-resistant organisms on patients considered for lung transplantation. *Inf Dis Clin North Am.* 2013;27(2):343–358.

20. Yazdani A, Singer LG, Strand V, et al. Survival and quality of life in rheumatoid-associated interstitial lung disease after lung transplantation. *J Heart Lung Transplant.* 2014;33:514–520.

21. Singer J, Chen J, Blanc PD, et al. A thematic analysis of quality of life in lung transplant: the existing evidence and implications for future directions. *Am J Transplant.* 2013;13(4):839–850.

22. All Kaplan-Meier Median Waiting Times for Registration Listed: 1999–2004. *Organ Procurement and Transplantation Network.* Available at www.optn.transplant.hrsa.gov. Accessed October 1, 2015.

23. OPTN/SRTR 2012 Annual Data Report: Lung. *OPTN/SRTR 2012 Annual Data Report: Lung.* Available at www.srtr.transplant.hrsa.gov/annual_reports/2012/pds/06_lung_13.pdf. Accessed October 1, 2015.

24. Smith PJ, Blumenthal JA, Trulock EP, et al. Psychosocial predictors of mortality following lung transplantation. *Am J Transplant.* 2016;16(1):271–277. doi: 10.1111/ajt.13447.

25. Rosenberger EM, Dew MA, DiMartini AF, et al. Psychosocial issues facing lung transplant candidates, recipients and family caregivers. *Thorac Surg Clin.* 2012;22(4):517–529.

26. Xu J. Adeboyejo O, Wagley E, et al. Daily burdens of recipients and family caregivers after lung transplant. *Prog Transplant.* 2012;22(1):41–47.

27. Cohen DG, Christie JD, Anderson BJ, et al. Cognitive function, mental health, and health-related quality of life after lung transplantation. *Ann Am Thorac Soc.* 2014;11(4):522–530.

28. Smits JM, Nossent GD, Vries ED, et al. Evaluation of the lung allocation score in highly urgent and urgent lung transplant candidates in Eurotransplant. *J Heart Lung Transplant.* 2011;30(1):22–28.

29. Braun AT, Dasenbrook EC, Shah AS, et al. Impact of lung allocation score on survival in cystic fibrosis lung transplant recipients. *J Heart Lung Transplant.* 2015;34(11):1436–1441. doi: 10.1016/j.healun.2015.05.020.

30. Organ Procurement and Transplantation Network. Policy 10: Allocation of Lungs. Available at http://optn.transplant.hrsa.gov/ContentDocuments/OPTN_Policies. Accessed September 29, 2015:134–150.

31. Snell GI, Westall GP. Selection and management of the lung donor. *Clin Chest Med.* 2011;32(2):223–232.

32. Moreno P, Alvarez A, Santos F, et al. Extended recipients but not extended donors are associated with poor outcomes following lung transplantation. *Eur J Cardiothorac Surg.* 2014;45(6):1040–1047.

33. Baran DA. The courage to push: donors and recipients. *J Heart Lung Transplant.* 2014;33(2):139–140.

34. Davis RD, Hartwig M. Lung transplantation procedure and surgical technique. In: Kirk AD, ed. *Textbook of Organ Transplantation.* New Jersey: Wiley-Blackwell; 2014:669–673.

35. Bae HY, Son HJ, Hahm KD, et al. Anesthetic considerations during heart lung transplantation in a patient with an unresectable pulmonary artery sarcoma. *Korean J Anesthesiol.* 2012;62(6):584–585.

36. Moten MA, Doligalski CT. Postoperative transplant immunosuppression in the critical care unit. *AACN Adv Crit Care.* 2013;24(4):345–350.

37. Rang HP, Ritter JM, Flower RJ, et al. *Rang & Dale's Pharmacolog.* 8th ed. Philadelphia, PA: Elsevier; 2015.

38. Floreth T, Bhorade SM. Current trends in immunosuppression for lung transplantation. *Semin Respir Crit Care Med.* 2010;31(2):172–178.

39. Afshar K. Future direction of immunosuppression in lung transplantation. *Curr Opin Organ Transplant.* 2014;19(6):583–590.

40. Carlin BW, Lega M, Veynovich B. Management of the patient: undergoing lung transplantation an intensive care perspective. *Crit Care Nurse Q.* 2009;32(1):49–57.

41. Evans CF, Iacono AT, Sanchez PG, et al. Venous thromboembolic complications of lung transplantation: a contemporary single-institution review. *Ann Thorac Surg.* 2015;100(6):2033–2039. doi: 10.1016/j.athoracsur.2015.05.095.

42. George EL, Guttendorf J. Lung transplant. *Crit Care Nurs Clin North Am.* 2011;23(3):481–503.

43. Coleman B, Blumenthal N, Currey J, et al. Adult cardiothoracic transplant nursing: an ISHLT consensus document on the current adult nursing practice in heart and lung transplantation. *J Heart Lung Transplant.* 2015;34(2):139–148.

44. Duarte RT, Linch GF, Caregnato RC. The immediate post-operative period following lung transplantation: mapping of nursing interventions. *Rev Lat Am Enfermagem.* 2014;22(5):778–784.

45. Solidoro P, Patrucco F, Bonato R, et al. Pulmonary hypertension in chronic obstructive pulmonary disease and pulmonary fibrosis: prevalence and hemodynamic differences in lung transplant recipients at transplant center's referral time. *Transplant Proc.* 2015;47(7):2161–2165.

46. Parmar B, Branch K, Mulligan M, et al. Clinical and procedural factors that predict post-operative atrial fibrillation among lung transplant patients. *J Am Coll Cardiol.* 2011;57(14):E157.

47. Kelly T, Buxbaum J. Gastrointestinal manifestations of cystic fibrosis. *Digest Dis Sci.* 2015;60(7):1903–1913.

48. Castor JM, Wood RK, Muir AJ, et al. Gastroesophageal reflux and altered motility in lung transplant rejection: gastroesophageal reflux and altered motility. *Neurogastroenterol Motil.* 2010;22(8):841–850.

49. Michaud GC, Channick CL, Marion CR, et al. ATS core curriculum 2015. Part I: adult pulmonary medicine. *Ann Am Thorac Soc.* 2015;12(9):1387–1397.

50. Atkins BZ, Petersen RP, Daneshmand MA, et al. Impact of oropharyngeal dysphagia on long-term outcomes of lung transplantation. *Ann Thorac Surg.* 2015;90(5):1622–1628.

51. Burguete S, Maselli D, Fernandez JF, et al. Lung transplant infection. *Respirology.* 2013;18(1):22–38.

52. Lee JC, Diamond JM, Christie JD. Critical care management of the lung transplant recipient. *Curr Respir Care Rep.* 2012;1(3):168–176.

53. Cason M, Naik A, Grimm JC, et al. The efficacy and safety of epidural-based anesthesia in a case series of patients undergoing lung transplantation. *J Cardiothorac Vasc Anesth.* 2015;29(1):126–132.

54. Arimura FE, Camargo PC, Costa AN, et al. Posterior reversible encephalopathy syndrome in lung transplantation: 5 case reports. *Transplant Proc.* 2014;46(6):1845–1848.

55. Stewart S, Fishbein MC, Snell GI, et al. Revision of the 1996 working formulation for the standardization of nomenclature in the diagnosis of lung rejection. *J Heart Lung Transplant.* 2007;26(12):1229–1242.

56. Hechem R. Antibody-mediated lung transplant rejection. *Curr Respir Care Rep.* 2012;1(3):157–161.

57. Sato M, Waddell T, Wagnetz D, et al. Restrictive allograft (RAS): a novel form of chronic lung allograft dysfunction. *J Heart Lung Transplant.* 2011;30(7):735–742.

58. Saito T, Horie M, Sato M, et al. Low-dose computed tomography volumetry for subtyping chronic lung allograft dysfunction (CLAD). *J Heart Lung Transplant.* 2016;35(1):59–66. doi: 10.1016/j.healun.2015.07.005.

59. Verleden S, Todd J, Sato M, et al. Impact of CLAD phenotype on survival after lung transplantation: a multicenter study. *Am J Transplant.* 2015;15(8):2223–2230.

60. Porteous MK, Diamond JM, Christie JD. Primary graft dysfunction: lessons learned about the first 72 h after lung transplantation. *Curr Opin Organ Transplant.* 2015;20(5):506–514.

61. Diamond JM, Lee JC, Kawut SM, et al. Lung transplant outcomes group. Clinical risk factors for primary graft dysfunction after lung transplantation. *Am J Respir Crit Care Med.* 2013;187(5):527–534.

62. Porhownik NR. Airway complications post lung transplantation. *Curr Opin Pulm Med.* 2013;19(2):174–180.

63. Mahida RY, Wiscombe S, Fisher AJ. Current status of lung transplantation. *Chron Respir Dis.* 2012;9(2):131–145.

64. Radzikowska E. Lymphangioleiomyomatosis: new treatment perspectives. *Lung.* 2015;194(4):467–475.

65. Lee HJ, Puchalski J, Sterman DH, et al. Secondary carina Y-stent placement for post-lung-transplant bronchial stenosis. *J Bronchology Interv Pulmonol.* 2012;19(2):109–114.

66. Mohanka MR, Mehta AC, Budev MM, et al. Impact of bedside bronchoscopy in critically ill lung transplant recipients. *J Bronchology Interv Pulmonol.* 2014;21(3):199–207.

67. Todd JL, Christie JD, Palmer SM. Update in lung transplantation 2013. *Am J Respir Crit Care Med.* 2014;190(1):19–24.

68. Hayes D Jr, Whitson BA, Ghadiali SN, et al. Influence of HLA mismatching on survival in lung transplantation. *Lung.* 2015;193(5):789–797.

69. Eberlein M, Reed RM, Bolukbas S, et al. Lung transplant outcomes group. Lung size mismatch and primary graft dysfunction after bilateral lung transplantation. *J Heart Lung Transplant.* 2015;34(2):233–240.

70. Martinu T, Dong-Feng C, Palmer SM. Acute rejection and humoral sensitization in lung transplant recipients. *Proc Am Thorac Soc.* 2009;6:54–65.

71. Mangi A, Mason D, Nowicki E, et al. Predictors of acute rejection after lung transplantation. *Ann Thorac Surg.* 2011;91(6):1754–1762.

72. Lowery E, Berniss B, Cascino T, et al. Low vitamin D levels are associated with increased rejection and infections after lung transplantation. *J Heart Lung Transplant.* 2012;31(7):700–707.

73. Nathan SD. The future of lung transplantation. *Chest.* 2015;147(2):309–316.

74. Dutau H, Vandemoortele T, Laroumagne S, et al. A new endoscopic standardized grading system for macroscopic central airway complications following lung transplantation: The MDS classification. *Eur J Cardiothorac Surg.* 2014;45(2):e33–e38.

75. Fernandez-Bussy S, Majid A, Caviedes I, et al. Treatment of airway complications following lung transplantation. *Arch Bronconeumol.* 2011;47(3):128–133.

76. Lari SM, Gonin F, Colchen A. The management of bronchus intermedius complications after lung transplantation: a retrospective study. *J Cardiothorac Surg.* 2012;7:8. doi: 10.1186/1749-8090-7-8.

77. Meyer KC, Raghu G, Verleden GM; ISHLT/ATS/ERS BOS Task Force Committee, ISHLT/ATS/ERS BOS Task Force Committee, et al. An international ISHLT/ATS/ERS clinical practice guideline: diagnosis and management of bronchiolitis obliterans syndrome. *Eur Respir J.* 2014;44(6):1479–1503.

78. Sammons C, Dolingalski C. Untility of procalcitonin as a biomarker for rejection and differentiation of infectious complications in lung transplant recipients. *Ann Pharmacother.* 2014;48(1):116–122.

79. Cupples SA, Dew MA, Grady KL, et al. Report of the Psychosocial Outcomes Workgroup of the Nursing and Social Sciences Council of the International Society for Heart Transplantation: present status of research on psychosocial outcomes in cardiothoracic transplantation: review and recommendations for the field. *J Heart Lung Transplant.* 2006;25:716–725.

80. Lanuza DM, McCabe M, Farcas GA, et al. Prospective study of functional status and quality of life before and after lung transplantation. *Chest.* 2000;188(1):115–122.

81. Toyoda Y, Toyoda Y. Heart–lung transplantation: adult indications and outcomes. *J Thorac Dis.* 2014;6(8):1138–1142.

SELF-ASSESSMENT QUESTIONS

1. The rationale for maintaining the pulmonary artery pressure within normal limits in the immediate postoperative period following lung transplantation is to:
   a. protect anastomosis sites.
   b. prevent immediate graft dysfunction.
   c. prevent pulmonary edema.
   d. a and c.
   e. all of the above.

2. Pulmonary artery pressures are maintained within normal limits with which of the following?
   a. Diuretic administration
   b. Administration of inhaled nitric oxide
   c. Intravenous administration of Nipride
   d. a and b
   e. All of the above

3. Administration of fluids to a lung transplant recipient in the immediate postoperative period should be done cautiously due to:
   a. the effect of high fluid volumes on anastomoses.
   b. increased capillary permeability in transplanted lung tissue.
   c. nephrotoxicity of anesthesias.
   d. hyporesponsiveness of alveoli in the immediate postoperative phase.

4. Cardiac dysrhythmias are not uncommon in the immediate postoperative period following lung transplantation. Atrial dysrhythmias are often associated with which of the following?
   a. Systemic inflammatory processes related to chest surgery
   b. Inflammation near the pulmonary vein and atrial cuff suture lines
   c. Early signs of hyperacute rejection
   d. Low levels of sodium related to dehydration

5. Tachycardia may be present in the immediate postoperative stages due to which of the following problems?
   a. Bleeding
   b. Use of nebulizers
   c. Pain, catecholamine release with stress
   d. Fluid loss, diuretic therapy
   e. a and b
   f. All of the above

6. With en bloc and sequential anastomoses of lung transplantation, pulmonary artery wedge pressures are usually not obtained because:
   a. increase in arterial pressure may precipitate rupture of the anastomoses sites.
   b. increase in venous pressure may precipitate rupture of the anastomoses sites.
   c. increases in atrial pressures may precipitate rupture of the anastomoses sites.
   d. increases in ventricular pressures may precipitate rupture of the anastomoses sites.

7. Warning signs of primary graft dysfunction include which of the following symptoms?
   a. Sudden rise in potassium levels
   b. Frequent oxygen desaturation
   c. Increased work of breathing
   d. b and c
   e. All of the above

8. Possible causes of primary graft dysfunction include which of the following?
   a. Increased capillary permeability
   b. Change in compliance and vascular resistance between donor and recipient
   c. Edema from extended ischemic time
   d. a and c
   e. All of the above

9. Acute rejection symptoms include which of the following?
   a. Dyspnea
   b. Elevation in temperature
   c. Decrease in FEV1
   d. a and c
   e. All of the above

10. Two major airway complications of lung transplantation are:
   a. bronchial dehiscence and tracheal stenosis.
   b. alveolar collapse and rejection.
   c. loss of surfactant and infections.
   d. increased production of CO_2 and an increase in reperfusion injury.

Correct Answers:
1.d 2.d 3.b 4.b 5.f 6.a 7.d 8.e 9.e 10.a

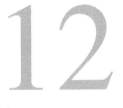

C H A P T E R 12

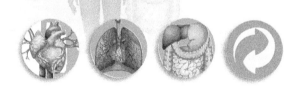

Liver Transplantation

Carolyn J. Driscoll, RN, PhD, FNP-C

Leslie Gallagher, RN, MS, ANP-BC

Margaret J. Schaeffer, RN, MS, MSHA, NE-BC

 I. PRETRANSPLANT CARE: END-STAGE LIVER DISEASE AND FAILURE

A. Overview

1. End-stage liver disease is a major health problem causing more than 30,000 deaths each year in the United States.[1] Medical management may be effective for short or even extended periods of time. However, liver transplantation is recognized as a successful therapy for patients for whom standard medical and surgical therapies have failed.

2. Liver transplantation has shown excellent results worldwide. In 2013, 6,455 liver transplants were performed and approximately 60,000 people worldwide were living with a transplanted liver.

   a. Five-year graft survival was 71.7% for recipients aged younger than 1 year, 74.9% for ages 1 to 5 years, 78.9% ages 6 to 10 years, 77.4% for ages 11 to 17 years, and 76.4% for adults.[2]

3. In the United States, the national Organ Procurement and Transplantation Network (OPTN) recognizes seven liver disease categories and lists 72 liver diagnoses as indications for transplantation.[3] Discussion of the major indications for liver transplantation follows. Box 12-1 lists the indications for and contraindications to liver transplantation.

   a. Chronic hepatitis C (viral disease) is the most common indication for liver transplantation in the United States.

   b. Alcoholic liver disease is the second leading indication for liver transplantation.

   c. Nonalcoholic fatty liver disease (NAFLD) is a prevalent form of disease caused by a variety of factors such as obesity, hyperglycemia, elevated serum lipids, and high blood pressure (BP).[4]

      i. The progression of disease leading to nonalcoholic steatohepatitis (NASH) can result in cirrhosis and is the third most common indication for liver transplantation in the United States.

BOX 12-1 **Indications and Contraindications for Liver Transplantation**

Indications for Liver Transplantation

Acute Liver Failure
- Viral
- Drug/medication toxicity
- Ischemia
- Wilson's disease
- Autoimmune
- Idiopathic

Cirrhosis and Decompensation
- Hepatitis B or C
- Alcohol
- Nonalcoholic steatohepatitis
- Cholestatic disease
- Autoimmune
- Metabolic
- Malignancy
- Cryptogenic

Absolute Contraindications
- Severe cardiopulmonary disease
- Anatomic abnormalities precluding adequate surgical reconstruction
- Uncontrolled human immunodeficiency virus
- Poorly controlled psychiatric illness
- Noncompliance with medical recommendations

Relative Contraindications
- Extrahepatic malignancy
- Hepatocellular carcinoma (exceeding Milan criteria)
- Acute substance or alcohol abuse
- Inadequate social or financial support

---

　　　　ii. NASH is estimated to become the leading indication for liver transplant in the next 10 to 20 years.[5]

　　d. Hepatocellular carcinoma (HCC) has become the fifth most common cancer in the world and is an indication for liver transplantation.

B. One of the largest barriers to transplantation is the shortage of available organs.

　　1. There are geographic disparities in the availability of organs for transplantation.

　　2. Consent rates for donation from deceased donors are not optimal.

　　3. Donation from a living donor is possible, although limited by the number of liver transplant programs that perform this procedure.

　　　　a. A living donor program is a component of an approved deceased donor transplant program within a transplant center.

　　　　b. In the United States, the Organ Procurement and Transplantation Network (OPTN), operated by the United Network for Organ Sharing (UNOS), must approve a program to perform living donor surgeries based on the OPTN criteria.

    c. OPTN criteria require very specific training and experience for all the transplant surgeons and physicians involved in living donor liver transplantation.[6]

C. The overall goal of liver transplantation is to prolong life and improve the patient's quality of life. Secondarily, there are economic benefits to the health care system as the cost of transplantation therapy is less of a burden on the system than care of a patient with liver failure.[7]

D. As of January 2015, approximately 16,000 patients were waiting for liver transplants in the United States.
    1. 6,455 liver transplants were performed in 2013, of which 252 were from living donors.
    2. During the same period, 6,322 patients were removed from the waiting list because of death.[8]

II. DISEASES THAT MAY LEAD TO HEPATIC FAILURE[9]

A. Hepatitis A viral infection is an acute, necroinflammatory disease of the liver.
    1. Virus is detectable in blood or feces for 2 weeks before the onset of jaundice and for up to 8 days afterward.
    2. Acquired through the oral-fecal route such as by ingestion of contaminated food or water.
    3. Symptoms may include malaise, fatigue, anorexia, low-grade fever, nausea, and vomiting.
    4. Most patients will have full recovery within 3 months.
    5. Acute liver failure occurs in approximately 1% of cases. Chronic infection is never seen.

B. Hepatitis B is an acute or a chronic liver disease.
    1. Most infections develop as a result of exposure to contaminated blood or body fluids including
        a. Vertical transmission from an infected mother to her newborn child
        b. Unprotected sexual contact with an infected person
        c. Blood and blood product infusions (rare since blood screening in 1971)
        d. Sharing of needles during intravenous (IV) drug use
    2. Exposure may lead to an acute infection, which usually resolves, although liver failure can occur. A number of adult patients fail to clear the virus and develop a chronic infection, which leads to cirrhosis and/or liver cancer. Conservatively, 54% of liver cancer cases are due to hepatitis B infection. An effective vaccination is available; however, hepatitis B remains a major health problem.[10]

C. Hepatitis C is the leading indication for liver transplantation in the United States.
    1. Viral disease can be transmitted by the following:
        a. Infected blood products or organs (uncommon since July 1992)
        b. Injection drug use
        c. Needlestick injuries in health care settings
        d. Less commonly from vertical transmission from an infected mother or sex with an infected person
    2. Chronic disease is related to chronic inflammatory process, reflective of an unresolved wound healing response, which causes fibrotic changes within the liver.[11]

3. 75% to 80% of people who become infected will develop chronic disease. Most cases progress asymptomatically and may be detected many years after infection. Approximately 20% develop cirrhosis and 4% of those will develop hepatocellular cancer (HCC).

D. Hepatitis D infection occurs only in the presence of concurrent or underlying chronic hepatitis B.
   1. Transmitted through percutaneous or mucosal contact with infected blood.
   2. Can be acute or chronic. Chronic hepatitis D may be completely asymptomatic or present with nonspecific symptoms like fatigue.
   3. Uncommon in the United States.

E. Hepatitis E may occur in epidemics or sporadic cases.
   1. Acquired similarly to hepatitis A and thought to be waterborne
   2. More serious for pregnant mothers and fetuses

F. Alcoholic liver disease[12]
   1. Alcoholic liver disease has a spectrum of presentation including fatty liver, alcoholic hepatitis, or cirrhosis.
   2. Fatty liver, which occurs after acute or chronic alcohol ingestion, is reversible with abstinence.
   3. Alcoholic hepatitis occurs with consumption of large amounts of alcohol over a prolonged period of time. It has a spectrum of severity that can lead to fulminant liver failure and death. Ability to reverse the process varies.
   4. Clinical manifestations of cirrhosis are similar to other etiologies. Complications of portal hypertension and liver failure can develop. It is not reversible.

G. Hepatocellular carcinoma (HCC)[13]
   1. HCC is a malignant cancer of liver cells, one of the most common cancers worldwide, and is responsible for >1 million deaths annually.
   2. Risk factors include male gender, cirrhosis, and chronic hepatitis B or C infection.
   3. Liver transplantation is an option in select patients. Patients are screened by the Milan criteria, which assess the suitability of patients and outcome based on tumor size and number that include the following:
      a. One lesion smaller than 5 cm
      b. Three lesions total each being <3 cm
      c. No extrahepatic manifestations
      d. No vascular invasion

H. Primary biliary cirrhosis (PBC) is a rare, chronic, progressive cholestasis (retention of bile) disorder.[14]
   1. Gradual destruction of the interlobular bile ducts leads to the development of cirrhosis.
   2. PBC is an autoimmune hepatitis.
   3. Pruritus and fatigue are common symptoms.
   4. The disease primarily affects middle-age women.

I. Primary sclerosing cholangitis (PSC) is a chronic progressive disease of unknown etiology.[15]
   1. Multiple fibrosing inflammatory strictures of the extra- and intrahepatic bile ducts

2. Progresses to cirrhosis, liver failure, and sometimes cholangiocarcinoma
3. Closely associated with inflammatory bowel disease, predominantly ulcerative colitis

J. Autoimmune hepatitis is a chronic inflammatory disease of the liver thought to be caused by a combination of autoimmunity, environmental triggers, and a genetic predisposition.[16]
1. More common in females. Can occur at any age and affects all ethnic groups.
2. Patients often have other autoimmune disorders, such as Crohn's disease, PSC, lupus, type 1 diabetes, or ulcerative colitis.
3. Treatment includes medications to suppress or slow the overactive immune system. May require liver transplantation.

K. Hemochromatosis is an inherited disease in which an excessive amount of iron is absorbed, cannot be excreted from the body, and is deposited in the liver and other organs. Eventually, cirrhosis may develop.[17]
1. Equally affects males and females
   a. Signs of the disease manifest in men in their 40s and 50s.
   b. Women typically demonstrate signs in their 60s and 70s.
2. More common in those of Northern European descent

L. Wilson's disease is a genetic disorder of copper metabolism.[18]
1. Copper is a component of many enzymes and plasma proteins.
2. Biliary excretion of copper and ceruloplasmin synthesis is impaired in Wilson's disease leading to the accumulation of copper in the liver and other organs, including the brain and eyes.
3. Wilson's disease can present as chronic liver disease or acute liver failure.

M. Alpha-1 antitrypsin deficiency (A1AT): A1AT is an enzyme made by the liver, which helps to break down trypsin and other tissue proteases.[19]
1. A1AT deficiency is an inherited disorder; structural abnormalities of the protein may disrupt normal cellular transport of A1AT in hepatocytes and accumulation of the defective protein results in potentially severe liver disease.
2. Lungs can also be affected, leading to emphysema and even lung transplantation.

N. Non-alcoholic Steatohepatitis (NASH) is an increasingly common liver disease.
1. Fatty changes (steatosis) and lobular infiltration in the liver develop in people who drink little or no alcohol. Liver damage can range from steatosis to cirrhosis.[20]
2. Associated with metabolic syndrome, obesity, diabetes, and dyslipidemia.

O. Cryptogenic cirrhosis is a term given to patients with cirrhosis where no diagnosis of the underlying liver disease can be established.

P. Drug-induced liver disease is a syndrome in which hepatotoxicity is caused by drugs, toxins, or other foreign chemicals. More than 900 drugs, toxins, and herbs have been reported to cause liver injury. Drugs account for 20% to 40% of fulminant liver failure.[21]
1. Presentation may be acute liver failure or fibrosis and cirrhosis that may develop over many years.
2. In the United States, United Kingdom, and Australia, acetaminophen (paracetamol) is one of the most common causes of acute liver failure, often resulting from deliberate or inadvertent overdoses.[22]

3. Other selected common drugs that cause hepatotoxicity include the following:
   a. Antimicrobials (i.e., amoxicillin/clavulanate)
   b. Dietary and herbal supplements
   c. Isoniazid
   d. Nonsteroidal anti-inflammatory drugs
   e. Antiseizure medication

Q. Budd-Chiari syndrome occurs as a result of thrombosis of the hepatic veins. Patients present with abdominal pain, ascites, and hepatomegaly. It is a rare disease and affects mainly young adults.[23]
   1. May develop in patients with underlying thrombotic conditions.
   2. When occlusion of the hepatic veins is more gradual, collateral vessels form and fibrosis develops leading to cirrhosis.
   3. When thrombosis occurs rapidly, acute liver failure may develop.

R. Liver diseases during pregnancy[24]
   1. Patients usually present in their third trimester of pregnancy. Symptoms vary from none to acute liver failure.
   2. Hyperemesis gravidarum presents with severe and persistent vomiting. Half of women who are hospitalized with this syndrome have liver disease.
   3. Intrahepatic cholestasis is reversible but possibly predictive of liver disease later in life.
   4. Acute fatty liver of pregnancy (AFLP) is rare but serious. The pathogenesis is largely unknown, and prompt recognition and delivery of the fetus is necessary to save the mother and child.
   5. HELLP syndrome is a cluster of symptoms that occur in pregnant women (1 to 2 in 1,000 pregnancies). The grouping includes hemolysis, elevated liver enzymes, and a low platelet count.
      a. H, hemolysis; EL, elevated enzymes; LP, low platelets
      b. Primary treatment is delivery of the baby.[25]

S. Acute liver failure[26]
   1. Rare and life-threatening critical illness, occurring most often in patients with no previous history of liver disease
      a. Types of acute liver failure:
         i. Hyperacute liver failure, defined by the development of encephalopathy within 7 days of becoming jaundiced.
         ii. Fulminant, defined by 2 weeks from jaundice to encephalopathy.
         iii. Subacute liver failure is often used to describe development of jaundice and encephalopathy over 5 to 12 weeks.
      b. Etiology of acute liver failure
         i. The etiologies for acute liver failure include viral hepatitis, drug-induced liver injury, autoimmune hepatitis, toxins, metabolic diseases, and others as listed above.

 III. WORSENING LIVER FUNCTION

A. Conditions that warrant concern and action
   1. Patients should be referred for transplant assessment when they develop or experience complications that are no longer managed successfully with treatment. For example:
      a. Ascites

      b. Variceal bleed
      c. Spontaneous bacterial peritonitis
      d. Hepatic encephalopathy

B. Objective and subjective indications of deterioration in liver failure include the following:

    1. Increasing jaundice: occurs as the liver fails to metabolize bilirubin normally.
    2. Increased risk of bruising and bleeding from decreased platelets (secondary to splenomegaly).
      a. There is decreased synthesis of coagulation proteins in the liver, which results in elevated prothrombin time (PT) and international normalized ratio (INR).
      b. In addition, there is decreased production of other components of the coagulation cascade, which help ameliorate the risk of bleeding.
    3. Pruritus: caused by increased concentration of bile salts or other chemicals in the blood due to impaired excretion of bilirubin.
    4. Peripheral edema: caused by low albumin (usually below 30 g/L SI units or 3 g/dL conventional units) and/or massive ascites blocking venous return.
    5. Prominent abdominal wall veins (caput medusa): collateral vessels bypass the scarred liver to carry portal blood to the superior vena cava.
    6. Hemorrhoids: internal veins dilate with increased portal hypertension.
    7. Anemia due to
      a. Gastrointestinal blood loss
      b. Erythrocyte destruction by pooling in enlarged spleen
      c. Decreased folic acid due to dietary deficiency
    8. Infection: leukopenia (low white cells) due to splenic sequestration.
    9. Emaciation: caused by malnutrition and hypoalbuminemia.
   10. Fatigue: mechanism is not well understood.
   11. Most patients are generally hemodynamically compensated while exhibiting some symptoms of volume overload. However, in more advanced cirrhosis, peripheral vasodilation can occur, manifested as decreasing BP.[26]

C. Complications of worsening liver failure include

    1. Portal hypertension
      a. Defined as the elevation of hepatic venous pressure gradient (HVPG) to >5 mm Hg
      b. Caused by increased resistance to the passage of blood flow through the liver and increased splenic blood flow secondary to vasodilation within the splenic vascular bed
    2. Ascites[27]
      a. Accumulation of fluid in the peritoneal cavity caused by portal hypertension and low albumin, leading to excess formation of fluid within congested hepatic sinusoids
      b. Treated with reduction in sodium intake, diuretics, and abdominal paracentesis
    3. Spontaneous bacterial peritonitis (SBP)
      a. Infection from bacterial translocation and diagnosed by analysis of ascites fluid.

b. Symptomatic patients should be admitted to the hospital and treated with a 10- to 14-day course of antibiotics, followed by a repeat peritoneal fluid analysis to assure declining polymorphonuclear (PMN) counts and sterilization of the ascetic fluid.[28]

4. Esophageal and gastric varices[29]

a. Abnormal and enlarged veins in the esophagus and stomach develop secondary to portal hypertension. Develop when normal blood flow to the liver is obstructed.

b. Treatments include non-selective beta blocker medications to reduce portal hypertension and "banding": the use of elastic bands to tie off veins that are bleeding or in danger of bleeding or rupture.

5. Encephalopathy and coma

a. Decreased excretion of ammonia and other toxins can lead to elevated levels that result in confusion and other mental status changes, including coma.

b. Treatment includes the following:

i. Lactulose and rifaximin are used to reduce ammonia levels.

ii. Lactulose should be titrated to obtain three to four bowel movements a day.

iii. Measurement of serum ammonia levels can be deceiving as results can be adversely affected by testing methods. Clinical examination of mental status and asterixis (hand tremor) is often sufficient to identify encephalopathy.

iv. Normal ammonia levels are <40 µmol/L.

v. Constipation, dehydration, infection, and hyponatremia may result in elevated ammonia levels and encephalopathy.[30]

c. Grades of encephalopathy

i. Minimal hepatic encephalopathy. No specific symptoms, but abnormal specialized testing results.

ii. Grade 1—Nonspecific changes without asterixis, with abnormal specialized testing results.

iii. Minimal hepatic encephalopathy and Grade 1 encephalopathy may be grouped together and called "covert hepatic encephalopathy."

iv. Grade 2—Drowsiness.

v. Grade 3—Confusion, reactive only to vocal stimuli.

vi. Grade 4—Presence of deep coma with absence of reaction to vocal stimuli.

vii. Grades 2, 3, and 4 can be grouped together and called "overt hepatic encephalopathy." No specialized testing is required for diagnosis.[31]

6. Hepatorenal failure involves a rapid decrease in renal function.

a. Occasionally precipitated by volume depletion

b. Often seen in patients with advanced liver disease

c. May need to be treated with dialysis

 IV. CHRONIC LIVER DISEASE

A. Definition: a gradual destruction of liver tissue over time

B. Clinical manifestations: Early symptoms may include the following:

1. Poor appetite, weight loss, and anorexia

2. Fatigue, weakness, and muscle loss

3. Right upper quadrant pain
4. Nausea and vomiting
5. Diarrhea
6. Jaundice
7. Liver enlargement and ascites

 V. LIVER TRANSPLANT ASSESSMENT[23]

A. Patients with liver disease undergo a thorough assessment before they are accepted for placement on the liver transplant waiting list.

1. Each transplant program has an individualized transplant evaluation process for patients. The evaluation may be done in an outpatient setting or, if the patient's condition dictates, while the patient is in the hospital.

2. Patient and family education is a major focus in the assessment process.

   a. At the first meeting, patients sign consents to participate in the evaluation process; the entire evaluation process is outlined for them at this time.

   b. National and center-specific liver transplant outcome data are given to patients to aid them in their decision making.

   c. See chapter on Patient Education for additional information

B. Assessment includes the following:

1. Laboratory tests.

2. Radiologic and other clinical tests.

3. Evaluation for suitability by an interdisciplinary transplant team.

   a. The Centers for Medicare and Medicaid (CMS) regulate specific roles of an interdisciplinary team in the assessment.

   b. The members of the team are defined by CMS and must include, at a minimum:

      i. Surgeon
      ii. Physician
      iii. Anesthesiologist
      iv. Pharmacist
      v. Registered dietician
      vi. Social worker
      vii. Transplant coordinator
      viii. Psychiatrist/psychologist

4. Evaluation of the patient's family/social situation is of major importance.

   a. This evaluation is the role of the social worker, psychologist, and transplant coordinator.

   b. Identifying the key caregiver for the patient both pre- and posttransplant is necessary in order to facilitate

      i. Adherence to the medical regimen, including keeping hospital appointments and medication management

      ii. A timely, effective, and safe hospital discharge

   c. Chronic illness, loss of employment, as well as travel to the transplant center, especially for patients living a long distance away, can have financial implications for individuals and the ability to comply with posttransplant requirements.

   d. Assessment by and involvement with social workers are needed to deal with these issues.

5. In some programs, patients with alcoholic cirrhosis will undergo a thorough assessment by a team of experts in addiction medicine.
   a. Data suggest that long-term posttransplant survival rates for patients with alcoholic cirrhosis are no different than survival rates for patients with other types of cirrhosis.
   b. In the United States, many transplant programs require 6 months of abstinence before a patient can be placed on the liver transplant waiting list. However, this time period is arbitrary and no studies to date have shown it to impact posttransplant survival.[32]
   c. Programs also have different criteria regarding whether or not patients must sign a contract or agreement that states they will participate in formal alcohol treatment programs and abstain from alcohol following transplantation.

C. Patients with acute liver failure can deteriorate rapidly. Therefore, the assessment process may be expedited so that these patients can be listed very quickly. In cases of acute and fulminant liver failure, family members may be interviewed to gather the patient's history and pertinent information.

D. The medical assessment of the patient for transplantation includes the following:
   1. Basic laboratory tests
      a. Hepatic panel (liver function tests [LFTs])
      b. Basic metabolic panel (creatinine, electrolytes, blood urea nitrogen [BUN])
      c. Complete blood count (CBC)
      d. PT, INR, and partial thromboplastin time (PTT)
      e. Antinuclear antibody (ANA) and antimitochondrial antibody (AMA)
      f. Alpha fetoprotein (AFP cancer marker)
      g. Blood type: per OPTN Policy 3 (Candidate Registrations, Modifications, and Removals)
         i. Transplant programs must determine each candidate's blood type by testing at least two candidate blood samples prior to registration on the waiting list. Transplant programs must test at least two blood samples from two separate blood draws taken at two different times.
         ii. After the candidate's blood type data are reported to UNOS, the candidate is added to the waiting list but is not registered as an active candidate until secondary reporting and verification of the candidate's blood type have been completed.
         iii. The secondary reporting and verification of the candidate's blood type must be completed by someone:
            ● Other than the individual who reported the candidate's blood type at registration on the waiting list
            ● Using source documents from the two blood samples used for the blood type testing
      h. Alcohol and drug toxicology levels
      i. Virology screen, may include the following:
         i. Hepatitis A virus
         ii. Hepatitis B virus
         iii. Hepatitis C virus
         iv. Human immunodeficiency virus (HIV)
         v. Cytomegalovirus (CMV), IgG/IgM
         vi. Epstein-Barr virus (EBV)
         vii. Varicella-zoster virus (VZV)

2. Other tests
   a. Liver biopsy.
   b. Chest radiograph.
   c. Electrocardiogram (ECG).
   d. Echocardiogram (ECHO) and/or cardiac stress testing: dynamic or nuclear.
   e. Pulmonary artery pressure and ejection fraction should be assessed. This may be done by echocardiogram or cardiac catheterization.
   f. Ultrasound (US) scan of liver to assess patency of portal and hepatic veins and look for the presence of mass lesions.
      i. If patency of portal vein cannot be documented on Doppler US, computed tomography (CT) imaging or magnetic resonance imaging (MRI) should be done.
      ii. Significant variation in normal anatomy of both the vascular and biliary trees in the liver may exist. This dictates the specific surgical approaches in transplantation; it is therefore important to map out these variations.
   g. Spirometry tests are usually an adequate screen of lung function.
      i. If readings are abnormal or lung function abnormality is suspected (e.g., alpha-1 antitrypsin or pulmonary fibrosis), formal lung function tests are required.
   h. Upper endoscopy: to observe for esophageal varices.
   i. Colonoscopy:
      i. Primary sclerosing cholangitis, as these patients are at increased risk of colon cancer
      ii. Inflammatory bowel disease (Crohn's disease or ulcerative colitis) to assess severity of disease or the presence of polyps or cancer
      iii. Age 50 or older who meet criteria for screening or diagnostic colonoscopy.
3. Interdisciplinary team consultations as indicated (e.g., infectious disease, oncology, etc.)

E. Candidate selection process
   1. Patients are presented at an interdisciplinary transplant team selection meeting. During this meeting, candidates for transplant are discussed and evaluated based on the program's inclusion and exclusion criteria.
   2. Reasons for not accepting a patient for liver transplantation vary by individual program and may include the following:
      a. HCC that is outside Milan criteria
      b. Active substance abuse
      c. Extrahepatic malignancy
      d. Advanced cardiac or pulmonary disease
      e. A demonstrated inability to be adherent with medication regimens and an overall lifestyle that is a barrier to successful transplant outcome.

 VI. LISTING FOR TRANSPLANTATION AND ORGAN ALLOCATION

A. Split or reduced-size livers may be used for transplantation because of the regenerative capacity of the liver.
   1. An adult patient can be listed to receive either a split or whole liver.
   2. Pediatric patients can receive a whole, split, or reduced-size graft. (See chapter on Pediatric Transplantation for additional information.)

B.   When a patient has been placed on the transplant waiting list in the United States, priority is based on the UNOS organ allocation policy.[33,34]

1. The current allocation is based either on the Model for End-Stage Liver Disease (MELD) scoring system for adults or the Pediatric End-Stage Liver Disease (PELD) scoring system, which are predictive models of death within a 3-month period.

   a. The MELD score is calculated using serum creatinine, serum bilirubin, INR, and serum sodium.

      i.   As of January 2016, the MELD score has been modified to incorporate serum sodium.

      ii. The score ranges from 6 to 40.

      iii. MELD score is calculated using the following formula: $0.957 \times \log_e$ (creatinine mg/dL) + 0. 378 × $\log_e$ (bilirubin mg/dL) + 1.120 × $\log_e$ (INR) + 0.643.

         • Laboratory values <1.0 will be set to 1.0 when calculating a candidate's MELD score.

         • The following candidates will receive a creatinine value of 4.0 mg/dL:

            ○ Candidates with a creatinine value >4.0 mg/dL

            ○ Candidates who received two or more dialysis treatments within the prior 7 days

            ○ Candidates who received 24 hours of continuous venovenous hemodialysis (CVVHD) within the prior 7 days

      iv. For candidates with an initial MELD score >11, the MELD score is then recalculated to include serum sodium. The MELD score is recalculated as follows: MELD = MELD(i) + 1.32 × (137-Na) − [0.033 × MELD(i) × (137-Na)]

         • Sodium values <125 mmol/L will be set to 125, and values >137 mmol/L will be set at 137.

   b. Candidates can also be assigned a priority status, within the MELD/PELD system, based on urgency of need: status 1A for adults and status 1A or 1B for pediatric patients

   c. Patients with HCC who have stage T2 lesions and meet all other criteria are initially registered at their calculated MELD/PELD scores for the first 3 months. In order for a candidate to maintain an HCC-approved exception, the transplant program must submit a new exception application every 3 months. (The median calculated MELD/PELD score as of November 2014 is 11). At 6 months (time of request for a second extension), the candidates are assigned a MELD/PELD score equivalent to a 35% risk of 3-month mortality. Then, an increase in the MELD score is given every 3 months until transplantation, to reflect a 10% increase in mortality risk. The score for HCC is capped at 34.

   d. Countries other than the United States may have different ways of organ allocation and do not necessarily use the MELD scoring system.

2. When an organ becomes available, the transplant coordinator will notify the patient of the organ offer. The patient has the right to turn down the offer at that time. If the patient is at home at the time of the organ offer and chooses to go forward with transplantation, he/she is sent to the hospital. Arrangements are made for the patient's admission and operating room (OR) time is secured. If the patient is already hospitalized and agrees to proceed with transplantation, the OR is secured.

VII. HOSPITAL ADMISSION

A. On admission to the hospital:
1. Vital signs are taken; an elevated temperature or any other signs of an infectious process are assessed. Some infections will prevent moving forward to transplantation at this time.
2. Weight is recorded as a baseline for drug dose calculations and maintenance of fluid balance following surgery.
3. Patients and families typically need psychological/emotional support and reassurance and may have many questions at this time.
4. Some patients and families may welcome an opportunity to meet with a hospital chaplain.

B. Preparation for surgery:
1. Laboratory tests:
    a. Complete blood count to review white blood cell count, platelet, and hemoglobin (Hgb) levels
    b. PTT and PT/INR
    c. Comprehensive metabolic panel
    d. Crossmatch may be done. (For additional information, see chapter on Transplant Immunology.)
2. Other tests:
    a. Chest radiograph: to look for any infection or new changes.
    b. ECG: to look for any cardiac changes.
    c. If patient is febrile, cultures should be obtained.
    d. If gross ascites is present, a diagnostic tap should be done to exclude spontaneous bacterial peritonitis.
3. If a patient is diabetic, a sliding scale insulin regimen and fluids should be given before surgery when the patient is taking nothing by mouth.
4. Blood products will be ordered for the surgery and may include packed red blood cells, platelets, and fresh frozen plasma (FFP).
    a. Amount will differ by program practice and patient circumstance.
5. Consent for the operation may have already been obtained by the transplant surgeon at listing but will likely be repeated upon admission to the hospital and prior to surgery.

 VIII. TRANSPLANT SURGERY

A. The liver transplant procedure typically takes between 4 and 12 hours.

B. The surgery consists of
1. The hepatectomy (removal of the native liver)
2. Implantation of the new liver, which involves
    a. Anastomosis of the inferior vena cava, portal vein, hepatic artery, and the biliary connection via a duct-to-duct anastomosis (choledochocholedochostomy).
    b. Some centers excise the vena cava with the native liver. Others preserve it and suture the donor cava and recipient cava as a piggyback.
    c. Some centers may use a T tube, which is placed in the bile duct before the anastomosis.
    d. If a Roux-en-Y choledochojejunostomy is performed where the bile duct is connected to the bowel, a T tube is not needed.

C. Intraoperative mortality remains very rare.

IX. ARRIVAL IN THE INTENSIVE CARE UNIT

A.   Patients may be fully ventilated for the first 12 to 24 hours.

B.   Drainage tubes: (to be included in output measurements)
1. Nasogastric (NG) drainage.
   a. All patients will return to the ICU with an NG tube in place to give medication or to use for aspiration of stomach contents if vomiting occurs.
   b. Once patients are able to tolerate oral fluids, the tube is removed.
   c. Any drainage from the NG must be included in output measurement.
2. A urinary catheter will be in place to enable close monitoring of urine output.
   a. A low urine output could be a sign of dehydration or renal compromise.
   b. If output does not improve with fluids or diuretics, dialysis may be necessary.
   c. The catheter is generally removed once a patient has been transferred out of the ICU.
3. Surgical drain or drains are inserted at the end of the transplant procedure.
   a. Different transplant programs have different practices, but in the United States, Jackson-Pratt drains are generally used and placed near the sites of vascular anastomosis.
   b. There can be three drainage sites:
      i.   Two in the right lower quadrant.
      ii. One in the left lower quadrant.
      iii. Other programs may only insert one drain on the right side.
      iv. The color and consistency of the drainage should be monitored and recorded for signs of bleeding or bile leakage (green).
4. T-tube drains are used routinely in some centers, but in other centers, T tubes are used only if the transplant was performed using a split liver.
   a. Amount and consistency of bile drainage should be monitored.
   b. T-tube drains may stay in for up to 3 months.
   c. T-tube cholangiogram may be performed to assess the intrahepatic bile ducts.

 X. POSTOPERTIVE MONITORING AND ASSESSMENT

A.   Hemodynamic monitoring
1. May be done via a pulmonary artery catheter, central venous catheter, and an arterial line.
2. A pulmonary artery catheter allows for measurements of
   a. Cardiac output (CO)
   b. Cardiac index (CI)
   c. Systemic vascular resistance (SVR)
   d. Pulmonary artery wedge (PAW) pressure
      i. The pulmonary artery catheter is the only accurate way to measure PAW pressure.
3. BP monitoring via an arterial line.

B.   Transesophageal echocardiogram
1. Use of pulmonary artery catheters is decreasing and patients are now often monitored with a transesophageal echocardiogram instead of a pulmonary artery catheter.
   a. A probe is inserted into the esophagus.
   b. Ultrasound technology enables visualization of the heart chambers and valves.
   c. The TEE provides information about left ventricular function and wall motion abnormalities.

C. Fluid balance
   1. For all posttransplant patients, IV maintenance fluid is generally necessary and will be titrated according to BP, central venous pressure (CVP), and urine output.
   2. Some centers may use $D_{10}W$ as maintenance to provide adequate glucose for the new stabilizing liver until gluconeogenesis is optimized and glycolysis can occur.
   3. Bowel sounds should be monitored closely and should be present before oral fluids are commenced.

D. Urine output: should be >30 mL/h or 1 to 2 mL/kg/h.

E. Daily weights are important to assess fluid accumulation or loss and malnutrition.

F. Laboratory tests are monitored per individual center protocol but often a minimum of once daily and will include the following:
   1. LFTs
      a. Aspartate transaminase (AST) and alanine aminotransferase (ALT) (should steadily decline over the first few days).
      b. Bilirubin levels (will decline initially; this decrease is not necessarily indicative of good graft function but rather a sign of hemodilution).
      c. Alkaline phosphatase (ALP).
         i. Often normal in the early postoperative period.
         ii. A rise in ALP can be a sign of biliary complications or cholestasis.
      d. Laboratory changes are indicative of graft dysfunction.
         i. In a nonfunctioning graft, a high AST and ALT will be seen.
         ii. AST elevations will be more pronounced and occur earlier than elevated ALT. These high values are a sign of liver parenchymal injury.
   2. Coagulopathy screen
      a. PT/INR should be measured every 8 hours.
         i. A decline in PT/INR is a sign of returning hepatic function.
         ii. FFP may be given to correct clotting and a platelet infusion may be given for low platelets.
      b. A PT that is elevated >25 seconds and that continues to rise following the administration of vitamin K or FFP is a sign of a nonfunctioning liver.
   3. Glucose level
      a. Low glucose levels should return to normal quickly after transplant if the liver is functioning.
         i. The liver is the primary source of blood glucose.
         ii. In a nonfunctioning liver, glucose levels will be low and support will be necessary with 50% dextrose.
      b. High glucose levels should be treated with insulin.
   4. Arterial blood gases (ABGs)
      a. ABGs will be monitored every 8 hours if the patient is stable but may need to be obtained every 2 to 4 hours in an unstable patient.
      b. Acid-base disturbances should resolve rapidly if the graft is functioning well.
      c. Lactate levels, high in the liver failure patient, should decline posttransplant.
      d. A high lactate level and acidosis is a sign of poor graft function.
   5. Kidney function tests
      a. Basic comprehensive panel (BUN and creatinine) along with close monitoring of urine output
   6. CBC

7. Immunosuppressant levels
   a. Levels of tacrolimus (Prograf) or cyclosporine (Gengraf, Neoral) should be monitored daily once immunosuppressive therapy is initiated.
   b. Target levels are based on a number of factors including
      i. Indication for the transplant
      ii. Use of induction therapy
      iii. Kidney function
      iv. Overall condition of the patient

G. Neurological assessment
   1. Neurologic complications after solid organ transplantation are not uncommon, affecting 15% to 30% of liver transplant recipients.[35]
      a. A decreased level of consciousness initially may be due to anesthetic agents. The rate of recovery will depend on the function of the new liver.
      b. Transplant patients with acute liver failure who had encephalopathy and cerebral edema pretransplant may also have a period of diminished consciousness postoperatively.
   2. Renal failure or sepsis posttransplant may lead to metabolic encephalopathy.
   3. Significant perioperative hypotension may lead to hypoxic ischemic encephalopathy.
   4. It is important to rule out an intracranial bleed in patients whose initial postoperative neurological course is normal but who subsequently have a sudden deterioration in their neurological status.
   5. De novo seizures can occur after liver transplant, and these can be caused by
      a. Electrolyte imbalances
      b. Reaction to cyclosporine or tacrolimus
      c. Intracerebral abscesses
      d. Intracranial hemorrhage or cerebral infarction
   6. An electroencephalogram (EEG) and CT/MRI brain scans should be considered.

H. Pain assessment and management
   1. Pain is initially controlled in the ICU by giving IV morphine or fentanyl in the first 24 to 48 hours.
   2. Pain medication is weaned to allow patients to breathe spontaneously and wean from the ventilator.
   3. Once the patient is able to tolerate oral analgesia agents, acetaminophen or oxycodone is begun. No more than 2 g/day of acetaminophen should be taken.[36]
   4. Nonpharmacologic methods of pain reduction should also be employed, to include
      a. Education of the patient prior to the transplant procedure regarding reasonable expectations of pain, the availability of pain medication, and the importance of taking pain medication following surgery
      b. Control of the hospital environment through decreased environmental stimuli and the use of music and/or aromatherapy
      c. Movement as soon as the patient is able, to include getting up in a chair and walking

XI. POSTTRANSPLANT COMPLICATIONS

A. The immediate postoperative course can vary greatly and is highly dependent on the acuity of illness, the overall physical condition of the patient prior to surgery, and the quality of the donor organ.

B. Primary nonfunction and early dysfunction
1. Overview
    a. Graft function can be visualized at the time of reperfusion in the OR.
    b. Primary nonfunction can lead to multisystem organ failure and death.
    c. Although the incidence of primary nonfunction will vary in different centers, the risk is about 4% to 6%.[37]
    d. In cases of initial poor function, recovery is usually seen by the third posttransplant day.
2. Potential etiology
    a. Preservation injury during the donor surgery can cause primary nonfunction of the new liver, preventing the organ from recovery immediately after transplantation.
    b. Donor-related factors:
        i.   Donor steatosis (fat in the liver)
        ii. Donor age (older donors)
        iii. Prolonged donor hospital stay with periods of hypotension
    c. Prolonged cold ischemic time
3. Early indicators of nonfunction
    a. A decrease in bile production as seen with minimal secretion in T-tube drain
    b. Extreme edema of the organ, identified by palpation
    c. Abnormal color of the organ upon reperfusion (mottled, pale, gray, etc.)
    d. Lack of reperfusion in the OR
    e. Urine output <30 mL/h
    f. Hemodynamic instability
    g. Glucose, potassium, and lactate abnormalities
    h. Coagulopathy
4. Treatment: retransplantation

C. Hepatic artery thrombosis (HAT)
1. Occurs in 3% to 4% of cases and can occur in early postoperative stage or many months later. Because the liver depends on hepatic artery flow, HAT can lead to massive necrosis.[37]
2. Clinical presentation:
    a. Dramatic or persistent increase in LFTs due to decreased blood flow through the hepatic artery to the new organ
    b. Delayed bile leak
    c. Persistent sepsis of unknown cause
3. Diagnosis: Angiography is the gold standard for diagnosis.
4. Treatment: Immediate return to the OR for revascularization of the organ

D. Bleeding
1. Bleeding is generally seen in the first 48 hours.
2. Potential etiology:
    a. Underlying coagulopathy, which may occur in the setting of poor graft function
    b. Technical problems in surgery
3. Monitor:
    a. Surgical drains for volume of output and color of drainage
    b. Patient:
        i.   Abdomen: increased swelling
        ii. Pallor
        iii. Clinical manifestations of hypovolemia

        c. Vital signs
           i.   BP
           ii. Heart rate
        d. Hemodynamic parameters
           i.   CVP: typically maintained between 6 and 8 cm H_2O
        e. Lab values:
           i.   Hgb: typically maintained between 11 and 14 mg/dL
           ii. INR
    4. Potential treatment options
        a. Administration of
           i.   Blood products
           ii. Clotting factors
        b. If the coagulopathy cannot be corrected, surgical re-exploration to determine if the etiology is due to a technical problem with the surgery itself

E. Fluid and electrolyte imbalances
    1. Potential etiology
        a. Hyperdynamic circulation conditions can exist in the population of liver transplant patients due to the etiology of their diseases and comorbidities involving the cardiovascular system. Massive shifts of fluid volume can occur during the surgical procedure.[38]
           i.   Low SVR and high CO and CI are often present in advanced liver disease and can continue in the early posttransplant stages.
           ii. May be treated with fluid management but may also require inotropic support. Adequate perfusion is necessary for the transplanted liver and other vital organs.
           iii. As liver function improves, the CO and CI will fall and the SVR will return to normal.
        b. Hypovolemia associated with rewarming
           i.   As the patient warms up, hypotension and a drop in CVP may develop due to hypovolemia.
           ii. Hypovolemia occurs less frequently with active patient warming.
        c. Hypovolemia due to bleeding
    2. Assessment and maintenance of fluid and electrolyte balance are essential components of the nurse's role.[38]
        a. Clinical manifestations of hypovolemia
           i.   Dry mucus membranes
           ii. Thirst
           iii. Poor skin turgor
           iv. Decreased urine output
           v. Mental status changes
           vi. Dizziness or feelings of light-headedness
           vii. Muscle aches/weakness
        b. Hypovolemia: abnormal lab values, for example:
           i.   Increased hematocrit
           ii. Increased serum BUN and creatinine level
           iii. Increased serum sodium
           iv. Increased urine specific gravity
        c. Clinical manifestations of hypervolemia
           i.   Dyspnea
           ii. Distended neck veins
           iii. Mental status changes

      iv. Edema (commonly seen in the extremities and/or scrotum)

      v. Ascites

   d. Hypervolemia: abnormal lab values, for example:

      i. Decreased hematocrit (due to hemodilution)

      ii. Decreased serum sodium (in some cases)

      iii. Decreased serum osmolality

3. Monitoring

   a. Daily weights

   b. Strict intake and output

   c. Lab tests:

      i. Electrolytes (sodium, potassium, magnesium, chloride, calcium)

      ii. Bicarbonate

      iii. BUN

      iv. Creatinine

      v. Glucose

4. Potential interventions

   a. Hypovolemia associated with rewarming

      i. Administration of colloids or blood

      ii. Albumin infusion in the setting of a low albumin level

   b. Hypovolemia due to bleeding

      i. Administration of with blood products as appropriate and FFP or platelets to correct abnormal coagulation

   c. Fluid replacement or restriction, as indicated

   d. Diuretics with/without salt-poor albumin replacement

   e. Electrolyte replacement as needed (oral or IV)

   f. Consultation with a registered dietician regarding potential dietary restrictions or supplements

E. Renal dysfunction[37]

1. Overview

   a. Chronic and acute renal dysfunction is a common complication after liver transplantation, seen in up to 95% of patients at some point.[37] It is associated with greater short-term and long-term patient mortality. Signs of renal failure are an indication for the initiation of dialysis.

   b. Renal dysfunction can be seen pretransplant but is most often seen in the postoperative phase, in the first 3 years.

   c. A patient with a low GFR (glomerular filtration rate <60 mL/min/1.73 m^2) after transplantation and within the first 3 months has a higher risk of developing renal failure in the long term.

2. Types of renal failure and clinical criteria

   a. Acute renal failure (ARF) criteria may include any of the following:

      i. Serum creatinine (SCr) increase by 1.5 times baseline and/or decrease of glomerular filtration rate (GFR) >25%

      ii. Doubling of SCr and/or a decrease in GFR >50%

      iii. Increase of SCr threefold and/or a decrease of GFR >75%

      iv. SCr >4 mg/dL

   b. Chronic renal failure (CRF) is defined by GFR <60 mL/min/1.73 m^2 for more than 3 months.

3. Potential etiology—immediate postoperative renal dysfunction:

   a. Hypotensive episodes

   b. Blood loss

   c. High renal vein pressure intraoperatively and postoperatively due to hemodynamic instability or sepsis

4. Treatment options
   a. Dialysis
      i. Signs of renal failure are an indication for the initiation of dialysis.
      ii. Although some patients may require dialysis for a period of time postoperatively, once liver function improves, renal function often recovers and dialysis may be discontinued.
   b. Kidney transplantation in the setting of end-stage renal disease

G. Hyperglycemia and hypoglycemia[38]
   1. Overview
      a. Hypo- and hyperglycemia may be seen post liver transplant as the liver plays a central role in regulation of whole body metabolism.
      b. Poor glycemic control is linked to allograft rejection, surgical site infection, and increased mortality.
      c. Once the new liver is able to convert glucose into glycogen and store it, the transplanted liver is functioning.
   2. Hyperglycemia
      a. Some degree of hyperglycemia is evident in the early postoperative phase.
      b. Potential etiology
         i. Pre-existing diabetes mellitus
         ii. Side effects of corticosteroids or tacrolimus
      c. Clinical manifestations: report immediately if noted.
         i. Polyuria
         ii. Polydipsia
         iii. Polyphagia
         iv. Blurred vision
         v. Poor wound healing
         vi. Recurrent infections
      d. Interventions
         i. Blood glucose monitoring
         ii. Administration of insulin
         iii. Oral hypoglycemic agents
         iv. Collaboration with the members of the interdisciplinary team as necessary with recommendations on dietary changes given by the registered dietician
         v. Reinforcement of the patient's education in the home setting by a home health nurse
   3. Hypoglycemia
      a. Potential etiology
         i. Compromised liver recovery
         ii. Dose of insulin or oral hypoglycemic agents that exceeds patient's metabolic requirements
         iii. Insufficient caloric intake
         iv. Factors that potentiate the action of hypoglycemic medications
            • Renal insufficiency
            • Certain medications (e.g., sulfonamides)
      b. Clinical manifestations: report immediately if noted.
         i. Cool clammy skin
         ii. Diaphoresis
         iii. Mental status changes

   iv. Fatigue

   v. Palpitations

   vi. Tremors

  4. Interventions

   a. Blood glucose monitoring

   b. Administration of oral or IV glucose (depending on severity of hypoglycemia)

   c. Decrease in dose of insulin or oral hypoglycemic agents

   d. Collaboration with the members of the interdisciplinary team as necessary with recommendations on dietary changes given by the registered dietician

   e. Reinforcement of the patient's education in the home setting by a home health nurse

H. Hypotension or hypertension

  1. Cardiorespiratory failure is the leading cause of non–graft-related death among liver transplant recipients. Patients must be closely monitored for changes in vital signs and level of consciousness.[37]

  2. Hypotension

   a. Potential etiology

    i. Dehydration

    ii. Bleeding

    iii. Sepsis

   b. Clinical manifestations

    i. Decreased BP

    ii. Increased heart rate

    iii. Dizziness or light-headedness

    iv. Signs or symptoms of bleeding

   c. Potential treatment options

    i. Hypotension is usually treated with fluid boluses or blood transfusions.

    ii. Hypotension due to sepsis may require inotropic therapy.

    iii. Hypotension due to sepsis will require appropriate antibiotic regimen

   d. Patient monitoring

    i. Monitor patient's electrolytes and CBC with differential each AM.

    ii. Patients' vital signs must be monitored frequently and evaluated for a response to any interventions performed.

  3. Hypertension

   a. Potential etiology

    i. Fluid overload

    ii. Pain

    iii. Immunosuppressants: calcineurin inhibitors or corticosteroids

   b. Clinical manifestations

    i. Increased BP and pulse

    ii. Headaches

    iii. Dizziness or light-headedness

   c. Potential treatment options

    i. Optimization of pain control

    ii. Diuretic therapy

    iii. Oral or IV antihypertensive agents

    iv. IV vasoactive therapy (possibly)

d. Patient monitoring
   i. Close observation during pharmacological treatments is required because calcium channel blockers used for BP control, such as diltiazem (Cardizem) or verapamil (Calan), may increase cyclosporine or tacrolimus levels and immunosuppression doses may need to be adjusted accordingly.
   ii. Vital signs must be monitored frequently and evaluated for a response to any interventions performed.
4. Education for patient and caregivers: instructions regarding
   a. Signs and symptoms of hypo- and hypertension
   b. BP medications
   c. Daily monitoring and recording of BP
   d. When to contact the postoperative transplant coordinator

I. Cholestasis (blockage of bile flow from the liver)
1. Cholestasis is common and is usually associated with rejection, sepsis, drug toxicity, or preservation injury. Most cases remain subclinical.
2. Physical manifestations:
   a. Clay-colored or white stools
   b. Dark urine
   c. Itching
   d. Pain in upper right quadrant
   e. Jaundice
   f. Inability to digest certain foods
   g. Nausea and vomiting
3. If preservation injury is the causative factor, LFTs start to normalize after 3 to 4 days.
4. There is no specific treatment for cholestasis. If severe, cholestasis may be associated with irreversible liver damage and requires retransplantation.

J. Bile duct complications[37]
1. Biliary complications are common and may be seen at any time post liver transplantation
2. Clinical manifestations include the following:
   a. Elevated alkaline phosphatase level
   b. Possibly elevated bilirubin, gamma glutamyltransferase (GGT), and transaminase levels
3. Types: biliary leaks and biliary obstructions
   a. Biliary leaks
      i. Bile leaks can occur in the following locations:
         - At the site of anastomosis
         - T-tube exit site
         - Along the T-tube tract at the time of removal
         - Within the liver as a result of bile duct destruction (bile leak)
         - From the cut surface in a split liver, living donor transplant, or after a liver biopsy
      ii. Anastomotic leak
         - If there is an anastomotic leak, bile-stained fluid may be seen in the surgical drain.
         - In severe cases, frank bile may even leak through the surgical wound.
         - The patient may develop peritonitis with signs of systemic sepsis.

- Blood tests frequently show elevated bilirubin and white cell count.
- In duct-to-duct anastomosis, small leaks may be treated with internal stents placed percutaneously or via endoscopic retrograde cholangiopancreatography (ERCP).
- Bile collections can be drained percutaneously and a pigtail drain inserted.
- Large leaks should be surgically repaired with construction of a Roux-en-Y choledochojejunostomy.

   iii. T-tube leaks

- A transient leak at the exit site of a T tube is quite common after T-tube removal and usually resolves spontaneously.
- Rarely, T-tube removal results in bile leaking into the peritoneal cavity, causing biliary peritonitis. This requires urgent radiological or surgical drainage.
- Delaying the removal of T tubes for up to 3 months posttransplant allows for the biliary tract to mature, but even after this time, leaks can occur.

  b. Biliary obstruction

    i. Bile duct obstruction is usually associated with technical complications at the anastomosis.

    ii. The earliest sign is an elevated serum alkaline phosphatase, followed by a rising bilirubin.

    iii. An ultrasound scan may show biliary dilatation and a cholangiogram will demonstrate the site of obstruction.

K. Anastomotic strictures[37]

1. An anastomotic stricture is a narrowing at the point where the donor bile duct has been sewn onto the recipient bile duct.
2. Potential etiology:
   a. Faulty surgical technique
   b. Local ischemia
   c. Scar tissue formation
   d. Hepatic artery thrombosis
3. Anastomotic strictures can be treated with ERCP, balloon dilatation, and a biliary stent.
4. Recurrent strictures often require surgical correction.
5. Nonanastomotic strictures may form at other sites, are usually secondary to ischemia, and are associated with:
   a. Hepatic artery thrombosis
   b. Prolonged cold ischemic time of the donor organ
   c. Livers from donation after cardiac death donors
   d. Recurrent cholangitis

L. Ascites[38]

1. Patients with preoperative ascites may continue to have this postoperatively as the sequelae of liver failure are not immediately resolved. However, persistent ascites for more than 4 months posttransplant is uncommon.
2. Diuretics and/or paracentesis may be required.
3. Good nutrition and low-sodium and high-protein diet are beneficial.
4. It is important to inform the patient that the ascites will decline as liver function improves.

M. Portal vein thrombosis[37]
1. Portal vein thrombosis is a very rare postoperative complication.
2. Typically occurs in the early postoperative period.
3. Potential etiology:
    a. Technical complication
    b. Inadequate restoration of portal flow in patients with a preoperative thrombosis
4. Manifests with abnormal LFTs and can lead to variceal hemorrhage, intestinal ischemia, and ascites.
5. Diagnosis is made by Doppler ultrasound scan. In the late posttransplant course, a patient may present with variceal hemorrhage due to portal hypertension caused by thrombosis.
6. Portal vein thrombosis is also associated with more complex surgical procedures in liver transplantation, but unlike HAT, it has no influence on overall morbidity and mortality.[37]

N. Impaired wound healing.[38]
1. Risk factors:
    a. Immunosuppressive therapy
    b. Poor nutritional status
2. Patient monitoring
    a. Daily comprehensive skin assessments should be done on every patient. Complete inspection of incisions, tube sites, and pressure areas helps to prevent complications.
3. Incisions
    a. Patients will often have an inverted Y incision, which is commonly called a Mercedes incision.
    b. Incisional edges should be well approximated without any signs of edge separation, necrosis, or dehiscence.
    c. There should be no sign of redness, swelling, or purulent drainage.
    d. If a local incision infection does occur, some incisions may require the removal of staples and remain opened for wet-to-dry dressings to promote wound healing.
    e. Depending on the wound appearance, a wound care nurse should be consulted for recommendations that might include an enzymatic debridement.
    f. Daily incision care should include cleaning the wound with normal saline or soap and water.
        i.   No lotions or powder should be applied directly to the incision.
        ii. Patients with fluid overload in the immediate postoperative period may require a dry dressing over the incision until drainage ceases.
4. Jackson-Pratt (JP) drains and/or T-tube drains
    a. These sites must be monitored for signs of redness, swelling, or purulent drainage.
    b. Once a drain is pulled, the site should still be cleaned daily and covered with a dry dressing until the site is healed.
    c. Generally, the T tube, whether it is open or capped off, remains for 3 to 4 weeks although timing will vary based on patient needs and center protocol.
5. Patient education is key to preventing wound infections.
    a. Patients and their families must be instructed on the importance of proper incision and drain care.

b. A home health nurse may be consulted as needed upon discharge from hospital.

c. Postoperatively and after discharge, mobility is an important strategy to promote healing.
    i. Physical and occupational therapists help to mobilize the patient, which is beneficial in preventing pressure ulcers and promoting wound healing.

d. A registered dietician should make recommendations to ensure the patient is receiving adequate nutrition, which is essential for wound healing.

O. Altered bowel function[38]

1. Constipation
    a. Constipation can be a common problem posttransplant, not unlike any postoperative/postanesthesia event.
    b. Assessment for bowel sounds and bowel movements should be done daily.
    c. Complaints of abdominal pain and distention should be reported to the physician/clinical provider.
    d. Encouraging an increase in fluid and fiber intake, in addition to increasing activity, may facilitate bowel movements.
    e. If the discomfort is too severe, it is unlikely that the patient can tolerate the mobility. In such a case, a stool softener such as docusate sodium (Colace) may be prescribed.
    f. If a stool softener is ineffective, a suppository may be needed (glycerin or Dulcolax suppositories are most commonly used).
    g. If the above are ineffective, an enema may be needed.

2. Diarrhea
    a. The frequency and consistency of the bowel movement should be assessed and documented.
    b. Note: Diarrhea may contribute to fluid imbalance.
    c. The physician/clinical provider should be notified and a specimen may need to be collected to rule out an infectious etiology.
        i. Watery, foul-smelling stool and more than three in 24 hours may indicate the presence of *Clostridium difficile*.
        ii. Isolation/contact precautions may be required.
        iii. Oral metronidazole (Flagyl) may be started until *Clostridium difficile* is ruled out.
    d. Dehydration should be of concern in a patient with diarrhea.
        i. Encourage oral fluid intake if possible.
        ii. Administer IV hydration if necessary.
    e. A review of the patient's medications should be done as some of the post–liver transplant medications can cause diarrhea. Changes in dose or type of medication may be considered.

P. Altered nutrition[38,39]

1. Overview
    a. During the initial posttransplant period, it is not uncommon for patients to be unable to meet their nutritional requirements.
    b. Protein-energy malnutrition is frequently seen in patients with end-stage liver disease because of the key role the liver plays in the regulation of nutritional state and energy. This causes a deterioration of the clinical condition prior to transplantation and affects posttransplant survival.[39]
    c. Assessment by a registered dietician is crucial.

2. Oral intake is usually started 1 to 3 days postoperatively with a clear liquid diet, advancing to solids as tolerated.
   a. Those patients who have had a Roux-en-Y anastomosis may take longer to start oral fluids and diet.
3. Appetite and caloric intake should be documented and assessed with each meal to ensure adequate intake of dietary needs.
   a. Patients should be assessed for low serum albumin levels and weight changes.
   b. Ideally, oral diets are the preferred method of nutrition.
   c. For patients who are unable to tolerate large meals, small, frequent, and high-calorie meals should be encouraged.
4. If nutritional goals are not met, it may be beneficial to start oral nutritional supplements.
5. If the goals are still not met, enteral tube feedings may be recommended by the registered dietician or provider.
6. In extreme cases of nonfunctioning gut, parenteral nutrition supplements may be instituted.
7. With collaborative interdisciplinary teamwork, including input from the registered dietician, a patient's nutritional needs can be met.
8. Ultimately good nutrition will help to prevent infection, promote adequate wound healing, and provide the metabolic support the patient requires.

Q. Altered mobility/self-care deficit[40]
1. Liver transplant recipients will initially have some degree of altered mobility or self-care deficit, often attributable to the aforementioned poor nutritional status prior to transplantation.
2. The efforts of an extended interdisciplinary team including physical therapy, occupational therapy, respiratory therapy, and, in extreme cases, speech therapy contribute to the patient's advancement.
3. Early assessment of level of independence with activities of daily living is essential for setting goals for discharge from the hospital setting.
4. The patient's pretransplant strength and activity may influence posttransplant recovery.
   a. The stronger the patient is going into the transplant, the quicker and easier the recovery should be.
5. Once a patient is off the ventilator and the organ is functioning, physical therapy should be initiated and respiratory therapy continued.
6. Patients should be encouraged on a daily basis to increase their progression to an independent level.
   a. Patients who are unable to reach their goals may need to be referred to an outpatient setting for further rehabilitation.
7. Patients and caregivers are key members of the interdisciplinary team.
   a. Caregivers play a vital role in the patient's recovery and should be included in the patient's hospital care and in all aspects of patient education and discharge preparation.

XII. INFECTION[37]

A. Infection is an important cause of posttransplant morbidity and mortality.

B. Factors predisposing a recipient to infection include those present in the recipient prior to the surgery and those that are secondary to intraoperative and posttransplant events.

C. Risk factors for infection
   1. Diabetes mellitus
   2. Higher pretransplant MELD scores
   3. Malnutrition

D. Fever
   1. In the first few postoperative days, a fever may possibly be due to infection, which can lead to sepsis if not treated promptly.
   2. In immunocompromised patients, a fever is typically defined at 38.2°C (lower than the fever threshold for other types of patients).
   3. However, it is important to note that hypothermia may also be suggestive of sepsis.

E. Evaluation of febrile patients
   1. Obtain blood cultures
      a. Note: Antibiotic therapy for potential bacterial infection may be started, but only after blood cultures are obtained.
   2. Obtain urine, sputum, and wound cultures to identify the site of the infection.
   3. Monitor C reactive protein (CRP), a protein present in acute inflammatory conditions and sepsis.

F. Types of infection
   1. Bacterial
      a. Bacterial infections involving the abdomen or surgical wound are not uncommon.
   2. Viral
      a. Cytomegalovirus (CMV)
         i. CMV is a common virus, carried in 50% to 80% of the population in the United States and can be transmitted through the donor liver.
         ii. CMV infection rarely occurs before 21 days but can be seen 1 to 4 months posttransplant.
         iii. Clinical manifestations
            • High fever
            • Rigors
            • Body aches
            • Night sweats
         iv. In immunocompromised patients, CMV can also cause pneumonia, hepatitis, gastrointestinal infection, pancreatitis, and retinitis.
         v. CMV prophylaxis
            • Valganciclovir (Valcyte) is used for 3 months posttransplant.
         vi. If active infection develops, IV ganciclovir (Cytovene) is administered until the virus has cleared.
         vii. Individual transplant center protocols may vary.

G. See chapter on Infectious Diseases for additional information.

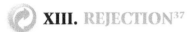

XIII. REJECTION[37]

A. Nurses are in a unique position to identify rejection in liver transplant recipients early in its course due to the daily observation and assessment of the patient's condition.

B. Rejection monitoring
   1. Daily monitoring of patient for signs and symptoms of rejection; suspected rejection is confirmed by biopsy.
      a. Temperature
      b. Sclera: yellowing of sclera (icterus)
      c. Skin: yellowing of skin (jaundice)
      d. Right upper quadrant pain
      e. Fatigue
      f. Malaise
      g. Pruritus
   2. Lab tests: typically drawn every morning
      a. Liver enzymes, bilirubin, and coagulation studies
         i. Increases in AST, ALT, and bilirubin above the patient's baseline may be indicative of rejection.
      b. Immunosuppression trough levels (to verify that levels are at the patient's individualized target therapeutic level)
   3. T-tube drainage
      a. Should be golden brown
      b. Immediately report any changes in bile such as:
         i. A lighter color
         ii. The presence of sludge
         iii. Thinning of bile
   4. Stools: Light-colored stools may be indicative of rejection.
   5. Urine: Dark-colored urine may be indicative of rejection.

C. Types of rejection: There are three types of rejection: hyperacute, acute (cellular and antibody mediated), and chronic.
   1. Hyperacute rejection is rare and is seen in the OR at the time of transplantation.
   2. Acute rejection
      a. Most common type of rejection, occurring in 10% to 30% of liver transplant recipients.[37]
      b. May be seen as early as 3 days after implantation. However, generally, it can occur from 7 to 10 days to 6 weeks postoperatively.
      c. Acute rejection is characterized as cellular (T-cell mediated) or antibody mediated.
      d. Clinical manifestations may include the following:
         i. Fever—continuous low-grade elevation
         ii. Listlessness
         iii. Loss of appetite
         iv. Irritability
         v. Fatigue
         vi. Liver pain
         vii. Abdominal distention
         viii. Jaundice
         ix. Abnormal transaminases[37]
      e. Recurrent episodes of acute rejection often lead to chronic rejection.

3. Chronic rejection:
   a. Occurs over a longer period of time
   b. Generally considered irreversible and not amenable to treatment, thus leading to the need for retransplantation
   c. Clinical manifestations of chronic rejection

D. Patient/caregiver education
   1. Patients and caregivers are educated to continue the same monitoring following discharge and contact their transplant coordinator/transplant team if they notice any signs or symptoms of rejection.

 XIV. LIVER BIOPSY

A. Some centers may routinely biopsy patients on day 7; however, most centers will only biopsy when there is a rise in LFTs suggesting a possible rejection episode.

B. Liver biopsies may be done in interventional radiology under guided imaging, percutaneously with ultrasound guidance in a gastroenterology suite or on the patient unit.

C. A very small piece of liver tissue is extracted.

D. Postbiopsy monitoring
   1. Vital signs are monitored for any signs that would indicate bleeding: low BP and tachycardia.
   2. If the patient has a T tube, the nurse must monitor for any blood in the bile.
   3. Hgb and hematocrit levels are typically checked 4 hours after the procedure and compared to the previously drawn levels to assess for any decrease.

E. Patients are typically kept on bed rest for 4 to 6 hours following the biopsy.

F. Patient education
   1. Patients are instructed to notify staff immediately should any of the following occur:
      a. Severe abdominal pain
      b. Dizziness or light-headedness
      c. Shortness of breath
      d. Bleeding from the biopsy site
   2. Patients are also given information regarding
      a. Reason for the biopsy
      b. The different levels of acute rejection—mild, moderate, and severe
      c. Possible interventions that may occur in the setting of rejection (note: interventions vary per transplant program)
         i.   Increase in dose of immunosuppressive agents
         ii. Administration of high-dose steroids
         iii. The potential need for longer hospitalization

 XV. POSTTRANSPLANT IMMUNOSUPPRESSION

A. Immunosuppression following liver transplantation addresses the central issue in organ transplantation: the suppression of rejection.[41]

1. Regimens vary from patient to patient and also among centers.
2. Patients and their support persons must be taught about their medication regimens and understand that these are lifelong medications.
3. Doses are adjusted to prevent rejection while minimizing side effects.

B. Types of therapy:
 1. Triple therapy may include a combination of
    a. A calcineurin inhibitor: tacrolimus (Prograf) or cyclosporine (Neoral or Gengraf)
    b. An antiproliferative agent: azathioprine (Imuran) or mycophenolate mofetil (CellCept) or mycophenolic acid (Myfortic)
    c. A corticosteroid: methylprednisolone (Solu-Medrol) IV or oral prednisone
 2. Double therapy may include the following:
    a. A calcineurin inhibitor: tacrolimus (Prograf) or cyclosporine (Neoral or Gengraf)
    b. A corticosteroid: methylprednisolone (Solu-Medrol) IV or oral prednisone
 3. Monotherapy—Some patients will be maintained on one immunosuppressant only; this is called monotherapy.

C. Other agents
 1. Sirolimus (rapamycin/Rapamune)
    a. Sirolimus (rapamycin/Rapamune) is now being used for some patients. It does not have the nephrotoxic side effects of calcineurin inhibitors.
    b. Used for continuing rejection, sirolimus has been shown to prevent chronic rejection; however, some centers are evaluating its use as a baseline immunosuppressant.
    c. Increases cholesterol levels, requiring close monitoring.
    d. May cause proteinuria.
 2. Induction agents
    a. Induction agents, in the form of antilymphocyte preparations, have not been widely used in liver transplantation.
    b. However, newer humanized induction agents are now being used in some patients. These include the following:
       i. Basiliximab (Simulect)
       ii. Daclizumab (Zenapax)
       iii. Alemtuzumab (Campath)
    c. Induction agents are to be given pre- or intraoperatively to
       i. Decrease the incidence of acute rejection
       ii. Delay first rejection
       iii. Delay the use of calcineurin inhibitors (tacrolimus or cyclosporine) due to their nephrotoxicity
    d. The long-term results of these newer agents are still under evaluation in liver transplantation.

D. Side effects of immunosuppression
 1. Patients are closely monitored for the side effects of immunosuppressive agents, particularly in the early postdischarge period.
 2. Calcineurin inhibitors (tacrolimus [Prograf] and cyclosporine [Neoral, Gengraf]) have side effects that include the following:
    a. Tremors
    b. Headaches
    c. Hypertension

    d. Nephrotoxicity

    e. Elevated blood glucose levels

    f. Hair growth or loss

    g. Increased risk of developing cancer

3. Corticosteroids (methylprednisolone or prednisone) have side effects, which include the following:

    a. Diabetes mellitus

    b. Hypertension

    c. High cholesterol levels

    d. Weight gain

    e. Fluid retention

    f. Indigestion

    g. Bone loss (with long-term use)

    h. Because of these side effects, some centers now prefer to use steroid-sparing regimens.

4. Azathioprine (Imuran): Side effects include the following:

    a. Low white blood cell count

    b. Joint pain

    c. Nausea and vomiting

    d. Dizziness

    e. Stomach upset

5. Sirolimus (rapamycin/Rapamune): Side effects include the following:

    a. Leukopenia

    b. Thrombocytopenia

    c. Anemia

    d. Hypertension

    e. Rash

    f. Acne

    g. Diarrhea

    h. Poor wound healing

6. Mycophenolate mofetil (CellCept): Side effects include the following:

    a. Low white cell count (especially low neutrophils)

    b. Diarrhea (this may be helped by splitting the dose)

    c. Vomiting

    d. Headaches

    e. Hypertension

7. Basiliximab (Simulect): Side effects include the following:

    a. Abdominal pain

    b. Sore throat

    c. Tremors

    d. Vomiting

    e. Swelling of ankles, body, face, and lower legs

    f. Loss of energy

8. Daclizumab (Zenapax): Side effects include the following:

    a. Dizziness

    b. Nausea and vomiting

    c. Rapid heart rate

    d. Chest pain

    e. Tremors

    f. Swelling of feet or lower legs

9. Alemtuzumab (Campath): Side effects include the following:
   a. Fever and chills shortly after infusion
10. See chapter on Pharmacology for additional information.

XVI. OTHER POSTTRANSPLANT MEDICATIONS

A. The following conditions may develop as a consequence of immunosuppressive therapy and require prophylaxis:
   1. *Pneumocystis carinii* pneumonia (PCP) prophylaxis:
      a. Sulfamethoxazole-trimethoprim (Bactrim)
   2. *Candida* prophylaxis
      a. Fluconazole (Diflucan)
      b. Nystatin (Mycostatin)
   3. Herpes virus prophylaxis
      a. Acyclovir (Zovirax)
   4. CMV prophylaxis
      a. Valganciclovir (Valcyte) (oral)
      b. IV ganciclovir (Cytovene)
   5. Gastritis/reflux associated with steroid use:
      a. H2 blockers:
         i. Ranitidine (Zantac)
         ii. Famotidine (Pepcid)
      b. Proton pump inhibitors:
         i. Omeprazole (Prilosec)
         ii. Lansoprazole (Prevacid)
         iii. Esomeprazole (Nexium)

B. See chapter on Infectious Diseases for additional information.

XVII. LONG-TERM COMPLICATIONS AND COMORBIDITIES[37]

A. Hypertension
   1. Approximately 75% of recipients develop elevated BP following transplantation.
   2. Cardiovascular disease is the leading cause of non–organ-related death post liver transplantation.

B. Dyslipidemia
   1. Many patients develop abnormal lipid levels. The incidence of dyslipidemia may be higher in patients on sirolimus (Rapamune).

C. Chronic renal insufficiency. Approximately 85% of recipients develop chronic renal insufficiency within 5 years of transplantation.

D. Diabetes
   1. The risk of developing diabetes varies depending on the underlying liver disease.
   2. Recipients who underwent liver transplantation for the following indications are at higher risk for developing posttransplant diabetes:
      a. HCV
      b. Alcoholic cirrhosis
      c. NASH

E. Metabolic bone disease

1. The greatest risk is immediately after transplantation when steroid doses are highest.

2. However, some recipients continue to be at risk long term even with lower or no steroid use.

F. Posttransplant malignancy

1. Second most common cause of late mortality.

2. Skin cancer is the most common cause of posttransplant malignancy with risk up to 20-fold higher than general population.

3. Increased risk of other solid organ malignancies such as head and neck, lung, and colon cancer.

4. Lymphoma. Higher risk in first 18 months posttransplant but can see late-onset development as well.[28]

G. See the chapter on Noninfectious Diseases for additional information.

 XVIII. PREVENTIVE HEALTH CARE

A. Preventive health care is extremely important for this patient group.

B. It is important to encourage patients to

1. Keep their follow-up appointments with their transplant program and primary care providers.

2. Undergo cancer screening as appropriate.

3. Obtain vaccinations as appropriate.

    a. Inactivated vaccines, such as the injectable influenza vaccine or the pneumococcal vaccine, should be encouraged when appropriate.

    b. Live vaccines, such as the shingles vaccine, are contraindicated.

REFERENCES

1. Heron M. Deaths: leading causes for 2010. *Natl Vital Stat Rep.* 2013;62(6):1–96.

2. Kim WR, Lake JR, Smith JM, et al. OPTN/SRTR 2013 Annual Data Report: liver. *Am J Transplant.* 2015;15(s2):1–28.

3. Health Resources and Services Administration. *Organ Procurement and Transplantation Network.* Available at http://optn.transplant.hrsa.gov/latestData. Accessed May 15, 2015.

4. Farrell GC, McCullough AJ, Day CP. *Non-Alcoholic Fatty Liver Disease: A Practical Guide.* 2nd ed. Oxford: Wiley-Blackwell; 2013.

5. Schwake JW, Torres DM, Harrison SA. *Non-Alcoholic Fatty Liver Disease: A Practical Guide.* 2nd ed. Oxford: Wiley-Blackwell; 2013.

6. United Network of Organ Sharing. UNOS. *Transplant Professionals.* Available at http://transplantpro.org. Accessed March 30, 2015.

7. Schnitzler MA, Skeans MA, Axelrod DA, et al. OPTN/SRTR 2013 annual data report: economics. *Am J Transplant.* 2015;15(s2):1–24.

8. United Network for Organ Sharing. UNOS. Available at www.unos.org. Accessed September 29, 2014.

9. Centers for Disease Control. CDC. Available at www.cdc.org. Accessed September 29, 2014.

10. Woller N, Kuhnel F. *Viruses and Human Cancer: From Basic Science to Clinical Prevention.* Berlin, Germany: Springer-Verlag; 2014.

11. Yamane D, McGivern D, Masaki T, et al. *Hepatitis C Virus: From Molecular Virology to Antiviral Therapy.* Berlin, Germany: Springer-Verlag; 2013.

12. Cleveland Clinic. Available at www.clevelandclinicmeded.com/medicalpubs/diseasemanagement/hepatology. Accessed September 29, 2014.

13. Saidi RF, Hejazi Kenuri SK. Liver transplantation for hepatocellular carcinoma: past, present and future. *Middle East J Dig Dis.* 2013;5:181–192.

14. Yarnell E. Primary biliary cirrhosis. *Altern Complement Ther.* 2012;18(3):148–151.
15. Lutz H, Trautwein C, Tischendorf J. Primary sclerosing cholangitis. *Dtsch Arztebl Int.* 2013;23(51): 67–74.
16. United States National Institutes of Health. National Institute of Diabetes and Digestive and Kidney Diseases. Available at www.digestive.niddk.nih.gov/health-information/health-topics/liver-disease/autoimmune-hepatitis/Pages/facts.aspx. Accessed September 29, 2014.
17. United States National Institutes of Health. National Institute of Diabetes and Digestive and Kidney Diseases. Available at www.digestive.niddk.nih.gov/ddiseases/pubs/hemochromatosis. Accessed September 29, 2014.
18. United States National Institutes of Health. National Institute of Diabetes and Digestive and Kidney Diseases. Available at www.digestive.niddk.nih.gov/ddiseases/pubs/wilson. Accessed September 30, 2014.
19. United States National Institutes of Health. National Library of Medicine. Available at www.ghr.nlm.nih.gov/condition/alpha-1antitrypsin-deficiency. Accessed September 29, 2014.
20. United States National Institutes of Health. National Institute of Diabetes and Digestive and Kidney Diseases. Available at www.niddk.nih.gov/health-information/health-topics/liver-disease/non-alcoholicsteatohepatitis/Pages/facts.aspx. Accessed September 29, 2014.
21. Mehta N. *Drug Induced Toxicity. Medscape.* Available at http://emedicine.medscape.com/article/169814. Accessed February 20, 2015.
22. Craig DG, Bates CM, Davidson JS, et al. Overdose pattern and outcome in paracetamol-induced acute severe hepatotoxicity. *Br J Clin Pharmacol.* 2011;71(2):273–282.
23. Brown K, Kazimi M. *Textbook of Organ Transplantation.* Oxford: Wiley-Blackwell; 2014.
24. Ahmed KT, Almashhrawi AA, Rahman RN, et al. Liver diseases in pregnancy: diseases unique to pregnancy. *World J Gastroenterol.* 2013;19(43):7639–7646.
25. United States National Institutes of Health. National Library of Medicine. Available at http://www.nlm.nih.gov/medlineplus/ency/article/000890.htm. *Accessed March 29, 2015.*
26. Stravitz RT, Carl DE, Biskobing DM. Medical management of the liver transplant recipient. *Clin Liver Dis.* 2011;15:821–843.
27. United States National Institutes of Health. National Library of Medicine. Available at http://www.ncbi.nlm.nih.gov/pmc/articles/PMC1860002. Accessed March 30, 2015.
28. Green TE. Available at http://www.emedicine.medscape.com/article/789105/treatment. Accessed March 30, 2015.
29. Mayo Clinic. *Esophageal Varices.* Available at http://www.mayoclinic.org/diseases-conditions/esophageal-varices/basics/treatment/con-20027505. Accessed March 30, 2015.
30. Kappus MR, Bajaj JS. Covert hepatic encephalopathy: not as minimal as you might think. *Clin Gastroenterol Hepatol.* 2012;10:1208–1219.
31. Johns Hopkins Medicine. *Health Library.* Available at http://www.hopkinsmedicine.org/healthlibrary/conditions/liver. Accessed May 15, 2015.
32. Shawcross DL, O'Grady JG. The 6-month abstinence rule in liver transplantation. *Lancet.* 2010;376:216.
33. United Network of Organ Sharing. UNOS. Available at http://www.transplantliving.org/before-the-transplant/about-organ-allocation. Accessed January 2016.
34. United States Health Resources Services Administration. *Organ Procurement and Transplantation Network.* Available at http://optn.transplant.hrsa.gov/ContentDocuments/OPTN_Policies.pdf#nameddest=Policy_09. Accessed January 2016.
35. Zivkovic SA. Neurologic complications after liver transplantation. *World J Hepatol.* 2013;5(8):409–416.
36. University of Pennsylvania Health System. Available at http//penn-medicine-liver-transplant.blogspot.com/2012/03/safe-acetaminophen-tylenol-doses-for.html. Accessed March 29, 2015.
37. Eghstesad B, Miller C, Fung J; Cleveland Clinic Center for Continuing Education. *Post-Liver Transplantation Management.* Available at http://www.clevelandclinicmeded.com/medicalpubs/diseasemanagement/hepatology/post-liver-transplantation-management. Accessed September 18, 2015.
38. Hasse JM. Nutrition and liver disease: complex connections. *Nutr Clin Pract.* 2013;28:12–14.
39. Murray EM, McCoy SM, Campbell KL, et al. Dieticians' practices and perspectives on nutrition priorities for liver transplant patients. *Nutr Diet.* 2014;71:86–91.
40. Zhang H, Chen L, Gu G, et al. Clinical observation and nursing care on the prevention of abdominal organ cluster transplantation rejection. *J Clin Nurs.* 2013;22:1599–1603.
41. Trotter JF. Rejection and immunosuppression trends in liver transplantation. In: Clavien P, Trotter JF, eds. *Medical Care of the Liver Transplant Patient.* 4th ed. Hoboken, NJ: Wiley-Blackwell; 2012:297–307.

SELF-ASSESSMENT QUESTIONS

1. Chronic hepatitis C is currently the leading cause of liver failure. What disease/syndrome is predicted to become the leading cause in the future?
   a. Hepatitis B
   b. Alcoholic cirrhosis
   c. Nonalcoholic fatty liver disease (NAFLD)
   d. Nonalcoholic steatohepatitis (NASH)

2. Patients with chronic liver disease may demonstrate which of the following hemodynamic states in the immediate transplant postoperative period?
   a. Elevated cardiac output
   b. Low systemic vascular resistance
   c. Elevated cardiac index
   d. a and b only
   e. b and c only
   f. All of the above

3. Bleeding may occur in the first 48 hours post liver transplantation due to which of the following factors?
   a. Poor functioning graft with underlying coagulopathy
   b. Improperly functioning drains
   c. Ascites developing from fluid mismanagement
   d. Poor renal function

4. Green-colored drainage post liver transplantation may be a sign of:
   a. bleeding into the GI tract.
   b. bile leakage.
   c. the development of a fistula to the gall bladder.
   d. ruptured gall bladder.

5. De novo seizures may occur post liver transplant and may be related to which of the following factors?
   a. Electrolyte imbalances
   b. Cyclosporine or tacrolimus
   c. Intracerebral abscesses
   d. a and b only
   e. b and c only
   f. All of the above

6. Early indicators of primary nonfunction of the new liver may include which of the following?
   a. The quantity and quality of bile production
   b. Extreme edema of the organ
   c. Hemodynamic instability
   d. a and b only
   e. b and c only
   f. All of the above

7. The risk for primary nonfunction of a liver after transplantation is:
   a. 10% to 15%.
   b. 15% to 20%.
   c. 1% to 2%.
   d. 4% to 6%.

8. Factors related to primary nonfunction of a new liver include which of the following?
   a. Prolonged ischemic time
   b. Donor age
   c. Prolonged donor management/hospital stay
   d. a and c only
   e. b and c only
   f. All of the above

9. Indicators of liver rejection posttransplantation include which of the following?
   a. A rise in AST, ALT, and bilirubin
   b. A rise in WBC
   c. Golden brown drainage from T tube
   d. b and c only
   e. All of the above

10. Hyperglycemia in the first few days post liver transplantation may be related to which of the following?
    a. Calcineurin inhibitors
    b. Steroids
    c. A normal functioning liver that is converting glucose into glycogen
    d. a and b only
    e. a and c only
    f. All of the above

11. In the immediate postoperative period, hypovolemia may be associated with rewarming. The patient may present with which of the following changes associated with hypovolemia?
    a. Hypertension and elevated urine output
    b. Hypotension and a decrease in CVP
    c. Increased urine output and drop in AST and ALT levels
    d. All of the above

Correct Answers:
1.d 2.f 3.a 4.b 5.f 6.f 7.d 8.f 9.a 10.f 11.b

CHAPTER 13

Intestine Transplantation

Beverly Kosmach-Park, RN, DNP, FAAN

Maria DeAngelis, MScN, NP

I. INTRODUCTION

A. Intestine transplantation was recognized in 2000 as the standard of care for adults and children with life-threatening intestinal failure in the United States. This was followed by an increased number of international cases being performed with the development of intestine transplantation becoming a successful procedure for patients with intestinal failure who could not be treated with long-term parenteral nutrition.[1]

B. History

1. First performed over 50 years ago, but clinical success has been challenging with improvements in survival and outcomes occurring only recently

2. First cohort: 1964–1972:
    a. Eight intestine transplants were performed internationally.
    b. Longest survival of this cohort was 6 months.
    c. Poor survival was attributed to technical complications, infection, and inability of available immunosuppressive protocols to control and treat rejection.[2]

3. Cyclosporine era: 1984–1989:
    a. Renewed attempts in intestine transplantation were based on the success of cyclosporine as the primary immunosuppressant for kidney, liver, and heart transplantation.
    b. Mean survival ($n = 6$) improved to 25.7 months.[3]
    c. Cyclosporine did not have a similar impact on survival in intestine transplantation as compared to other solid organs.
    d. There is one surviving recipient from this cohort who received an isolated intestine transplant in 1989; however, immunosuppression is now maintained with tacrolimus (Francis Lacaille, *personal communication*, March 31, 2015).[4]

4. Significantly improved patient and graft survival has been achieved since the early eras of intestine transplantation due to
    a. Improved immunosuppressive strategies

      i. Tacrolimus was first used in 1990 as the primary immunosuppressant in intestine transplantation with significantly improved survival.

      ii. Induction therapy: The use of preconditioning protocols with antilymphoid medications such as alemtuzumab and antithymocyte globulin has been shown to decrease the incidence of early rejection and improve survival.[5]

  b. Innovative surgical techniques

  c. Improved infection surveillance and treatment

C. Current Data

  1. Intestine Transplant Registry (ITR):

    a. Registry of worldwide data from intestine transplant centers since 1985.

    b. Data reflects global trends because case volumes are low within each transplant center.

  2. 2013 ITR Registry Report[5]:

    a. The 2013 Registry Report contains data from 82 contributing centers.

    b. As of February 2, 2013: 2,887 transplants have been performed in 2,699 patients. The majority of these transplants (76%) have been performed in North America.

    c. Although the number of cases had increased annually since 1985, there has been a steady decline in intestinal transplantation since 2009. This can be partially attributed to improvements in the multidisciplinary care and treatment of patients with intestinal failure–associated liver disease (IFALD), thus decreasing the need for concomitant liver transplant and/or intestine transplant.

    d. Isolated intestine transplantation, without the liver component, is now the most common type of intestine transplant.

      i. Inclusion of the liver with the intestine graft is associated with significantly better graft survival ($p = 0.017$).

    e. Transplantation of the colon is performed more frequently.

    f. Length of stay has been reduced to a median of 44 days.

    g. Induction therapy is used in a majority of patients (72%).

    h. Tacrolimus is the primary immunosuppressant medication used for maintenance immunosuppression (92%).

    i. Actuarial patient/graft survival for transplants performed since 2000:

      i. 77/71% at 1 year

      ii. 58/50% at 5 years

      iii. 47/41% at 10 years

    j. Retransplantation:

      i. 8% of patients have received a second or third transplant.

      ii. Survival of the second or third graft is 56% at 1 year and 35% at 5 years.

    k. Leading causes of graft loss:

      i. Sepsis (>50%)

      ii. Rejection (13%)

      iii. Cardiovascular events (8%)

    l. Improved graft survival related to

      i. Waiting at home at time of transplant

      ii. Younger recipient age

      iii. Maintenance therapy with rapamycin

      iv. Presence of a liver component

m. Outcome:
  i.   At >6 months posttransplant, most recipients (63%) are well or have only minor issues and have returned to normal activities.
  ii. TPN has been discontinued in 67% of recipients.

 II. INTESTINAL FAILURE

A. Intestinal Failure (IF): Defined as "the reduction of gut function below the minimum necessary for the absorption of macronutrients and/or water and electrolytes, such that intravenous supplementation is required to maintain health and/or growth."[6]

1. Classifications of IF based on gastrointestinal or systemic diseases[6]:
   a. Short bowel: due to extensive surgical resection or congenital disease including mesenteric infarction, Crohn's disease, intestinal volvulus, or necrotizing enterocolitis.
   b. Intestinal fistula: abnormal communication between two parts of the gastrointestinal tract, between the GI tract and other organs, or the GI tract and the skin. Etiology may be inflammatory, neoplastic, iatrogenic, infectious, or due to trauma.
   c. Intestinal dysmotility: motility disorder leading to poor propulsion through the intestine in the absence of any occlusions (chronic intestinal pseudo-obstruction).
   d. Mechanical obstruction: due to a physical abnormality that affects the intestine (tumors, bowel lesions).
   e. Extensive small-bowel mucosal disease (microvillus inclusion disease, tufting enteropathy, radiation enteritis).

2. Intestinal failure results in alterations in absorption so that the patient is unable to gain or sustain weight and/or maintain fluid balance. Growth and development are affected in the pediatric population.

3. Prognosis depends on residual bowel length, anatomy, and residual bowel function.
   a. Indications for poor prognosis[7]:
     i.   Length <10% of normal age-expected bowel length
     ii.   Absence of the ileocecal valve or colon
     iii. Prematurity
     iv.   Presence of bacterial overgrowth
     v.   Presence of persistent liver disease

4. Common causes of intestinal failure (Table 13-1)

TABLE 13-1 Common Causes of Intestinal Failure

Adult	Pediatric
• Ischemia	• Midgut volvulus
• Crohn's disease	• Necrotizing enterocolitis
• Desmoid tumor	• Gastroschisis
• Trauma	• Congenital atresias
• Volvulus	• Hirschsprung's disease
• Pseudo-obstruction	• Chronic intestinal pseudo-obstruction
• Gardner's disease	• Microvillus inclusion disease

III. INTESTINAL REHABILITATION

A. Goals of Intestinal Rehabilitation and Treatment[8]

1. Maximize the absorptive capacity of the intestine remnant.
2. Minimize symptoms of malabsorption.
3. Eliminate the need for parenteral nutrition.

B. Rehabilitation Strategies

1. Intravenous nutrition:
   a. Nutritional requirements are maintained through total parental nutrition (TPN) via central venous lines (CVLs).
      i. Macronutrients, micronutrients, and/or fluid requirements are provided through daily infusions.
      ii. Patients with intestinal failure require 30% to 70% more calories to compensate for malabsorption.[9]
      iii. Patients require long-term venous access.
      iv. Patients are at great risk for developing life-threatening complications:
         - Hepatotoxicity
         - Sepsis
         - Loss of venous access
   b. Interventions to improve or preserve liver function in patients who are TPN dependent[10]:
      i. Decrease the dextrose and lipid load of the TPN solution when possible.
      ii. TPN cycling with enteral feedings may be helpful to preserve liver function in patients who will tolerate at least minimal enteral feedings.
      iii. Patients with normal intestinal motility of their existing gut should receive enteral nutrition to avoid intestinal stasis. Enteral nutrition is the most important intervention for preventing and treating TPN-induced cholestasis.[10]
      iv. Omega-3 lipid formulation (Omegaven):
         - Short-chain fish oil–based lipid emulsion may be helpful in preserving liver function.
         - Although sample sizes are small, some studies report cholestasis to be reversed and that progressive liver disease is halted, while others suggest that although serum bilirubin levels are significantly reduced, the degree of hepatic fibrosis is not affected.[11-14]
      v. Ursodiol may be helpful in facilitating bile secretion in patients with cholestasis.
2. Enterocyte growth factors used with nutritional support to promote intestinal adaptation:
   a. Recombinant growth hormone (rGH):
      i. The use of rGH with glutamine and an optimal diet has been shown to significantly reduce the volume, calories, and frequency of parenteral nutrition in adults.[15]
      ii. Reported to increase absorption with improved uptake of carbohydrates, protein, sodium, and water; decreases stool output.
      iii. The experience of rGH use in pediatrics is limited.
   b. Teduglutide:
      i. Approved in the United States and Europe as a treatment for adults with short-bowel syndrome–associated intestinal failure.[16]

      ii. May promote mucosal growth, reduce gastric emptying and secretion, decrease fecal losses, and increase absorption.

      iii. Has been shown to increase citrulline levels, a biomarker for mucosal mass.

      iv. Reduces the number of days and volume of parenteral nutrition required in adult patients with intestinal failure.

      v. Optimal results depend on the length of remaining intestine, the presence of the colon, and less volume of TPN.[8]

      vi. Approval for use in pediatrics is pending.

3. Surgical interventions:

  a. Autologous reconstruction:

    i. Potential intervention for patients with a disconnected GI tract and multiple enterocutaneous fistulae.[17]

    ii. Intestinal segments exhibiting normal motility should be reconnected, closing all stomas, whenever possible.

    iii. When reanastomosed, dysmotile segments increase the risk of bacterial translocation due to intestinal stasis.[10]

  b. Bowel lengthening techniques:

    i. Bianchi procedure: Longitudinal Intestinal Lengthening and Tailoring (LILT)[18]:

      • A type of longitudinal lengthening procedure that has been most successful in patients who have had a period of normal adaptation following intestinal resection.

      • The bowel is divided along the longitudinal axis into two tubes with independent blood supply. Bowel division is possible because the mesenteric vasculature bifurcates to provide the blood supply for half of the bowel circumference. The two tubes are then connected to form a segment that is nearly double the length and half the circumference of the preoperative intestine.

      • Good outcomes and survival are associated with bowel length, liver function, and the ability to wean from parenteral nutrition.[19]

    ii. Serial transverse enteroplasty procedure (STEP):

      • Performed in patients with dilated bowel loops.

      • Near-doubles the length of the intestine through serial transverse stapling from opposite directions that creates a zigzag appearance.

      • The International STEP Data Registry reports that 47% of patients attained full enteral nutritional support. Results were less favorable for patients with a higher direct bilirubin and shorter bowel length.[20]

4. Medical issues and interventions:

  a. Bacterial overgrowth:

    i. Characterized by an increased number and/or abnormal type of bacteria in the small intestine.

    ii. Intestinal stasis provides the opportunity for bacteria to proliferate.

    iii. Value suggested is a finding of $\geq 1 \times 10^3$ colony-forming units (cfu) per milliliter of proximal jejunal aspiration.[21]

    iv. Most common causes: gastric achlorhydria due to long-term use of proton pump inhibitors, anatomic abnormalities of the small intestine with intestinal stasis, motility disorders, and gastrocolic or coloenteric fistula.[21]

    v. Symptoms: bloating, flatulence, abdominal pain, diarrhea, weight loss, and steatorrhea. May lead to systemic infection and sepsis syndrome.[22]

vi. Diagnosis[21]:
- Quantitative culture of jejunal aspirate (suggested $\geq 1 \times 10^3$ cfu/mL).
- Hydrogen breath test (older children and adults).
- Stool studies to confirm steatorrhea.
- Lab tests: B_{12} deficiency, anemia, low serum prealbumin, elevated serum folate, and vitamin K levels.
- Barium studies and CT enterography are used to identify mechanical causes.

vii. Treatment:
- Goals: treat the underlying condition, eliminate bacterial overgrowth, and address nutritional deficiencies.
- No consensus in regard to antibiotic regimen. Options include trimethoprim/sulfamethoxazole, rifaximin, ciprofloxacin, metronidazole, gentamicin, neomycin, and/or colistimethate.[21,22]
- Antibiotics are given continuously or for a short intermittent course, such as every other week or 2 weeks on/2 weeks off.[22]

b. Central venous line (CVL) infections[23]:
i. Patients are at risk for developing systemic infections leading to hemodynamic instability and death.
ii. Goals: eradicate the organism(s) and preserve the CVL.
iii. Symptoms: fever, reduced enteral tolerance, and irritability (infants).
iv. Diagnosis: blood cultures.
v. Treatment:
- Based on patient's history
- Start with broad-spectrum coverage until organisms with sensitivities are confirmed, and then modify antimicrobial therapy.
- Remove the CVL if
  - The organism continues to be cultured positive despite antimicrobial therapy.
  - The CVL is cultured with *S. aureus* or yeast.
  - The patient becomes hemodynamically unstable.

c. Lock therapy:
i. Antimicrobial lock therapy (ALT):
- Strategy to preserve catheters and decrease the incidence of infection
- Used when there are >2 days of persistently positive cultures in the setting of appropriate antimicrobial therapy[22]
- Catheter salvage reported to be increased with the use of antimicrobial lock therapy[24]
- Procedure[25]:
  - An antibiotic solution is instilled into the hub of the CVL when it is not in use to achieve a concentration of antibiotic that is greater than the minimal inhibitory concentration (MIC) for the cultured organism.
  - The antibiotic dwells in the catheter for a minimum of 8 to 12 hours and then is removed.
  - The lock is instilled daily for a minimum of 1 to 4 weeks based on the organism and antimicrobial agent.

ii. Ethanol lock therapy:
- Used in combination with antimicrobial lock therapy and after antimicrobial treatment to reduce the incidence of line infections

- Ethanol[26]:
  - ◦ Antimicrobial and fibrinolytic agent
  - ◦ Reported to be effective in preventing and treating CVL infections
  - ◦ Also an anticoagulant and can maintain line patency
- Procedure[24]:
  - ◦ Hospital guidelines vary, but usually, 0.8 to 3 mL (based on catheter size) of 74% ethanol is instilled for a minimum of 2 hours from three times weekly to daily.
  - ◦ Following the required dwell time, the ethanol is withdrawn and discarded and the line is flushed with saline.
  - ◦ Compromised line integrity in polyurethane catheters from exposure to ethanol has been reported.

5. Outcomes of intestinal failure patients:
   a. Rehabilitation through medical and surgical interventions based on the patient's age, bowel length, absorptive capacity, and transit time.
   b. If nutritional autonomy cannot be achieved, intestinal transplantation should be considered as a treatment for intestinal failure.

IV. PRETRANSPLANT CARE AND ASSESSMENT

A. Objective Measures of Intestinal Failure
   1. Vital signs: temperature:
      a. Monitor routinely as indicated and more frequently with complaints of illness and malaise.
      b. Fever is usually a symptom of infection, which requires immediate attention.
      c. Increased risk for sepsis:
         i. Central venous lines
         ii. Intestinal stasis due to impaired motility of the residual intestine, which contributes to bacterial overgrowth and translocation
   2. Vital signs: blood pressure/heart rate:
      a. Hypotension and tachycardia may indicate
         i. Dehydration
         ii. Sepsis
         iii. Bleeding in patients with impaired synthetic function from hepatic dysfunction
      b. Hypertension may occur with impaired renal function secondary to prolonged and frequent administration of aminoglycosides and antifungals in patients with recurrent sepsis.
   3. Laboratory tests (Table 13-2):
      a. Assessment through laboratory tests varies in patients with intestinal failure based on
         i. Disease etiology
         ii. Effect on other organ systems
         iii. Organ deterioration
         iv. Infection history
         v. Amount, type, and macro-/micronutrient content of parenteral nutrition
      b. Lab tests are obtained weekly or every other week to monitor abnormalities and to make appropriate adjustments in contents of TPN solution and volume.

(*text continues on page 556*)

TABLE 13-2 **Electrolyte Imbalances in Intestinal Failure and Postintestinal Transplantation**

Electrolyte	Alteration	Cause	Symptoms	Treatment
Sodium	Hypernatremia Na >150 mEq/L	• Water loss secondary to diarrhea and vomiting • Increased evaporative water loss: fever • Excess sodium intake: increased oral or IV source	Nonspecific: thirst, irritability, lethargy, increased deep tendon reflexes, seizures	• Reduce serum sodium slowly through administration of appropriate IV fluids and volumes.
	Hyponatremia Na <130 mEq/L	• Edema-associated states: hepatic failure leading to third spacing of fluid • Hyperglycemia • GI losses: vomiting, ostomy losses, tube drainage, diarrhea • Diuresis; thiazides and loop diuretics	Nonspecific: headache, lethargy, nausea weakness, encephalopathy, seizures	Dependent on cause • Restore intravascular volume. • Edematous state (low albumin)—do not restrict water intake but restrict NA intake. • Hyperglycemia: resolve hyperglycemia.
Potassium	Hyperkalemia K+ >5.5 mEq/L	• Metabolic acidosis • Increased K+ intake: supplements, blood transfusions • Decreased renal excretion: K+ sparing diuretics, calcineurin immunosuppression • Increased tacrolimus levels post transplant	Cardiac arrhythmias (V fib and asystole) Muscle weakness, decreased tendon reflexes, ileus, anorexia, tingling of mouth and extremities, malaise, tetany	Dependant on cause and severity. May include administration of: • Kayexalate • Lasix • Sodium Bicarbonate • Insulin • Salbutamol • Dialysis • Calcium gluconate • Administer K+ supplementation (oral/IV).
	Hypokalemia K+ <3.5 mEq/L	• Increased GI losses: vomiting, diarrhea, ostomies, tube drainage • Increased renal losses: drug-related aminoglycoside toxicity	Cardiac arrhythmias (bradycardia, V tac, AV block, premature atrial and ventricular beats), fibrillation, muscle paralysis, ileus, tetany, confusion, hypotension, polyuria, polydipsia	

(continued)

TABLE 13-2 Electrolyte Imbalances in Intestinal Failure and Postintestinal Transplantation (*Continued*)

Electrolyte	Alteration	Cause	Symptoms	Treatment
Magnesium	Hypermagnesemia Mg >2.5 mEq/L	• Excess magnesium intake (i.e., oral prep, via TPN) • Decreased renal excretion; assess GFR	Decreased deep tendon reflexes; weakness, confusion, lethargy, and hypotension with levels >7 mEq/L, bradycardia	• Remove excess source. • Administer calcium. • Dialysis.
	Hypomagnesemia Mg <1.5 mEq/L	• GI losses: diarrhea, prolonged NG drainage • Malnutrition: ↓ calories, ↓ protein • Fat malabsorption • Increased renal losses: renal tubular acidosis, diuretic therapy, drugs (aminoglycosides, amphotericin, calcineurin inhibitors) • Pancreatitis • Refeeding	Weakness, tremors, anorexia, seizures, cardiovascular manifestations (widening QRS complex, prolonged PR interval, ventricular arrhythmias), increased susceptibility to digitalis toxicity	• Administer magnesium supplement (IV/PO).
Phosphate	Hypophosphatemia (varies by age)	• Decreased intestinal absorption (diarrhea, vitamin D deficiency, antacid abuse, fat malabsorption) • Internal redistribution (recovery from malnutrition, sepsis, rickets) • Decreased phosphate intake • Hyperventilation	Muscle weakness, bone pain, arthralgias, hemolytic anemia, anorexia, nausea, vomiting, confusion, rhabdomyolysis	• Low phosphate associated with hypercalcemia; treating high calcium often resolves low phosphate • Administer phosphate once calcium and renal function assessed.
	Hyperphosphatemia (varies by age)	• Increased external load (IV/oral) • Increased endogenous load (bowel infarction) • Reduced renal excretion (Mg deficiency, bisphosphonate therapy) • Hypocalcemia	With associated hypocalcemia, tetany can occur. Ectopic calcification in vessels and wall tissues	• Restrict phosphate intake. • Administer phosphate binding salts (aluminum, calcium, magnesium). • Saline diuresis if normal renal function
Calcium	Hypocalcemia (varies by age)	• Low albumin • High phosphate • Low magnesium • Vitamin D–deficient rickets • Pancreatitis	Muscle weakness, numbness, and tingling in extremities, cramps, hyperreflexes, tetany, seizures, prolonged QT interval	• Correct other electrolyte imbalances. • Administer calcium (IV/oral). • Vitamin D therapy

	Assessment	Causes	Signs & Symptoms	Treatment
Hypercalcemia		• Excess vitamin D administration • Thiazide drug therapy	Renal etiology: polyuria, polydipsia, nephrocalcinosis, renal insufficiency Nonrenal etiology: fatigue, weakness, nausea, vomiting, constipation, symptoms of pancreatitis, headache, pruritus, bone pain, hypotonia, hypertension, arrhythmias, short QT interval, heart block	• Correct dehydration. • Saline diuresis • Loop diuretics • Steroids • Calcitonin • Bisphosphonates
Metabolic Acidosis	Assessed on blood gas • Low pH • Reduced HCO_3	• GI losses: diarrhea, intestinal fluid loss from ileostomy, NG drainage • Excess acid via TPN • Renal losses: drugs (spironolactone, amphotericin)	Vomiting, nausea, diarrhea, hyperventilation, headache, lethargy	• Treat underlying cause. • Bicarbonate • Correct fluid balance.
Metabolic alkalosis	Assessed on blood gas • High pH • Elevated HCO_3	• GI losses: vomiting, NG drainage, chloride losing diarrhea • Renal losses: diuretics, penicillins • Low chloride intake • Refeeding syndrome • Hypocalcemia • Hypokalemia • Massive blood transfusions (excessive citrate)	Related to underlying cause. Refer to hypokalemia. Refer to hypocalcemia. If volume depleted: thirst, lethargy, muscle cramps, irritability	• Treat underlying cause. • Correct K+ deficit. • Correct calcium deficit. • Correct chloride deficit. • Correct fluid imbalances.

    c. Lab tests commonly obtained include
- i. Electrolyte panel (calcium, magnesium, phosphorus, sodium, potassium, carbon dioxide, chloride)
- ii. Renal function tests (blood urea nitrogen, creatinine)
- iii. Cholesterol and triglycerides
- iv. Nutritional status: micronutrient deficiencies are common in intestinal failure. Albumin, protein, trace elements, zinc, copper, selenium, iron, and vitamins A, D, E, K, and B_{12} are monitored routinely.[27]
- v. Absorption: D-xylose testing and fecal fat testing

    d. Assess electrolyte imbalances:
- i. Patients are at risk for increased fluid losses with electrolyte imbalances due to
  - Development of a hypersecretory state, bacterial overgrowth, infection, and/or intrinsic deficits
  - Interruptions in ability to provide optimal TPN because of venous access problems

    e. Monitor liver function:
- i. Monitored by liver function tests (ALT, AST, GGTP, and bilirubin)
- ii. Markers for synthetic function (PT/PTT and INR), platelets, and hemoglobin
- iii. Ammonia level (NH_3)

    f. Monitor for infection:
- i. Infection should be considered with an increase in the white blood cell count, sedimentation rate (ESR), and platelet count.
- ii. If infection is suspected, blood cultures should be obtained to identify the specific organism causing infection.
- iii. Stool, sputum, and/or urine cultures are obtained as indicated.

4. Radiology tests:

    a. Completed during the evaluation for intestine transplantation or as complications arise related to disease etiology

    b. Upper GI with small-bowel follow-through[28]:
- i. Used to assess the residual native bowel and any abnormalities:
  - Test completed with water-soluble contrast or barium
  - Observe for dilated loops of bowel, strictures, or narrowing of the bowel
  - Provides an estimate of bowel length and transit time
- ii. Structural etiologies[28]:
  - Assess for short-bowel length:
    - Adults: <200 cm[10]
    - Pediatrics: <25% of the predicted length for age at primary surgery[29]
- iii. Functional etiologies[28]:
  - Normal or near-normal length
  - Distended bowel loops may be present
  - Hyper- or hypomotility of native intestine:
    - Motility testing performed in patients with Hirschsprung's disease or chronic intestinal pseudo-obstruction to assess transit time
  - Gastric emptying scan to assess gastric function

    c. Barium enema:
- i. Used to assess anatomy and function of the remaining colon

    d. Vascular patency[28,30]:
       i. Ultrasound of great vessels to assess patency of internal jugular, subclavian, and iliac veins.
      ii. Important to identify any occlusions of common central venous access sites because access may be required for prolonged parenteral nutrition in intestinal failure or for up to a year or more posttransplant.
     iii. Angiography may be indicated in some cases.
     iv. An MRI is used to confirm any reported occlusions of the primary vasculature.
    e. Abdominal ultrasound[28,30]:
       i. Used to visualize and identify vascular anatomy, preexisting conditions, and any variants that may affect the surgical approach.
      ii. Is not specific or exact enough to replace cross-sectional imaging in intestinal failure patients, but may provide additional information for a patient in no immediate danger.
     iii. Minimizes radiation exposure from CT angiography.
     iv. The aorta, bilateral common iliac arteries and veins, and IVC are assessed:
        • IVC thrombosis or stenosis may preclude intestine transplant depending on the location of the variant.
        • The portal venous system, IVC, and liver inflow and outflow are assessed in liver/intestine transplant candidates.
      v. CT angiography is completed if the ultrasound cannot adequately visualize vessels.
     vi. CT also used to assess for hepatomegaly, splenomegaly, and/or ascites.
    f. Liver biopsy:
       i. Performed in patients with deteriorating liver function to determine the extent and severity of liver disease.
      ii. Evidence of bridging fibrosis or cirrhosis is an indication for concomitant liver transplantation.
     iii. The extent of liver disease, rate of progression, and estimated waiting time to transplant are also considered in listing for liver transplant.
    g. Cardiac assessment:
       i. Completed to rule out cardiac anomalies and contraindications for surgery.
      ii. Tests:
        • Electrocardiogram (ECG)
        • Echocardiogram (ECHO)
        • Chest radiograph (CXR):
          ○ Used to assess for respiratory complications, particularly in candidates with cystic fibrosis or in premature infants with history of bronchopulmonary dysplasia
5. Physical assessment:
    a. Widely variable from relatively healthy to critically ill:
       i. Will vary by age, indication for transplant, severity, and duration of intestinal failure and associated complications
      ii. Observe for the general state of health or distress, skin color, height/weight, mobility, energy, and mood
    b. Skin:
       i. Jaundice and bruising are present in patients with concomitant liver disease.

    ii.   Skin irritation, lesions, and breakdown secondary to pruritus, particularly in pediatric patients.

    iii.   Decreased skin turgor or edema due to nutritional deficits and fluid imbalances.

    iv.   Dry, scaling skin that lacks elasticity.

    v.   Poor nail growth or thin nails.

    vi.   Thinning, dull hair.

    vii.   Potential for ulcers, rash, and skin breakdown around catheter sites, drainage or feeding tube sites, stomas, mucous fistulas, ostomies, and around the buttocks/diaper area.

    viii.   Assess scarring from previous surgeries for any breaks in skin integrity or keloid formations.

    ix.   Skin mottling may be a sign of sepsis.

c. HEENT:

    i.   Abnormalities occur based on the indication for intestinal failure and complications.

    ii.   Icteric sclerae are usually present in concomitant liver disease.

    iii.   Patients who have received repeated courses of parenteral aminoglycosides should be assessed for hearing deficits.[31]

        • Aminoglycosides are associated with ototoxicity.

        • Deficit is related to the duration of treatment and amount of drug administered.

        • Infants are particularly at risk and often have high-range hearing deficits.

    iv.   Cervical lymphadenopathy may be associated with infection.

    v.   Dentition is affected by nutritional status.

        • Assess for the presence\absence of teeth, staining, obvious caries, gingivitis, and gum integrity.

        ○ Tooth eruption may be delayed in nutritionally impaired infants.

    vi.   Dehydration is assessed through skin turgor, decreased or absent tearing, sunken eyes, dry oral mucosa, and cracked lips.

    vii.   Atrophic glossitis:

        • Smooth glossy appearance of the tongue with a red or pink background

        • May indicate a nutritional deficiency (iron, folic acid, B_{12}, riboflavin, niacin)[32]

d. Cardiac:

    i.   There are no specific cardiac abnormalities directly related to intestinal failure; however, cardiac-related symptoms can occur as a result of complications related to intestinal failure.

    ii.   Baseline cardiac assessment is completed to determine any cardiac illness or anomaly that may be a contraindication to the surgical procedure.

    iii.   Signs and symptoms of compromised cardiac function may include

        • Tachycardia due to blood loss and/or volume depletion.

        • Arrhythmias secondary to electrolyte imbalances.

        • Murmurs from anemia or fluid imbalance.

        • Hypotension may be associated with bleeding, volume depletion, and sepsis.

e. Respiratory:
   i.   Abnormalities are secondary to comorbidities or secondary diagnoses.
   ii. Tachypnea may be associated with metabolic acidosis, hypoglycemia, fever, and/or anxiety.
   iii. Rales and tachypnea may be present with fluid overload related to hypoalbuminemia.
   iv. Decreased breath sounds may be due to atelectasis, effusions, and/or pneumonias.
f. Gastrointestinal:
   i.   GI assessment determines the extent and function of the existing intestine and any associated abdominal anomalies.
   ii. Abdominal assessment:
        - Observation:
          ○ Surgical scars
          ○ Enteral tubes: gastrostomy tube, jejunostomy tube, and gastrojejunostomy tube
          ○ Fistulas
          ○ Ostomies
          ○ Abdominal protuberance suggests ascites and/or organomegaly
          ○ Distended abdominal veins and telangiectasis (spider angioma) are indicative of liver disease with vascular obstruction
          ○ Herniations
        - Auscultation:
          ○ Hyperactive bowel sounds may be indicative of diarrhea or an early obstruction.
          ○ Hypoactivity, followed by absent bowel sounds, may indicate an ileus and/or peritonitis.
        - Palpation:
          ○ Hepatomegaly in patients with TPN-induced liver disease can be evaluated by palpating in the right upper quadrant and assessing the size of liver below the costal margin.
          ○ With splenomegaly, the spleen may be palpated well below the costal margin due to portal hypertension; tenderness may be present.
          ○ Epigastric and rebound tenderness are associated with pancreatitis.
          ○ Generalized discomfort may indicate peritonitis.
g. Musculoskeletal assessment:
   i.   Fractures:
        - Increased risk due to malabsorption of fat-soluble vitamins (A, D, E, and K).
        - Malabsorption of vitamin D may cause rickets and lead to fractures.
   ii. Joint abnormalities:
        - Assess for swollen, painful, and reddened joints.
        - May indicate arthritis-associated liver disease.
   iii. Muscle atrophy:
        - Decreased muscle tone, decreased muscle mass, and muscle atrophy may develop due to malabsorption and poor nutrition.
        - Disuse atrophy occurs from inactivity related to chronic illness and compromised mobility.

h. Neurologic and mental status:
   i. Neurologic changes are associated with hyperammonemia in patients with liver disease.
   ii. Symptoms may include altered sleep patterns (day-night reversal), extreme lethargy, behavioral changes, confusion, obtundation, ataxia, asterixis, and clonus.
i. Growth and development:
   i. Infants and young children with intestinal failure usually display some degree of growth failure.
   ii. Growth failure is associated with a small-bowel length of <50 cm and is due to inadequate absorption of nutrients.[33]
   iii. Height and weight curves are often less than the 25th percentile; growth along the curve is not commonly achieved with early-onset disease.[33]
   iv. Growth and development is closer to the norm in children or adolescents with a later onset of short gut, such as a spontaneous volvulus or trauma, or with diseases having a slower, chronic impact, such as Crohn's disease or pseudo-obstruction.
   v. Developmental milestones may not be achieved due to frequent illnesses, poor nutrition, decreased muscle mass and strength, repeated hospitalizations with impaired socialization, and isolation from the family environment.
   vi. Oral aversion is common in children who have been limited in their oral intake or who have had frequent extended periods of nothing by mouth.

V. PRETRANSPLANT CARE

A. Subjective Complaints of Intestinal Transplant Candidates
   1. Subjective complaints are variable, depending on patient age and duration of illness, the severity of intestinal failure, nutritional status and associated complications.
   2. Common subjective complaints related to intestinal failure include
      a. Weight loss
      b. Poor growth (pediatrics)
      c. Intractable diarrhea
      d. Dry, scaling skin
      e. Skin breakdown
      f. Thinning hair
      g. Abdominal distention
      h. Flatus
      i. Malaise
      j. Lethargy
      k. Weakness
      l. Abdominal pain
      m. Complaints related to mental status and mood changes
   3. Additional complaints of patients with concomitant liver disease:
      a. Bruising
      b. Extreme tiredness
      c. Confusion and mood changes
      d. Abdominal distention
      e. Bleeding

      f. Abdominal pain

      g. Pruritus

      h. Acholic stools

  4. Emotional issues:

      a. Time-consuming care routine

      b. Limitations in activity

      c. Frequent hospitalizations

      d. Inability to work/attend school

      e. Social isolation

      f. Impaired family support

      g. Financial stressors

      h. Sleep disturbances

      i. Fear of dying before an organ is available

      j. Mental health or mood disorders, particularly anxiety and depression

VI. PREPARING THE PRETRANSPLANT PATIENT FOR SURGERY

A. Pretransplant Period

  1. Transplant evaluation (Table 13-3):

      a. Protocols vary by center, adult versus pediatric candidates, and etiology of intestinal failure.

      b. Essential to complete a comprehensive medical and psychosocial assessment of the intestine transplant candidate with intestinal failure and associated comorbidities[30]:

         i. The evaluation is completed through a 3 to 5 day inpatient admission or as an outpatient over several days.

        ii. Focus of the evaluation:

            • Anatomy of the GI tract

            • Nutritional status

            • Liver function

            • Venous access and patency

            • Infection history

            • Cardiovascular system

        iii. History:

            • Birth history (pediatrics or as applicable for congenital defects)

            • Etiology of intestinal failure

            • Surgical history

            • Intestinal anatomy:

                ○ Remaining length of small intestine and colon

                ○ Presence of ileocecal valve

                ○ Continuity status

                ○ Stomas and fistulas

            • Appliances: feeding tubes, ostomies, drainage tubes, and intravenous lines

            • Stool consistency and pattern, emesis, nausea, and abdominal distention

            • Central venous lines: number of lines, access, and infections

            • Infection history and response to antimicrobial treatment

            • Nutritional history and current status: enteral and parental feeding history, oral aversion, and incidence of hypoglycemia when off TPN

TABLE 13-3 Evaluation for Intestinal Transplantation

Assessment	Testing/Procedures
Routine assessment	Complete history and physical CXR ABO compatibility
Gastrointestinal assessment	Upper and lower barium studies to assess bowel length, anatomy, and abnormalities Motility testing and gastric emptying as indicated for functional indications D-xylose testing and fecal fat testing to assess absorption
Nutritional assessment	Laboratory testing: electrolytes, blood urea nitrogen, creatinine, calcium, magnesium, phosphorus, zinc, trace elements, cholesterol, triglycerides, vitamin levels (A, D, E, K, B$_{12}$) Feeding history to assess tolerance, absorption, weight gain, growth (children) Caloric intake: enteral and parenteral Growth parameters: height, weight, skin folds, head circumference (infants) Assess for oral aversion, abnormal eating behaviors, pica
Hepatic function	Liver function tests including ALT, AST, GGT, direct and indirect bilirubin, albumin, prothrombin time, partial thromboplastin time, alpha-fetoprotein, platelets, ammonia, and factors V and VII Physical exam to assess for hepatomegaly, splenomegaly, ascites, caput medusae Liver ultrasound to further assess liver size, vasculature, and any evidence of portal hypertension Liver biopsy if indicated to establish baseline hepatic injury
Vascular patency	Catheter history with number of line placements, location, duration, and reason for replacement Ultrasound of the great vessels to assess vascular access and to evaluate the splanchnic venous anatomy and internal jugular, subclavian, and iliac veins Angiography if indicated MRI to confirm any reported occlusions of the primary vasculature
Infection history and immunology assessment	History of infections to assess etiology and frequency of infection, pathogens, response to treatment, resistant organisms Screening cultures of blood, urine, stool, throat, or ascitic fluid for bacterial, fungal, or viral organisms as indicated Complete blood count and differential Tissue typing and crossmatch Screening for hepatitis B and C and HIV IgG and IgM titers for CMV, EBV, herpes zoster, and MMR Quantitative immunoglobulins in patients with intestinal atresia
Cardiac assessment	EKG, ECHO Rule out cardiac anomalies and contraindications for surgery.
Respiratory assessment	CXR Obtain pulmonology consult for patients with a history of BPD, cystic fibrosis, or other respiratory complications.
Neurologic assessment	Obtain neurology consult in patients with seizure disorders or neurologic impairments.
Development and physical functioning	Further evaluation as indicated for developmental delays, impairments in physical functioning, oral aversion, behavioral issues Consults may include physical therapy, speech therapy, occupational therapy, and neurodevelopment. Child life, child development in pediatrics

TABLE 13-3 Evaluation for Intestinal Transplantation (*Continued*)

Assessment	Testing/Procedures
Psychological evaluation	To assess patient (age-appropriate) and parent/family's psychological status and history for psychopathology, coping skills, responses to stress, family support
	Assess for alcohol or substance abuse in adults, adolescent patients, and parents.
	Adherence history
	Referrals for psychotherapy, counseling
Social work evaluation	Assess patient and family psychosocial functioning.
	Provide psychosocial care and support during the evaluation and in preparation for transplant.
	Guide families in referrals for financial assistance programs and supportive services.
	Assist in referrals to volunteer pilot associations if needed for transport to the transplant center when organs are available.
	Assist family in preparing for temporary relocation needs to the transplant center.
Clinical nurse specialist	Addresses the educational needs of the patient and family pre- and posttransplant
	Provides clinical information and psychosocial support throughout the transplant process
	Consultation to assess developmental needs, patient or family psychosocial functioning, adherence
Transplant coordinator	Maintains outpatient communication with candidate and referring physician following evaluation
	Lists patient according to UNOS requirements
	Provides information to the patient and family about the transplant process
	Maintains updated medical information on the candidate to the team during the waiting period
	Follows patient post transplant to facilitate medical management and follow-up; with physician, assesses for problems or complications through lab testing and procedures; communicates medication changes and assesses for medication adherence
Financial counselor	Works with the family and insurer to obtain insurance coverage for transplantation
	Provides guidance in fund raising for personal expenses related to relocation

Adapted from Kosmach-Park B. Intestinal transplantation in pediatric patients. *Prog in Transplant.* 2002;12(2):97–113.

iv. Physical examination.
v. Patient-specific consultations:
- Based on associated medical issues and pediatric versus adult evaluation.
- Consultations may include, but are not limited to, anesthesia, neurology, immunology, pulmonology, genetics, nephrology, endocrine, infectious disease, physical, and occupational therapy.
vi. Psychosocial evaluation:
- Completed by social work, psychology/psychiatry, and child development (pediatrics).
- Assessment includes the patient's psychological status, history of psychopathology and medications, coping skills, responses to stress, family support, drug and alcohol use, adherence history, and pain history and treatment.
vii. Transplant education (Table 13-4):
- Patient and family education is an essential component of the evaluation.

TABLE 13-4 Educational Topics Pretransplant

Basic anatomy and physiology of the intestine
- Indication for intestinal failure
- Intestinal rehabilitation
- Intestinal transplant

Listing for intestine transplant
- Listing status
- United Network for Organ Sharing (US) or other organ procurement organization

Waiting period
- Patient responsibilities
- Anxiety, stress, and coping mechanisms
- Staying healthy
- Communicating with your transplant coordinator and the transplant center

Surgical procedure
- Type of intestinal transplant
- Duration of surgery

What to expect in the intensive care unit
- Unit routine
- Length of stay
- Appliances and drains
- Procedures
- Goals for transfer to the transplant unit

Pain
- Current pain status
- Pain control
- Postoperative pain
- Treatment

Surgical complications

Immune system basics

Rejection
- Incidence
- Symptoms
- Diagnosis
- Treatment
- Outcome
- Retransplantation

Infection
- Incidence
- Most common infections
- Symptoms
- Diagnosis
- Treatment
- Outcomes

TABLE 13-4 Educational Topics Pretransplant (*Continued*)

Medications (most commonly prescribed)
- Immunosuppressants
- Anti-infective agents
- Antimotility medications
- Electrolyte supplements
- Antacids

Posttransplant Care
- Follow-up care/appointments
- Labs
- Developmental issues (pediatrics): OT/PT, oral aversion, developmental delay, early intervention
- Returning to work/school
- Reproductive health
- Activity and exercise
- Nutrition
- Family support
- Psychosocial stressors

Long-Term Outcomes
- Patient and graft survival
- Psychosocial functioning
- Quality of life

- Each member of the multidisciplinary team is responsible for presenting appropriate information about their respective area of focus; additionally, a comprehensive education session is usually provided by a transplant coordinator, clinical nurse specialist, or nurse practitioner during the evaluation period.

2. Nursing interventions:
    a. Provide patients and families with a schedule for the evaluation with a list of appointments, tests, and consultations.
    b. Provide education regarding test procedures and examinations through written and/or electronic media.
    c. Support the patient and family throughout the evaluation by answering questions to clarify and reinforce information and by reviewing results presented by the transplant team and other consultants.
    d. Facilitate discussions with the respective transplant team members for specific information and results.
        i. A core group from the team may be responsible for providing an overview of the results, the immediate plan for listing and medical management, long-term management, and reinforcement of teaching.
        ii. The core group usually includes the transplant surgeon(s), GI physician, pretransplant coordinator, advanced practice nurse (CNS or CRNP), physician assistants, psychologist, and/or social worker.

3. Listing for intestine transplant:
    a. Multidisciplinary meeting to review outcome of the evaluation.
    b. A patient is accepted or rejected as a candidate for intestine transplantation based on the results of a comprehensive medical and psychosocial

        evaluation as well as the patient's risk of developing life-threatening complications with a high risk for death without transplantation.

    c. Current listing criteria[34]:

       i. Advanced cirrhosis

      ii. Loss of ≥2 central venous catheter sites related to thrombosis

      iii. ≥2 episodes of sepsis annually, especially fungal sepsis

      iv. High risk of death secondary to the underlying disease

    d. If accepted for transplantation, financial clearance must be obtained through the patient's medical insurance plan.

    e. After financial clearance is obtained, the patient is listed for intestine, intestine/liver, or multivisceral transplant through the United Network of Organ Sharing (UNOS).

    f. Each organ is listed separately and by status:

       i. Liver allocation: based on the candidate's score as calculated by the Model for End-Stage Liver Disease (MELD) and the Pediatric End-Stage Liver Disease (PELD) as for isolated liver transplantation

      ii. Intestine candidates:

         • Status I: deteriorating liver function and decreased/limited venous access

         • Status II: normal liver function and adequate venous access

    g. Waiting time may range from several months to years based on the candidate's UNOS status/score, organ(s) required, patient weight, blood type, severity of illness, current medical status, and accrued waiting time.

    h. Patients must have a plan for transportation to arrive at the transplant center within the appropriate time frame, usually within 6 hours of being contacted by the transplant coordinator.

4. The waiting period:

    a. Medical management is usually maintained by the referring local physician.

    b. The patient will return to the transplant center as requested for medical follow-up, consultations, and/or education or if there is deterioration in their condition.

    c. This is an extremely stressful time for the patient and family as the patient's health status deteriorates.

    d. Nursing interventions:

       i. Develop a supportive relationship with the patient and family during repeated hospitalizations.

      ii. Identify the patient's fears and clarify misconceptions:

         • Recognize that the patient has increased fear and anxiety as the waiting period extends.

         • Acknowledge fears: death due to organs not being available, potential surgical and postoperative complications, pain, and prolonged hospitalizations.

      iii. Encourage patients to verbalize concerns to lessen anxiety.

      iv. Facilitate referrals for psychological, psychiatric, and/or spiritual counseling and support.

      v. Be aware of patient and family's cultural needs and religious practices:

         • Acknowledge and discuss cultural considerations regarding coping strategies, family, diet, blood products, and religious practices.

         • Facilitate care conferences to better understand cultural differences and to design appropriate supportive interventions.

TABLE 13-5 **Preoperative Orders**

Maintain NPO status.

Obtain vital signs, height, weight, abdominal girth.

Obtain labs: complete blood count and differential, liver function tests, calcium, magnesium, phosphate, urea, BUN, creatinine, glucose, electrolytes, PT/PTT, INR, protein, albumin.

Type and cross for specified amount of packed red blood cells and fresh frozen plasma.

Obtain viral serologies for cytomegalovirus (CMV), Epstein-Barr virus (EBV).

Chest x-ray

Infuse fluids and/or TPN as ordered.

Administer preoperative broad-spectrum antibiotics.

Administer methylprednisolone.

Administer induction immunosuppression per center protocol.

5. Preparation for surgery
   a. Preoperative orders and protocols are center specific.
      i. Orders vary according to the patient's medical status prior to intestine transplant, organs transplanted, and concurrent complications
   b. Standard preoperative orders (Table 13-5).
   c. Nursing interventions.
      i. Ensure that informed consent has been given and that the consent forms are signed.
      ii. Establish where the family will be waiting during surgery and confirm contact information so they can be available if and when needed throughout the surgical procedure.
      iii. Reinforce previous teaching:
         • Duration of surgery and brief overview of the procedure
         • What to expect when seeing the patient in the intensive care unit
         • Description of the early postoperative period and the most common complications

 VII. INTESTINE TRANSPLANTATION

A. Intestine Transplant Variants

There are several variants of intestinal transplantation. The surgical procedure and organ(s) are based on the indication for intestinal failure, the extent of organ deterioration, anatomic anomalies, and dysfunction of other abdominal organs.
1. Isolated intestine transplant:
   a. Intestinal failure without associated liver disease or other organ involvement
   b. Indications: extreme short gut, motility disorders, malabsorption syndromes, and gastrointestinal neoplasms
2. Combined intestine and liver transplantation:
   a. Performed for patients with irreversible intestinal and hepatic failure
   b. Usually includes the donor pancreas to allow for hepatobiliary continuity
3. Multivisceral transplantation:
   a. Various combinations of intestine, liver, stomach, and/or pancreas
   b. Modified multivisceral without the liver is performed if minimal cholestasis with good liver function

      c. Recommended based on the etiology of intestinal failure and associated organ dysfunction

      d. Indications: massive gastrointestinal polyposis, mesenteric desmoid tumors, chronic intestinal pseudo-obstruction, hollow visceral myopathy, and extensive splanchnic vascular thrombosis

    4. Intestinal transplantation including the colon[35]:

      a. Included as part of the intestinal graft in those patients with loss of colonic segments or dysmotility including necrotizing enterocolitis, chronic intestinal pseudo-obstruction or megacystis microcolon syndrome, volvulus, Hirschsprung's disease, and Gardner's syndrome

      b. May include the donor ileocecal valve

B. Surgical Procedures

    1. Donor selection[36]:

      a. Hemodynamically stable

      b. ABO-compatible, brain-dead donor

      c. BMI ≤25 that matches the recipient

      d. ICU stay ≤5 days with minimal vasopressor requirements

      e. Crossmatch negative

      f. Cold ischemia time of ≤6 hours to prevent irreversible intestinal mucosal injury

    2. Recipient surgery[36]:

      a. Operative time ranges from 6 to 18 hours or more depending on

        i. Type of transplant

        ii. Surgically related risk factors:

          • Abdominal adhesions

          • Loss of abdominal domain due to multiple previous surgeries

        iii. Presence of underlying diseases

        iv. Recipient's current health status

      b. Patients are prepared in the usual fashion, sedated and intubated.

      c. Placement of lines and tubes:

        i. Require several peripheral intravenous lines in addition to the existing central venous line (CVL)

        ii. Arterial line

        iii. Nasogastric drainage tube

        iv. Urinary catheter

      d. Midline abdominal laparotomy incision with unilateral or bilateral transverse extensions as needed.

      e. Isolated intestine transplantation[37-40] (Figures 13-1 and 13-2):

        i. Diseased intestine removed proximally from the ligament of Treitz and distally to the ileocecal valve or ileocolic anastomosis in patients with neoplasms and functional disorders.

        ii. Healthy residual intestine is usually preserved in patients with structural disorders.

        iii. Patient may present with previous enterectomy of native residual intestine related to pretransplant complications.

        iv. Donor intestine, including the jejunum and ileum, is implanted using the appropriate vascular anastomoses.

          • Vascular anastomoses vary based on the patient's anatomy and usable vessels.

        v. Arterial reconstruction: the donor's superior mesenteric artery (SMA) is anastomosed to the recipient's infrarenal aorta using a small aortic patch.

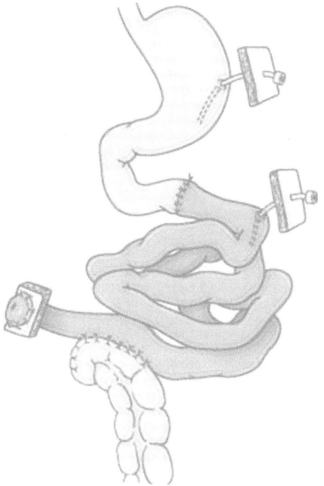

FIGURE 13-1 Isolated intestine transplant. (Adapted from the Department of Transplant Surgery, Children's Hospital of Pittsburgh of the University of Pittsburgh Medical Center.)

vi.   Venous reconstruction: the donor's superior mesenteric vein (SMV) is drained into the recipient's portal vein, recipient SMV or splenic vein, or the recipient IVC.

vii. Intestinal reconstruction:
- The proximal end of the donor jejunum is anastomosed to the most distal segment of the recipient's residual intestine (native jejunum or duodenum).
- The distal end is fashioned as a permanent end ileostomy or joined to the native colon with a short portion brought out as a temporary ileostomy.
  - The ileostomy is used to facilitate frequent surveillance endoscopies in the early postoperative period.
  - The distal anastomosis varies depending on the underlying disease, motility issues, length of remnant colon, and method of ileostomy creation.

viii. Jejunal feeding tubes with or without gastrostomy tubes are inserted.

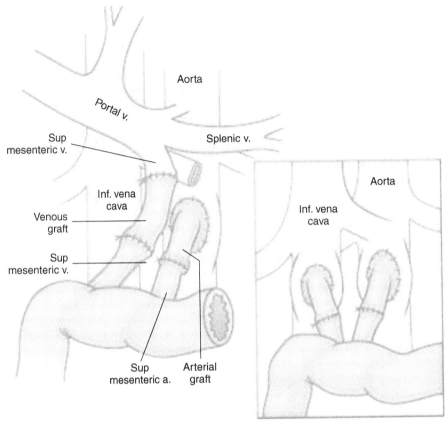

FIGURE 13-2 Vascular implantation of an isolated intestine graft using vascular conduits to the mesenteric vessel or to the aorta and IVC. (Adapted from the Department of Transplant Surgery, Children's Hospital of Pittsburgh of the University of Pittsburgh Medical Center.)

    f. Combined liver and intestine transplant[37-40] (Figure 13-3):

        i. Native liver is removed preserving the native retrohepatic vena cava in the standard piggyback fashion.

        ii. The healthy residual intestine (duodenum with or without a portion of the jejunum), stomach, and native pancreas are usually preserved in patients with structural disorders.

        iii. A duodenal C-loop and pancreas are also included with the combined liver and intestine graft to maintain hepatobiliary continuity so that a Roux-en-Y jejunal allograft loop is not needed to drain the bile duct.

        iv. Venous outflow of the native foregut is achieved through a permanent portocaval shunt. Venous outflow from the entire graft is from the donor suprahepatic cava to the confluence of the recipient hepatic veins and cava.

        v. Arterial inflow to the graft is from the recipient infrarenal aorta.

        vi. Intestinal reconstruction:

           • Similar to isolated intestine transplantation with the proximal anastomosis between the end of the remnant native intestine and the donor jejunum.

           • Distal end is fashioned as a permanent end ileostomy or joined to the native colon with a short portion brought out as a temporary ileostomy.

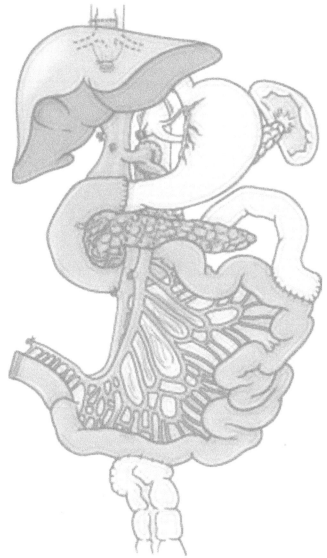

FIGURE 13-3 Combined liver and intestine transplant. (Adapted from the Department of Transplant Surgery, Children's Hospital of Pittsburgh of the University of Pittsburgh Medical Center.)

   g. Multivisceral transplantation[17,37–40] (Figures 13-4 and 13-5):
      i. The entire GI tract is removed including a majority of the stomach.
      ii. Vascular anastomosis is similar to combined liver and intestine transplant:
         • Aortic inflow is from the recipient infrarenal aorta or supraceliac artery.
      iii. The graft stomach is anastomosed proximally to the recipient gastric cuff or abdominal esophagus.
      iv. The distal anastomoses is as described with isolated intestine transplantation.
      v. A modified multivisceral transplant is performed in patients with a healthy liver, excluding the donor liver as part of the multivisceral graft. The native liver, pancreas, and a C-loop of the duodenum are retained.

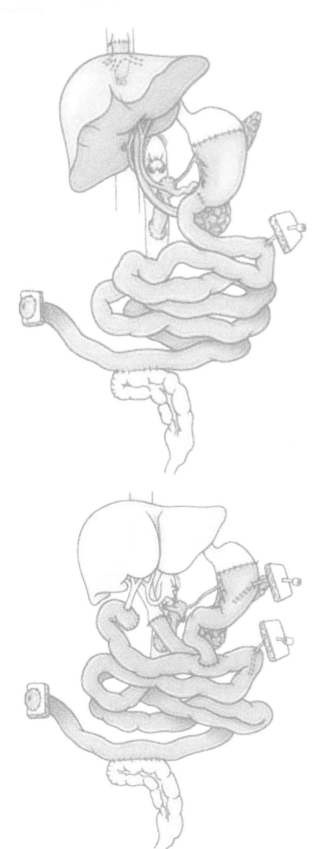

FIGURE 13-4   Complete multivisceral
transplant. (Adapted from the Department
of Transplant Surgery, Children's Hospital
of Pittsburgh of the University of Pittsburgh
Medical Center.)

FIGURE 13-5   Modified multivisceral
transplant. (Adapted from the Department
of Transplant Surgery, Children's Hospital
of Pittsburgh of the University of Pittsburgh
Medical Center.)

Isolated bowel with colon

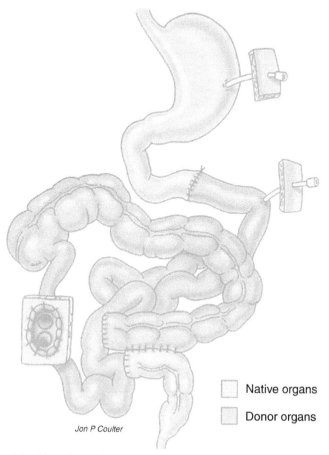

Native organs

Donor organs

Jon P Coulter

FIGURE 13-6 Combined intestine and colon transplant. (Adapted from the Department of Transplant Surgery, Children's Hospital of Pittsburgh of the University of Pittsburgh Medical Center.)

   h. Inclusion of the colon[34,37–40] (Figure 13-6):
      i. The inclusion of the colon was reported to be a potential risk factor for morbidity and mortality in the early era of intestine transplant.[41]
      ii. More recent series report that the inclusion of the ileocecal valve and right hemicolon is safe and is associated with less watery stools, resulting in a decreased incidence of dehydration and fewer hospital readmissions.[5,35,42]
   i. Retransplantation[37]:
      i. Associated with a higher incidence of morbidity and mortality.
      ii. Primary indication for retransplantation is rejection.[17]
      iii. The overall retransplantation rate is 8% as reported by the ITR:
         • Survival of the second or third graft is 56% at 1 year and 35% at 5 years.[5]
         • Mortality is highest in the early postoperative period, but the 5-year survival rate for retransplantation is similar to those alive with a primary graft at 5 years posttransplant.[43]

        iv. Improved outcomes for retransplantation are related to improved immunosuppressive protocols, desensitization protocols, technical modifications, and improved infection surveillance, and treatment.[37,44]

- rATG has been associated with improved patient and graft survival in those patients previously transplanted using steroid induction and maintenance tacrolimus.[45]
- Important to assess donor-specific antibodies, panel reactive antibodies, and crossmatch in patients who are being considered for retransplantation to assess the risk of rejection and to plan the immunosuppressive regimen.[37,44,45]

    j. Living donor intestine transplantation:

        i. Treatment option for intestinal failure, particularly for pediatric patients in a life-threatening situation.

        ii. Experience remains limited; ITR reports that 37 living donor transplants were performed in 2001 to 2011, which is 1.8% of the total transplants performed during that era.[5]

        iii. Advantages that may contribute to fewer postoperative complications[46]:

- Optimal timing
- HLA matching

        iv. Long-term outcomes comparable to transplantation with deceased donors.[47,48]

3. Reperfusion:

    a. Donor organs reperfused following completion of all vascular anastomoses

4. Ileostomy:

    a. Created following completion of intestinal anastomoses and reperfusion:

        i. Variants: end ileostomy, loop ileostomy, or diverting proximal ileostomy[39]

    b. Provides direct access for frequent surveillance endoscopies in the early postoperative period.

    c. The ileostomy is usually closed between 3 and 6 months posttransplant if the patient has stable graft function, is maintaining adequate nutritional intake, and does not require frequent endoscopic monitoring.

    d. Permanent ileostomies may be necessary in some patients. The distal end of the donor ileum is fashioned as a permanent ileostomy.

5. Enteral tube placement:

    a. Enteral feeding is often necessary to maintain appropriate caloric intake and nutrition because oral intake, particularly in pediatrics, is not dependable in the early postoperative period.

    b. The type of enteral tube varies based on the organs transplanted, underlying disease, and complications. May include

        i. Gastrostomy (GT): used in patients who do not receive a stomach as part of a multivisceral transplant.

        ii. Jejunostomy (JT): used in grafts containing the stomach; some centers prefer separate jejunostomy tubes with gastrostomy tubes.

        iii. Gastrojejunostomy (G-J): a "2-in-1" tube with the gastric portion in the stomach and the jejunal portion in the transplanted proximal jejunum.

        iv. Nasogastric tubes (NG): rarely used because long-term access to the gastrointestinal tract is usually required.

    c. Enteral tubes are also used for decompression in the early postoperative period.

6. Abdominal wall management[37,39]:
   a. Primary fascial closure is the goal, but usually not possible in most patients.
   b. Closure is complicated by the loss of abdominal domain due to the presence of a complex incision, extensive adhesions, abdominal scars from previous surgeries, enteral feeding tubes, ostomies, fistulas, the shortage of recipient-size-matched donors, and/or graft edema.
   c. The abdominal wall cannot be closed under tension. Strategies for closure include
      i. Use of pretransplant abdominal tissue expanders.
      ii. Staged closure with abdominal mesh to provide temporary coverage and flexibility as the patient recovers and graft edema resolves; closure is usually achieved with a second surgery.
      iii. Perform a skin-only closure. The patient will have an abdominal hernia that may require surgical correction in the future.
      iv. Use of reduced-size grafts (pediatrics).
      v. Use of bioengineered skin equivalents or split- or full-thickness skin grafts.
      vi. Abdominal wall transplantation as a vascularized composite graft has been performed in patients with extreme abdominal wall defects.
   d. Skin closure is achieved with sutures or staples, which can usually be removed in 2 to 3 weeks depending on complications and the progression of wound healing.
   e. Placement of Jackson-Pratt (JP) drainage tubes:
      i. Closed suction drainage device that is inserted in the abdominal cavity to promote drainage of residual fluid to prevent infection, abscess formation, and disruption of the wound.
      ii. Two to four drainage tubes are placed in the abdomen.
      iii. The drains are removed when drainage decreases, usually within a week of surgery.

C. Posttransplant Monitoring
   1. Requires an in-depth understanding of the patient's responses to the surgical procedure, potential complications, and effects of immunosuppression:
      a. Detailed medical management is essential.
      b. Requires timely and appropriate response to signs and symptoms of infection, rejection, and/or fluid and electrolyte imbalance.
   2. Hospital course:
      a. Patients are usually transferred directly from the operating room to intensive care.
      b. ICU length of stay ranges from a few days to weeks depending on center-specific protocols and complications.
      c. Patients are transferred to a dedicated transplant unit or surgical unit when stable for further recovery and monitoring of graft function, rejection, infection, and electrolyte balance.
      d. Length of stay:
         i. Ranges from 2 weeks to several months depending on center-specific protocols, intensity of daily medical management and routines, postoperative surgical complications, and the severity and incidence of rejection and infection.
         ii. Length of stay has significantly decreased over time to a median duration of 44 days.[5]

  e. Readmission after initial discharge:
      i.   Common occurrence in first 6 months posttransplant.
      ii. The incidence of readmission is 86.1% within 6 months posttransplant
           for those receiving intestine transplants between 2007 and 2012 and is
           nearly 100% by 1 year posttransplant.[49]
  f. Patients usually reside in the transplant center area for 2 to 6 months prior
      to returning home, but this period may be prolonged in some cases.
  g. Goals for discharge to local area (vary by center):
      i.   Stable graft function without recent rejection (usually two consecutive
           negative pathology reports)
      ii. Stable levels of immunosuppression
      iii. No evidence of infection
      iv. Have attained or are progressing well toward nutritional goals
3. Postoperative complications[50]:
  a. Complications are common and are to be expected.
  b. May be due to challenges present from previous surgeries and
      comorbidities.
  c. Common complications: hemorrhage, vascular thrombosis, wound
      dehiscence, intra-abdominal sepsis, obstruction, anastomotic leak, stoma
      prolapse, abdominal abscess, graft volvulus, hematoma evacuation, and
      perforation.[50-52]
  d. Postoperative hemorrhage[30,50]:
      i.   Usually a technical problem from an anastomotic leak, peritoneal
           bleeding, or vascularized adhesions from previous surgeries.
      ii. Preexisting coagulopathy and portal hypertension may predispose
           patients with hepatic dysfunction to bleed.
      iii. Hemostasis must be achieved to minimize the development of
           hematomas that may become infected.
      iv. Symptoms:
           • Pallor.
           • Tachycardia.
           • Hypotension.
           • Increased serosanguineous drainage through Jackson-Pratt
             drains.
           • Reduction in serial hemoglobin levels.
           • Abnormal serum pH and lactate levels may indicate intestinal
             ischemia or tissue injury.
      v.   Treatment:
           • Surgical reexploration and repair.
           • Administer blood products as required.
           • Improved liver function following liver transplantation for those
             with hepatic dysfunction pretransplant contributes to the resolution
             of bleeding.
           • Accumulated blood in the abdomen may become infected and
             require surgical exploration, irrigation, and drainage.
  e. Gastrointestinal bleeding in the later postoperative period:
      i.   Etiology:
           • Mucosal sloughing from rejection
           • Infectious etiology: *Clostridium difficile*, CMV, rotavirus
           • Localized trauma postintestinal biopsy

    ii. Symptoms:
- Sanguineous ileostomy drainage or rectal bleeding
- Tachycardia
- Hypotension
- Abdominal pain
- Decreasing hemoglobin levels

    iii. Diagnosis:
- Endoscopy with biopsy is useful to determine if there is an infectious etiology versus rejection

    iv. Treatment:
- Surgical intervention if technical etiology
- Increased immunosuppression per treatment protocols if bleeding is related to mucosal damage from rejection
- Antimicrobials and/or reduced immunosuppression if etiology is infection

f. Vascular thrombosis[30,50]:

    i. Thrombosis of the central veins is common due to complications from previous line placements. Subsequent line placements that may be required during and after intestine transplantation can be challenging and time consuming during surgery.

    ii. Acute vascular thromboses of the graft can significantly compromise graft function and is a major emergency; may result in necrosis of the organs provided by that arterial supply.

    iii. Acute onset of symptoms; patients present with general clinical deterioration depending on the location of the thrombus:
- Stoma may become pale, dusky, edematous, or friable
- Decreased stomal output
- Blood in stool or stoma output
- Abdominal distention
- Malaise, nausea/vomiting, and lethargy
- Bacteremia

    iv. Complete obstruction:
- Can lead to ascites and infarction of the mesentery
- Requires enterectomy of graft

    v. Thromboses affecting the liver vasculature:
- Results in significantly elevated liver function tests
- May lead to fulminant hepatic failure

    vi. Diagnosis of vascular thrombosis:
- Ultrasound
- Endoscopy
- CT angiogram of abdomen
- Angiogram
- Abdominal exploration

    vii. Prevention/treatment:
- Surgical intervention if vascular thrombosis is confirmed.
- Anticoagulant therapy:
  - Protocols vary by center.
  - Heparin bolus followed by a continuous infusion is commonly used.
  - Therapy goal is a partial thromboplastin time (PTT) of 70 to 80 seconds.

- Enterectomy with retransplantation may be required in the setting of complete thrombosis and large segment ischemia.

g. Intestinal anastomotic leaks[30]:

- i. Etiology:
  - Technical complications
  - Poor wound healing due to malnutrition pretransplant and/or the effect of high-dose steroids
- ii. Symptoms:
  - Abdominal distention and tenderness
  - Fever
  - Peritonitis
  - Leukocytosis
  - Presence of bile in abdominal drains
- iii. Diagnosis:
  - Upper GI series with contrast
  - Abdominal CT scan with contrast
- iv. Prevention/treatment:
  - Important to maintain decompression of the stomach and intestine through the gastrostomy, jejunostomy, ileostomy, and/or nasogastric tube to minimize risk of leaks
  - Exploratory laparotomy performed to revise the affected segment of intestine and remove infected peritoneal fluid
  - Intravenous antibiotics and/or antifungal agents administered as indicated based on cultures and sensitivities

h. Intestinal obstruction[30,50]:

- i. Etiology:
  - Early postoperative period: surgical technique or ischemic damage
  - Later causes: rejection, electrolyte abnormalities, peritonitis, or posttransplant lymphoproliferative disease (PTLD)
- ii. Signs and symptoms:
  - Decreased or absent stool/stoma output
  - Abdominal distention and pain
  - Vomiting and diarrhea
- iii. Diagnosis:
  - Abdominal x-ray
  - Upper GI with small-bowel follow-through
  - Abdominal CT scan
  - Labs: electrolytes and EBV PCR
  - Endoscopy with biopsy
- iv. Treatment:
  - Based on etiology of obstruction
  - Decompression with nasogastric tube

i. Wound dehiscence:

- i. Can occur from tension on the abdominal wall due to loss of abdominal domain
- ii. Partial thickness wounds involve the epidermis and may include some of the dermal layer. Treatment is with moist dressings that aid in reepitheliazation.[53]
- iii. Full-thickness wounds are deep into the fascia or bone and heal very slowly. Wound packing is used to help the wound heal from the bottom up.[53]

4. Complications of the transplanted intestine[30,50,54]:
   a. Intestinal dysmotility:
      i. Extrinsic innervation to the transplanted intestine is absent following procurement.
      ii. Peristalsis begins when the intestine is reperfused, but can be erratic.
      iii. Hypermotility is common.
      iv. Fluid and electrolyte balance must be accurately maintained by monitoring intake and output, daily weight, and serum electrolytes.
   b. Absorption of the transplanted intestine:
      i. Generally absorbs well posttransplant as evidenced by serum immunosuppressive levels, particularly tacrolimus
      ii. Carbohydrate absorption:
         • Determined by D-xylose testing
         • Normalizes within the first several months posttransplant
      iii. Protein absorption:
         • Appears to be adequate in the early posttransplant period
         • Measured by prealbumin levels
      iv. Fat absorption:
         • Fats commonly malabsorbed due to surgical disruption of the lymphatic drainage of the donor intestine
         • May take several months for the intestinal lymphatic drainage to be reestablished allowing for better absorption of medium chain triglycerides[54]

5. Vital signs:
   a. Continually monitored during the intensive care phase to assess for complications
   b. Obtained less frequently, every 4 to 8 hours, when the patient is on the transplant unit
   c. Obtained more frequently, per individual hospital protocol, during certain medication administrations or postprocedures
   d. Temperature:
      i. Temperature elevation related to infection:
         • ≥38.5°C/101°F in early postoperative period.
         • Usually related to surgical complications, the patient's pretransplant status, or postoperative complications.
         • Source of fever must be identified quickly through pan cultures (blood, urine, sputum, wound, stool), chest x-ray, and/or CT scan.
         • Appropriate broad-spectrum antimicrobials administered until the source of infection and sensitivity of the organism(s) is identified.
         • Aggressive pulmonary toilet required in patients with atelectasis and pneumonia.
         • Antipyretics usually ordered for comfort.
         • Cooling blankets may be used adjunctively for high fevers.
      ii. Temperature elevation related to rejection:
         • Less common in the very early posttransplant period.
         • Fever, in conjunction with a change and/or increase in stool output and consistency, and/or abdominal pain and distention, may be related to rejection; however, an infectious etiology should also be ruled out.

e. Tachycardia:
   i.   Etiology:
       * Fluid imbalance
       * Fever
       * Pain or anxiety
   ii. Differential diagnoses:
       * Hypernatremia
       * Anemia
       * Hypoglycemia
       * Hyperthyroidism
       * Effect of medications: albuterol, pseudoephedrine, and antiarrhythmics
   iii. A sustained heart rate greater than the upper limits of normal for age or subjective complaints of palpitations should be reported.
   iv. Treatment:
       * Tachycardia due to dehydration is corrected by administration of IV fluids.
       * An EKG should be obtained if arrhythmias are suspected.
       * Tachycardia due to postoperative pain is controlled through administration of pain medications and supportive nursing care.

f. Bradycardia:
   i.   A low heart rate sustained at less than the lower limits of normal for age
   ii. Associated with a disruption of the electrical impulses generated by the sinoatrial or atrioventricular node
   iii. Etiology:
       * Associated with coronary artery disease and myocarditis
       * Hypothyroidism
       * Hyperkalemia
       * Side effect of narcotics
       * Side effect of some cardiac medications including beta-blockers, calcium channel blockers, antiarrhythmic, and digoxin

g. Hypotension:
   i.   Etiology:
       * Fluid imbalance
       * Electrolyte abnormalities
       * Sepsis
       * Bleeding
       * Narcotics
       * Other medications associated with hypotension: diuretics, beta-blockers, calcium channel blockers, angiotensin-converting enzyme (ACE) inhibitors, nitrates, antipsychotics, antianxiolytics, and tricyclic antidepressants
   ii. Symptoms:
       * Sustained low systolic blood pressure for age/height
       * Weak pulse
       * Decreased capillary refill
       * Output greater than intake
       * Fever
       * Signs/symptoms of bleeding
       * Decreased hematocrit

   iii. Treatment:
- Dehydration corrected through administration of IV fluids.
- If bleeding is suspected, the source of blood loss is identified with appropriate treatment/intervention.
   h. Hypertension:
   i. Etiology:
- Nephrotoxicity from immunosuppressant medications (corticosteroids and calcineurin inhibitors) and other nephrotoxic medications (aminoglycosides, ganciclovir)
- Fluid and electrolyte imbalance
- Hepatorenal syndrome
- Preexisting diabetes
- Postoperative pain
   ii. Symptoms:
- Sustained high blood pressure >95th percentile for age and gender.
- Decreased urinary output.
- Rising creatinine and increased creatinine clearance.
- Patient may not have any physical complaints.
   i. Treatment:
- Varies based on etiology of hypertension.
- Scheduled or PRN antihypertensive medications.
- If hypertension is related to nephrotoxicity from sustained high tacrolimus levels or high-dose steroids, dosages of these medications may be decreased while balancing the risk of rejection.
- Fluid and electrolyte imbalances are corrected by balancing intake and output, infusing or restricting fluids, and administering electrolyte additives in parenteral fluids or enteral feedings.
   j. Tachypnea:
   i. Patients are ventilated until able to sustain a normal respiratory rate and appropriate oxygenation.
   ii. Is present with fever and infection, particularly pneumonias and septicemia.
   iii. Pain.
   k. Hypoxia:
   i. Usually related to the effects of anesthesia and/or narcotics
   ii. Symptoms:
- Decreased respiratory rate and effort
- Decreased oxygen saturation
- Need for supplemental oxygen
- Decreased PaO_2 and/or increased $PaCO_2$
   iii. Treatment:
- Supportive oxygenation as needed to maintain adequate oxygen saturation
- Decrease or discontinue narcotics
   l. Neurologic assessment:
   i. Neurotoxicities vary by patient.
   ii. Assess neurologic status every 2 hours in early postoperative period, then less frequently as the patient recovers.

      iii. Assess pupils and reaction to light, facial symmetry, reflexes, response to stimuli, speech, and bilateral strength of the extremities related to the patient's level of consciousness.

      iv. Neurotoxic side effects may be related to high tacrolimus levels, usually ≥15 ng/mL.

- Tacrolimus has been associated with headache, tremor, insomnia, photophobia, confusion, and seizures.
- Accurately obtain tacrolimus trough levels at the appropriate time (10 to 12 hours after the previous dose) and monitor levels.
- Observe for side effects related to a high trough level, usually ≥15 ng/mL.
- Higher tacrolimus levels are associated with an increased risk of significant neurotoxicities, particularly seizures.

      v. In addition to high tacrolimus trough levels, an increased risk of seizure is also associated with hyperglycemia, hypomagnesemia, and hyponatremia.

D. Postoperative Appliances and Drains

1. Venous/arterial access:
   a. Adequate venous access is required due to fluid needs.
   b. Central venous lines.
      i. Double- or triple-lumen catheters are preferred.
      ii. Access via the internal/external jugular veins, subclavians, or inguinal veins.
      iii. Patients with a paucity of sites may have a transhepatic or an azygous line.
   c. Additional peripheral intravenous lines for increased access:
      i. If intravenous tacrolimus is being administered, a dedicated line must be used for tacrolimus administration only and not used for lab draws so that an accurate trough level is obtained. Tacrolimus may be adsorbed by the tubing resulting in a higher level if drawn from that line.
   d. Arterial line:
      i. Inserted to monitor blood gases and central venous pressure
      ii. Discontinued following extubation.
   e. Meticulous nursing care of central venous lines is essential.
      i. Minimize entry when possible to prevent infection.
      ii. Maintain patency to save access for potential long-term intravenous needs.
2. Respiratory support:
   a. Ventilated for 12 to 24 hours or more depending on the length of surgery, pretransplant status, and postoperative complications:
      i. Monitor blood gases and central venous pressure while intubated.
   b. Supportive oxygenation as needed following extubation:
      i. Oxygen via cannula or face mask to maintain oxygen saturations of ≥92%
      ii. Oxygenation monitored through continual or intermittent pulse oximetry readings
3. Gastrointestinal appliances (prefeeding):
   a. The stomach and intestine must be decompressed to avoid gastric or intestinal perforation at the anastomotic lines or within the intestine.
   b. Decompression is achieved through suction and drainage from a nasogastric tube, gastrostomy tube, and/or jejunostomy tube and the ileostomy.

4. Enteral feeding appliances:
   a. Enteral feedings are initiated after the upper gastrointestinal contrast study confirms the absence of any intestinal leaks.
   b. Feedings are administered through a gastrostomy tube (GT), jejunostomy tube (JT), or gastrojejunostomy tube (G-JT).
5. Abdominal drainage appliances:
   a. Jackson-Pratt (JP) drains:
      i. Remove residual fluid in abdominal cavity.
      ii. Two drains are usually inserted intraoperatively in pediatric patients; adults may have up to four drains.
      iii. Drainage is emptied, recorded, and monitored every 4 hours or as needed.
      iv. Fluid is initially serosanguineous, becoming less serous by 3 to 5 days posttransplant:
         • Increased serous drainage may be a sign of bleeding from the vascular anastomoses.
         • Hematocrit of the fluid may be obtained to assess intra-abdominal hemorrhage.
         • Site of bleeding determined through abdominal ultrasound or CT scan.
      v. Drains usually removed within 7 days after surgery as drainage decreases.
   b. Biliary drain or percutaneous transhepatic catheter (PTC):
      i. Uncommon in patients receiving a composite liver and intestine graft
      ii. Used to dilate an occluded bile duct and maintain bile flow
   c. Urinary catheter:
      i. An accurate measurement of intake and output is imperative in the early postoperative period.
      ii. The urinary catheter provides a drainage method to accurately assess urinary output.
      iii. To avoid infection, the urinary catheter is removed as soon as possible.
   d. Ileostomy:
      i. Created to provide easy access to the transplanted intestine for routine surveillance for rejection.
      ii. Stooling from the rectum occurs in patients with an intact large intestine, although most of the output will drain from the ileostomy.
      iii. Drainage is emptied and recorded every 4 hours or as needed.
      iv. Stool is assessed for amount, color, and consistency.
      v. The desired stool output is 1 to 2 L/day for adults and 40 to 60 mL/kg/d for pediatric recipients.
      vi. Stomal output varies depending on intake, NPO status, the presence of infection or rejection, absorption, and/or dysmotility.
      vii. Stool color ranges from yellow to deep brown.
      viii. Stool consistency is often watery due to hypermotility and because the large intestine is bypassed. A thicker consistency may be achieved through diet change, antimotility medications, and/or the addition of fiber, as the motility of the transplanted intestine normalizes.

E. Fluid and Electrolyte Balance (see Table 13-2)
   1. Fluid and electrolyte imbalances and related complications are common, particularly in the early postoperative period, during rejection, and with infections affecting the transplanted intestine.

2. Intravascular volume is depleted while the patient is retaining fluids due to increased interstitial fluid accumulation in the peripheral tissue, the intestinal graft, and lungs from leakage of the mesenteric lymphatics.
3. Hypermotility is common until the graft adapts due to the disruption of extrinsic innervation resulting in
   a. Increased transit time
   b. Decreased enteral absorption
   c. Increased output with subsequent electrolyte imbalances
4. Nursing interventions[55]:
   a. Maintain strict record of intake and output.
   b. Observe for symptoms of electrolyte imbalance, fluid overload, or dehydration (see Table 13-2).
   c. Obtain electrolytes and renal function tests as ordered.
   d. Notify the physician of any abnormal levels.
   e. Administer IV maintenance fluids or boluses to correct imbalances as ordered.
   f. Obtain repeat lab values to evaluate resolution of electrolyte imbalance.
5. Alterations in blood glucose levels:
   a. Hyperglycemia:
      i. Presents as a complication of calcineurin inhibitors and high-dose steroids, particularly intravenous Solu-Medrol or methylprednisolone.
      ii. Monitor blood glucose levels as ordered, usually four to six times daily.
      iii. Administer insulin as ordered.
      iv. Provide patient education regarding the signs and symptoms of hyper- and hypoglycemia and treatment.
      v. Consult the diabetic educator for comprehensive instruction on insulin administration if the patient requires insulin at discharge for an extended period of time.
6. Daily weights:
   a. Important element to assess fluid overload and the absorptive capacity of the graft.
   b. Weigh patient at approximately the same time every day, in the same manner, and on the same scale.
   c. Weight gain with edema may be a sign of fluid overload and/or renal dysfunction.
   d. Weight loss:
      i. May occur in the early postoperative period as TPN and enteral feedings are adjusted to meet the patient's caloric needs.
      ii. Occurs in the longer term as a result of inadequate calories, poor absorption, hypermotility with a high output, nonadherence to enteral feeds/diet, and chronic rejection.

F. Pain Management
1. The goal of pain management is satisfactory control of pain from the patient's perspective.
2. Most patients experience some degree of pain in the immediate postoperative period, but do not require narcotics in the long term.
3. Pain management education is an essential part of preoperative teaching for transplant nurses to help patients prepare for postoperative pain control.
   a. Facilitate understanding of patient's ability to control the pain experience.
   b. Understand the patient's beliefs and attitudes about pain and be aware of sociocultural factors that affect coping, pain, and pain management.

    c. Explain the use of an age-appropriate and/or developmentally appropriate pain scale to the patient and confirm understanding of how to report the level of pain that is being experienced.

    d. Investigate alternative methods for coping with pain:

       i. Deep breathing

       ii. Relaxation techniques

       iii. Imagery

4. Pain management interventions[56]:

    a. Continuous intravenous infusion of opioids are usually administered during the early postoperative period.

    b. Intravenous patient-controlled anesthesia (PCA):

       i. Provides the patient with the ability to control pain with demand doses

       ii. Can be used in children as young as 5 to 7 years of age

       iii. Provides sustained pain relief

    c. Pain management medications:

       i. Acetaminophen for mild-moderate pain (score of 1 to 5)

       ii. Opioids IV or PO for moderate to severe pain (>4):

          • Oxycodone, fentanyl, hydromorphone, and morphine.

          • Oral narcotics are prescribed when patients are tolerating enteral feeds.

          • Transitioning to long-acting medications, such as OxyContin or methadone, is helpful in some patients.

       iii. Opioid tapering must be monitored closely for signs of withdrawal.

          • Opioid use for <3 days does not require tapering.

          • Longer-term use requires slow dose tapering and the addition of methadone.

          • After the opioid is discontinued, initiate a methadone wean.

    d. Chronic pain:

       i. Defined as pain that extends >3 months beyond the early postoperative period

       ii. Uncommon, but may develop in patients with significant postoperative complications or related to the indication for transplant and pretransplant pain control needs:

          • Includes neuralgias from entrapped nerves, musculoskeletal pain, or neuropathic pain without identified pathology

       iii. Must identify and quantify pain to plan for effective pain management:

          • Rating pain from scale of 1 to 10 (adults)

          • Visual Analogue Scale (VAS)

          • Wong-Baker FACES Pain Rating Scale

          • FLACC Behavioral Pain Assessment Scale

          • CRIES Scale (0 to 6 months of age)

       iv. Pain management with opioids, alpha-2 agonists (clonidine), and anticonvulsants (gabapentin)

    e. Consultations:

       i. Pain service/palliative care should be consulted in the immediate postoperative period.

       ii. Psychiatry/psychology intervention and counseling may be therapeutic for patients with chronic pain.

       iii. Supportive service therapies such as pet therapy, art therapy, massage therapy, and music therapy are helpful when available.

        iv. Child life specialists play an essential role in pediatrics to help assess and intervene in pain management through therapeutic play therapy, distraction techniques, relaxation techniques, and guided imagery.

    f. Dependency on pain medications:

        i. Some intestine transplant candidates have chronic pain and/or pain control issues prior to transplant depending on the etiology of intestinal failure and comorbidities.

        ii. Concerns of dependency must be investigated prior to transplant during the evaluation period. A postoperative plan should be discussed and confirmed with the patient during the pretransplant period so they will experience good pain control with narcotic weaning as they recover.

    g. Nursing considerations in administering narcotics:

        i. Assess the patient for excessive sedation, respiratory depression, bradycardia, and hypotension.

        ii. Assess the graft for dysmotility.

           • Constipation is a side effect of narcotics. Motility of the transplanted intestine may be further compromised with prolonged narcotic use.

G. Graft Function

    1. Early graft function[57]:

      a. Preservation injury or a positive crossmatch may lead to an edematous graft and intestinal mucosal congestion.

      b. Peristalsis begins immediately but motility may be intermittent and/or rapid because the graft is denervated.

      c. Malabsorption is common in the early postoperative period due to mucosal disruption.

      d. Early graft nonfunction (postoperative day 1 to 3) is rare and, if it occurs, is usually due to a technical complication.

    2. Monitoring graft function[54,58,59] (Table 13-6):

      a. Clinical surveillance through endoscopy with biopsy

      b. Monitoring protocols:

        i. Protocol endoscopy intervals vary by center

        ii. Surveillance endoscopies may be scheduled as frequently as twice weekly for 4 to 6 weeks, weekly for 4 to 6 weeks, and then every other week until the risk of rejection has decreased in the setting of stable immunosuppressive levels.

TABLE 13-6 Nursing Assessment of Graft Function

Observe for abdominal distention and signs of discomfort or pain.
Auscultate for hypoactive bowel sounds.
Palpate to assess any firmness or abdominal rigidity.
Assess stoma output for changes in: • Volume: a trend or acute increase in stoma output • Color: from yellowish-brown to melena and/or frank blood • Consistency: increased watery fluid with little consistency
Observe for presence of blood.

iii. After 3 to 6 months, endoscopies are usually only performed when clinically indicated based on center protocols, patient history, and patient risk factors.

iv. Long-term stable patients are usually assessed annually.

c. Monitoring nutritional status:

  i. Goal: obtain full nutritional needs from oral and/or enteral nutrition.

  ii. Carbohydrate absorption normalizes within the first few months posttransplant as measured by D-xylose testing.

  iii. Protein absorption normalizes within the first several months.

   • Hypoalbuminemia (serum albumin <2.5 g/dL) may occur.
     ○ Symptoms: edema, diarrhea, increased output, and ascites
     ○ Treatment:
       ▪ Intravenous albumin 25% every 12 to 24 hours and to replace ascitic drainage
       ▪ Optimize enteral/parenteral nutrition
       ▪ Antimotility agents are to treat diarrhea if rejection or an infectious etiology has been ruled out
       ▪ Follow albumin levels daily

  iv. Fat absorption is compromised until the intestinal lymphatic drainage is reestablished.

   • Symptoms of fat malabsorption: increased stool output, change in stool consistency, greasy stool, and weight loss
   • Diagnosis
     ○ Fecal fat collection for 24 to 72 hours (normal fat excretion is 0.8% to 5%)
     ○ Serum triglyceride level >3 mmol/L
     ○ Low-fat–soluble vitamin levels (A, D, E, K)
   • Treatment:
     ○ Low-fat diet
     ○ Pancreatic enzymes
     ○ Short-term lipid infusions in cases of severe and/or prolonged fat malabsorption with weight loss and/or poor growth

H. Immunosuppression after Intestine Transplantation

1. Intestinal grafts have a high immunogenic load, containing a large amount of gut-associated lymphoid tissue.

  a. Initially thought to require higher levels of immunosuppression than other solid organs

  b. Resulted in an era of overimmunosuppression in the mid-1990s that was associated with a high incidence of posttransplant lymphoproliferative disease (PTLD) and, less commonly, graft-versus-host disease (GVHD)[60]

  c. Was later understood that immunosuppressive therapy in intestine transplantation was a delicate balance in maintaining a healthy graft while preventing rejection and infection.

2. Immunosuppressant protocols vary by center, but standard practice includes induction therapy combined with tacrolimus for maintenance immunosuppression.[5]

3. Induction therapy:

  a. Use of induction therapy in intestine transplantation has become standard practice with over 75% of recipients receiving induction therapy and has significantly improved graft survival.[5,17,49]

   b. Used to reduce the initial alloimmune response and provides polyclonal lymphocyte depletion of the intestine transplant recipient.[61]
   c. Accelerates the elimination of donor-specific T-cytotoxic cells by apoptosis; may reduce the need for long-term high-dose immunosuppression.[62]
   d. Induction agents:
      i.   Antithymocyte globulin (rATG)
      ii. Alemtuzumab
      iii. Basiliximab
4. Maintenance immunosuppression:
   a. Tacrolimus is the primary immunosuppressant agent used in intestine transplantation.
      i.   Oral tacrolimus is begun on the first postoperative day with induction therapy.
      ii. Intravenous tacrolimus:
         * Not commonly used in the early postoperative period since the use of induction therapy.
         * May be used for brief periods to optimize low tacrolimus levels or to maintain adequate levels if GI absorption is compromised.
      iii. Minimum trough levels in the *early* postoperative period are usually maintained at 12 to 15 ng/mL in whole blood. Trough levels vary based on
         * Use of induction therapy
         * Renal function
         * Concomitant nephrotoxic medications
         * Time posttransplant
         * Presence of rejection or infection
         * Center-specific protocols
   b. Corticosteroids:
      i.   Steroid therapy varies by center.
      ii. Long-term versus short-term therapy.
      iii. Steroids may be weaned to discontinuation in some patients.
         * Due to chronic rejection affecting graft loss in the long term, some centers have reintroduced low-dose steroids in the immunosuppressive protocol.[61]
      iv. Used in treatment of rejection.
   c. Adjunctive agents:
      i.   Mycophenolate mofetil
      ii. Sirolimus (rapamycin):
         * Maintenance therapy with rapamycin is associated with improved survival ($p = 0.005$).[5]
      iii. Azathioprine

I. Rejection
   1. Common complication following intestine transplantation because of the large amount of lymphoid tissue associated with the graft.[63]
   2. Pre- and/or posttransplant donor-specific antibodies (DSA) are associated with rejection and graft loss.[64,65]
      a. Preformed DSAs are present in nearly one-third of intestine transplant recipients and de novo DSAs develop in up to 40% of patients.[64]

  b. Reports suggest that with the optimal use of induction and maintenance immunosuppressive agents, the impact of DSAs on the graft may be insignificant.

3. Incidence:
  a. Nearly 50% of recipients develop at least one episode of rejection in the first year after transplant.[49]
  b. Most commonly occurs within the first 90 days posttransplant.
  c. Pediatric intestine transplantation:
    i. Incidence of rejection is 60%.[43]
    ii. Severe rejection occurs in over 30% of this group and effects long-term survival.[43]

4. Symptoms:
  a. No single symptom is a clear indicator; presents as a combination of clinical signs[30]:
    i. Fever
    ii. Significant increase or decrease in stool output
    iii. Change in stool consistency
    iv. Abdominal distention
    v. Cramping and abdominal pain
    vi. Nausea and vomiting
    vii. Dusky appearance of the stoma
    viii. Poor appetite and weight loss
    ix. Melena
    x. Bacteremia due to disruption of the intestinal mucosal barrier
    xi. Hypoalbuminemia

5. Diagnosis through surveillance endoscopic biopsies[30,66]:
  a. Surveillance endoscopy:
    i. Mild to moderate rejection:
- Ischemic or dusky mucosa
- Edema
- Granularity
- Ulcerations
- Absent or decreased peristalsis

    ii. Severe rejection:
- Diffuse ulcerations
- Nodular mucosa
- Exfoliation of the mucosa with bleeding
- Aperistalsis

  b. Histology[63,66]:
    i. Four to six sites biopsied throughout as much of graft as possible
    ii. Histologic findings:
- Crypt apoptosis
- Lymphocytic infiltration
- Loss of goblet cells
- Blunted villi
- Ulceration

    iii. Severe rejection:
- Crypt loss
- Epithelial sloughing

6. Treatment[30,66,67]:
   a. Mild to moderate rejection (Table 13-7):
      i. Optimize tacrolimus levels (Table 13-8).
      ii. Administer intravenous methylprednisolone as a bolus dose with decreasing cycled dosing over a short period of time, usually 5 days.
      iii. Adjunctive agents (azathioprine, sirolimus, or mycophenolate mofetil) may be added to the baseline immunosuppressive regimen.
      iv. Repeat endoscopy with biopsy every 3 to 5 days to assess effect of treatment and determine further immunosuppressant management.
   b. Severe rejection (see Table 13-7):
      i. Antilymphocyte antibody treatment with alemtuzumab or rATG is used in severe rejection or if rejection is refractory to steroids.
         • Administered for 5 to 7 days depending on response to treatment and complications
         • Monitor for cytokine release syndrome[61]:
            ○ Occurs due to the excessive production of certain cytokines: TNF-α and IL-1.
            ○ Premedicate with methylprednisolone, diphenhydramine, and acetaminophen.
            ○ Symptoms include fever, respiratory distress, photophobia, and tachycardia.
      ii. Rituximab is administered in patients with B-cell–mediated rejection:
         • Anti-CD20 monoclonal antibodies
         • Weekly dose for 4 weeks

TABLE 13-7 Nursing Interventions to Assess Rejection

Administer immunosuppressive medications as ordered.
Assess the patient for the clinical signs of rejection: • Fever • Significantly increased or decreased stool output • Change of consistency of stool to a more watery fluid • Abdominal pain • Distention • Bleeding from the stoma or rectum • Change in stoma color • Hypoactive bowel sounds
Notify the physician in the event of any of these symptoms.
Be aware of the desired tacrolimus level for the patient and any changes in that level. Notify the physician immediately for levels outside of the desired range.
Facilitate the endoscopy procedure as required in the GI suite or at bedside and provide postprocedure care per center protocol.
Administer immunosuppressive medications as ordered to treat rejection. Monitor for drug toxicities secondary to increased levels.
Provide education for the family and patient in regard to the diagnosis of rejection, treatment, and potential side effects of treatment.
Provide emotional support for the patient/family in expressing anxiety and fear related to rejection.
Reassure the patient that rejection is a common complication of transplantation and can usually be treated.

TABLE 13-8 Nursing Interventions: Effective Tacrolimus Administration and Monitoring

Administer tacrolimus as ordered and on time, usually every 12 h.

Administer doses within an hour of the prescribed time unless there is an order to hold a dose.

Achieve stable levels with consistency of administration.

Administer whole capsules.

Use alternative administration strategies in pediatric patients as required, but identify and record a consistent method for that patient.

Obtain tacrolimus trough levels 10–12 h after the previous dose.

Do not draw blood for the tacrolimus level through lines where tacrolimus has previously infused or is currently infusing if the patient has received tacrolimus intravenously.

Be aware of the desired tacrolimus level for the patient and alert the physician immediately to an inappropriate level.

Monitor patient for the most common side effects of tacrolimus:

- Neurotoxicities: insomnia, headache, burning or tingling of the hands and feet, tremors, photophobia, aphasia, confusion, seizures
- Nephrotoxicities: hyperkalemia, hypomagnesemia, hypertension, renal dysfunction
- GI distress: abdominal distress, nausea, vomiting, diarrhea
- Increased risk of infection: fever
- Hyperglycemia

Be aware of drug interactions that increase or decrease tacrolimus levels.

     iii. Consider graft enterectomy if refractory to prolonged treatment and If there are significant complications related to a high immunosuppressive load
     iv. Retransplantation may be considered.
   c. Adjunctive treatments/therapies during periods of high immunosuppression:
     i. Monitor for hypertension and hyperglycemia associated with high-dose steroids and increased tacrolimus levels.
     ii. Provide prophylactic antibacterial therapy due to the risk of translocation-induced sepsis from severe mucosal breakdown and sloughing.
     iii. Maintain pneumocystis prophylaxis with SMX-TMP.
     iv. Provide prophylactic antiviral therapy.
- Monitor CMV and EBV PCRs weekly to every 2 weeks during periods of high immunosuppression.
- Ganciclovir is administered daily as prophylaxis during periods of increased immunosuppression.

     v. Monitor for oral candidiasis (thrush) and provide antifungal prophylaxis with nystatin or clotrimazole.
     vi. Maintain acid suppression with a proton pump inhibitor to decrease the risk of stomach upset and development of gastric ulcers from increased steroids.
     vii. Maintain electrolyte balance with intravenous replacement fluid for high output.

7. Chronic rejection:
   a. Generally characterized by a gradual decrease in graft function or may present as sudden graft loss following an acute dehydrating condition.[67]
   b. Early stages of chronic rejection are not easily recognized; median time for development is 39 months (range: 22 to 67 months).[61]
   c. Incidence: 8% to >10%.[5,61]
   d. Occurs more frequently in patients with isolated intestine transplants than in composite liver/intestine grafts.[5]
   e. Symptoms[30,67]:
      i. Prolonged increased output
      ii. Progressive weight loss
      iii. Intermittent fevers
      iv. Abdominal pain (can be due to graft strictures or obstruction)
      v. GI bleeding
   f. Endoscopic findings:
      i. Tubular appearance
      ii. Thickened mucosal folds
      iii. Pseudomembranes
      iv. Chronic ulcers
   g. Histology:
      i. Mucosal biopsies:
         • Biopsies are not diagnostic of chronic rejection because the pathology is in the vessels of the graft mesentery and larger arteries within the intestinal wall, rather than the graft mucosa.[67]
         • Histology of the mucosa is less specific in chronic rejection, but may reveal evidence of previous injury and regeneration with irregular crypt and villus architecture, mucosal fibrosis, and granulation tissue with continued crypt apoptosis.[68]
      ii. Confirmation is through full-thickness biopsy:
         • Completed on graft enterectomies
         • Reveal thickening or obliteration of the intestinal arterioles causing compromised oxygenation of the intestinal mucosa, blunted villi, loss of the lamina propria, and expansion of stromal tissue.[61]
   h. Treatment:
      i. Increased immunosuppression does not improve graft function and may increase the risk of infection.
      ii. Partial resection of the graft may be helpful in some cases.
      iii. Complete enterectomy is usually performed; retransplantation may be considered.
8. Graft-versus-host disease (GVHD)[51,69,70]:
   a. Although a common complication after bone marrow transplantation, GVHD is a rare occurrence in solid organ transplantation.
   b. Incidence is highest in intestine transplant recipients when compared to other solid organ transplants (5 to 10 times higher incidence) due to the abundance of lymphoid tissue in the intestine graft.[70]
   c. Occurs in approximately 5% to 10% of patients postintestine transplant and leads to significant morbidity and mortality.[69,70]
   d. Presents most commonly as a skin rash, but also may involve the liver and gastrointestinal tract.

e. Can occur from days to years posttransplant.

f. Etiology[68,70]:

    i. The large lymphoid cell population of the intestine is replaced by cells from the recipient after transplant. The immune responses of recipients against donor result in rejection, but if the immune responses is that of donor against recipient, GVHD is induced.

g. Diagnosis through tissue biopsy[68-70]:

    i. Histopathology.

    ii. Keratinocyte necrosis.

    iii. Epithelial apoptosis of the native intestine or oral mucosa.

    iv. In sex mismatches, donor cell infiltration is observed by fluorescence in situ hybridization for X and Y chromosomes (FISH).

h. Treatment[69-71]:

    i. Methylprednisolone with decreased tacrolimus dosing.

    ii. Steroid dose is adjusted based on patient response.

    iii. Most cases respond to high-dose steroids, but if refractory to treatment, mortality is very high.

    iv. New therapies for steroid-refractory GVHD are difficult to evaluate due to the patient being critically ill with multisystem complications.

J. Patient Monitoring during the Endoscopic Procedure

1. Surveillance endoscopies (see Tables 13-9 and 13-10):

a. Obtained routinely and more frequently during the first 3 months posttransplant and whenever rejection is suspected.

b. Ileostomy is created to facilitate frequent endoscopies and maintained until the graft is stable, usually for 6 to12 months posttransplant.

TABLE 13-9 Nursing Interventions Prior to Endoscopy

Maintain NPO status as ordered: usually NPO for 4 h prior to procedure if endoscopy is performed through the ileostomy and patient is sedated

Obtain labs within 3 d prior to the procedure or per center protocol: hemoglobin and hematocrit, platelet count, and PT/PTT

Notify the transplant physician or GI physician with any abnormalities.

Administer appropriate blood products or medications as ordered to correct abnormal levels.

Repeat labs after interventions are performed to assess correction.

Perform the ordered bowel preparation:
- Protocols vary by center.
- Preparation for a lower endoscopy may include:
  - Clears for 12 h then NPO
  - Administer GoLYTELY on the evening prior to endoscopy
  - Normal saline enemas as needed
- No bowel preparation for an upper endoscopy or ileoscopy

Administer intravenous bacterial prophylaxis if ordered.

Explain procedure and postprocedure care to patient/family.

Provide emotional support for fears or concerns they may have about the procedure, particularly if rejection is suspected.

TABLE 13-10 Nursing Interventions Postendoscopy

Monitor vital signs frequently as ordered until awake. Notify the physician for fever, tachycardia, or hypotension.

Obtain postprocedure hemoglobin and hematocrit levels if ordered. Notify the physician with abnormal results.

Assess for postprocedure complications:
- Bleeding from the ileostomy due to intestinal perforation
- Abdominal discomfort or pain
- Hypoactive bowel sounds
- Firm abdomen secondary to an ileus

Assess for abdominal distention.
- Some distention is normal because air is inserted into the intestine to facilitate viewing and to obtain the biopsy.
- Distention should decrease within hours as patient passes gas from the ileostomy or rectum and as physical activity is resumed.
- Notify the physician for:
  - Prolonged or increased distention
  - Hypoactive or absent bowel sounds
  - Vomiting
- Bleeding

Encourage intake of the ordered diet and fluids when fully awake.

Resume preprocedure activity level when fully awake or as ordered.

Review the findings of the study with the patient/family, as explained by the transplant physician or gastroenterologist.

Assess understanding of the outcome and any required treatment.

c. If sedation is not required:
   i. Resume preprocedure care.
   ii. Resume ordered diet.
   iii. Resume preprocedure activity.
d. If patient is sedated:
   i. Monitor vital signs per hospital protocol.
   ii. Resume diet and activity when recovered.
e. Hospitalized patients:
   i. Monitor as above for possible complications.
   ii. Frequent vital signs are not usually ordered.
f. Outpatient endoscopies:
   i. Outpatient procedure for patients in the later postoperative period or during annual assessment
   ii. Usually monitored in the GI suite then discharged
g. Patient education:
   i. Signs and symptoms of postprocedure complications
   ii. How to contact their transplant coordinator and/or physician in event of fever, discomfort, or bleeding

K. Infection
   1. Significant cause of morbidity and mortality in intestine transplant recipients, with over 90% of patients developing an infection, usually bacterial in origin[72]:
      a. Sepsis is the leading cause of graft loss in over 50% of patients.[5]

b. Pediatric patients who are <1 year of age have a significantly greater incidence of mortality.[73]

c. Medical management requires a delicate balance between the risk of infection from a highly immunosuppressed state and the risk of rejection from decreased immunosuppression.

2. Risk factors for infection[74]:

a. Prolonged operative time

b. Preoperative status and the presence of liver disease

c. Surgical complications

d. Multiple surgeries

e. Sepsis prior to transplant

f. Inability to close the abdominal wall following implantation of organ(s)

g. Presence of multiple invasive lines and indwelling catheters that compromise the skin barrier

3. Timing of infections[74,75]:

a. Early postoperative period (0 to 2 months):

  i. Usually due to preexisting conditions, surgical and technical complications, pneumonia, and indwelling catheters[76]

  ii. Most common pathogens:

   • Bacteria

   • Candida organisms

b. Middle period (2 to 6 months):

  i. Opportunistic infections related to immunosuppression:

   • Cytomegalovirus (CMV)

   • Epstein-Barr virus (EBV) and posttransplant lymphoproliferative disease (PTLD)

   • Adenovirus

c. Long-term infectious complications (>6 months):

  i. Continued risk if requiring higher levels of immunosuppression:

   • EBV/PTLD and CMV may present any time there is a significant increase in immunosuppression during treatment for rejection.[76]

   • Bacteremia can occur during episodes of severe rejection and in the setting of PTLD.

  ii. Community-acquired infections are most common in the later period:

   • Usually tolerated well in the long term if the patient's overall health is improved and immunosuppression is at baseline:

    ○ Influenza

    ○ Respiratory syncytial virus (RSV)

    ○ Rotavirus

4. Bacterial infections:

a. Can occur at any time, but most commonly seen during the first 1 to 2 months posttransplant

b. Predisposing factors: prolonged operative time, reexplorations, blood transfusions, technical problems, presence of CVLs, and preoperative status.[74]

c. Common organisms[72,74,76,77]:

  i. Gram-negative bacteria:

   • Enteric organisms: *Staphylococcal* species, enterococci, enteric gram-negative rods (*E. coli, Klebsiella, Enterobacter*):

    ○ Usually associated with technical complications, rejection, PTLD, and enteritis

    ○ Treatment with piperacillin-tazobactam or cefepime

- *Pseudomonas* species:
  - Most common gram-negative bacteria found in postoperative pneumonias
  - Usually treated with piperacillin-tazobactam or a carbapenem (meropenem or imipenem)
  - May also be used in conjunction with an aminoglycoside

  ii. Gram-positive bacteria:
  - *Staphylococcus epidermidis* (coagulase negative *Staphylococcus*) is the most common bloodstream isolate.
    - Associated with CVL infections
    - Treatment with vancomycin
  - *Staphylococcus aureus:*
    - Antibiotic therapy with oxacillin, nafcillin, or daptomycin for minimum of 2 weeks; may require longer treatment with more complicated infection.
    - Remove the infected CVL.
    - Patients infected with *S. aureus* are at risk for endocarditis.

  iii. Vancomycin-resistant *Enterococcus* (VRE) is an increasingly problematic infection:
  - Associated with prior antibiotic use, multiple abdominal surgeries, and biliary complications in liver transplant recipients.
  - Linezolid is used to treat VRE.

d. Bacterial overgrowth:
  i. Characterized by an increased number and/or abnormal type of bacteria in the small intestine with >105 colony-forming units per milliliter of proximal jejunal aspiration[78]
  ii. High correlation between bacteria identified in stool and those in the blood
  iii. Can lead to translocation when the intestinal mucosa is damaged through ischemia, reperfusion injury, or rejection
  iv. Symptoms[30]:
  - Increased stool output
  - Abdominal distention or pain
  - Frothy and/or foul-smelling stools
  - Bacteremia with an enteric organism
  - Ulcerations of the mucosa that are not associated with rejection, EBV, or CMV

  v. Treatment:
  - IV antibiotics are administered in patients with bacteremias from enteric organisms.
  - IV fluids with additives administered as needed for dehydration secondary to diarrhea.
  - Intestinal decontamination:
    - Treatment protocols vary by center.
    - A common protocol includes giving oral metronidazole twice daily for 2 weeks every month followed by 1 week of colistimethate and 1 week without antimicrobial therapy.

e. Bacterial translocation:
  i. Intestinal epithelium may be damaged if there is preservation injury to the graft resulting in bacterial translocation into the splanchnic venous system causing bacteremia.[54]

      ii. Bacteria translocate from the graft and travel to the peritoneal cavity through leakage from division of the lymphatics during procurement.

      iii. Associated with antibiotic therapy, TPN, ischemia/reperfusion injury, bacterial overgrowth, intestinal motility disorders, hepatic insufficiency, and an immunosuppressed state.[72]

      iv. Patient at risk for peritonitis and sepsis.

  f. Signs and symptoms of bacterial infection:

      i. Fever, usually ≥101°F or 38.5°C

      ii. Flu-like symptoms: malaise, lethargy, decreased appetite, irritability, or change in behavior (pediatrics)

      iii. Catheter or tube insertion sites that are erythematous, swollen, and tender

      iv. Wound site abnormalities: erythema, purulent drainage, tenderness, and swelling

      v. Wound dehiscence

      vi. Changes in respiratory status: tachypnea, decreased breath sounds, and cough

      vii. Changes in drainage or output: purulence, cloudy urine, stool consistency, amount, and odor

  g. Diagnosis:

      i. Central and peripheral blood cultures

      ii. Cultures of the wound, throat, urine, sputum, JP drainage, and/or stool

      iii. Chest x-ray particularly in the setting of respiratory symptoms

      iv. Abdominal CT scan to assess for fluid collections

  h. Treatment:

      i. Broad-spectrum antibiotics administered after cultures are obtained based on the apparent or suspected etiology of fever:

- If a CVL is present, begin vancomycin until the organism is identified.
- If the patient is colonized with VRE, linezolid should be considered.

      ii. Antibiotic treatment is adjusted based on the sensitivities of the identified bacteria.

      iii. Immunosuppression may be decreased, but with caution, particularly in the setting of severe polymicrobial infections.

- Closely monitor tacrolimus levels and report any levels that are not within the desired therapeutic range.
- Observe the patient for symptoms of rejection.

      iv. Wound infections:

- Administer appropriate antibiotics as determined through culture and sensitivities.
- Wound treatment varies based on type of wound, extent and depth, amount of drainage, progression of granulation tissue, and location.

      v. Bacterial pneumonia:

- Administer appropriate antibiotics as determined through culture and sensitivities.
- Auscultate routinely for changes in respiratory assessment.
- Facilitate administration of inhalation therapy and/or percussive therapy.
- Encourage deep breathing and coughing.

- Provide and monitor supplemental oxygen flow, oxygen saturation, and/or blood gases.
- Reposition the patient every 2 hours; encourage activity if ambulatory.
- Mechanical ventilation is required for severe respiratory compromise.
  - Perform endotracheal suction per hospital protocol if ventilated.
  - Monitor blood gases for changes in oxygenation.

vi. Central venous line (CVL) infections:
- Administer appropriate antimicrobial medications as determined through culture and sensitivities.
- Blood cultures are drawn daily until negative.
- Depending on the organism, treatment usually continues for 10 to 14 days from the first negative blood culture.
- Removal of the CVL may be necessary
  - The CVL may be changed over a guide wire and a temporary line inserted in patients with limited access.
  - The temporary line will be replaced with a permanent line following antimicrobial therapy.

5. Fungal infections:
  a. Less common than bacterial infections
  b. Usually occur in the early postoperative period
  c. Risk factors[74]:
     i.   Deteriorating health status prior to transplant
     ii. Surgical complications (particularly intestinal leaks)
     iii. Surgical reexplorations
     iv. Polymicrobial therapy
     v.   High levels of immunosuppression
     vi. Disruption of the mucosal barrier leading to translocation
     vii. Indwelling venous catheters
  d. *Candida albicans* (noninvasive)[74,79]:
     i.   Most common fungal species following intestinal transplantation
     ii. Most commonly presents in the oropharynx, esophagus, or genitalia
     iii. Symptoms:
          - White plaques on oral mucosa, tongue, or throat
          - Red pinpoint rash of the buttocks or genitalia (pediatrics)
          - Vaginal discharge and itching
     iv. Treatment:
          - Prophylaxis with oral/topical nystatin or clotrimazole:
            - During the first 3 months posttransplant
            - When receiving higher doses of steroids
            - When immunosuppression is increased during episodes of rejection
          - If receiving prophylaxis, dosage frequency may be increased and/or a second agent added.
          - Oral fluconazole may be prescribed if the infection is refractory to nystatin or clotrimazole.
            - Fluconazole increases tacrolimus levels.
            - Tacrolimus levels must be monitored carefully and the dose adjusted as needed during fluconazole therapy.

e. *Candidemia*[74,79]:
    i. Significant infection associated with high mortality and graft loss
    ii. Symptoms:
        * Fever
        * Lymphadenopathy
        * Rash
    iii. Diagnosis:
        * Blood culture and sensitivities
        * CT scan to rule out abscess formation
        * ECHO to rule out cardiac vegetations in patients with CVLs
    iv. Treatment:
        * Intravenous liposomal amphotericin B:
            ○ Monitor renal function closely due to the increased risk of nephrotoxicity from concomitant use with tacrolimus.
        * Caspofungin:
            ○ Can be used in patients with renal insufficiency
        * Fluconazole:
            ○ Adjust tacrolimus dose
            ○ Can be used in patients with renal insufficiency
f. *Aspergillus*[74,79]:
    i. Later infection, occurring 6 months or more posttransplant.
    ii. Lungs are the most common site of a primary infection followed by the sinuses.
    iii. Metastatic disease seen in central nervous system (CNS), liver, and/or kidneys.
    iv. Risk factors:
        * Extended operative time >12 hours
        * Reexplorations
        * Retransplantation
        * Neutropenia
        * High immunosuppressive load
        * Prolonged use of broad-spectrum antibiotics
    v. Symptoms:
        * Isolated fever without symptoms of rejection
        * Dyspnea/hypoxia
        * Sinusitis: headache, facial pain, and facial edema
        * GI: abdominal pain, dysphagia, melena, and intestinal perforation with hemorrhage
        * CNS symptoms: headache, lethargy, hemiparesis, and seizure
    vi. Diagnosis:
        * CXR and CT scan to observe for nodular pneumonias with indistinct margins
        * CT scans of the sinuses or brain
        * Tissue biopsies
    vii. Treatment:
        * Intravenous liposomal amphotericin B
        * Additional or alternative therapies with caspofungin or voriconazole
        * Prolonged treatment up to 6 months

TABLE 13-11 Nursing Interventions: Monitoring for CMV Infection

Monitor for fever and report temperatures >101°F/38.5°C.

Monitor for increased stool output and GI symptoms.

Obtain serial CMV PCRs, CBC, and other laboratory tests as ordered.

Monitor serial CMV PCRs for response to treatment.

Monitor CBC results for leukopenia and thrombocytopenia.

Provide postendoscopy care per protocol.

Administer intravenous antiviral therapy as ordered.

Monitor for signs and symptoms of nephrotoxicity.

Be aware that changes may be made in the level of immunosuppression during treatment for CMV. Notify the physician of any tacrolimus levels that are not within the desired range.

Provide patient/family with information about CMV disease, lab tests, endoscopy findings, and treatment. Reinforce teaching as necessary.

6. Viral infections:
   a. Cytomegalovirus (CMV)[72,74,80] (Table 13-11):
      i. Etiology:
         * Most common viral infection in intestine transplant recipients with majority of infections being asymptomatic reactivation of a CMV-seropositive recipient
         * Usually occurs within first 3 months posttransplant
      ii. Risk factors:
         * Donor-recipient CMV serology mismatch:
            ⊙ CMV-negative recipient receiving a CMV-positive graft is at risk for developing invasive CMV disease.
         * High levels of immunosuppression
         * Use of antilymphocyte antibodies
      iii. Signs and symptoms:
         * May be asymptomatic
         * CMV syndrome: fever, leukopenia, atypical lymphocytosis, and thrombocytopenia
         * Enteritis
         * Anorexia
         * Nausea and vomiting
         * Elevated liver function tests
         * Pneumonitis
         * Rash
      iv. Diagnosis:
         * CMV PCR:
            ⊙ Measurement of CMV DNA in peripheral blood with polymerase chain reaction (PCR).
            ⊙ Elevated or increasing CMV PCR is associated with the risk or presence of CMV disease.
         * Invasive disease most commonly found in the gastrointestinal tract and liver:

○ An endoscopy with biopsy is performed if invasive disease is suspected and enteritis persists:
- Ulcerations within normal intestinal mucosa seen on endoscopy
- Histology reveals CMV inclusion bodies with inflammatory changes[68]

○ If hepatitis is suspected, a liver biopsy is performed.

- Although rare, may also present as CMV pneumonitis, retinitis, or as central nervous system disease

v. Treatment:

- Intravenous ganciclovir is administered twice daily until the CMV viral load is negative, usually on two consecutive tests.
  ○ CMV PCR may be followed weekly to monitor response to treatment.
  ○ Clinical response usually seen within a week of treatment.
- CMV-IVIG (CytoGam) may be beneficial in treating CMV enteritis or pneumonitis, but is not necessary in all cases.[74]
- Baseline immunosuppression is usually maintained, but may be decreased in the setting of a very high viral load or if the patient is deteriorating.
- Ganciclovir-resistant CMV is treated with foscarnet. If resistant to foscarnet, CMV is treated with cidofovir.
- Monitor renal function closely during treatment due to the nephrotoxicity of these agents and concomitant use of tacrolimus.
- Following treatment, the CMV viral load is monitored per center protocol. A common protocol is every other week for 3 months, every month for month 4 to 6 posttransplant, every 3 months for month 6 to 12 posttransplant, and then discontinue at 12 months.

vi. Prophylactic strategies:

- Most commonly used for CMV D+/R− recipients and in CMV R+ recipients
- Treatment for CMV D+/R− recipients:
  ○ Intravenous ganciclovir is administered twice daily for 14 days followed by valganciclovir for 3 months or longer depending on center protocol.
  ○ Valganciclovir is not used in the early postoperative period because drug absorption is not optimal due to ischemia of the graft.[81]
  ○ CMV-IVIG is given within 72 hours of transplantation and at 2, 4, 6, and 8 weeks and then at a lower dose at 12 and 16 weeks posttransplant.

vii. Nursing considerations:

- Be aware of the individual patient's risk factors for developing CMV:
  ○ CMV D+/R− recipients
  ○ The patient's immunosuppressive load
  ○ Use of antilymphocyte antibodies
- Keep in mind that the symptoms of CMV enteritis appear similar to those of rejection of the intestine.

b. Epstein-Barr virus (EBV) and EBV-associated lymphoproliferative disease (PTLD)[72,74,76,82,83] (Table 13-12):

i. Includes a range of illnesses from a nonspecific viremia to polyclonal or monoclonal disease and, ultimately, lymphoma.

TABLE 13-12 Nursing Interventions: Monitoring for EBV/PTLD

Be aware of the patient's unique risk factors for EBV/PTLD.

Monitor for fever and report temperatures □40°C.

Monitor for clinical symptoms of EBV:
- Diarrhea
- Bloody stools
- Tonsillar enlargement (often with exudate)
- Peripheral lymphadenopathy
- Fatigue
- Malaise
- Decreased appetite

Obtain an EBV PCR, CBC, and other laboratory tests as ordered.

Monitor serial EBV PCRs for response to treatment.

Monitor CBC results for pancytopenia, leukopenia, and atypical lymphocytosis.

Facilitate procedures such as CT scan and endoscopy.

Provide postendoscopy care per protocol.

Administer intravenous antiviral therapy as ordered.

Be aware that changes may be made in the level of immunosuppression during treatment for EBV/PTLD. Notify the physician of any tacrolimus levels that are not within the desired range.

Provide the patient/family with information about EBV/PTLD, lab tests, endoscopy findings, and treatment. Reinforce teaching as necessary.

Provide supportive care to the patient and family during diagnosis and treatment.

    ii. Significant cause of morbidity and mortality following intestine transplantation.

    iii. Risk is highest in the first year posttransplant, but PTLD can occur at any time.

    iv. Intestine recipients have the highest risk of developing PTLD of all solid organ transplants due to the need for prolonged elevated levels of immunosuppression.

    v. Risk factors:
- Induction therapy with T-cell–depleting agents.
- EBV mismatch: seropositive donor organ transplanted into a seronegative recipient (D+/R−):
  - Pediatric recipients at greater risk because they are usually seronegative
- Recipient splenectomy is associated with a higher incidence of PTLD.[76]
- Increased risk of GI tract involvement in intestine transplant recipients.

    vi. Symptoms of EBV:
- High fever (40°C) for at least 3 days
- Diarrhea
- Bloody stools
- Peripheral lymphadenopathy
- Fatigue and malaise

- Decreased appetite
- Elevated liver function tests
- Pancytopenia
- Leukopenia
- Atypical lymphocytosis

vii. Diagnosis:
- Measurement of EBV viral load in peripheral blood with polymerase chain reaction (PCR):
  - Serial EBV PCRs are monitored frequently during the first year posttransplant in patients who are at greater risk.
  - There is an association of elevated EBV viral loads and PTLD.[82]
- Endoscopy with biopsy
- Lymph node excision with biopsy when indicated
- Diagnosis confirmed through tissue histology
- CT scan of the neck, chest, abdomen, and pelvis

viii. Treatment[83]:
- Primary treatment strategy: decrease the level of immunosuppression and provide vigilant surveillance.
- Tacrolimus levels may be decreased by 25% to 50% to maintain levels of 5 to 7 ng/mL.
- If receiving steroids, dosage may be decreased to a lower baseline dose.
- Antiviral therapy is administered per transplant center protocol:
  - Intravenous ganciclovir
  - Cytomegalovirus immune globulin (CytoGam)
  - Rituximab (anti-CD20 antibody)
  - Chemotherapy is used in cases that do not respond to rituximab
- Close surveillance through weekly endoscopies with biopsy and serial EBV PCRs.
- Treatment is maintained until there is clinical and virological evidence that EBV/PTLD has resolved.
- Other therapies if refractory to standard management:
  - Cytotoxic chemotherapy
  - Radiation
  - Surgical resection
  - Graft enterectomy in isolated intestine transplant recipients with discontinuation of immunosuppression
- Preemptive antiviral therapy and minimization of posttransplant immunosuppression have significantly reduced the morbidity and mortality of PTLD, even in the setting of induction therapy.[84]
- With recent strategies, patient survival has improved to 91% at 1 year and 75% at 5 years following diagnosis.[84]
- Prognosis is poor in patients who have disease involving more than one site, CNS involvement, monoclonal disease, EBV-negative PTLD, T- or NK-cell PTLD, or the presence of tumor suppressor genes.[82]

L. Nutrition (Table 13-13)
1. Goal of intestinal transplantation is to provide the patient's nutritional requirements enterally without TPN support.
2. Total parental nutrition:

TABLE 13-13 Nursing Interventions Related to Nutritional Needs

Provide enteral and/or oral feedings as ordered.

Encourage oral intake.

Maintain an accurate calorie count if ordered.

Assess tolerance to feeds by observing the patient for:
- Change in stool consistency and output
- Weight gain or loss
- Abdominal distention
- Cramping
- Nausea
- Emesis

Maintain strict intake and output records.

Report changes in stool output.

Administer motility agents as ordered.

Monitor albumin levels.

Encourage oral intake.

Obtain the patient's weight at the same time, same scale, and in the same way every day.

Facilitate testing as ordered and per hospital protocols for:
- Fecal fat collection
- D-xylose testing
- Calorie counts

Facilitate team consultations related to nutritional needs:
- Nutrition services (transplant dietitian)
- Physical therapy
- Speech therapy
- Occupational therapy

     a. Required by most patients for the first few weeks posttransplant, depending on complications.

     b. ITR reports that 67% of patients are completely free of TPN within 6 months posttransplant.[5]
- The rate of enteral autonomy was 5% higher in patients who received a colon segment.[5]

     c. Intravenous nutritional support may be needed during episodes of severe rejection or prolonged infection.

     d. Pediatric patients may require intermittent periods of partial TPN to support growth and development.

  3. Enteral feeding[30,67,85]:

     a. Upper gastrointestinal contrast study is completed to evaluate the integrity of the intestinal anastomoses before starting feeds.

     b. Enteral feedings initiated if

       i. No confirmed intestinal leaks.

      ii. Peristalsis has resumed with the presence of gas and stomal output; usually occurs as the ileal inflammation response to ischemia/reperfusion injury decreases.

   c. Feeding routines vary by center, the type of intestine transplant, and postoperative complications.
      i. Usually begun within the first postoperative week.
      ii. Administered directly into the stomach through a gastrostomy tube or through a jejunostomy tube into the jejunum.
      iii. Transpyloric feeding via a jejunostomy tube is often required due to delayed gastric emptying.
   d. Formulas:[85]
      i. Ideal formula is low fat and hypo-osmolar and provides maximal calories with a minimal volume to reduce the risk of chylous ascites due to poor lymphatic drainage of the graft.
      ii. Should contain medium chain triglycerides as fat content.
      iii. A low osmolality isotonic dipeptide formula containing medium chain triglycerides and glutamine is preferred for children.
   e. Feedings initiated with diluted formula (15 to 20 kcal/oz) at a low rate,[67] usually 5 mL/hour in children and 10 mL/hour in adults and then slowly increased by 5 to 10 mL/hour increments every 12 to 24 hours as tolerated.
   f. After the goal rate is achieved, the formula strength is increased to ¾ strength and then to full strength.
   g. Oral feedings can be introduced as tube feedings are being advanced.
   h. Jejunostomy feeds can be transitioned to gastrostomy feeds in those patients receiving enteral feedings through the jejunostomy.
   i. Some centers limit high sugar-containing foods, which may increase output in the early postoperative period.
   j. Vitamins A, D, E, and K may be used to provide water-soluble forms of fat-soluble vitamins, water-soluble vitamins, and zinc due to fat malabsorption in the early postoperative period.[86]
   k. Additional zinc may be required in patients with high outputs at 1 to 1.5 times the recommended dietary allowance (RDA).[86]
   l. Nutrition consults and continued monitoring by a dietician dedicated to the patient's nutritional needs are essential.
   m. Common complaints as enteral feedings are optimized include abdominal pain, nausea, vomiting, or increased output.
      i. Discontinue or reduce rate of feeding until the etiology of the symptoms is identified
      ii. Patients who received all nutrition parentally prior to transplant with minimal oral intake may be uncomfortable with GT feedings because they are not accustomed to a large gastric volume.
      iii. Decreased gastric motility may occur due to
         • Etiology of intestinal failure
         • Disuse of the stomach prior to transplant
         • Dysmotility of the transplanted stomach as part of a multivisceral graft
      iv. Interventions for abdominal discomfort in the absence of rejection:
         • Administer enteral feeds at a slower rate over a longer period of time.
         • Administer metoclopramide intravenously or orally to improve gastric motility.
         • Change the enteral formula.
4. Management of stool output[30]:
   a. Considered excessive if >1 to 2 L/day for adults or 40 to 60 mL/kg/d or children in the absence of rejection, infection, or other pathology.

b. High stool output may be caused by rejection, bacterial overgrowth, infection (*Clostridium difficile*, rotavirus, EBV, CMV), food allergies, medication side effects, feeding intolerance, hypoalbuminemia, fat malabsorption, or parasites.
  i. Signs and symptoms:
   - Increased stool output (>60 mL/kg in pediatrics; >2 L in adults)
   - Abdominal distention and pain
   - Weight loss
   - Electrolyte abnormalities
   - Dehydration
   - Fatty stools
  ii. Diagnosis: testing based on history and symptoms:
   - Viral and bacterial stool cultures
   - EBV and CMV PCRs
   - RAST panel for allergy testing
   - Serum IgE for allergy testing and parasites
   - Stool electrolytes
   - Fecal fat collection
   - Serum albumin
  iii. Treatment depends on etiology of hypermotility:
   - Hypermotility in the absence of rejection:
     ○ A single motility agent is used, then combination therapy until an acceptable stool output is achieved.
     ○ Medications for diarrhea and increased stool output:
       ▪ Loperamide (Imodium)
       ▪ Diphenoxylate hydrochloride and atropine (Lomotil)
       ▪ Hyoscyamine (Levsin)
       ▪ Clonidine
       ▪ Cholestyramine
       ▪ Tincture of opium
       ▪ Fiber supplements (pectin, Benefiber)
     ○ Intravenous or subcutaneous somatostatin used when output is extremely high and refractory to oral antidiarrheal medications.
     ○ Intravenous hydration required to stabilize electrolyte levels until output decreases.
   - Infection:
     ○ Metronidazole is used to treat *Clostridium difficile*.
     ○ Bacterial overgrowth:
       ▪ Treatment varies by center.
       ▪ Metronidazole (2 weeks per month) alternating with colistimethate (1 week per month) and 1 week without treatment.
   - Electrolyte imbalances:
     ○ Corrected by administration of IV maintenance and replacement fluids with appropriate additives:
       ▪ Bicarbonate and magnesium levels are usually low with diarrhea
   - Hypermotility associated with enteral feedings:
     ○ May need to adjust feedings in the setting of diarrhea.
     ○ Dilute feedings to ½ or ¼ concentration.
     ○ If on bolus feeds, change to continuous infusion.
     ○ If on enteral infusion, decrease the rate of tube feedings and increase the hours of infusion.
     ○ TPN may be required for the short term if there is continued weight loss and electrolyte imbalances.

5. Oral aversion:
   i. Common problem both pre- and postintestine transplantation, particularly in pediatric intestinal recipients
   ii. Factors contributing to oral aversion:
      - Early age of onset of intestinal failure with initiation of TPN and limited/no oral feedings
      - Intermittent and/or extended periods of nothing by mouth
      - Development of a hyperactive gag reflex
      - Changes in taste
      - Hospital environment
      - Behavioral issues
      - Limited experience with food textures, tastes, and aromas
   iii. Interventions/treatment:
      - Early consultation prior to transplant with occupational and speech therapy
      - Inpatient or outpatient feeding rehabilitation programs
      - Psychological counseling
      - Behavioral modification
6. Food allergies[30]:
   i. Symptoms:
      - Increased stool output
      - Changes in stool consistency
      - Abdominal distention/pain
      - Cramping
      - Eosinophilia
      - Weight loss
      - Failure to thrive
      - Rash
   ii. Diagnosis:
      - Serum IgE levels.
      - Intestinal tissue biopsy showing eosinophilia.
      - Serum radioallergosorbent testing (RAST):
        ○ Reported as class 0 (no allergy) to class 4 (high allergy).
        ○ Class 3 and 4 foods are restricted from diet.
      - Most common food allergies are milk protein, lactose, wheat, peanuts, and eggs.[87]
   iii. Treatment[30,85,87]:
      - Limited to symptomatic patients with class 3 and 4 allergens and intestinal eosinophilia on biopsy or peripherally.
      - Limit exposure to allergens through dietary restrictions.
      - A short course of low-dose prednisone may be prescribed.
      - Antihistamines may be of value in some patients.
7. Nutritional outcomes:
   i. Long-term nutritional goal is ability to tolerate a regular oral diet that maintains appropriate growth/weight without intravenous fluids, enteral nutrition, or parenteral supplementation.
   ii. Weight gain and growth may be affected by repeated or prolonged episodes of rejection and infection.
   iii. Many adults achieve nutritional goal within a year.
   iv. May take pediatric recipients longer to achieve goal:
      - Improvements are seen but attaining linear growth is challenging in the majority of patients.[87]

TABLE 13-14 Nursing Interventions: Compromised Skin Integrity

Monitor abdominal wound routinely for bleeding, infection, dehiscence, and evisceration.

Instruct patient on abdominal splinting techniques when coughing, sneezing, or vomiting to decrease pressure on the site.

Assess wound site when cleaning and changing the dressing.

Pack wounds with wet to dry dressings and change twice daily or as ordered.

Monitor wound site for signs of infection including erythema, edema, wound separation, localized pain, and purulent drainage.

Obtain cultures of wound drainage as ordered.

Report abnormalities to the surgeon.

Monitor nutritional intake.

Administer antibiotics as ordered for positive wound cultures.

Consult the enterostomal nursing specialist as needed for skin care concerns.

- Routinely monitor height and weight.
- Adjust and maintain calorie requirements based on the absorptive ability of the graft.

M. Impaired Wound Healing (Table 13-14)
1. Impaired or delayed wound healing common in the early postoperative period
2. Contributing factors:
   a. Pretransplant nutritional status
   b. Concomitant liver disease
   c. Posttransplant complications
   d. Surgical reexplorations
   e. Staged closing of the abdominal wound secondary to surgical complications
   f. Inadequate nutritional intake posttransplant
   g. Prolonged use of steroids
3. Compromised skin integrity:
   a. Extensive abdominal incision
   b. Ileostomy
   c. Puncture wounds:
      i. Jackson-Pratt drain sites
      ii. Enteral feeding tube insertion sites
      iii. Central lines
      iv. Venous catheters
   d. Other wound sites related to complications:
      i. Chest tubes to drain pleural effusions
      ii. Percutaneous transhepatic catheter for biliary duct complications
      iii. Abdominal fistulas
      iv. Skin ulcerations/pressure ulcers
4. Wound healing:
   a. Achieved through optimizing nutrition:
      i. Maximize calories
      ii. May require short-term TPN in cases of serious wound complications
      iii. Increased protein requirements
   b. Provide meticulous wound care.
   c. Minimize/eliminate steroids when possible.

TABLE 13-15 **Nursing Interventions Related to Output and Ileostomy Care**

Monitor the patient for any subjective complaints of cramping, abdominal pain, or nausea.

Examine the patient for abdominal distension and auscultate for bowel sounds.

Maintain accurate intake and output records.

Administer intravenous fluids as ordered to maintain electrolyte and fluid balance secondary to an increased output.

Administer antidiarrheal medications as ordered.

Examine ileostomy output for color and consistency.

Monitor stoma tissue for changes in color, texture, and size.

Report bleeding or changes in output to the physician.

Provide the appropriate ileostomy appliance and meticulous skin care.

Facilitate consultation with the enterostomal therapy nurse.

Provide teaching sessions on ileostomy care.

Facilitate ordering and delivery of ostomy supplies prior to discharge with the ET nurse or discharge planner.

N. Ileostomy Care[53] (Table 13-15)
   1. Pretransplant education regarding ileostomy care is essential.
      a. Rationale for ileostomy
      b. Basic ileostomy care
      c. View stoma appliances or pictures of appliances
      d. Provide emotional support:
         i. Partner the patient with another recipient who has an ileostomy.
         ii. Refer to the United Ostomy Associations of America (www.ostomy.org) for additional peer support.
      e. If the ileostomy is temporary, discuss the plan for ileostomy closure with the patient.
   2. Reinforce teaching posttransplant through collaborative effort by the enterostomal therapy (ET) nurse and staff nurse to design an individualized nursing care plan to meet the patient's needs:
      a. An enterostomal therapy (ET) nurse is an invaluable resource in choosing appliances for an optimal and comfortable fit and to help with wound care.
      b. Adults and older children should be able to provide self-care of the ileostomy prior to discharge from the hospital.
      c. A support person, parent, or spouse should also be taught ileostomy care.
   3. Stoma surveillance:
      a. Routine surveillance may lead to early detection of complications.
      b. Normal stoma is comparable in color and moistness to oral mucosa.
      c. Monitor stoma site for changes in tissue color, texture, or size:
         i. Change in color, particularly a deeper red or dusky appearance, may indicate rejection, an internal obstruction, or a prolapse.
         ii. Texture change may indicate rejection or infection.
         iii. Size changes may be due to inflammation from rejection, obstruction, or prolapse.
      d. Other abnormal findings:
         i. Ulcerations
         ii. Stomal prolapse

   iii. Bleeding:
- Bleeding is of concern and may be a sign of rejection or infection.
- Can occur following an intestinal biopsy and is usually self-limiting.
- Superficial bleeding of the stoma tissue may occur from localized trauma when cleaning the site or when changing the ostomy appliance.

4. Stool assessment:
 a. Assess stool color. Ranges from deep brown to light yellow depending on the patient's diet and medical status.
 b. Monitor stool amount. Varies depending on
  i. Presence of rejection or infection
  ii. Oral/enteral intake
  iii. Diet
  iv. Absorption/motility issues
  v. Intestinal obstruction or ileus
 c. Monitor stool consistency; ranges from a very thick fluid to a watery effluent:
  i. Watery diarrhea may be associated with rejection, infection, dysmotility, allergens, and diet.
  ii. Consistency is variable based on
- Diet
- Amount of oral/enteral intake
- Presence of rejection or infection

  iii. Treatments to improve consistency:
- Antidiarrheal medications administered to slow transit time and increase absorption
- Fiber added to enteral feedings to decrease transit time and improve absorption

 d. In the absence of rejection, output changes should be correlated to formula or diet changes and enteral infusion rate or route:
  i. Accepted output: adults 1 to 2 L/day; children 40 to 60 mL/kg/d.
  ii. Maintain accurate intake and output records.
  iii. Be aware of the patient's normal output range.
  iv. Administer intravenous replacement fluids as ordered to prevent fluid and electrolyte imbalance in cases of high output.

O. Self-Care Deficit
 1. Learn self-care routines:
  a. The patient and family should participate in formal and informal teaching sessions with the transplant nurse to reinforce previous education. Topics include
   i. Immunosuppression: rationale for use, importance of stable trough levels, side effects, and risks of immunosuppression
   ii. Transplant medications: rationale for use, dose, times, side effects, and any special instructions
   iii. Signs and symptoms of rejection
   iv. Signs and symptoms of infection
   v. Ileostomy care
   vi. Care of feeding tubes
   vii. Central line care

        viii. Maintaining records of intake and output, vital signs, and weight

        ix. Importance of routine medical follow-up

        x. Long-term care issues

        xi. Potential long-term complications

  b. Collaborate with the patient and family to schedule and implement a medication schedule that will optimize adherence.

  c. Adherence can be affected by

        i. Perceived or actual side effects

        ii. Inability to obtain medications due to physical limitations

        iii. Distance from the pharmacy

        iv. Availability of medications

        v. Insurance coverage

  d. Encourage discussions with the patient and family to assess factors that may affect their adherence.

  e. Facilitate consultations with social work, psychology/psychiatry, a financial counselor, or pastoral care as needed.

2. Activity:

  a. Recuperation can be challenging for many patients, particularly when critically ill and debilitated prior to transplant.

  b. Activity is increased as tolerated by the patient postoperatively.

  c. Physical therapy should be consulted early in the postoperative period to improve strength and endurance as the patient recovers.

  d. Patients with an extended postoperative course and multiple complications may benefit from more extensive rehabilitation in an inpatient setting.

REFERENCES

1. Abu-Elmagd K, Bond G, Reyes J, et al. Intestinal transplantation: a coming of age. *Adv Surg.* 2002;36:65–101.
2. Pritchard TJ, Kirkman RL. Small bowel transplantation. *World J Surg.* 1985;9:860–886.
3. Asfar S, Atkinson P, Ghent C, et al. Small bowel transplantation. *Transplant Proc.* 1966;28:2751.
4. Goulet O, Frederique S, Dominique C, et al. Intestinal transplantation in children: Paris report. Abstract 0–96. IXth International Small Bowel Transplantation Symposium. Brussels, July 2, 2005.
5. Grant D, Abu-Elmagd K, Mazariegos GV, et al. Intestinal Transplant Registry Report: global activity and trends. *Am J Transplant.* 2015;15:210–219.
6. Pironi L, Arends J, Baxter J, et al. ESPEN endorsed recommendations: definition and classification of intestinal failure in adults. *Clin Nutr.* 2014;34(2):171–180. http://dx.doi.org/10.1016/j.clnu.2014.08.017
7. Quirós-Tejeira RE, Ament ME, Reyen L, et al. Long-term parenteral nutritional support and intestinal adaptation in children with short bowel syndrome: a 25-year experience. *J Pediatr.* 2004;145(2):157–163.
8. Jeppesen PB, Pertkiewwicz M, Messing B, et al. Teduglutide reduces need for parenteral support among patients with short bowel syndrome with intestinal failure. *Gastroenterology.* 2012;143:1473–1481.
9. Nightingale J, Woodward JM; Small Bowel and Nutrition Committee of the British Society of Gastroenterology. Guidelines for management of patients with a short bowel. *Gut.* 2006;55(suppl 4):iv1–iv12.
10. Pirenne J. *Advances in intestinal Transplantation: Report from the VII International Small Bowel Transplant Symposium.* Medscape Transplantation, 2002. Available at www.medscape.com/Medsapre/transplantation/journal/2002/v03.n01/
11. Diamond IR, Sterescu A, Pencharz PB, et al. Changing the paradigm: omegaven for the treatment of liver failure in pediatric short bowel syndrome. *J Pediatr Gastroenterol Nutr.* 2009;48(2):209–215.
12. Malone FR, Javid PJ, Davis C, et al. Impaired glucose production and b-cell dysfunction contribute to the disturbed metabolism in children with protein-energy malnutrition. *J Pediatr Gastroenterol Nutr.* 2009;49(suppl 1):E38.
13. Diamond IR, Pencharz PB, Wales PW. Omega-3 lipids for intestinal failure associated liver disease. *Semin Pediatr Surg.* 2009;18:239–245.
14. Seida JC, Mager DR, Hartling L, et al. Parenteral w-3 fatty acid lipid emulsions for children with intestinal failure and other conditions: a systemic review. *JPEN J Parenter Enteral Nutr.* 2013;37:44–55.

15. Byrne TA, Wilmore DW, Iyer K, et al. Growth hormone, glutamine and an optimal diet reduces parenteral nutrition in patients with short bowel syndrome. *Ann Surg.* 2005;242:655–661.
16. Jeppesen PB. New approaches to the treatments of short bowel syndrome-associated intestinal failure. *Curr Opin Gastroenterol.* 2014;30(2):182–188.
17. Abu-Elmagd K. The concept of gut rehabilitation and the future of visceral transplantation. *Nat Rev Gastroenterol Hepatol.* 2015;12:108–120.
18. Sommovilla J, Warner B. Surgical options to enhance intestinal function in patients with short bowel syndrome. *Curr Opin Pediatr.* 2014;26(3):350–355.
19. Reinshagen K, Kabe C, Wirth H, et al. Long term outcome in patients with short bowel syndrome after longitudinal intestinal lengthening and tailoring. *J Pediatr Gastroenterol Nutr.* 2008;47:573–578.
20. Jones BA, Hull MA, Potanos KM, et al. Report of 111 consecutive patients enrolled in the International Serial Transverse Enteroplasty (STEP) Data Registry: a retrospective observational study. *J Am Coll Surg.* 2013; 216:438–446.
21. Sachdev AH, Pimentel M. Gastrointestinal bacterial overgrowth: pathogenesis and clinical significance. *Ther Adv Chronic Dis.* 2013;4(5):223–231.
22. Horslen S. Management of the patient with intestinal failure. In: Remaley L, McGhee W, Reyes J, et al., eds. *The Pediatric Transplant Manual.* 2nd ed. Hudson, OH: Lexi-Comp; 2009:37–45.
23. Harrison E, Allan P, Ramu A, et al. Management of intestinal failure in inflammatory bowel disease: small intestinal transplantation or home parenteral nutrition? *World J Gastroenterol.* 2014;20(12):3155–3163.
24. Vassallo M, Dunais B, Roger PM. Antimicrobial lock therapy in central-line associated bloodstream infections: a systematic review. *Infection.* 2015;43(4):389–398.
25. O'Grady NP, Alexander M, Burns LA, et al. Guidelines for the prevention of intravascular catheter-related infections. *Clin Infect Dis.* 2011;39(4 suppl 1):S1–S34.
26. Oliveira C, Nasr A, Brindle M, et al. Ethanol locks to prevent catheter-related bloodstream infections in parenteral nutrition: a meta-analysis. *Pediatrics.* 2012;129(2):318–329.
27. Yang CF, Duro D, Zurakowski D, et al. High prevalence of multiple micronutrient deficiencies in children with intestinal failure: a longitudinal study. *J Pediatr.* 2011;159(1):39–44.
28. Phillips G, Bhargava P, Stanescu L, et al. Pediatric intestinal transplantation: normal radiographic appearance and complications. *Pediatr Radiol.* 2011;41:1028–1039.
29. Avitzur Y, Wang JY, de Silva NT, et al. The impact of intestinal rehabilitation program and its innovative therapies on the outcome of intestine transplant candidates. *J Pediatr Gastroenterol Nutr.* 2015;61(1):18–23.
30. Fazzolare T, Remaley L, Mazariegos G. Pediatric intestinal and multivisceral transplantation. In: Remaley L, McGhee W, Reyes J, et al., eds. *The Pediatric Transplant Manual.* 2nd ed. Hudson, OH: Lexi-Comp; 2009:79–91.
31. Xie J, Talaska AE, Schacht J. New developments in aminoglycoside therapy and ototoxicity. *Hear Res.* 2011;281(1–2):28–37.
32. Stoopler ET, Kuperstein AS. Glossitis secondary to vitamin B12 deficiency anemia. *CMAJ.* 2013;185(12):E582.
33. Kyle U, Shekerdemian L, Coss-Bu J. Growth failure and nutrition: considerations in chronic childhood wasting diseases. *Nutr Clin Pract.* 2015;30:227–238.
34. Kaufman SS, Atkinsin JV, Bianchi A, et al. Indications for pediatric intestinal transplantation: a position paper of the American Society of Transplantation. *Pediatr Transplant.* 2001;5:80–87.
35. Kato T, Selvaggi G, Gaynor J, et al. Inclusion of donor colon and ileocecal valve in intestinal transplantation. *Transplantation.* 2008;86(2):293–297.
36. Wunderlich H, Brockman JG, Voight R, et al. DTG procurement guidelines in heart beating donors. *Transpl Int.* 2011;24:733–757.
37. Nickkholgh A, Contin P, Abu-Elmagd K, et al. Intestinal transplantation: review of operative techniques. *Clin Transplant.* 2013;27(suppl 25):56–65.
38. Soltys K, Bond G. Surgical procedures in pediatric abdominal transplantation. In: Remaley L, McGhee W, Reyes J, et al., eds. *The Pediatric Transplant Manual.* 2nd ed. Hudson, OH: Lexi-Comp; 2009:Appendix II.
39. Farmer DG. Isolated small bowel transplantation and combined liver-small bowel transplantation. In: Lagnas A, Goulet O, Quigley E, et al., eds. *Intestinal Failure: Diagnosis, Management and Transplantation.* Malden, MA: Blackwell Publishing; 2008:254–269.
40. Sudan D. The current state of intestine transplantation: indications, techniques, outcomes and challenges. *Am J Transplant.* 2014;14:1976–1984.
41. Todo S, Reyes J, Furukawa H, et al. Outcome analysis of 71 clinical transplantations. *Ann Surg.* 1995; 222(3):270–282.
42. Matsumoto CA, Kaufman SS, Fishbein TM. Inclusion of the colon in intestinal transplantation. *Curr Opin Organ Transplant.* 2011;16:312–315.
43. Abu-Elmagd K, Costa G, Bond GJ, et al. Five hundred intestinal and multivisceral transplantations at a single center: major advances with new challenges. *Ann Surg.* 2009;250:567–581.
44. Mazariegos GV, Soltys K, Bond GJ, et al. Pediatric intestinal retransplantation: techniques, management, and outcomes. *Transplantation.* 2008;86(12):1777–1782.

45. Reyes J, Mazariegos GV, Abu-Elmagd KM, et al. Intestinal transplantation under tacrolimus monotherapy after perioperative lymphoid depletion with rATG. *Am J Transplant.* 2005;5:1430–1436.

46. Tzvetanov IG, Oberholzer J, Benedetti E. Current status of living donor small bowel transplantation. *Curr Opin Organ Transplant.* 2010;15(3):346–348.

47. Benedetti E, Panaro F, Testa G. Living donor intestinal transplantation. In: Lagnas A, Goulet O, Quigley E, et al., eds. *Intestinal Failure: Diagnosis, Management and Transplantation.* Malden, MA: Blackwell Publishing; 2008:262–269.

48. Gangemi A, Tzvetanov IG, Beatty E, et al. Lessons learned in pediatric small bowel and liver transplantation from living-related donors. *Transplantation.* 2009;87(7):1027–1030.

49. Smith JM, Skeans MA, Horslen SP, et al. OPTN/SRTR 2012 data report. *Intest Am J Transplant.* 2014;14 (suppl 1):97–111.

50. Grant WJ. Surgical complications of intestinal transplantation. In: Lagnas A, Goulet O, Quigley E, et al., eds. *Intestinal Failure: Diagnosis, Management and Transplantation.* Malden, MA: Blackwell Publishing; 2008:290–296.

51. Kato T, Tzakis A, Selvaggi G, et al. Intestinal and multivisceral transplantation in children. *Ann Surg.* 2006; 243:756–766.

52. Goulet O, Sauvat F, Ruemmele F, et al. Results of the Paris program: ten years of pediatric intestinal transplantation. *Transplant Proc.* 2005;37:1667–1670.

53. Harris P. Skin, incision and ostomy care in the pediatric transplant patient. In: Remaley L, McGhee W, Reyes J, et al., eds. *The Pediatric Transplant Manual.* 2nd ed. Hudson, OH: Lexi-Comp; 2009:99–105.

54. Fryer J. Intestine transplantation. In: Stuart F, Abecassis M, Kaufman D, eds. *Organ Transplantation.* 2nd ed. Georgetown, TX: Landes Bioscience; 2003:244–460.

55. Palocaren M. An overview of intestine and multivisceral transplant. *Critical Care Nurs Clin N Am.* 2011;23:457–469.

56. Cladis F. Pain management following kidney, liver, intestine and multivisceral transplantation. In: Remaley L, McGhee W, Reyes J, et al., eds. *The Pediatric Transplant Manual.* 2nd ed. Hudson, OH: Lexi-Comp; 2009:92–98.

57. Hauser GJ, Plotkin J, Fishbein T. Immediate postoperative care of the intestinal transplant recipient. In: Lagnas A, Goulet O, Quigley E, et al., eds. *Intestinal Failure: Diagnosis, Management and Transplantation.* Malden, MA: Blackwell Publishing; 2008:283–289.

58. Horslen S. Optimal management of the post-intestinal transplant patient. *Gastroenterology.* 2006;130 (suppl):163–169.

59. Remaley L, Fazzolare T, Mazariegos G. Daily management and care of the pediatric transplant recipient. In: Remaley L, McGhee W, Reyes J, et al., eds. *The Pediatric Transplant Manual.* 2nd ed. Hudson, OH: Lexi-Comp; 2009: 150–175.

60. Garcia-Roca R, Gruessner R. Immununosuppression after intestine transplantation. In: Lagnas A, Goulet O, Quigley E, et al., eds. *Intestinal Failure: Diagnosis, Management and Transplantation.* Malden, MA: Blackwell Publishing; 2008:305–310.

61. Nayyar N, Mazariegos G, Ranganathan S, et al. Pediatric small bowel transplantation. *Semin Pediatr Surg.* 2010; 19:68–77.

62. Starzl TE, Murase N, Abu-Elmagd K, et al. Tolerogenic immunosuppression for organ transplantation. *Lancet.* 2003;3:1502–1510.

63. Newell K, Fryer J. Immunology of intestinal allograft rejection. In: Lagnas A, Goulet O, Quigley E, et al., eds. *Intestinal Failure: Diagnosis, Management and Transplantation.* Malden, MA: Blackwell Publishing; 2008:314–321.

64. Kaneku H, Wozniak LJ. Donor-specific human leukocyte antigen antibodies in intestinal transplantation. *Curr Opin Organ Transplant.* 2014;19(3):261–266.

65. Kubal CA, Mangus RS, Vianna RM, et al. Impact of positive flow cytometry crossmatch on outcomes of intestinal/multivisceral transplantation: role of anti-IL-2 receptor antibody. *Transplantation.* 2013;95:1160–1166.

66. Mazariegos G, Reyes J, Abu-Elmagd K, et al. Intestinal and multiple organ transplantation. In: Shoemaker WC, Ayers SM, Grenvik A, et al., eds. *Critical Care Medicine.* Philadelphia: Lippincott Williams & Wilkins; 2004.

67. Malone F, Horslen SP. Long-term management of intestinal transplant recipients. In: Lagnas A, Goulet O, Quigley E, et al., eds. *Intestinal Failure: Diagnosis, Management and Transplantation.* Malden, MA: Blackwell Publishing; 2008:331–334.

68. Wu T, Abu-Elmagd K, Bond G, et al. A schema for histologic grading of small intestine allograft acute rejection. *Transplantation.* 2004;75:1241–1248.

69. Mazariegos GV, Abu-Elmagd K, Jaffe R, et al. Graft versus host disease in intestinal transplant. *Am J Transplant.* 2004;4:1459–1465.

70. Vianna, RM Mangus RS, Fridell JA, et al. Induction immunosuppression with thymoglobulin and rituximab in intestinal and multivisceral transplantation. *Transplantation.* 2008;85:1290–1293.

71. Andres A, Santamaria M, Ramos E, et al. Graft-vs-host disease after small bowel transplantation in children. *J Pediatr Surg.* 2010;45:330–336.

72. Freifeld A, Kalil A. Infections in small bowel transplant recipients. In: Lagnas A, Goulet O, Quigley E, et al., eds. *Intestinal Failure: Diagnosis, Management and Transplantation.* Malden, MA: Blackwell Publishing; 2008:297–304.

73. Gaynor JJ, Kato T, Selvaggi G, et al. The importance of analyzing graft and patient survival by cause of failure: an example using pediatric small intestine transplant data. *Transplantation.* 2006;81:1133–1140.

74. Gonzalez I, Green M. Infections of the pediatric liver, intestine and multivisceral transplant recipient. In: Remaley L, McGhee W, Reyes J, et al., eds. *The Pediatric Transplant Manual.* 2nd ed. Hudson, OH: Lexi-Comp; 2009:111–129.

75. vanDelden C. Timeline of infections after organ transplantation. In: Kumar D, Humar A, eds. *The AST Handbook of Transplant Infections.* Hoboken, NJ: Wiley-Blackwell; 2011:3.

76. Reyes J, Green M. Risks and epidemiology of infection. In: Bowden R, Ljungman P, Paya C, eds. *Transplant Infections.* 2nd ed. New York, NY: Lippincott Williams & Wilkins; 2004:132–139.

77. Sigurdsson L, Reyes J, Kocoshis S, et al. Bacteremia after intestinal transplantation in children correlates temporarily with rejection or gastrointestinal lymphoproliferative disease. *Transplantation.* 2002;70:302–305.

78. Bures J, Cyrany J, Kohoutova D, et al. Small intestinal bacterial overgrowth syndrome. *World J Gastroenterol.* 2010;16(24):2978–2990.

79. Morris M. Management of selected fungal infections after transplantation. In: Kumar D, Humar A, eds. *The AST Handbook of Transplant Infections.* Hoboken, NJ: Wiley-Blackwell; 2011:68–72.

80. Guaraldi G, Cocchi S, Codeluppi M, et al. Outcome, incidence and timing of infectious complications in small bowel and multivisceral organ transplantation patients. *Transplantation.* 2005;80:742–1748.

81. Florescu D, Abu-Elmagd K, Mercer D, et al. An international survey of cytomegalovirus prevention and treatment practices in intestinal transplantation. *Transplantation.* 2014;97(1):78–82.

82. Green M, Webber S. Post-transplantation lymphoproliferative disorders. *Pediatr Clin N Am.* 2003;50:1471–1491.

83. Madan R, Herold B. Epstein-Barr virus and post-transplant lymphoporliferatice disorders. In: Kumar D, Humar A, eds. *The AST Handbook of Transplant Infections.* Hoboken, NJ: Wiley-Blackwell; 2011:42–44.

84. Abu-Elmagd KM, Mazariegos G, Costa G, et al. Lymphoproliferative disorders and de novo malignancies in intestinal and multivisceral recipients: improved outcomes with new outlooks. *Transplantation.* 2009;88(7):926–934.

85. Strohm S. Parenteral and enteral nutrition in the pediatric transplant patient. In: Remaley L, McGhee W, Reyes J, et al., eds. *The Pediatric Transplant Manual.* 2nd ed. Hudson, OH: Lexi-Comp; 2009:106–110.

86. Kowalski L, Nucci A, Reyes J. Intestinal transplantation. In Rolandelli RH, Boullata J, Compher C, eds. *Clinical Nutrition: Enteral and Tube Feeding.* 4th ed. Philadelphia, PA: Elsevier; 2005: 523–529.

87. Nucci A, Barksdale E, Beserock N, et al. Long-term nutritional outcomes after pediatric intestinal transplantation. *J Pediatr Surg.* 2002;37(3):460–463.

SELF-ASSESSMENT QUESTIONS

1. Which of the following is *not* descriptive of intestinal failure?
   a. Inadequate gut mass to maintain fluid and nutritional requirements
   b. Always includes liver disease
   c. Can be due to motility or absorptive disorders
   d. Nutrition supplied primarily by TPN

2. Which of the following treatments/therapies could be used in a patient with intestinal failure?
   1. Omega-3 lipid formulation
   2. Teduglutide
   3. Serial transverse enteroplasty procedure
   4. Ethanol locks
   a. 1, 3, 4
   b. 2, 3, 4
   c. 1, 2, 3
   d. 1, 2, 3, 4

3. You are caring for a 23-year-old female who is listed for a multivisceral transplant. She is ill but stable and is hospitalized for supportive care as she waits for an organ. Which of the following would preclude transplant when an organ is offered?
   a. Positive blood cultures with *Klebsiella*
   b. History of nonadherence to medications and medical care
   c. Ammonia level of 200 µmol/L
   d. Seizure disorder controlled with phenytoin

4. You are caring for a 10-year-old boy following isolated intestine transplant on postoperative day 2. He has become increasingly tachycardic and his blood pressure is 80/55. JP drainage has increased serosanguineous fluid. The abdomen is mildly distended. His hemoglobin is 9.2 g%. The ileostomy drainage is 40 mL/kg/d and watery brown. He is afebrile. What do you suspect?
   a. Vascular thrombosis
   b. Postoperative hemorrhage
   c. Acute rejection
   d. Perforation of the intestine graft

5. During the early postoperative period (weeks 1 to 6), surveillance endoscopies are usually performed:
   a. when the stool output is 1 to 2 L/day in an adult.
   b. if tacrolimus levels are <10 ng/mL.
   c. twice weekly.
   d. only if febrile.

6. Your patient is a 35-year-old female at 2 weeks postintestine transplant. Enteral feedings via a GT are ordered at 40 mL/hour continuously. Her complaints of nausea are increasing, and she has vomited a large amount of formula. She is afebrile. What is your first nursing intervention prior to informing the physician?
   a. Stop the infusion of formula.
   b. Decrease the rate to 20 mL/hour.
   c. Increase the IV fluid rate.
   d. Assess the ileostomy drainage.

7. In this patient (#6), what other issue might be considered in regard to nausea and vomiting?
   a. Rejection
   b. Decreased gastric motility
   c. Food allergies
   d. Oral aversion

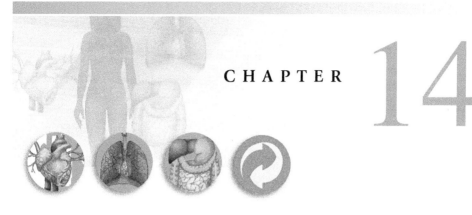

C H A P T E R

14

Kidney Transplantation

Wendy Escobedo, RN, MSN, PHN, CCTN

Ashley H. Seawright, DNP, ACNP-BC

 I. INTRODUCTION

   A. Transplantation provides an opportunity to leave the rigors of dialysis behind and improve the quality of life for chronic kidney disease patients.

      1. Thousands of patients in countries worldwide are awaiting a new kidney.

      2. Table 14-1 provides data on patients awaiting renal transplantation in the United States, Australia, Eurotransplant, and the United Kingdom.[1-4]

      3. In the United States, there are also 1,971 individuals awaiting simultaneous kidney-pancreas transplantation.[1]

      4. Thousands of others throughout the world are in the process of being evaluated or scheduled for living donor transplantation.

      5. Economically, transplantation is the most cost-effective treatment for chronic kidney disease.[5-7]

   B. This chapter provides information on the evaluation and preparation for kidney transplantation and the complex postoperative nursing care required.

      1. To have a clear understanding of both the pre- and the postrenal transplant process, it is necessary to have knowledge of renal function, causes of chronic kidney disease (CKD), and the manifestations of abnormal renal function.

      2. In most cases, early kidney disease is a silent and insidious process.

         a. Patients accommodate to their worsening physiological condition without realizing they are doing so and often without being aware they have a health problem.

         b. Renal failure often is not recognized until the patients have irreversibly lost a significant percentage of their kidney function and have multiple manifestations of renal disease.

         c. The state where all or most kidney function has been lost and dialysis is indicated has traditionally been referred to as end-stage renal disease (ESRD).

         d. The current term used to describe this state is chronic kidney disease (CKD), and this term will be used throughout this chapter.

TABLE 14-1 **Patients Awaiting Renal Transplant (as of August 2015)**

Country	Number of Patients
United States[1]	101,021
Australia[2]	1,073
Eurotransplant[3]	11,080
Austria, Belgium, Croatia, Germany, Hungary Luxembourg, the Netherlands, and Slovenia	
United Kingdom[4]	5,465

C. The kidneys:
1. Are paired organs
2. Sit behind the peritoneum at approximately the level of the first lumbar vertebra
3. Receive their blood supply via the renal arteries and are drained via the renal veins
   a. It is not uncommon to have two to three renal arteries supplying each kidney.
   b. It is less common to have multiple renal veins.
4. Perform numerous functions (see Table 14-2)[8]
   a. Primary product, urine, is drained via the ureters into the urinary bladder.
      i.   On occasion, there may be two ureters from a single kidney.
      ii. The bladder is a hollow muscular organ that is readily distensible and has a capacity of 500 mL.
   b. The urine produced contains waste products, electrolytes, and other substances outlined in Table 14-3.[8]
   c. Abnormalities in the urine composition such as the presence of protein, blood cells, glucose, or other substances can indicate renal or systemic disease.
   d. The nephron is the basic structural and functional unit of the kidney, with each kidney having approximately 1 million nephrons.[9]
      i.   Each nephron is capable of carrying out all of the functions of the kidney.
      ii. About 50% of the nephrons must be impaired before the creatinine will rise.
   e. When the kidneys fail, dialysis or transplantation is required to sustain life.

TABLE 14-2 **Major Kidney Functions**

- Excretion of most metabolic end products of the body
- Control of fluid and electrolyte balance
- Maintenance of acid-base balance
- Production of erythropoietin for stimulation of red blood cell production
- Activation of vitamin D to facilitate calcium absorption
- Production of renin as part of the renin/angiotensin system for blood pressure control

From Hall JE. *Guyton & Hall Textbook of Medical Physiology.* 13th ed. Philadelphia, PA: WB Saunders; 2015; Briggs JP, Kriz W, Schnermann JB. Overview of kidney function and structure. In: Gilbert SJ, Weiner DE, Gipson DS, et al., eds. *National Kidney Foundation's Primer on Kidney Diseases.* 6th ed. Philadelphia, PA: Elsevier Saunders; 2014:2–18.

TABLE 14-3 Urine Composition

Common Substances Found in Urine

Water

Nitrogenous waste products: creatinine, urea, uric acid, ammonia

Electrolytes: sodium, potassium, ammonia, chloride, bicarbonate, phosphate, sulfate, minerals

Hormones

Other: drug metabolites, bacterial toxins, pigments

Abnormal substances: glucose, albumin, protein, red blood cells, white blood cells, casts, calculi

From Hall JE. *Guyton & Hall Textbook of Medical Physiology*. 13th ed. Philadelphia, PA: WB Saunders; 2015; Briggs JP, Kriz W, Schnermann JB. Overview of kidney function and structure. In: Gilbert SJ, Weiner DE, Gipson DS, et al., eds. *National Kidney Foundation's Primer on Kidney Diseases*. 6th ed. Philadelphia, PA: Elsevier Saunders; 2014:2–18.

 II. CHRONIC KIDNEY DISEASE

    A. Etiology

        1. The causes of CKD are many (Table 14-4), but diabetes mellitus (DM), hypertension, and glomerulonephritis account for the majority of patients with CKD.

          a. These three diseases account for almost 80% of all patients on dialysis.[10]

          b. DM is the most common cause of CKD.

        2. Although all forms of glomerulonephritis may recur, focal segmental glomerulosclerosis has the highest rate of recurrence.

        3. Other causes of CKD that may recur include Henoch-Schönlein purpura, amyloidosis, hemolytic-uremic syndrome, and oxalosis.[11]

TABLE 14-4 Major Causes of Chronic Kidney Disease

Most common causes of CKD:
- Diabetes mellitus
- Hypertension
- Glomerulonephritis

Cystic disorders:
- Polycystic kidney disease
- Medullary cystic disease
- Acquired cystic diseases

Urinary tract abnormalities:
- Reflux nephropathy
- Posterior ureteral valves
- Neurogenic bladder

Tubular disorders:
- Renal tubular acidosis
- Fanconi's syndrome

Obstructive disorders:
- Renal calculi
- Retroperitoneal fibrosis
- Prostatic hypertrophy

(continued)

TABLE 14-4 Major Causes of Chronic Kidney Disease (*Continued*)

Autoimmune disorders:
- Goodpasture's disease
- Wegener's disease
- Systemic lupus erythematosus
- IgA nephropathy

Hemolytic disorders:
- Hemolytic-uremic syndrome
- Thrombotic thrombocytopenic purpura

Nephrotoxic agents:
- Cyclosporine
- Gentamicin
- Nonsteroidal anti-inflammatory drugs
- Analgesics
- Intravenous contrast dyes

Cancers:
- Multiple myeloma
- Renal cell cancer

Congenital disorders:
- Renal agenesis
- Renal aplasia

Others:
- Amyloidosis
- Oxalosis
- Henoch-Schönlein purpura
- Interstitial nephritis
- Nephrotic syndrome
- Focal segmental glomerulosclerosis
- Human immunodeficiency virus nephropathy
- Pyelonephritis

HIV, human immunodeficiency virus.
From Whittier WL, Lewis EJ. Pathophysiology of chronic kidney disease. In: Gilbert SJ, Weiner DE, Gipson DS, et al., eds. *National Kidney Foundation's Primer on Kidney Diseases*. 6th ed. Philadelphia, PA: Elsevier Saunders; 2014:448–457; Jennette JC, Falk RJ. Glomerular clinicopathologic syndromes. In: Gilbert SJ, Weiner DE, Gipson DS, et al., eds. *National Kidney Foundation's Primer on Kidney Diseases*. 6th ed. Philadelphia, PA: Elsevier Saunders; 2014:152–163.

4. Patients with polycystic kidney disease may require bilateral nephrectomy before or at the time of transplant if the cysts are large, cause frequent infection or bleeding, impinge on surrounding structures, or fail to allow sufficient room for the new kidney.

B. Chronic kidney disease stages
   1. In most cases, CKD occurs over months to years, although some diseases such as rapidly progressive glomerulonephritis can cause permanent damage within weeks or months.
   2. CKD is differentiated from acute disease in that the damage to the kidney lasts for more than 3 months in CKD.

TABLE 14-5 **Stages of Chronic Kidney Disease**

Stage	Description	GFR (mL/min)
1	Kidney damage with normal or increased GFR	≥90
2	Kidney damage with mild decrease in GFR	60–89
3	Moderate decrease in GFR	30–59
4	Severe decrease in GFR	15–29
5	Kidney failure	<15 (or dialysis)

Data from National Kidney Foundation (NKF). K/DOQI Clinical Practice Guidelines For Chronic Kidney Disease: Evaluation, Classification, and Stratification. Available at http://www.kidney.org/professionals/kdoqi/guidelines_ckd/toc.htm. Accessed September 29, 2014.

3. Gradual loss of kidney function is described in five stages (Table 14-5) that have been clearly defined in the clinical practice guidelines by the Kidney Disease Outcomes Quality Initiative (KDOQI).[12]
   a. The staging of CKD enables clinical practice guidelines and performance measures to be used as tools for improving the evaluation and management of CKD.
   b. The two primary markers used to define the stages of disease are
      i. Damage to the kidneys as manifested by abnormalities in blood and/or urine (BUN, creatinine, etc.)
      ii. Level of kidney function as measured by the glomerular filtration rate (GFR)
   c. The stages also indicate how soon renal replacement therapy may be required.
   d. Those in stage 4 should be preparing for dialysis by having access placed or seeking a living donor for preemptive transplant.
   e. Those who have reached stage 5 are in need of immediate renal replacement therapy.

C. Manifestations of chronic CKD
   1. As it progresses, CKD leads to a syndrome known as uremia, which literally means urine in the blood and refers to the buildup of waste products, excess electrolytes, and toxins in the blood.
   2. Physical signs and symptoms develop due to the presence of unfiltered waste products and the loss of kidney function.
      a. CKD can affect the most elemental of patient parameters, the vital signs.
         i. Despite an increased susceptibility to infection, CKD patients may have a subnormal temperature as BUN acts as a hypothermic agent.
         ii. Tachycardia is often present in response to cardiac and volume changes.
         iii. Tachypnea can be present as a compensatory response to metabolic acidosis.
         iv. Blood pressure (BP) can be normal but is often elevated due to the cardiovascular changes that occur in many diseases that cause kidney disease.
      b. CKD disease evolves into a multisystem disease affecting many aspects of bodily function.
      c. Table 14-6 describes clinical symptoms that may develop with a diagnosis of CKD.[8,13–15]

TABLE 14-6 Systemic Effects of Chronic Kidney Disease

System	Effect of Disturbance
Cardiovascular disturbances	Hypertension
	Left ventricular hypertrophy
	Congestive heart failure
	Pericarditis
	Pericardial effusion
	Pericardial tamponade
	Edema of extremities
Gastrointestinal disturbances	Uremic fetor
	Nausea
	Vomiting
	Gastritis
	Diarrhea
	Anorexia
	Gastrointestinal bleeding
	Stomatitis
	Gastritis
	Peptic ulcer disease
Musculoskeletal disturbances	Renal osteodystrophy
	Osteitis fibrosa/osteomalacia
	Muscle wasting
	Muscle irritability
	Bone pain
	Bone fractures
Pulmonary disturbances	Pulmonary edema
	Pleuritis
	Dyspnea
	Pneumonia
	Tachypnea
Hematologic disturbances	Anemia
	Impaired platelet function
	Infection
Neurologic disturbances	Drowsiness, fatigue
	Muscle twitching
	Headache
	Confusion
	Delirium
	Tremors
	Seizures
	Coma
	Peripheral neuropathy
	Sleep disturbances
	Paresthesias
	Restless legs syndrome
	Motor weakness

TABLE 14-6 Systemic Effects of Chronic Kidney Disease (*Continued*)

System	Effect of Disturbance
Genitourinary disturbances	Oliguria Anuria Urinary tract infections Proteinuria
Metabolic/electrolyte/acid-base disturbances	Hyperkalemia Hyperlipidemia Acidosis Hypo-/hypercalcemia Hypoalbuminemia Hyperphosphatemia Carbohydrate intolerance Waste product accumulation
Endocrine disturbances	Altered insulin metabolism Reduced insulin requirements Peripheral insulin resistance Thyroid abnormalities Hyperparathyroidism
Reproductive disturbances	Amenorrhea Impotence Infertility
Integumentary disturbances	Uremic frost Pallor, pigmentation changes Pruritus, dry/scaly skin Ecchymosis Excoriations Calcium-phosphate deposits
Psychologic disturbances	Anxiety Depression Noncompliance Denial Psychosis

From Hall JE. *Guyton & Hall Textbook of Medical Physiology*. 13th ed. Philadelphia, PA: WB Saunders; 2015; Patton KT, Thibodeau GA. *Anatomy and Physiology*. 7th ed. St. Louis, MO: Mosby; 2010; Inker LA, Levey AS. Staging and management of chronic kidney disease. In: Gilbert SJ, Weiner DE, Gipson DS, et al., eds. *National Kidney Foundation's Primer on Kidney Diseases*. 6th ed. Philadelphia, PA: Elsevier Saunders; 2014:458–466; Hain DJ, Haras MS. Chronic kidney disease. In: *Core Curriculum for Nephrology Nursing*. 6th ed. Pitman, NJ: ANNA; 2015:153–182.

3. Although dialysis can improve fluid and electrolyte balance and remove waste products, other measures are necessary to prevent and treat the many symptoms and complications of CKD:
   a. Dietary restrictions/modifications
   b. Antihypertensive therapy
   c. Iron replacement
   d. Stimulation of red blood cell production
   e. Control of calcium and phosphate levels

D. Radiologic and invasive testing for CKD
1. As described earlier, CKD is defined by stages that enable the application of guidelines for treatment and management.
   a. In order to determine the stage of CKD and the underlying cause of the CKD, patients typically undergo radiologic and invasive testing in addition to routine lab work.
   b. Imaging of the kidneys provides information on the size and structural abnormalities of the kidneys:
      i. Renal or abdominal ultrasound
      ii. Computed tomography (CT)
      iii. Magnetic resonance imaging (MRI)
   c. A renal biopsy provides tissue for histological classification of the disease.
   d. A 24-hour urine for creatinine and protein may be collected. This test provides information regarding the severity of the kidney disease.
   e. An excellent test to determine the degree of renal dysfunction is a nuclear medicine glomerular filtration rate.
   f. These diagnostic studies provide information regarding the potential causes and reversibility of the kidney disease and help guide treatment and prevention of further loss of function.

III. EVALUATION FOR KIDNEY TRANSPLANTATION

A. The evaluation process and acceptance criteria for renal transplant candidates differ from program to program and from country to country. The evaluation should be tailored according to patient-specific conditions.
1. Patients who may be considered acceptable candidates by one program may be deemed unacceptable by another.
2. There is no one set of definitive acceptance or rejection criteria or methodology for assessment.

B. Physical assessment
1. Physiologically, the potential candidate must be able to undergo and withstand the transplant procedure itself and have a low risk of long-term morbidity and mortality.
2. Cardiovascular function, respiratory status, body mass index, and the absence of defined contraindications form the basis of the assessment.
3. Major contraindications are listed in Table 14-7.[16]
4. Although some of these criteria and/or contraindications will exclude a patient at the time of initial assessment, if they can be resolved, the patient can be reassessed.
   a. Examples of this would be obese patients who complete a weight reduction program or patients with symptomatic coronary artery disease who undergo coronary artery bypass graft surgery.
5. Older age, in itself, is not a definitive contraindication because physiologic age is more important than chronologic age.
6. Physical assessment is aimed at determining a patient's potential morbidity and mortality in both the short term and long term.
7. A battery of laboratory, tissue and blood-typing, and radiologic and diagnostic tests are required to determine the state of a potential candidate's health (see Table 14-8).
8. Certain patients may require additional tests and procedures depending on their medical history.

TABLE 14-7 **Contraindications to Kidney Transplantation**

- Active or current malignancy
- Active infection
- Significant peripheral vascular disease (that would interfere with surgical anastomoses)
- Untreatable end-stage diseases of other organs, for example, inoperable coronary artery or valvular disease, severe cardiomyopathy, end-stage emphysema
- Active inflammatory disease (systemic)
- Noncompliance
- Active substance abuse; current recreational drug abuse
- Untreated psychiatric illness or mental incapacity without an adequate support system
- Active peptic ulcer disease
- Irreversible rehabilitative potential
- Primary oxalosis

From Bunnapradist S, Danovitch GM. Evaluation of adult kidney transplant candidates. In: Danovitch GM, ed. *Handbook of Kidney Transplantation*. 5th ed. Philadelphia, PA: Lippincott Williams & Wilkins; 2010:157–180.

9. Based on the evaluation results, the interdisciplinary team members will determine if a candidate falls within the range of acceptable risk.
10. It must be understood that if a patient is deemed not a candidate on one occasion, periodic reevaluation may be considered to determine if there have been changes such that the patient may now meet physiological and/or psychosocial eligibility criteria for transplantation.

C. Psychosocial assessment
1. The psychosocial assessment of patients is of particular importance to the long-term success of kidney transplantation.
   a. Major components of the psychosocial evaluation include
      i. Psychiatric history
      ii. Adherence history
      iii. Substance abuse history
      iv. Mental status
      v. Social history
      vi. Availability of social support
      vii. Family social and mental health history
      viii. Perceived health, coping style, and quality of life[17]
      ix. Presence of any religious or cultural concerns
         - Are there any objections to receiving blood or blood products?
            ○ Certain religious faiths such as Jehovah's Witnesses do not accept blood products under any circumstances.
            ○ The risks associated with this belief must be carefully discussed before proceeding.
         - Consideration must be given as well to cultural norms and values.
      x. When the nursing assessment indicates that cultural or religious norms could be a concern, they should be fully investigated, seeking experts as needed to ensure that no cultural norms or values are violated. Examples include
         - Dietary restrictions
         - Use of herbal or alternative therapies

TABLE 14-8 Pretransplant Tests and Investigations for Potential Kidney Transplant Recipients

Laboratory tests: blood and urine	*Hematology:*
	• Complete blood count (CBC) with differential
	• PT, INR, PTT
	Chemistry panel:
	• Sodium, potassium, carbon dioxide, chloride, creatinine, blood urea nitrogen, blood glucose
	Liver function tests
	Urine: (If patient is able to produce urine)
	• Culture, urinalysis, 24-hour urine for protein and creatinine
	Serology:
	• Hepatitis B surface antigen and antibodies
	• Hepatitis C PCR
	• CMV, EBV, HSV, VZV
	• HIV
	• VDRL
	Others:
	• Papanicolaou (PAP) smear
	• Prostate-specific antigen (men 50 or older)
	• PPD
	• Hemoglobin A1C (diabetics)
	• Pregnancy test (females)
Tissue- and blood-typing tests	• ABO blood typing
	• Tissue typing
	• Panel reactive antibodies (PRA)
	• Crossmatch
Radiologic/diagnostic tests	• Chest x-ray
	• Electrocardiogram
	• Pulmonary function tests*
	• Mammogram (women 40 or older)
	• Cardiac echocardiogram*
	• Stress test*
	• Cardiac catheterization*
	• Abdominal computed tomography*
	• Magnetic resonance imaging*
	• Noninvasive vascular studies*
	• Voiding cystourethrogram (VCUG)
Physical exams	• Full history and physical by a transplant nephrologist and surgeon
	• Psychosocial assessment by CSW
	• Gynecologic exam (females)
	• Prostate exam (males)

*If indicated by exam or other studies.
aPTT, activated partial thromboplastin time; CMV, cytomegalovirus; EBV, Epstein-Barr virus; HIV, human immunodeficiency virus; HSV, herpes simplex virus; INR, international normalized ratio; PCR, polymerase chain reaction; PPD, purified protein derivative; PT, prothrombin time; VDRL, venereal disease research laboratories; VZV, varicella-zoster virus.
From Bunnapradist S, Danovitch GM. Evaluation of adult kidney transplant candidates. In: Danovitch GM, ed. *Handbook of Kidney Transplantation*. 5th ed. Philadelphia, PA: Lippincott Williams & Wilkins; 2010:157–180.

  b. Psychosocial support

   i. Patients need to be able to care for themselves posttransplant or have a support network in place that is capable of assisting them.

   ii. Posttransplant self-care is critical to graft and, at times, patient survival.

   iii. Regular attendance at posttransplant clinics, adherence to all aspects of the posttransplant medical regimen, and awareness of the signs and symptoms of rejection and infection are all a shared responsibility among the transplant center, the patients, and their support network.

  c. Adherence

   i. As well as assessing patients' and their support systems' ability to cope with the rigors of posttransplant life, an assessment of patients' history of adherence to medical management must be done.

   ii. Patients should demonstrate reliability in this regard before being allowed to proceed.

   iii. For patients who have not been able to demonstrate consistent adherence, contracts of varying lengths can be established. These contracts provide detailed criteria patients must meet to be accepted for transplantation in the future.

    • This may not be an accepted practice at all centers and in all countries.

  d. Patients who are actively abusing illegal or legal substances or have an untreated psychiatric disorder do not meet eligibility criteria for transplantation.[18]

  e. For all patients, ensuring that they have a current and long-term source of income to cover hospitalization, their medications, and posttransplant costs is essential.

   i. In a large number of Western countries, organ transplant services and medications are provided to patients either free of charge or with minimal charge through National Health Services or National Social Insurance Plans.

   ii. In the United States, the coverage for transplantation and posttransplant medications can be provided by a wide variety of private and governmental insurance programs.

    • For those patients with adequate insurance, the appropriate approvals and authorizations are obtained.

    • Patients who are uninsured or underinsured are assisted in completing the paperwork necessary to obtain adequate coverage.

    • No kidney patients are ever refused transplantation on the basis of inability to pay.

2. Psychosocial evaluations must be completed by a trained professional such as a licensed social worker.

3. Additional assessment by a psychologist or psychiatrist familiar with transplantation may be necessary in cases where the initial assessment is equivocal or for individuals with a history of significant psychiatric or compliance issues.

  a. In the United States, there are regulatory standards that require the availability of psychiatric and social support services in transplant programs.

4. For additional information, see chapters on Solid Organ Transplantation: The Evaluation Process and Psychosocial Issues in Transplantation.

IV. PRETRANSPLANT EDUCATION AND THE EVALUATION PROCESS

A. Not only is the patient assessment process a time when the transplant team evaluates patients, it is also a time to educate patients and members of their support system.

B. Clear, concise, understandable, and structured education sessions should be provided to all potential transplant patients and members of their support system.

C. Topics should include
   1. The transplant evaluation process
   2. Responsibilities while awaiting transplant
   3. National and center-specific transplant outcome data
   4. Transplant surgery
   5. Posttransplant management and responsibilities
   6. Importance of adherence with the medical regimen
   7. Potential complications
   8. Options of living versus deceased donor transplantation
   9. Options such as Kidney Paired Donation, blood type incompatible transplant, or desensitization protocols if the patient has a willing but incompatible donor

D. These sessions ideally should occur at the first stage of the patient evaluation process and be repeated as necessary throughout the evaluation process.
   1. Early education provides benefits to both the patients and the transplant team.

E. Additionally, it is important to:
   1. Introduce patients and families to other patients who have undergone transplantation
   2. Provide patients with ample time to ask questions
   3. Provide patients and families with information on support groups and continuing education on transplantation

F. Table 14-9 describes benefits of early patient education.

G. For additional information, see chapter on Education for Transplant Patients and Caregivers.

TABLE 14-9 Benefits of Early Patient Education

- Ensures patients have a solid understanding of what is required of them
- Allows patients and their support system to make informed decisions regarding their willingness to proceed to transplant before they and the program commit resources to their evaluation
- Introduces the concept of living donor transplant early in the process, thereby enabling early identification of potential live donors and possible early transplant
- Allows the program to assess the cognitive ability of the patients and their supporters

V. LIVING VERSUS DECEASED DONOR TRANSPLANTATION

A. For those patients who are accepted as transplant candidates and have potential live donors, efforts should be directed toward early live donor transplantation.

1. Living donor assessment may entail the evaluation of a number of potential donors.
2. The general assessment requirements for living donor transplantation are provided in Table 14-10.
3. See Chapter 7 on Care of Living Donors for additional information.

 ## VI. DECEASED DONOR WAITING LIST PATIENT MAINTENANCE

A. If a living donor transplantation is not an option, patients will be placed on the deceased donor transplant waiting list.

B. Waiting times can vary widely depending on patient location, blood type, age, severity of disease, panel reactive antibodies (PRA), and other factors.

C. In the United States, median waiting times range from 3 to 5.3 years.[19]

D. It is necessary to have a process whereby the physical and psychosocial status of listed patients is reviewed on a regular basis to ensure their ongoing suitability for transplantation.

TABLE 14-10 Required Testing for Living Donors As per United Network of Organ Sharing (UNOS)/OPTN Policies optn.transplant.hrsa.gov/ Accessed August 14, 2015

- History and physical: complete medical and social history
- Physical exam to include height, weight, BMI, vital signs, and exam all major organ systems
- Routine blood tests: complete blood count (CBC), platelet count, PT, PTT, chemistry panel (metabolic testing to include electrolytes, BUN, creatinine, transaminase levels, albumin, calcium, phosphorus, alkaline phosphatase, bilirubin), liver function tests, lipid panel, glucose tolerance test (GTT)
- Serology: hepatitis B and C screening, HIV, CMV, EBV, tuberculosis
- Urine tests: urinalysis, urine culture, 24-hour urine for protein and creatinine clearance, HCG quantitative pregnancy testing (premenopausal women without surgical sterilization)
- ABO typing, tissue typing, and crossmatch
- Nephrology/urologic evaluation
- Chest x-ray
- Electrocardiogram
- Cardiac stress test (if >50 years old)
- Magnetic resonance imaging (MRI), angiography, or 3D computed tomography
- Cancer screening
- Psychosocial assessment by LCSW including an evaluation for the presence of behaviors that may increase risk for disease transmission as defined by the U.S. Public Health Service (PHS) 2013 Guidelines
- Donor advocate evaluation
- Informed consent/education

CMV, cytomegalovirus; EBV, Epstein-Barr virus; HIV, human immunodeficiency virus.

E. Close liaison with dialysis programs is important to ensure timely communication of changes in candidates' conditions.

F. Additionally, regular blood work results must be provided to the tissue-typing laboratory for periodic reassessment of the candidate's PRA and, depending on local protocols, pretransplant (prospective) donor/recipient crossmatch.

VII. TRANSPLANT SURGERY

A. Preparation for surgery
1. Kidney transplantation is considered an elective procedure although it may be considered an urgent procedure in deceased donor transplantation.
2. Live donor transplantation has a number of advantages over deceased donor transplantation.
    a. The condition of the candidate can be maximized prior to transplantation.
    b. Organ cold ischemic time is minimized prior to the transplant.
    c. Incidence of delayed graft function is decreased.
    d. Short- and long-term outcomes are better.
    e. The organ is not subjected to the physiological insults that accompany brain death.
    f. The candidate can be dialyzed prior to final preparation for surgery.
    g. Allows for a planned date that is mutually convenient for both the donor and candidate who will receive the organ.
    h. All relevant tests and investigations can be completed.
3. Deceased donor transplantation, in comparison, provides a much shorter time for patient preparation.
    a. When an organ becomes available, the candidate is contacted and detailed information is obtained regarding recent medical history, date of last dialysis, and whether the patient has received any recent blood transfusions.
    b. Questions are directed at ascertaining if there are any impediments to transplantation:
        i.   Any cardiovascular events (myocardial infarction, stroke)
        ii. Recent infections or fevers
        iii. New diagnoses of cancer or any other major medical or surgical events
4. If no contraindications are identified, the patient is asked to proceed to the hospital.
5. Upon admission:
    a. Vital signs are checked.
    b. Blood samples are taken.
    c. If not anuric, a urine sample is sent for analysis and culture.
    d. Full history and physical.
    e. Chest radiograph.
    f. Electrocardiogram (EKG).
    g. The patient is dialyzed, if necessary.
    h. Table 14-11 provides a list of preoperative tests for kidney transplantation.
6. Careful attention should be paid to the results that are critical to patient survival and transplant outcome.
    a. If the patient is febrile or has an elevated white blood cell count, infection must be ruled out before proceeding to transplantation.

TABLE 14-11 Preoperative Tests for Kidney Transplantation

- History and physical including vital signs, weight, height, and oxygen saturation
- Routine blood tests: CBC, chemistry panel, calcium, phosphate, magnesium, liver function tests, PT, INR, aPTT
- Routine urine tests: urinalysis, pregnancy test (females)
- Type and crossmatch for blood (2–4 units)
- ABO typing
- Tissue typing and final crossmatch with donor
- Chest x-ray
- Electrocardiogram

aPTT, activated partial thromboplastin time; CBC, complete blood count; INR, international normalized ratio; PTT, partial thromboplastin time.

    b. If the potassium level is elevated, dialysis will be required to prevent intraoperative arrhythmias.

    c. Coagulation study results such as the partial thromboplastin time (PT), international normalized ratio (INR), and activated partial thromboplastin time (aPTT) must be reviewed given that clotting dysfunction may be present.

        i. A prolonged PT, INR, or PTT may necessitate the use of vitamin K or fresh frozen plasma to minimize intraoperative bleeding.

        ii. Anticoagulants and antiplatelet agents such as warfarin (Coumadin), aspirin, and clopidogrel (Plavix) must be discontinued and reversed when possible.

    d. Although a low hemoglobin level is common in renal failure patients, a hemoglobin level of 8 to 8.5 g/dL may predispose patients to cardiac ischemic events and necessitate preoperative transfusion.

    e. Untreated pneumonias or suspicious lesions on the chest radiograph or serious EKG abnormalities may result in cancellation of the case.

    f. The candidate's cytomegalovirus (CMV) status should also be determined as more aggressive antiviral therapy may be needed postoperatively for CMV-negative recipients who receive kidneys from CMV-positive donors.

    g. Confirmation of tissue typing, compatibility of ABO blood group between donors and recipients, and a negative donor/recipient crossmatch result is of utmost importance to a successful outcome.

    h. Incompatibility of ABO blood groups and/or a positive crossmatch can lead to an immediate hyperacute rejection of the organ.

        i. These results must be ascertained and promptly reported prior to going to surgery.

        ii. It is important to note, however, that there are different degrees of positivity and treatments are available to desensitize patients who have high levels of preformed cytotoxic antibodies, thereby making transplant possible.

    i. If all assessments indicate that the patient is in good health and the crossmatch with the donor is negative, the final preparation for surgery is initiated.

    j. As with any surgical procedure, the patients are not to have any oral intake from the moment they are called in for the transplant.

        i. Critical medications can be given by mouth with sips of water.

        ii. Several units of blood should be typed and crossed for the unlikely event of intraoperative bleeding.

       iii. Generally, patients are given a third- or fourth-generation cephalosporin as a preoperative medication.

       iv. Tacrolimus (Prograf) and/or mycophenolate mofetil (CellCept) or a similar immunosuppressant drug may be given prior to surgery. This may vary by center.

       v. An intravenous corticosteroid such as dexamethasone or methylprednisolone may be given just prior to or early in the transplant surgery.
- Both of these drugs induce suppression of the immune system to prevent rejection.

       vi. If a graft or native fistula is present, the affected extremity should be labeled "no procedures."

       vii. Abdominal scrubs may be done to decrease the risk of infection.

       viii. For peritoneal dialysis patients, the abdomen should be drained just prior to going to surgery and the peritoneal catheter capped.

  k. Throughout the preparation for surgery, close attention should be given to the emotional state of the patient, family, and other members of the patient's support system, as this is a time of great anxiety and uncertainty.

B. Surgical procedure[20]

  1. Upon arrival in the operating room (OR), the patient is placed in a supine position on the OR table and is prepared for surgery by the anesthesia team.

    a. A central venous catheter is inserted, and an arterial line may be placed.

    b. The patient is then anesthetized.

    c. Prophylactic antibiotics are usually given at this time if they were not given on call.

    d. Once the patient is asleep, a bladder catheter is placed and several hundred milliliters of normal saline or antibiotic solution are instilled into the bladder.

       i. Antibiotic solutions help decontaminate the bladder.

       ii. The instilled fluid also distends the bladder thereby facilitating location of the bladder and completion of the ureteric anastomosis.

    e. The operative site is shaved and prepared with a topical anti-infective cleansing agent such as povidone-iodine, and the patient is draped.

  2. The usual placement of the kidney is extraperitoneal in the iliac fossa.

    a. Allows easy access to the iliac vessels and the urinary bladder.

    b. Provides easy access if a biopsy is required.

    c. Alternative placements may be used and are indicated by the recipient size or if both donor kidneys are to be used in the recipient.

       i. If the donor kidneys are from a small child, then both kidneys may be implanted en bloc in the abdomen (Figure 14-1).

       ii. Intra-abdominal placement may also be used if the patient has had previous transplants and multiple abdominal surgeries or the iliac vessels are unsuitable for anastomosis due to vessel disease.

    d. A curved incision is made beginning near the iliac crest and ending above the symphysis pubis in the left or right lower abdomen (Figure 14-2).

       i. The side chosen depends on:
- The donor kidney
- Surgeon's assessment
- Previous surgery
- Future plans for pancreas transplant: use left side if pancreas transplant is anticipated

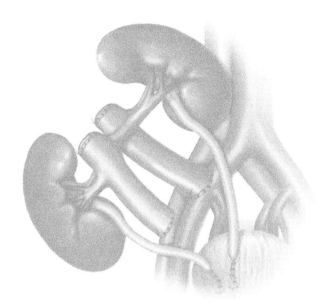

FIGURE 14-1 Illustration of donor kidneys implanted en bloc.

ii. Muscle layers are divided, and the peritoneum is retracted superiorly.
iii. Iliac vessels (external, internal common) are identified.
iv. Selected vessels are dissected out, slung with vascular slings, and clamped proximal and distal to the chosen anastomosis site.
v. The anastomoses may be end-to-end or end-to-side.
vi. The anatomy of the kidney and the quality of both the donor and recipient vessels determine the method of anastomosis.

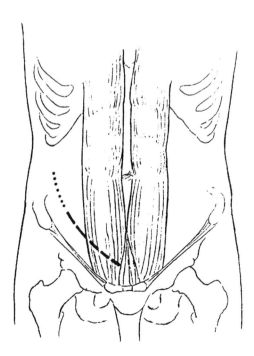

FIGURE 14-2 Illustration of standard incision for adult kidney transplant.

vii. When venous and arterial anastomoses are completed, the clamps are released.
  - The kidney should turn pink and produce urine.
  - Furosemide (Lasix) or mannitol may be given at this time to stimulate urine production.
  - Each vascular anastomosis is checked carefully for leaks.
  - If none are noted, the surgeon will proceed to the bladder anastomosis.

viii. In most cases, the bladder dome is exposed and the muscle is divided along a length of about 4 to 5 cm.
  - A small incision at the distal end of the muscle incision is used to open the bladder mucosa.
  - A small cut is made in the end of the donor ureter to open it out or splay it and it is anastomosed to the mucosa.
  - At many institutions, the anastomosis is over a ureteric stent to ensure patency and facilitate healing of the vesicoureteral anastomosis.
  - The muscle is then closed over the ureter forming a tunnel that acts as an antireflux valve compressing the ureter as the bladder fills.

ix. A final check for hemostasis and the positioning of the vessels is done before closure.

x. One or two low-pressure drains may be placed in the surgical bed.

xi. A standard wound closure is performed using staples or sutures, and anesthesia is reversed.

VIII. POSTTRANSPLANT CARE: MONITORING AND MAINTENANCE

A. Transfer from the OR

  1. Once the surgical transplantation procedure is completed, transplant recipients will be transferred to the ICU or transplant unit for close monitoring and care.
  2. Recipients transferred to the ICU can expect to be there for approximately 24 hours and then transfer to the inpatient transplant unit. Recipients will arrive with:
     a. Urinary catheter.
     b. Central line.
     c. Possibly one or more wound drains.
     d. An arterial line.
     e. Endotracheal tube is typically removed in the OR or postanesthesia care unit.

B. Postoperative management and nursing includes assessing the following:

  1. Vital signs: Parameters should be followed at least hourly for 12 hours, then every 3 hours for 8 hours, and then every 4 hours for stable patients[21] who may then transfer to the general transplant floor.
     a. Temperature
        i. If elevated, may indicate postoperative atelectasis, dehydration, infection, and/or rejection.

    ii. Transplant recipients may not be able to mount a normal fever response due to the effects of immunosuppressant drugs.[22]

   iii. Therefore, nurses must assess the patient for other indicators of infections as well.

   iv. Suspected atelectasis should be addressed with aggressive pulmonary toilet and dehydration with increased fluid infusion.

    v. Possible infections should be evaluated by obtaining blood and urine cultures and a chest radiograph.

   vi. Suspected rejection will require a biopsy for confirmation.

b. Heart rate

    i. Bradycardia may indicate a cardiac problem such as heart block or excessive beta blockade (e.g., with a beta-blocker such as metoprolol [Lopressor]) being used for rate or blood pressure control.

   ii. Tachycardia can be a sign of febrile illness, rebound tachycardia due to the rapid discontinuation of alpha-adrenergic stimulators (e.g., clonidine [Catapres]), or volume status changes such as hypovolemia related to bleeding or dehydration.

c. Respiratory rate

    i. Decreased respirations may be a sign of oversedation or cardiopulmonary problems.

   ii. Rapid respirations may be a response to acidosis or fluid overload.

   iii. Abnormal respiratory patterns should be further investigated by monitoring oxygen saturation levels and, if indicated, arterial blood gases.

d. Blood pressure

    i. Both hypotension and hypertension are detrimental to renal function.

   ii. Causes of hypotension include
- Bleeding
- Dehydration
- Sepsis
- Medications
- Adrenal insufficiency
- Neuropathy
- Can lead to poor perfusion of the renal transplant resulting in:
  - Acute tubular necrosis (ATN)
  - Delayed graft function (DGF)
  - Vascular thrombosis

   iii. Causes of hypertension are[23]
- Persistent chronic hypertension
- Rebound hypertension due to cessation of an adrenergic agent
- Volume overload

   iv. Hypertension can be worsened postoperatively due to:
- Steroids
- Calcineurin inhibitors such as tacrolimus (Prograf)
- Development of renal artery stenosis
- Pain and hypoxia[21]

    v. Persistent hypertension can damage the new kidney, increase the risk of vascular leaks, and increase the chance of cerebrovascular events.[21]

TABLE 14-12 **Hypotension: Monitoring and Maintenance**

Etiology	Associated Signs and Symptoms	Treatment
Postoperative bleeding	Dizziness Decreased level of consciousness Tachycardia	*Bleeding:* Surgical exploration to identify and ligate source Red blood cell transfusions Fluid boluses Administration of vasoconstrictive agents (e.g., Neo-Synephrine)
Dehydration related to postoperative osmotic diuresis		*Dehydration:* Fluid boluses Maintenance intravenous fluids (IV) Replacement of urine output cc for cc with ½ normal saline or 0.9% normal saline
Sepsis	Increased temperature (in sepsis) Tachycardia	*Sepsis:* Fluid boluses Cultures Antibiotics Administration of vasoconstrictive agents, if indicated
Antihypertensive medications		*Antihypertensive-induced:* Withhold antihypertensives Adrenal insufficiency/autonomic neuropathy Midodrine or Florinef administration
Adrenal insufficiency autonomic neuropathy		*General treatment for all etiologies:* Limit activity Frequent vital signs Renal ultrasound to assess blood flow to kidney Evaluate response Consultation with physician

From Hinkle JL, Cheever KH. *Brunner & Suddarth's Textbook of Medical–Surgical Nursing.* 13th ed. Philadelphia, PA: Lippincott Williams & Wilkins; 2013.

      vi.   Systolic BP that exceeds 180 mm Hg should receive immediate treatment.

     vii.   Systolic BP should be kept above 110 mm Hg to avoid complications associated with poor perfusion.

    viii.   The etiology, associated symptoms, and treatments for hypotension and hypertension are varied. See Tables 14-12 and 14-13 for additional information.

2. Laboratory/blood work

    a.   Basic laboratory values provide excellent information regarding kidney function, electrolyte balance, metabolic function, and the presence of postoperative bleeding or infection.[24]

    b.   The transplant procedure can cause electrolyte imbalances such as hyponatremia related to IV infusion of ½ normal saline as a replacement fluid.

TABLE 14-13 **Hypertension: Monitoring and Maintenance**

Etiology	Associated Signs and Symptoms	Treatment
Persistent chronic hypertension	Can be asymptomatic Headache	Resume preoperative antihypertensives as ordered.
Rebound hypertension due to stopping alpha-adrenergic receptor stimulator		If patient was on alpha-adrenergic agent, resume to prevent rebound hypertension. Add additional agents (IV and oral) as ordered.
Volume overload		If volume related, reduce IV infusion rates and/or replacement fluids.
Pain		Pain control
Hypoxia		Oxygenation to maintain oxygen saturation >92% Frequent vital signs and consultation with health care provider as status changes

From Hinkle JL, Cheever KH. *Brunner & Suddarth's Textbook of Medical–Surgical Nursing.* 13th ed. Philadelphia, PA: Lippincott Williams & Wilkins; 2013.

    c. CKD patients have significant lab value abnormalities before transplantation, such as hypocalcemia and anemia, many of which can persist for a time postoperatively, especially if the kidney does not function immediately.

    d. Careful attention to lab values can prevent or allow for the early treatment of complications.

    e. Laboratory indicators of ATN or early nonfunction of the kidney include:

        i. Hyponatremia related to the dilutional effect of fluid retention when the kidney is unable to excrete body water

        ii. Indicators that the kidney is unable to excrete waste products include

- Hyperkalemia
- Increased BUN
- Increased serum creatinine
- Hypermagnesemia
- Hyperphosphatemia
- Decreased carbon dioxide level
- Carbon dioxide is an indirect measure of bicarbonate.
- Levels fall when acid accumulates in renal failure.

    f. If the new kidney works immediately, it is expected that the BUN and creatinine will begin to fall.

        i. Hyponatremia may occur related to aggressive fluid replacement and can usually be corrected by:

- Decreasing the amount of fluid infused
- Increasing the sodium content

        ii. Hypokalemia, hypophosphatemia, and hypomagnesemia may develop as the kidney begins to function and significant diuresis occurs.

        iii. A decreased carbon dioxide level may persist.

    g. All of these values require assessment to determine if the recipient is in ATN or experiencing rejection so the appropriate treatment can be initiated.

    h. See Table 14-14 for normal values for common electrolytes/metabolites.

TABLE 14-14 Normal Values for Common Electrolytes/Metabolites

Electrolyte	Normal Range
Sodium	135–148 mEq/L
Potassium	3.5–5.0 mEq/L
Chloride	96–109 mEq/L
Creatinine	0.5–1.2 mg/dL
Blood urea nitrogen	7–22 mg/dL
Glucose	60–109 mg/dL
Phosphate	2.7–4.5 mg/dL
Calcium	8.4–10.5 mg/dL
Magnesium	1.3–2.0 mEq/L
Carbon dioxide	21–30 mEq/L

    i. See Table 14-15 for electrolyte/metabolic disorders in kidney transplant recipients.[25-28]

    j. Lab work can also provide indications of postoperative bleeding.

       i. CKD patients have chronic anemia related to their kidney failure.

- Many patients at the time of transplant can have a hematocrit of 25% or less.
- After transplantation, it is essential to assess the trend of the hematocrit (Hct) and hemoglobin (Hgb) in reference to the patient's preoperative levels.
- If there is a significant decrease in the Hct/Hgb, then a full workup to assess for bleeding should be initiated including serial Hct/Hgb testing, renal ultrasound, and CT scan.
- Attention should also be given to the platelet (PLT) count to ensure that it is in the normal range and is not contributing to a bleeding episode.
- The prothrombin (PT) and activated partial thromboplastin (aPTT) times should also be reviewed to determine if they are abnormal.

    k. Blood work abnormalities can also provide an early warning of infection in transplant recipients.

       i. An elevated white blood cell count (WBC), erythrocyte sedimentation rate (ESR), and C-reactive protein can indicate an infection.

       ii. An elevated WBC may also develop in response to high doses of steroids.

       iii. An elevation of any of these parameters warrants further investigation.

3. Hemodynamic status

    a. Hemodynamic monitoring is of paramount importance for kidney transplant recipients as the success of the transplant and prevention of complications revolves around tight control of fluid balance and BP.

    b. The nursing assessment should include[21,24]

       i. Vital signs as discussed above

       ii. Cardiovascular assessments

TABLE 14-15 **Electrolyte/Metabolic Disorders in Kidney Transplant Recipients**

Abnormality	Etiology	Clinical Presentation	Treatment
Hypernatremia	Dehydration Osmotic diuresis posttransplantation Large-volume NS infusions IV sodium bicarbonate	Fever Thirst Dry mucous membranes Flushing Restlessness Agitation Confusion Weakness Twitching Seizures Coma Decreased urine output If due to water loss: decreased weight, BP, CVP, and increased pulse If due to Na^+ excess: increased weight, BP, CVP, edema, weak pulse	If due to water losses: rehydration with D_5W or hypotonic saline If due to Na^+ excess: restrict Na^+, administer D_5W and diuretics Gradual correction of hypernatremia essential to prevent cerebral and pulmonary edema
Hyponatremia	Fluid overload Osmotic diuresis with impaired concentrating ability posttransplantation Large-volume hypotonic saline infusions (e.g., ¼ or ½ NS) Diuretics Gastrointestinal losses: vomiting, NG suction, diarrhea	If due to water excess: headache, weakness, confusion Muscle weakness, seizures, coma, nausea, vomiting, increased weight, BP, CVP, HR, and edema If due to Na^+ losses: irritability, confusion, anxiety Thirst, dry mucous membranes Muscle weakness, tremors, seizures, decreased weight, BP, CVP, and increased HR	If due to water excess: fluid restriction and careful use of diuretics Dialysis If due to Na^+ losses: stop hypotonic infusions and NS infusion Stop diuretics, if indicated In life-threatening situations: 3%–5% hypertonic NS with great caution Rapid overcorrection of hyponatremia can cause central pontine myelinolysis
Hyperkalemia	Renal insufficiency/ failure Acute tubular necrosis (ATN) Calcineurin inhibitors Beta-blockers Angiotensin-converting enzyme inhibitors (ACEI) Oral PO_4 supplements Potassium-sparing diuretics (e.g., spironolactone) Bleeding/cell damage Metabolic acidosis	Lethargy Confusion Muscle irritability, muscle cramps, muscle weakness, flaccid paralysis, paresthesias, hyperactive reflexes, abdominal cramps Nausea Diarrhea EKG changes: tall peaked T waves, prolonged PR interval, ST segment depression, widened QRS Tachycardia that can proceed to bradycardia Ventricular fibrillation Cardiac arrest	Eliminate IV/drug sources of K^+ (e.g., beta-blockers, ACEI, oral PO_4 supplements, and spironolactone) Restrict dietary intake of K^+ Diuretics Sodium polystyrene sulfonate (Kayexalate) if no ileus Dextrose 50% and insulin Keep calcineurin inhibitor levels within therapeutic range Calcium gluconate or chloride to increase threshold for arrhythmias Sodium bicarbonate if metabolic acidosis present Dialysis

(continued)

TABLE 14-15 Electrolyte/Metabolic Disorders in Kidney Transplant Recipients (*Continued*)

Abnormality	Etiology	Clinical Presentation	Treatment
Hypokalemia	Osmotic diuresis posttransplantation Diuretics GI losses Magnesium depletion Alkalosis Renal tubular acidosis Steroid therapy	Fatigue Confusion Dizziness Muscle weakness Leg cramps Paresthesias Decreased reflexes Respiratory paralysis Nausea, vomiting Ileus Constipation EKG changes: ST depression, flattened or inverted T waves, U wave present Cardiac arrest	IV or oral K^+ supplements Increase dietary intake of K^+. Stop diuretics, if possible. Magnesium supplementation, if indicated Correct alkalosis
Hypermagnesemia	Renal insufficiency/ failure Excessive supplementation Mg-containing laxatives or antacids	Lethargy Fatigue Drowsiness Confusion Muscle weakness, decreased/absent reflexes Flaccid paralysis, seizures Depressed resp. Respiratory muscle paralysis Bradycardia Weak pulse Hypotension Heart block Cardiac arrest	Restrict dietary Mg Avoid Mg-containing products Dialysis Hydration and diuretics IV Ca gluconate to oppose cardiotoxic effects of Mg
Hypomagnesemia	Calcineurin inhibitor induced Excessive urine output Diuretics GI losses: diarrhea, vomiting, or NG suction Malnutrition	Dizziness, lethargy, confusion Twitching, tremors, seizures, coma Muscle weakness Leg/foot cramps EKG: flat or inverted T waves, ST segment depression, prolonged QT interval	Increase dietary intake of Mg (fish, green vegetables) Oral Mg supplements IV Mg supplements
Hyperphosphatemia	Renal insufficiency/ failure Secondary hyperparathyroidism with hypocalcemia PO_4-containing enemas	Muscle weakness Muscle cramping Tetany Seizures Hypocalcemia Ca-PO_4 deposits in the soft tissues, blood vessels, skin, and organs (heart, brain, eyes) Joint pain related to deposits	Restrict dietary PO_4 (dairy products) Phosphate binders (e.g., calcium acetate, sevelamer) Activated vitamin D (IV and oral) Ca supplements Dialysis

TABLE 14-15 Electrolyte/Metabolic Disorders in Kidney Transplant Recipients (*Continued*)

Abnormality	Etiology	Clinical Presentation	Treatment
Hypophosphatemia	Increased posttransplant urinary excretion Phosphaturia due to glucocorticoid-induced gluconeogenesis PO_4 binders Hypercalcemia Poor oral intake	Fatigue Confusion Muscle weakness, tremor Paresthesias Diaphragmatic weakness Cardiac arrhythmias Osteomalacia	Increase dietary intake of PO_4. Oral PO_4 supplements (e.g., K phos neutral) IV PO_4 supplementation (sodium phosphate)
Hypocalcemia	Chronic kidney disease Hyperphosphatemia Vitamin D deficiency Inadequate oral intake of Ca and vitamin D Loop diuretics Citrate in blood products	Depression Lethargy Confusion Irritability Fatigue Perioral and extremity numbness/tingling Hyperactive reflexes Muscle cramps + Chvostek's sign + Trousseau's sign Tetany Seizures Bone pain Abdominal cramps Constipation Nausea, vomiting EKG changes: prolonged ST and QT, ventricular tachycardia	Increase dietary intake of Ca and vitamin D. Oral calcium supplements IV calcium supplements (Ca gluconate or chloride) Vitamin D supplements (IV and oral) High Ca dialysate
Decreased carbon dioxide	Renal insufficiency/failure Diabetic ketoacidosis Diarrhea Malnutrition	Drowsiness, confusion Headache Coma Deep, rapid resp. (Kussmaul) arrhythmias, if K+ elevated Nausea, vomiting, diarrhea	Sodium bicarbonate (IV or oral) Correct hyperkalemia Dialysis

BP, blood pressure; Ca, calcium; CVP, central venous pressure; EKG, electrocardiogram; GI, gastrointestinal; HR, heart rate; IV, intravenous; K+, potassium; Mg, magnesium; Na+, sodium; NG, nasogastric; NS, normal saline; PO_4, phosphate; Resp, respirations. Data from Stark, JL. The renal system. In: Alspach JG, ed. *Core Curriculum for Critical Care Nursing*. 6th ed. Philadelphia, PA: WB Saunders; 2006:525–610; Weil S. Nutrition in the kidney transplant recipient. In: Danovitch GM, ed. *Handbook of Kidney Transplantation*. 5th ed. Philadelphia, PA: Lippincott Williams & Wilkins; 2010:416–431; Verbalis JG. Hyponatremia and hypoosmolar disorders. In: Gilbert SJ, Weiner DE, Gipson DS, et al., eds. *National Kidney Foundation's Primer on Kidney Diseases*. 6th ed. Philadelphia, PA: Elsevier Saunders; 2014:62–70.

  iii. Assessment of fluid balance (see below)

  iv. Pulmonary assessments (see below)

 c. Cardiovascular assessment

  i. The heart must be functioning properly to ensure adequate fluid management.

  ii. Cardiac monitoring is the standard of care for immediate posttransplant recipients in order to:

   • Assess effects of fluid alterations

   • Observe for EKG indications of electrolyte abnormalities such as hyperkalemia

   • Identify life-threatening arrhythmias

  iii. A central venous pressure (CVP) of 6 to 12 cm H_2O should be adequate to prevent hypotension and hypoperfusion of the kidney or hypertension and fluid overload.[24]

  iv. Absence of lower extremity pulses particularly on the side of the transplant could herald a serious vascular complication and requires immediate attention.

4. Assessment of fluid balance

 a. The function of the allograft influences posttransplant fluid balance.

  i. Recipients who received a living donor transplant or a deceased donor organ with a short cold ischemia time (CIT, cold storage time) may anticipate immediate graft function.

  ii. Delayed graft function may be expected for a deceased donor recipient with a prolonged CIT or technical problems. The nursing care can be very different in each situation.

 b. An estimate of an acceptable hourly output takes into consideration donor characteristics, operative history, and the patient's preoperative output (if any).

  i. If patients do not achieve this goal, the health care provider (physician and/or nurse practitioner) should be notified to discuss strategies to increase the output.[24]

 c. Assessment of fluid balance includes

  i. Strict intake and output (I and O)

   • Record the patient's entire oral and IV fluid intake.

    ◦ Most transplant patients will receive maintenance IV fluids, a carrier for patient-controlled analgesia, and hourly urine replacements.

    ◦ In addition, fluid boluses may be ordered for patients whose urine outputs are inadequate.

  ii. Daily weights

  iii. Daily CVP levels

  iv. Monitoring patient for peripheral edema

   • The presence of truncal and lower extremity edema provides clues as to the fluid status of a patient.

   • Peripheral edema and pulses in the lower extremities should be assessed at least once every 8 hours.

   • Edema that is greater in the extremity on the side of the transplant could simply be related to the surgery or could indicate a deep vein thrombosis or lymphocele.

 d. IV infusion rates are carefully adjusted according to the patient's hemodynamic status.

 e. If fluid balance is not maintained, volume-related complications can develop rapidly with serious consequences.

5. Alterations in fluid balance: hypervolemia
   a. Hypervolemia is quite common both in patients with immediate and delayed function. Causes include
      i. Intraoperative overhydration
      ii. Cardiac dysfunction
      iii. Primary nonfunction of the kidney
      iv. Simple obstruction of the urinary catheter
   b. Clinical manifestations
      i. Dyspnea
      ii. Decreased oxygenation
      iii. Rales, rhonchi, wheezing
      iv. Pulmonary and/or peripheral edema
      v. Increased weight
      vi. Hypertension
      vii. Elevated CVP
      viii. Distended neck veins
      ix. Presence of an S_3 on cardiac auscultation[23,24]
      x. Pleural effusions
      xi. Decreased oxygen saturation
   c. When a patient demonstrates hypervolemia with a decreased urine output, assess the urinary catheter to determine
      i. If it is patent
      ii. If there are any clots or hematuria
         • Clots may be occluding the catheter, particularly if the urine output has dropped off suddenly.
   d. Examine the patient's abdomen for distention and/or pain over the bladder.
   e. Notify the provider of all assessment findings.
   f. If ordered, gently flush the catheter with 30 mL of normal saline.[24]
   g. If there are no noticeable clots flushed through the catheter and the urine output remains low, treatment for hypervolemia is typically initiated.
      i. Administration of diuretics
      ii. Decreasing IV infusion rate
      iii. Dialysis[23,24]
6. Alteration in fluid balance: hypovolemia
   a. Hypovolemia can lead to hypotension, hypoperfusion, and ATN.
      i. Hypovolemia regardless of cause should be reported to the transplant team immediately.
   b. Common etiologies of hypovolemia are
      i. Inadequate IV or oral intake of fluids
      ii. Osmotic diuresis
      iii. Bleeding
   c. BP and CVP can provide vital information regarding intravascular fluid status.
      i. CVP levels below 6 and systolic BP readings of <110 mm Hg warrant immediate attention.
   d. Clinical manifestations
      i. Decreased urine output
      ii. Decreased BP
      iii. Decreased weight
      iv. Tachycardia

       v.   Increased bleeding from the wound and the drain

       vi. Pallor

       vii. Hypoxia

       viii. Poor skin turgor

       ix. Dry mucous membranes

       x.   Weakness

       xi. Mental status changes

  e. Diagnosis:

       i.   A renal ultrasound may be ordered to assess the blood flow to the kidney.[21]

  f. Potential treatment options depend on the etiology.

       i.   Fluid depletion: If a patient is simply fluid depleted, fluid boluses are a quick, effective means of rehydration.

       ii. Discontinuation of diuretics.

       iii. Holding antihypertensive drugs until the BP stabilizes.

       iv. Bleeding confirmed by a precipitous fall in the Hct/Hgb: Administration of red blood cell transfusions.

       v.   Active bleeding: May require return to the OR for exploration.

7. Pulmonary assessment and management

  a. Respiratory assessment also provides information regarding the hemodynamic status.

  b. The patient should be assessed for rales, rhonchi, wheezing, and any other indicators of difficult air passage due to the presence of fluid.

  c. Through auscultation and radiologic studies, the potential presence of effusions should be assessed.

  d. The oxygen saturation level should be monitored.

  e. Most patients receive oxygen for the first 24 hours postoperatively and should be able to maintain oxygen levels in excess of 92% or higher.

  f. Oxygen can be weaned when the patient is able to maintain this level on room air.

  g. Essential components of care to prevent infection include

       i.   Turning, coughing, and deep breathing

       ii. Use of assist devices such as the incentive spirometer

  h. Patients should be out of bed by the first postoperative day and spend as much time as possible ambulating or sitting in the chair to prevent respiratory infections related to atelectasis and inactivity.[29]

8. Neurologic assessment

  a. Renal transplant recipients should be neurologically intact postoperatively, but the effects of anesthesia, narcotics, and immunosuppressants can have a negative impact.

  b. All patients should be examined for level of consciousness, orientation, and motor and cognitive function.

  c. Altered level of consciousness, disorientation, agitation, and inability to follow commands or move the extremities should be reported immediately.

  d. Special attention should be paid to the presence of tremors particularly of the hands associated with tacrolimus toxicity.[29]

  e. Potential neurological complications

       i.   Leukoencephalopathy is a rare toxicity associated with tacrolimus and can cause significant mental status changes and usually requires cessation or reduction of the dose of the drug.[30]

  ii. Delirium is not uncommon following transplantation, has been associated with immunosuppressant agents, and can be worsened by advanced age and concomitant medical conditions.[31]
  - When possible, the offending agent should be discontinued or used at the lowest possible dose.
  - When acute delirium occurs, haloperidol (Haldol) is usually effective but must be used cautiously.
  - Narcotics should be discontinued as early as possible.
  iii. Seizures have been reported with calcineurin inhibitor toxicity as well as hyponatremia.
 f. It is important to make sure the patient is neurologically intact before initiating patient education.
9. Assessment of the gastrointestinal (GI) tract
 a. Assess the patient every 8 hours for:
  i. Bowel sounds
  ii. Abdominal distention
  iii. Eructation, flatus
  iv. Bowel movement (including consistency of stool)
  v. Ability to tolerate fluids
 b. If the patient has an ostomy, the stoma should be examined and the quantity of stool should be recorded.
 c. Common GI problems reported postoperatively include nausea and vomiting, constipation, diarrhea, and anorexia.
  i. Nausea, vomiting, and constipation are generally due to the effects of residual renal disease, anesthesia, and narcotic usage.
  - Nausea and vomiting generally abate after several days but can be treated acutely with antiemetics such as ondansetron (Zofran) or promethazine (Phenergan) or motility agents such as metoclopramide (Reglan).
  - Constipation can be treated by eliminating narcotics as early as possible, increasing fluid intake, ambulation, a high-fiber diet, stool softeners, laxatives, and enemas.
    ○ The dietitian can be consulted regarding a high-fiber diet.
  ii. Diarrhea is usually medication related, but cultures should always be sent to confirm the absence of infection.
  - Mycophenolate mofetil (CellCept), phosphate supplements, and magnesium oxide can cause diarrhea.
  - For persistent diarrhea, the patient's provider may consider
    ○ Decreasing the dose of mycophenolate mofetil
    ○ Discontinuing mycophenolate mofetil
    ○ Discontinuing oral magnesium oxide and phosphate supplements and substituting IV magnesium and phosphate
  - If stool cultures are positive, consultation by infectious disease specialist should be considered and appropriate antibiotics should be initiated.
  - If the stool cultures are negative and the diarrhea persists, antimotility agents such as loperamide (Imodium) may be administered.
  - Until the diarrhea is controlled, adequate hydration is essential to maintain the BP and prevent hypoperfusion of the new kidney.

      iii. Some patients complain of stomach discomfort and anorexia.
- Both mycophenolate mofetil (CellCept) and steroids can irritate the GI tract.
- Generally, these side effects can be managed with the prescription of an H_2 blocker such as omeprazole (Prilosec) or pantoprazole (Protonix).

10. Hematologic assessment
    a. There are two major hematologic concerns: infection and anemia.
    b. Infection: elevated WBC
        i. As previously discussed, transplant recipients are at increased risk for infection associated with:
- The surgical procedure itself
- Immunosuppressive therapy
- Comorbid illnesses[32]

        ii. Of note, transplant recipients typically have a urinary catheter in place for 3 to 4 days after surgery to allow the bladder anastomosis to heal.
- Observe for clinical manifestations of a urinary tract infection (UTI):
    ○ Urethral burning
    ○ Cloudy, foul-smelling urine
    ○ Frequency
    ○ Pain on urination
    ○ Dribbling
    ○ Difficulty initiating a stream
- A urinalysis and urine culture/sensitivity should be obtained if a UTI is suspected.
- It is important to assess the patient for a UTI after the catheter is removed.

        iii. See chapter on Transplant Complications: Infectious Diseases for additional information.

    c. Anemia
        i. CKD causes anemia as the failed kidneys are no longer able to produce the erythropoietin necessary to stimulate the bone marrow to produce new red blood cells (RBCs).
        ii. Pretransplant anemia persists following transplantation and can be worsened by operative blood losses.
        iii. Assess the patient's Hct/Hgb, ferritin, transferrin percent saturation (TSAT), and reticulocyte count.
        iv. The Kidney Disease Outcomes Quality Initiative (KDOQI) recommends that the:
- Hct be maintained between 33 and 36 g/dL.
- Hgb be maintained between 11 and 12 g/dL.[33]

        v. Darbepoetin alfa (Aranesp) and epoetin alfa (Epogen) stimulate RBC production and can be used to increase the Hct/Hgb.
        vi. It is essential that iron stores be adequate for erythropoiesis to take place.
- Iron, if required, can be supplemented orally or by the IV route (iron dextran, iron gluconate, iron sucrose)
- TSAT should be ≥20%.
- Ferritin ≥ or equal to 100 ng/mL.[33]

        vii. Correction of anemia is essential to prevent fatigue, improve quality of life, and reduce morbidity and mortality.

11. Wound and drainage assessment
    a. Transplant recipients are at risk for impaired wound healing due to:
        i. Steroid therapy, which can interfere with tissue healing
        ii. Increased risk of infection associated with immunosuppressants
    b. Observe wounds for:
        i. Abnormal wound drainage
        ii. Evidence of infection
        iii. Dehiscence
    c. Wound assessment: Drainage
        i. Observe any drain for the volume, consistency, and color of the effluent.
            * The drain should be emptied and the bulb recompressed every 8 hours and as needed.
        ii. If there is excessive serosanguineous or bloody drainage from the wound or the wound drain, check the patient's vital signs and Hct/Hgb.
        iii. If a significant Hct/Hgb drop is noted and the vital signs are consistent with bleeding (decreased BP, tachycardia), the transplant team should be notified and the appropriate radiologic testing performed.
            * A renal ultrasound or CT scan may be ordered.
        iv. If active bleeding is occurring, the patient will likely return to the OR for exploration.
            * While the patient waits for transfer to the OR, fluid boluses and RBC transfusions may be required to stabilize the patient.
            * To alleviate their anxiety, patients should be kept informed of what is happening and reassured that all the appropriate measures are being taken.
        v. Excessive clear or yellow fluid drainage from the wound can indicate a urine leak, lymphocele, or seroma.
            * It is important to have the fluid analyzed (including creatinine and cell count).
            * A fluid creatinine level well in excess of the serum creatinine may be indicative of a urine leak.
            * Suspicion of a urine leak will require a renal scan for confirmation and urinary catheter placement to decompress the bladder.
            * Lymphocytes present in the fluid may be indicative of a lymphocele.
            * Fluid with a normal creatinine and no cells may be indicative of a seroma.
        vi. Notify the transplant team of any abnormal findings.
        vii. If the fluid drainage is not deemed to be abnormal, frequent dressing changes with meticulous skin care may be the only care required until the excessive drainage abates.
    d. Wound assessment: Infection
        i. Most transplant recipients receive IV antibiotics for 24 hours perioperatively to minimize the risk of wound infections.
        ii. Nevertheless, wound infections can occur. Therefore, it is important to assess the primary wound and drain site(s) at least twice a day for clinical manifestations of infection (purulent drainage, erythema, pain, tenderness) or necrosis and promptly notify the transplant team accordingly.

iii. The nurse can expect to send wound cultures, initiate antibiotics, and provide wound care.
- Simple wounds
  - May require cleaning with normal saline and the application of a dry sterile dressing.
  - The wound can be left open to air when drainage ceases.
  - The wound drain should have a dry drain dressing around it until it is removed.
- Infected wounds
  - May be opened and packed with normal saline gauze or an agent designed to:
  - Disinfect the wound such as chlorpactin
  - Debride the wound such as an enzymatic ointment
- Complex wounds
  - Will require consultation with a wound care specialist who has knowledge of state-of-the-art treatments.
  - Pulse lavage (use of a small stream of fluid to debride the wound) may be needed for wounds with a large amount of nonviable tissue.
  - At the time of discharge, if complex wound care is still required, a home nursing referral should be initiated.

e. Wound assessment: Dehiscence
   i. A final assessment parameter for wounds is the intactness of the sutures, both external and fascial.
   ii. The wound edges should be observed for any separation or evidence of fascial dehiscence.
   iii. Separation of wound edges must be promptly reported to the transplant team.
   iv. If the separation is due to infection, wound care can be initiated as described above.
   v. If bowel is noted through the wound opening appearing as a moist, shiny, tubular structure, the surgeon should be notified immediately as this is a medical emergency that could result in herniation or obstruction of the bowel.
   vi. Dehiscence occurs when the fascial sutures break.
   vii. The exposed bowel should be covered with a nonadherent dressing, an abdominal binder applied, and the patient placed on strict bed rest.
   viii. As soon as possible, the patient should return to the OR for exploration and fascial closure.

f. The dietitian should also be consulted to provide a diet that will promote wound healing.

12. Pain assessment and management
a. Assessment
   i. Pain is expected after any major surgical procedure.
   ii. The nursing assessment for pain should include a subjective pain scale rating, visual inspection, and physical examination.
   iii. Severe and rapidly escalating pain is unusual and is indicative of a serious complication such as bleeding or fascial dehiscence.
   iv. Typical pain manifests as discomfort directly over the transplant surgical site that worsens with movement.

  b. Pain management

    i. Most patients will receive patient-controlled anesthesia (PCA) where the patient can deliver IV pain medication (typically morphine or fentanyl) independently.

      • Morphine and fentanyl are metabolized by the liver.

    ii. Meperidine (Demerol) is contraindicated in renal disease.

      • Meperidine is metabolized by the liver but is dependent on the kidneys for the excretion of metabolites.

      • Retained metabolites can cause seizures.[34]

    iii. Ketorolac (Toradol)[34] and other nonsteroidal anti-inflammatory drugs should be avoided as they can block vasodilatory prostaglandins and impair renal perfusion.

    iv. Within 24 to 48 hours, most patients are ready to transition to oral pain medication such as oxycodone.

    v. Because of the constipating effects of narcotics, a bowel regimen should be initiated that includes docusate sodium to soften the stool, ambulation, fluids, and a high-fiber diet.

    vi. Laxatives and enemas can be administered as required. However, it is important to remember that if the new kidney has limited function, phosphate- and magnesium-containing laxatives and enemas should be avoided.

13. Nutrition assessment

  a. Adequate nutrition is essential for carrying out activities of daily living and wound healing.[26]

  b. As noted above, transplant patients may experience anorexia and other complications that reduce their caloric intake.

  c. As the GI tract is minimally disturbed during renal transplant surgery, patients typically can begin a clear liquid diet on postoperative day 1 and then advance as tolerated.

  d. The nutritional assessment typically includes the following:

    i. Daily caloric intake, particularly if inadequate oral intake is suspected[26]

    ii. Daily weight (factoring in fluid shifts)

    iii. Albumin and prealbumin levels

    iv. Transferrin percent saturation

    v. Total protein

  e. If any of these values are subtherapeutic or a patient has a special need such as DM or weight or lipid reduction, the provider and dietitian must be notified so that a tailored dietary plan can be developed.

  f. Medications that may facilitate eating should be administered including antiemetics, motility agents, and H_2 blockers.

  g. For the rare transplant patient who cannot consume sufficient calories orally, calories should be provided enterally or parenterally.

14. Assessment of mobility and self-care capability

  a. One of the goals of transplantation is to enable transplant recipients to resume as normal a life as possible.

  b. It is important to assess the patient's

    i. Mobility and ambulation skills

    ii. Ability to carry out activities of daily living independently

    iii. Motivation to participate actively in care

c. Mobility
    i. Activity should be encouraged to the level that is ordered by the provider, and in most cases, this will be ambulation early on postoperative day 1.
    ii. Patients should remain out of bed for as much of the day as possible. Assess frequently and monitor for safety.
    iii. Deep vein thrombosis (DVT) is a postoperative risk that may be ameliorated by early activity.
       • The use of support stockings, automatic compression devices, and subcutaneous heparin can also help prevent DVTs.
d. Self-care
    i. The incentive spirometer and flutter valve should be used every hour while awake.
    ii. Activity and respiratory devices will help prevent postoperative atelectasis and respiratory infections.
e. If a patient is debilitated or has other physical impairments, physical, occupational, and speech therapy consults should be obtained as needed.
f. Family members and friends should be encouraged to participate in the care, and the primary caregiver at home should be identified.

15. Psychosocial assessment
a. The psychosocial status of new transplant recipients must be closely monitored as patients and caregivers adjust to this life-changing event and the effects of anesthesia, narcotics, new immunosuppressant medications, and a complex posttransplant regimen.
b. Attention should be given to the frequency and quality of assistance from patient's support system, particularly in regard to the patient's needs following discharge.
c. Social workers and mental health providers.
    i. Assess patients throughout the transplant continuum
    ii. Are key participants in the interdisciplinary discharge planning process
d. See chapter on the Psychosocial Issues in Transplantation for additional information.

IX. IMMUNOSUPPRESSION

A. Nurses have an important role in:
1. Administering immunosuppressive agents
2. Obtaining and reporting blood drug levels
3. Collaborating with providers regarding dose adjustments
4. Monitoring patients for side effects and toxicities
5. Educating patients and caregivers about the medication regimen

B. Most renal transplant recipients are on a triple drug regimen including:
1. A calcineurin inhibitor (tacrolimus [Prograf] or cyclosporine [Neoral, Gengraf])
2. Prednisone
3. An antiproliferative agent (e.g., mycophenolate mofetil [CellCept])

C. Sirolimus (Rapamune) is at times substituted for one of these drugs if a patient is intolerant although care must be taken especially in the early post-op phase as one of the side effects of sirolimus is delayed wound healing.

D. Blood level monitoring is available for tacrolimus, cyclosporine, sirolimus, and mycophenolate mofetil.

E. Induction therapy
1. Some patients will receive induction therapy starting just before or immediately after the transplant procedure (e.g., antithymocyte globulin [Thymoglobulin]).
2. Induction therapy can continue daily for days to a week.

F. See chapter on Transplant Pharmacology for additional information.

 X. POSTTRANSPLANT COMPLICATIONS

A. Acute tubular necrosis (ATN)
1. Refers to the condition where the newly transplanted kidney does not function in the absence of rejection or obstruction.
2. Potential etiology:
   a. Prolonged cold ischemic time (CIT)
   b. Prolonged warm ischemia time
   c. Hypoperfusion
   d. Hypotension[21,29]
3. Contributing factors: premortem donor incidents such as:
   a. Hypotension
   b. Cardiac or respiratory arrest[21,35]
4. Clinical manifestations:
   a. ATN presents as renal failure with:
      i. Elevated BUN, creatinine, potassium, phosphate, and magnesium
      ii. Anuria or oliguria
      iii. Increased weight
      iv. Shortness of breath
      v. Pulmonary edema
      vi. Lower extremity edema
      vii. Decreased oxygenation
   b. Severity of the signs and symptoms depends on the severity of the ATN.
5. Potential treatment options
   a. If there are no life-threatening electrolyte abnormalities such as hyperkalemia or fluid overload causing pulmonary edema, watchful waiting will be the treatment strategy.
   b. There is no direct treatment for ATN, but if it is expected at the time of transplant, induction therapy may be initiated.
      i. An induction agent such as antithymocyte globulin (Thymoglobulin) may be used so that calcineurin inhibitors can be withheld, thus avoiding the introduction of a nephrotoxin that could further impair function in the immediate postoperative period.
   c. Throughout this period, the patient will remain on a renal diet and phosphate binders.
6. Patient monitoring
   a. Recovery from ATN can take days to weeks.
   b. Renal ultrasounds and renal scans should be done periodically to ensure adequate flow, absence of collections or hydronephrosis, or absence of a urine leak.[21]

c. The patient will be observed closely waiting for the kidney function to improve or the need for dialysis to become apparent.
    i. This is a very frustrating time for the patient as the expectation is that the new kidney will function immediately.
d. If ATN persists for more than 5 to 7 days, a kidney biopsy should be done to ensure there is not a concurrent episode of rejection.[21]

B. Rejection
    1. Despite advances in immunology, tissue-typing and crossmatching techniques, surgical strategies, and immunosuppressive agents, rejection remains a major cause of graft dysfunction and loss.
    2. Types of rejection based on etiology and time of onset (Table 14-16):
        a. Hyperacute
        b. Accelerated

TABLE 14-16 Types of Kidney Transplant Rejection and Treatment Options

Type	Onset	Etiology	Clinical Presentation	Treatment
Hyperacute rejection	Occurs within minutes or hours of transplantation	B cell Ab-mediated, humoral preformed cytotoxic B cells attack the new kidney.	Graft becomes cyanotic, can rupture irreversible condition anuria *Bx findings:* Fibrinoid necrosis, fibrin thrombi, marginating neutrophils, ischemic necrosis, marked interstitial hemorrhage	None Transplant nephrectomy Wound is usually not even closed before damage occurs
Accelerated rejection	Occurs 24 h to 5 d posttransplantation	B cell Ab-mediated humoral due to presensitization from prior exposure to one or more of the donor's antigens May have a cellular component	Fever Edema Abdominal pain or tenderness over graft site Increased BUN, Cr Increased weight and BP Decreased UOP + XM or antibody screen + for DSA *Bx findings:* +C4D, marginating neutrophils	Plasmapheresis: Removes all Ab IVIG: replenishes good Ab and modulates immune system over time so that Ab is no longer made or responded to
Acute rejection	Occurs days to weeks after transplantation	T cell Cell-mediated cellular inflammatory response	Fever Myalgias/arthralgias Edema Gross hematuria Abdominal pain or tenderness over graft site Increased BUN, Cr Increased weight and BP Decreased UOP *Bx findings:* Interstitial edema, tubulitis, mononuclear infiltration, arteritis, fibrinoid necrosis, Banff grades 1–3.	*Mild–Moderate:* Banff grades 1–2: IV steroids *Moderate–Severe:* Banff grades 2–3: antithymocyte globulin

TABLE 14-16 **Types of Kidney Transplant Rejection and Treatment Options (Continued**

Type	Onset	Etiology	Clinical Presentation	Treatment
Chronic Rejection	Months to years after transplantation, insidious	Not well defined Immune and nonimmune mechanisms involved	Chronic renal failure Elevated BUN, Cr Electrolyte abnormalities Edema Increased BP and weight Decreased UOP *Bx findings:* Tubular atrophy, glomerulosclerosis, interstitial fibrosis	None Progression may be slowed by discontinuing calcineurin inhibitors Retransplant

Ab, antibody; BUN, blood urea nitrogen; Bx, biopsy; Cr, creatinine; XM, crossmatch; DSA, donor-specific antibody; IVIG, intravenous immune globulin; +, positive; UOP, urine output.
From Wilkinson A. The "first quarter:" the first three months after transplantation. In: Danovitch GM, ed. *Handbook of Kidney Transplantation*. 5th ed. Philadelphia, PA: Lippincott Williams & Wilkins; 2010:198–216; Colaneri J, Neyhart C. Kidney transplantation. In: *Core Curriculum for Nephrology Nursing*. 6th ed. Pitman, NJ: ANNA; 2015:3–25; Nankivell BJ, Alexander SI. Rejection of the kidney allograft. *N Engl J Med*. 2010;363:1451–1462; Nast CC, Cohen AH. Pathology of kidney transplantation. In: Danovitch GM, ed. *Handbook of Kidney Transplantation*. 5th ed. Philadelphia, PA: Lippincott Williams & Wilkins; 2010:311–329.

    c. Acute
    d. Chronic[21,29]
  3. Types of rejection based on primary mediator:
    a. T-cell (cell-mediated, cellular) rejection
    b. B-cell (antibody-mediated, humoral) rejection
  4. Diagnosis of rejection
    a. Diagnosis is based on the clinical presentation of the patient and biopsy findings.[36]
    b. A renal scan that indicates decreased flow further confirms the diagnosis.
  5. Acute rejection due to T-cell activation
    a. Most common type of rejection.
    b. Most episodes occur within the first 3 months after transplantation.[37]
    c. The severity is determined by the degree of tubulitis and arteritis.
    d. The severity of T-cell rejection is rated using the Banff 97 Classification System, with 2005 and 2007 updates.[37–39]
      i. The grades are borderline, IA, IB, IIA, IIB, or III.
      ii. Borderline is the mildest form and easiest to reverse, whereas grade III is the most severe and most difficult to reverse.
      iii. Treatment is based on the rejection grade.
  6. B-cell rejection (antibody mediated)
    a. Characterized on biopsy by marginating neutrophils and a positive C4D that is an end product of complement degradation.
  7. Treatment of rejection
    a. Treatment varies based on the primary cause and severity of the rejection episode.
    b. The diagnosis of rejection is frightening for most patients and their caregivers.
      i. Patients may experience anxiety due to uncertainty regarding whether or not the treatment will be successful.
      ii. It is important to reassure patients that rejection is often reversible.
      iii. Providing information to patients often helps to alleviate their concerns.

8. Kidney biopsy
   a. Preparation for kidney biopsy
      i. It is important to establish that coagulation studies and the platelet count are within normal limits before attempting a kidney biopsy.
      ii. Prior to the biopsy, patients must be educated about its purpose, how the results will guide treatment, potential treatment options, and postbiopsy monitoring.
         • Patients can expect to have some pain over the biopsy site and to be on bed rest for several hours lying on the biopsy site with a pressure roll to facilitate hemostasis and prevent postbiopsy bleeding.
   b. Postbiopsy monitoring includes
      i. Frequent vital signs
      ii. Hct/Hgb to assess for significant bleeding
      iii. Observation of urine for and prompt reporting of any new-onset hematuria or the presence of clots in the urine
   c. If postbiopsy bleeding is suspected, a repeat ultrasound will be done to check for evidence of bleeding.

C. Surgical complications
   1. Potential complications are listed in Table 14-17.
   2. Because the clinical manifestations of surgical complications may be similar, it is important to monitor the patient for subtle changes, which are key to establishing the correct diagnosis.
   3. The most common early complications include
      a. Urine leaks
      b. Lymphoceles
      c. Renal vein thrombosis
      d. Ureteral obstruction
      e. Wound infections and bleeding (discussed above)
      f. Infectious complications (see chapter on Transplant Complications: Infectious Diseases for additional information)
   4. Renal artery stenosis is a late complication.

D. Endocrine and metabolic dysfunction
   1. Bone disease related to hyperparathyroidism and medications (see chapter on Transplant Complications: Noninfectious Diseases for additional information).
   2. DM
      a. DM is the major cause of end-stage renal disease in the United States, so many patients who undergo transplantation had this disease prior to transplantation.[10]
      b. Other patients may develop type 2 DM following transplantation.
      c. Effect of immunosuppressants:
         i. Immunosuppressants may make preexisting DM more difficult to manage or cause de novo DM.[26]
            • Insulin requirements will likely increase for patients with preexisting DM.
            • Patients with de novo disease will have the additional burden of learning about and managing DM.
         ii. Steroids increase peripheral insulin resistance and alter pancreatic beta cell secretion.
         iii. Calcineurin inhibitors alter peripheral insulin sensitivity and decrease islet cell function.

TABLE 14-17 Surgical Complications of Kidney Transplantation

Complication	Etiology	Clinical Presentation	Diagnostic Studies	Treatment
Urine leak	Ureteroneocystostomy (anastomotic) leak Necrosis of ureter due to interrupted blood supply Tight ureteral stenosis	Sudden loss of kidney function Decreased UOP Increased BUN/Cr Pain over transplant site Drainage of yellow fluid from wound in large quantities	Cr on drain fluid Cr of fluid is higher than serum Cr Renal scan shows extravasation of dye outside urinary tract Renal US shows fluid collection or mass CT cystogram shows extravasation of dye	*Conservative for small leak:* Insertion of urinary catheter to decompress bladder Nephrostomy tube placement *Larger leaks or necrotic ureter:* Surgical repair
Lymphocele	Severed lymphatics in iliac region without ligation resulting in fluid collecting around transplanted kidney	Decreased kidney function Decreased UOP Increased BUN/Cr Pain over transplant site Leg swelling on the side of the transplant due to compression of iliac vessels Incontinence, frequency due to pressure on the bladder	Renal US: round, septated collection CT scan: collection Needle aspiration of collection: a high-protein content is consistent with lymphocele	Watchful waiting for small noncompressive collections Percutaneous drainage for large collections Instillation of sclerosing agent via drain (e.g., Betadine or tetracycline) Surgical drainage with marsupialization into the peritoneum for persistent recurrent collections
Graft thrombosis	Can be arterial or venous Due to clots and anastomotic problems	Sudden cessation in urine production Graft tenderness and swelling Elevated BUN/Cr Hematuria with venous thrombosis	Renal US with high impedance through artery with reversed diastolic flow Renal scan: no flow	Immediate return to the operating room for surgical exploration Nephrectomy if kidney is thrombosed

(continued)

TABLE 14-17 **Surgical Complications of Kidney Transplantation (Continued)**

Complication	Etiology	Clinical Presentation	Diagnostic Studies	Treatment
Ureteral obstruction	Blood clots Anastomotic complications Ureteral sloughing Ureteral fibrosis due to infection or ischemia Lymphocele Hematoma	Impaired renal function Hydronephrosis Decreased UOP Pain over transplant site Elevated BUN/Cr	Renal US Intravenous pyelogram Retrograde pyelogram Percutaneous antegrade pyelogram Renal scan	Percutaneous balloon dilatation, if stricture present Nephrostomy tube placement Surgical repair Correction of lymphocele, if present (as described above) Percutaneous or surgical drainage, if hematoma present
Renal artery stenosis	Technical complications at anastomosis Occurs months to years after transplantation	Uncontrolled hypertension Impaired renal function Bruit over anastomosis	Arteriogram with minimal dye	Angioplasty to dilate stenotic area Surgical repair if not amenable to angioplasty

BUN, blood urea nitrogen; Cr, creatinine; UOP, urine output; US, ultrasound.
Data from Veale JL, Singer JS, Gritsch HA. The transplant operation and its surgical complications. In: Danovitch GM, ed. *Handbook of Kidney Transplantation*. 5th ed. Philadelphia, PA: Lippincott Williams & Wilkins; 2010:181–197; Wilkinson A. The "first quarter:" the first three months after transplantation. In: Danovitch GM, ed. *Handbook of Kidney Transplantation*. 5th ed. Philadelphia, PA: Lippincott Williams & Wilkins; 2010:198–216; Colaneri J, Neyhart C. Kidney transplantation. In: *Core Curriculum for Nephrology Nursing*. 6th ed. Pitman, NJ: ANNA; 2015:3–25; Ponticelli C. *Medical Complications of Kidney Transplantation*. Abington, Oxon: Informa UK, CRC Press; 2007.

      d. Clinical manifestations of hyperglycemia
         i.   Blood glucose levels consistently > 110
         ii. Polydipsia
         iii. Polyuria
         iv. Polyphagia
         v.   Blurred vision (possibly)
      e. Patient monitoring
         i.   Blood glucose readings should be checked before each meal and at bedtime
         ii. Clinical manifestations of hypoglycemia (typically present when the blood glucose falls below 60 to 70 mg/dL)
            • Cool, clammy skin
            • Diaphoresis
            • Nausea and vomiting
            • Decreased mental status
            • Agitation
            • Feeling of impending doom
      f. Potential treatment options
         i.   Regimen designed to keep blood glucose levels in the normal range using a combination of diet, oral antihypoglycemic agents, insulin, and exercise.
         ii. When possible, doses of steroids and calcineurin inhibitors should be reduced to the lowest possible dose to prevent rejection.
      g. Patient/caregiver education
         i.   Both the diabetes educator and dietitian should be consulted for patients with a new diagnosis of DM.
         ii. Education includes, but is not limited to, the following:
            • Prescribed diet
            • Medications
            • Blood glucose monitoring
            • Signs and symptoms of hyperglycemia and hypoglycemia
            • Management of hypoglycemia
            • Weight loss instructions (overweight patients)
      h. Postdischarge follow-up
         i.   A home care referral will be crucial to patient's success in managing DM and the posttransplant regimen.
         ii. The hemoglobin A1C should be followed to assess the patient's long-term adherence to and efficacy of the prescribed DM regimen.

   E. See chapter on Transplant Complications: Noninfectious Diseases for additional information.

XI. DISCHARGE PLANNING AND EDUCATION

   A. Preparing transplant patients and their families for discharge is a major undertaking.

   B. Patients are not just learning about their new organ(s) but how to manage numerous medications and observe for and report complications such as infection and rejection.

   C. See chapter on Patient Education for the Transplant Patient for additional information.

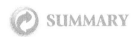

SUMMARY

A. Kidney transplantation is a multifaceted and ever-changing process. It begins with careful evaluation of the patient and continues for as long as the patient has a viable transplant.

B. The success of transplantation depends on the quality of the organ provided, the patient's ability to actively participate in care, presence of complications and comorbid conditions, and close follow-up care.

C. Transplantation presents significant challenges for kidney disease patients, their families, and the transplant team, but it also provides these patients the opportunity to transform their lives and escape many of the complications of CKD and dialysis.

REFERENCES

1. Organ Procurement and Transplantation Network (OPTN). Kidney and Kidney–Pancreas Waiting List Statistics. Available at http://optn.transplant.hrsa.gov/latestData/rptData.asp. Accessed August 11, 2015.
2. ANZDATA. Waiting List Data. Available at http://www.anzdata.org.au/anzod/v5/waitinglist2014.html. Accessed August 14, 2015.
3. Eurotransplant website. Active Recipient ORGAN Needs Per Year End 2014 in ET. Available at http://statistics.eurotransplant.org/index.php?search_type=waiting+list&search_organ=&search_region=All+ET&search_period=by+year&search_characteristic=&search_text=. Accessed August 15, 2015.
4. Organ Donation and Transplantation Activity Data: United Kingdom. Available at http://www.odt.nhs.uk/uk-transplant-registry/. Accessed August 15, 2015.
5. Klarenbach SW, Tonelli M, Chui B, et al. Economic evaluations of dialysis therapies. *Nat Rev Nephrol.* 2014;10:644–652.
6. Domingos M, Gouveia M, Pereira J, et al. A prospective assessment of renal transplantation versus haemodialysis: which therapeutic modality is good value for society? *Port J Nephrol Hypert.* 2014;28(4):300–308.
7. Wong G, Howard K, Chapman JR, et al. Comparative survival and economic benefits of deceased donor kidney transplantation and dialysis in people with varying ages and co-morbidities. *PLoS ONE.* 2012;7(1):1–9. Accessed September 18, 2014.
8. Hall JE. *Guyton & Hall Textbook of Medical Physiology.* 13th ed. Philadelphia, PA: WB Saunders; 2015.
9. Briggs JP, Kriz W, Schnermann JB. Overview of kidney function and structure. In: Gilbert SJ, Weiner DE, Gipson DS, et al., eds. *National Kidney Foundation's Primer on Kidney Diseases.* 6th ed. Philadelphia, PA: Elsevier Saunders; 2014:2–18.
10. Whittier WL, Lewis EJ. Pathophysiology of chronic kidney disease. In: Gilbert SJ, Weiner DE, Gipson DS, et al., eds. *National Kidney Foundation's Primer on Kidney Diseases.* 6th ed. Philadelphia, PA: Elsevier Saunders; 2014:448–457.
11. Jennette JC, Falk RJ. Glomerular clinicopathologic syndromes. In: Gilbert SJ, Weiner DE, Gipson DS, et al., eds. *National Kidney Foundation's Primer on Kidney Diseases.* 6th ed. Philadelphia, PA: Elsevier Saunders; 2014:152–163.
12. National Kidney Foundation (NKF). K/DOQI Clinical Practice Guidelines for Chronic Kidney Disease: Evaluation, Classification, and Stratification. Available at http://www.kidney.org/professionals/kdoqi/guidelines_ckd/toc.htm. Accessed September 29, 2014.
13. Patton KT, Thibodeau GA. *Anatomy and Physiology.* 7th ed. St. Louis, MO: Mosby; 2010.
14. Inker LA, Levey AS. Staging and management of chronic kidney disease. In: Gilbert SJ, Weiner DE, Gipson DS, et al., eds. *National Kidney Foundation's Primer on Kidney Diseases.* 6th ed. Philadelphia, PA: Elsevier Saunders; 2014:458–466.
15. Hain DJ, Haras MS. Chronic kidney disease. In: Counts CS, ed. *Core Curriculum for Nephrology Nursing.* 6th ed. Pitman, NJ: ANNA; 2015:153–188.
16. Bunnapradist S, Danovitch GM. Evaluation of adult kidney transplant candidates. In: Danovitch GM, ed. *Handbook of Kidney Transplantation.* 5th ed. Philadelphia, PA: Lippincott Williams & Wilkins; 2010:157–180.
17. Rifkin MH. Psychosocial and financial aspects of transplantation. In: Danovitch GM, ed. *Handbook of Kidney Transplantation.* 5th ed. Philadelphia, PA: Lippincott Williams & Wilkins; 2010:432–440.

18. Heinrich TW, Marcangelo M. Psychiatric issues in solid organ transplantation. *Harv Rev Psychiatry.* 2009;17(6):398–406.
19. Organ Procurement and Transplantation Network. Kaplan–Meier median Waiting Times for Registrations Listed: 1999–2004. Available at http://optn.transplant.hrsa.gov/latestData/rptStrat.asp. Accessed May 12, 2016.
20. Veale JL, Singer JS, Gritsch HA. The transplant operation and its surgical complications. In: Danovitch GM, ed. *Handbook of Kidney Transplantation.* 5th ed. Philadelphia, PA: Lippincott Williams & Wilkins; 2010:181–197.
21. Wilkinson A. The "first quarter:" the first three months after transplantation. In: Danovitch GM, ed. *Handbook of Kidney Transplantation.* 5th ed. Philadelphia, PA: Lippincott Williams & Wilkins; 2010:198–216.
22. Pegues DA, Kubak BM, Maree CL, et al. Infections in kidney transplantation. In: Danovitch GM, ed. *Handbook of Kidney Transplantation.* 5th ed. Philadelphia, PA: Lippincott Williams & Wilkins; 2010:251–279.
23. Hinkle JL, Cheever KH. *Brunner & Suddarth's Textbook of Medical–Surgical Nursing.* 13th ed. Philadelphia, PA: Lippincott Williams & Wilkins; 2013.
24. Urden LD, Stacy KM, Lough ME. *Critical Care Nursing Diagnosis and Management.* 6th ed. St. Louis, MS: Mosby Elsevier; 2010:1080–1083.
25. LaCharity LA. Care of patients with acute renal failure and chronic kidney disease. In: Workman I, ed. *Medical–Surgical Nursing.* 6th ed. St. Louis, MI: Saunders Elsevier; 2010.
26. Weil S. Nutrition in the kidney transplant recipient. In: Danovitch GM, ed. *Handbook of Kidney Transplantation.* 5th ed. Philadelphia, PA: Lippincott Williams & Wilkins; 2010:416–431.
27. Verbalis JG. Hyponatremia and hypoosmolar disorders. In: Gilbert SJ, Weiner DE, Gipson DS, et al., eds. *National Kidney Foundation's Primer on Kidney Diseases.* 6th ed. Philadelphia, PA: Elsevier Saunders; 2014:62–70.
28. Stark JL. The renal system. In: Alspach JG, ed. *Core Curriculum for Critical Care Nursing.* 6th ed. Philadelphia, PA: WB Saunders; 2006:525–610.
29. Colaneri J, Neyhart C, Carlson L. Kidney transplantation. In: Counts CS, ed. *Core Curriculum for Nephrology Nursing.* 6th ed. Pitman, NJ: ANNA; 2015:3–25.
30. Crowder CD, Guyure KA, Drachenberg CB, et al. Successful outcome of a progressive multi-focal leukoencephalopathy in a renal transplant recipient. *Am J Transplant.* 2005;5:1151–1158.
31. Danovitch I. Psychiatric aspects of kidney transplantation. In: Danovitch GM, ed. *Handbook of Kidney Transplantation.* 5th ed. Philadelphia, PA: Lippincott Williams & Wilkins; 2010:389–408.
32. Karuthu S. Common infections in kidney transplant recipients. *Clin J Am Soc Nephrol.* 2012;7(12):2058–2070.
33. National Kidney Foundation. K/DOQI Clinical Practice Guidelines for anemia of chronic kidney disease. *Am J Kid Dis.* 2006;47(5):S11–S28.
34. Sarinkapoor H, Kaur R, Kaur H. Anaesthesia for renal transplant surgery. *Acta Anaesthesiol Scand.* 2007;51:1354–1367. Accessed August 25, 2015.
35. Ponticelli C. *Medical Complications of Kidney Transplantation.* Abington, Oxon: Informa UK, CRC Press; 2007.
36. Mandelbrot DA, Sayegh MH. Transplantation immunobiology. In: Danovitch GM, ed. *Handbook of Kidney Transplantation.* 5th ed. Philadelphia, PA: Lippincott Williams & Wilkins; 2010:19–35.
37. Nankivell BJ, Alexander SI. Rejection of the kidney allograft. *N Engl J Med.* 2010;363:1451–1462.
38. Nast CC, Cohen AH. Pathology of kidney transplantation. In: Danovitch GM, ed. *Handbook of Kidney Transplantation.* 5th ed. Philadelphia, PA: Lippincott Williams & Wilkins; 2010:311–329.
39. Gill JS. Post transplantation monitoring and outcomes. In: Gilbert SJ, Weiner DE, eds. *National Kidney Foundation's Primer on Kidney Disease.* 6th ed. Philadelphia, PA: Elsevier Saunders; 2014:556–558.

SELF-ASSESSMENT QUESTIONS

1. The most common causes of chronic kidney disease (CKD) include which of the following disorders?
   1. Hypertension
   2. Congestive heart failure
   3. Diabetes
   4. Glomerulonephritis
   a. 1, 2, 3
   b. 2, 3, 4
   c. 1, 3, 4
   d. All of the above

2. Clinical systemic symptoms that may develop with CKD include which of the following?
   1. Amenorrhea, impotence
   2. Pallor, pruritus
   3. Hyperkalemia, acidosis
   4. Muscle twitching, seizures
   a. 1, 3, 4
   b. 1, 2, 3
   c. 1 and 3 only
   d. All of the above

3. The severity of T-cell rejection is rated using the Banff 97 with 2007 update Grading System. The severity of T-cell rejection is determined by the degree of:
   a. proliferating B cells.
   b. circulating donor antibodies.
   c. tubulitis and arteritis.
   d. tubular atrophy.

4. Acute tubular necrosis (ATN) may occur in kidney recipients during the immediate postoperative phase. Donor factors that may affect the development of ATN in the newly transplanted kidney include which of the following?
   1. Hypotension during the donor management phase
   2. Cardiac or respiratory arrest
   3. Ventilator-associated pneumonia
   4. Fluid overload during donor management
   a. 1 and 3
   b. 1 and 2
   c. 2 and 3
   d. 3 and 4

5. ATN presents as renal failure in the absence of rejection or obstruction. Signs of ATN include which of the following?
   1. Increased BUN and creatinine
   2. Anuria or oliguria
   3. Pulmonary edema
   4. Elevated potassium and magnesium levels
   a. 1, 2, 3
   b. 1, 2, 4
   c. 1 and 2
   d. All of the above

6. Potential complications following renal transplantation during the immediate postoperative phase include which of the following?
   1. Urine leaks, ATN
   2. Ureteral obstruction
   3. Infections
   4. Lymphoceles
   a. 1 and 4
   b. 1, 2, 3
   c. 1 and 3
   d. All of the above

7. To prevent hypoperfusion of the kidney during the immediate postoperative phase, the central venous pressure (CVP) should be maintained:
   a. between 4 and 6 mm H_2O.
   b. between 6 and 8 mm H_2O.
   c. between 6 and 12 mm H_2O.
   d. >12 mm H_2O.

8. Edema in the lower extremity on the same side of the renal transplant could indicate which of the following problems?
   a. Acute rejection
   b. Deep vein thrombosis (DVT)
   c. Lymphocele
   d. b and c
   e. All the above

9. Prior to a renal biopsy, which of the following tests should be evaluated?
   a. Platelet count
   b. Coagulation studies
   c. Hematocrit
   d. a and b
   e. b and c

10. Following a renal biopsy, the most important nursing intervention(s) are:
    a. ensuring that the patient is lying on the opposite side of the biopsy site.
    b. applying pressure to the biopsy site by having the patient lie on that side.
    c. checking for new-onset hematuria or the presence of clots in the urine.
    d. a and c.
    e. b and c.

Correct Answers:
1.c 2.d 3.c 4.b 5.d 6.d 7.c 8.d 9.d 10.e

CHAPTER 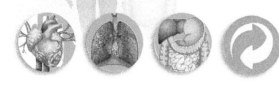 15

Pancreas and Kidney-Pancreas Transplantation

Michelle James, RN, MS, APRN-CNS, CCTN

 I. INTRODUCTION

A. Overview
1. The World Health Organization estimates that approximately 347 million people have been diagnosed with diabetes, worldwide.[1]
2. In the United States, there are approximately 29 million people, or 9.3% of the population, who have diabetes.[2]
3. Diabetes is classified into two main types: type 1 and type 2.
   a. Type 1 diabetes results from cellular-mediated autoimmune destruction of pancreatic islet beta cells causing the loss of insulin production.
      i. Type 1 diabetes (insulin dependent) affects 5% of those with diabetes, and although disease onset can occur at any age, it peaks in mid teenage years.[2]
   b. Type 2 diabetes (non–insulin dependent) is the more common type, affecting 95% of those with diabetes.[2]
      i. Type 2 diabetes usually occurs in adulthood and is characterized by insulin resistance. As resistance rises, the beta cells are eventually unable to produce the necessary amount of insulin to lower and maintain normal blood glucose levels.
      ii. In recent years, there has been an increase in type 2 diabetes diagnosed in children and adolescents.
      iii. Diet and obesity, older age, family history of diabetes, history of gestational diabetes, impaired glucose metabolism, physical inactivity, and race/ethnicity are associated with development of type 2 diabetes.
4. Pancreas transplantation has been performed since 1966.[3]
5. Goals of pancreas transplantation are
   a. To restore normoglycemia in patients with labile diabetes
   b. To halt or prevent secondary complications of diabetes[3]
6. The International Pancreas Transplant Registry (IPTR) reports[3]:
   a. Greater than 35,000 pancreas transplants were performed between 1966 and 2011.

TABLE 15-1 Patient and Graft Survival by Type of Pancreas Transplant

Procedure	1-Year Patient Survival*	1-Year Graft Survival*	5-Year Graft Survival*
Pancreas transplant alone (PTA)	>95%	77.8%	82%
Simultaneous pancreas-kidney (SPK) transplant	>95%	Pancreas: 85.5% Kidney: 93.4%	Pancreas: 72% Kidney: 80%
Pancreas after kidney (PAK) transplant	>95%	79.9%	78%

*Per 2011 IPTR data. Data from Gruessner AC. 2011 Update on pancreas transplantation: comprehensive trend analysis of 25,000 cases followed up over the course of twenty-four years at the International Pancreas Transplant Registry (IPTR). *Rev Diabet Stud.* 2011;8:6–16.

      i. More than 24,000 transplants were performed in the United States during this period.

      ii. More than 12,000 pancreas transplants were performed outside the United States during this period.

  b. Table 15-1 depicts patient and graft survival by type of pancreas transplant.

  c. Distribution of pancreas transplant volume by type of transplant is displayed in Figure 15-1.

7. Patients with severe or "brittle" diabetes are very limited in their ability to pursue normal activities of daily living due to

  a. Frequent problems with high and/or low blood glucose

  b. Hyperglycemia, which causes microvascular, macrovascular, and autonomic complications:

      i. Microvascular complications:

        • Diabetic nephropathy

          ⟩ Diabetic nephropathy is the leading cause of end-stage renal disease (ESRD), accounting for more than 44% of all new cases annually in the United States.[4]

        • Diabetic retinopathy

      ii. Macrovascular complications:

        • Accelerated cardiovascular disease including myocardial infarction (MI), cerebrovascular accidents (CVA), and peripheral arterial disease (PAD).

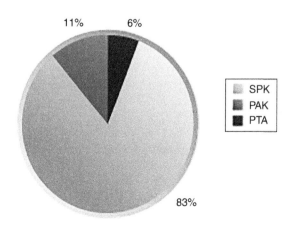

FIGURE 15-1 Distribution of transplant volume by type of transplant.

iii. Autonomic complications:
- Gastroparesis
- Peripheral neuropathy
- Neurogenic bladder
- Sexual dysfunction
- Orthostatic hypotension

c. Hypoglycemia, reoccurring over time, causes a shift in the threshold for symptoms and counterregulatory responses to occur, referred to as hypoglycemic unawareness.

i. If not corrected, hypoglycemia may progress to diabetic coma and cause brain cell death or injury as the brain is the only organ that requires glucose for function.[5]

8. Most patients tend to do very well with a pancreas transplant.[6–9]
a. Quality of life may be dramatically enhanced.
b. Progression of complications of diabetes (neuropathy, nephropathy, and retinopathy) may be arrested.

 II. INDICATIONS[10]

A. Pancreas transplant alone (PTA) or pancreas after kidney (PAK) transplant
1. Diagnosis of diabetes:
a. Most candidates for pancreas transplantation have had type 1 diabetes manifested by poor metabolic control, especially hypoglycemic unawareness, for many years.
b. Candidates must meet the following criteria[10]:
i. On insulin and C-peptide $\leq$ 2 ng/mL OR
ii. On insulin and C-peptide $\geq$2 ng/mL AND a body mass index (BMI) less than or equal to the maximum allowable BMI (currently $\leq$28 kg/m^2)
2. Pancreatic exocrine insufficiency
3. Patients with type 2 diabetes are seldom evaluated for pancreas transplantation and account for only 7% of all pancreas transplant recipients in 2010.[3]

B. Simultaneous pancreas-kidney (SPK) transplantation
1. Diagnosis of diabetes or pancreatic exocrine insufficiency with renal insufficiency

 III. CANDIDATE SELECTION CRITERIA

A. Eligibility criteria can vary widely at each transplant center.

B. Objective measures of end-organ failure include
1. C-peptide deficiency
2. Frequent or severe metabolic complications:
a. Hypo- or hyperglycemia
b. Ketoacidosis
c. Hypoglycemic unawareness despite optimized medical management
3. Evidence of secondary complications such as
a. Peripheral neuropathy
b. Retinopathy
c. Gastroparesis
d. Coronary artery disease

C. Subjective measures of end-organ failure:
   1. Numbness, tingling, or loss of perception in extremities
   2. Lethargy
   3. Nausea
   4. Dizziness
   5. Blurred vision, low vision, or blindness

 IV. PREOPERATIVE PHASE

A. Candidate evaluation testing:
   1. Evaluation protocols vary by institution and are individualized according to patient's medical history and physical examination.
      a. Table 15-2 lists typical evaluation tests.

B. Patient and caregiver education
   1. Principles of patient education
      a. Before providing education, assess the patient for
         i. Readiness to learn

TABLE 15-2 Typical Evaluation Tests

Laboratory	Cardiovascular
• Electrolyte panel	• 12-lead EKG
• Phosphate and magnesium	• Chest radiograph
• Uric acid	• Echocardiogram
• Liver function tests	• Ultrasound of carotid arteries
• Hgb A-1C	• Nuclear stress test/or cardiac catheterization
• C-peptide	• Doppler ultrasound of peripheral vessels to detect vascular disease
• Fasting lipid panel	• Letter of clearance from cardiologist
• Amylase and lipase	
• CBC with differential	
• Coagulation profile	
• Serologies (CMV; HIV; EBV; HBV surface antigen, antibody, and core antibody; HCV antibody; and HAV IgG)	
• Urinalysis	
• 24-hour protein/creatinine clearance	
• Glomerular filtration rate	
• Thyroid function studies (T_3, T_4, TSH)	
• FANA (flourescent) and/or ANA	
• Blood type (ABO)	
• Prostate-specific antigen	
• PAP smear	
Immunogenetics	**Radiology**
• PRA	• Bone density scan
• HLA typing/tissue typing	• Mammogram
	• Sigmoidoscopy/barium enema or colonoscopy
Dental exam	**Psychosocial and financial consultation**

CBC, complete blood count; Hgb A-1C, glycosylated hemoglobin; CMV, cytomegalovirus; EBV, Epstein-Barr virus; HCV, hepatitis C; HBV, hepatitis B; HLA, human leukocyte antigen; T_3, triiodothyronine; T_4, thyroxine; TSH, thyroid-stimulating hormone; FANA, fluorescent antinuclear antibody; ANA, antinuclear antibody; PRA, preformed reactive antibody; HLA, human lymphocyte antibody; EKG, electrocardiogram.

    ii. Level of health literacy

    iii. Potential barriers to learning, for example:

- Physiological (e.g., visual impairment)
- Psychological (e.g., anxiety)

    iv. Preferred learning style

2. Education begins with the initial referral and continues throughout the transplant continuum. Topics discussed at one point in the continuum will often need to be reemphasized at subsequent time points. For the purposes of this chapter, key transplant phase-specific educational topics will be highlighted in the discussion of each particular phase.

3. Preoperative phase: key education topics include, but are not limited to, the following:

    a. Topics required by the Centers for Medicare and Medicaid:

       i. Evaluation process:

- Results of physical exam, labs, and diagnostic testing
- Patient selection criteria and suitability for transplant
- Relationship of psychosocial issues to transplant success
- Financial responsibilities for transplant
- Requirement to follow a strict medical regimen
- Outcome of the evaluation

       ii. Surgical procedure:

- Detailed discussion of surgical procedure
- Anesthesia risk; other potential risks
- Risk related to the use of blood or blood products
- Expected postsurgical course
- Benefits and risk of transplant surgery relative to other alternatives

       iii. Alternative treatment options

       iv. Potential medical risks of transplantation:

- Wound infection
- Pneumonia
- Blood clot formation
- Organ rejection, failure, or retransplant
- Lifetime immunosuppression therapy
- Arrhythmias
- Cardiovascular collapse
- Multiorgan failure
- Death

       v. Potential psychosocial risks:

- Depression.
- Posttraumatic stress disorder.
- Generalized anxiety.
- Feelings of guilt.
- Future health problems may not be covered by insurer.
- Alternative financial resources.
- Future attempt to obtain medical, life, or disability may be affected.

       vi. National and transplant program outcomes from most recent Scientific Registry of Transplant Recipients center report:

- 1-year patient survival.
- 1-year graft survival.
- Transplant program does or does not meet outcomes.

- If center does not meet outcomes, Medicare B will not pay for immunosuppression medications.
- Web sites for additional information www.ustransplant.org and www.optn.org.

    vii. Organ donor risk factors:
- Health risk of donor could affect organ related to donor.
- Medical and social history and age of donor.
- Condition of the organ.
- Risk of disease transmission including
  - Human immunodeficiency virus, hepatitis B, and hepatitis C
  - Cancer
  - Malaria
  - Disease not detectable at time of donor recovery

    viii. Right to refuse transplantation; right to withdraw consent for transplantation

    ix. Medicare B coverage for immunosuppressive medications:
- Transplant must be performed at a Medicare-approved facility for Medicare to pay for immunosuppressive medications

  b. United Network for Organ Sharing required topics:

    i. Right to be listed at more than one transplant center and the ability to transfer accumulated wait time between transplant centers

    ii. Coverage plan for transplant program medical and surgical provider

    iii. Increased donor risk: advise patient at time of organ offer

  c. Other potential topics:

    i. Patient's expectations regarding transplantation

    ii. Role of interdisciplinary team members

    iii. Waitlist and organ allocation

    iv. Preoperative or intraoperative immunosuppression

    v. Posttransplant immunosuppression
- The standard immunosuppression for pancreas transplant recipients typically includes
  - Tacrolimus (Prograf; FK506)
  - Mycophenolate mofetil (CellCept)
  - Prednisone (steroid)

  4. See chapter on Patient Education for additional information.

V. SURGICAL APPROACH[7,11]

A. Native kidneys or pancreas are not removed during the transplant operative procedure.

  1. Allows the exocrine function of the native pancreas to be preserved.

  2. There are two surgical approaches to handle exocrine secretions produced by the transplanted pancreas.

  a. Exocrine secretions are generally drained into

    i. Enteric drainage (ED): bowel drainage:
- When the pancreas is drained enterically, much of the approximate 2 L of exocrine enzymatic fluid and bicarbonate produced by the pancreas is reabsorbed in the bowel.
- The donor portal vein is anastomosed to the side of the recipient's superior mesenteric vein.

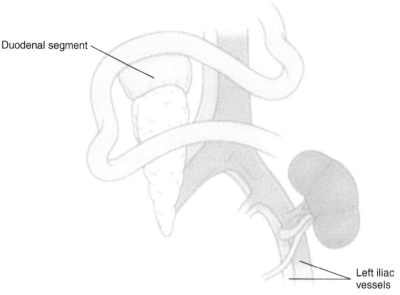

FIGURE 15-2 Enteric drainage technique.

- The transplanted donor duodenal segment is attached to the recipient's jejunum to establish exocrine drainage.
- The enteric drainage technique is shown in Figure 15-2.
- The benefit of ED is that no fluid and electrolyte changes occur posttransplant due to its similarity to natural anatomy.

ii. Bladder drainage (BD)[12]:

- The systemic-bladder drainage technique directs venous outflow and insulin drainage into the iliac vein.
- Exocrine drainage is via anastomosis of a donor duodenal segment to the recipient's urinary bladder.
- The bladder drainage technique is shown in Figure 15-3.

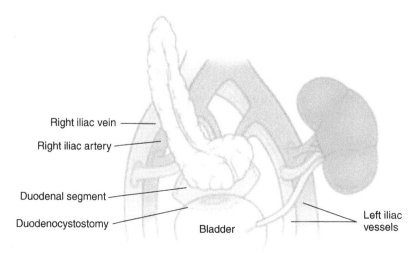

FIGURE 15-3 Technique of a combined pancreas-kidney transplantation through a lower midline approach.

* The benefit of bladder drainage is that rejection episodes in the pancreas can be detected more readily by measuring the exocrine enzyme (amylase) in the urine.
        * Bladder drainage may predispose the patient to
            ○ Dehydration
            ○ Recurrent urinary tract infections (UTIs), especially if patient has a history of neurogenic bladder with poor bladder emptying.
            ○ Cystitis
            ○ Metabolic acidosis (large amounts of sodium bicarbonate are emptied into the bladder)
            ○ Reflux pancreatitis
            ○ Hematuria
    b. IPTR data indicate that there is no significant difference in the success rates between ED and BD techniques in SPK recipients.[3]
        i. Most centers use the ED technique.
        ii. Approximately 10% to 25% of BD recipients undergo a surgical procedure called "enteric conversion" in the first 5 years following transplant due to recurrent UTIs, large duodenal leaks, severe or recurrent hematuria, or significant cystitis.[7,11]
            * Enteric conversion moves the duodenal segment (and as such, exocrine drainage) from the bladder to the bowel
    c. When the pancreas is transplanted simultaneously with a kidney from the same donor, the kidney can serve as the early rejection detection mechanism.
  B. Average length of surgical procedure:
    1. 4 to 8 hours for combined kidney-pancreas transplant
    2. 3 to 4 hours for isolated pancreas transplant

VI. POSTTRANSPLANT PHASE

  A. Posttransplant course (Table 15-3)
    1. Average length of stay: 7 to 14 days
    2. May require 24- to 48-hour stay in intensive care unit for cardiac monitoring, depending on individual transplant center policy

  B. Postoperative tubes, drains, and devices may include
    1. Nasogastric (NG) tube in place for approximately 1 to 2 days, or until bowel function returns.
    2. Foley catheter in place for generally 2 to 3 days.
    3. Compression stockings or device to prevent deep vein thrombosis.
    4. Incentive spirometer; coughing/deep breathing 10 times an hour while awake.
    5. Central venous catheter for parenteral medications and fluid management until diet is advanced.
    6. Surgical drain, if indicated.
    7. Insulin infusion may be utilized to address hyperglycemia for the first 24 to 48 hours posttransplantation to "rest" the insulin-producing islet cells.[7]

  C. Pain management:
    1. It is important to continually assess the patient's level of pain and response to analgesia throughout hospitalization.
    2. Strategies to manage pain are guided by institutional protocols.

TABLE 15-3 Potential Complications and Appropriate Interventions

Potential Complication	Report Signs and Symptoms	Intervene as Ordered by Provider and Evaluate Patient's Response	Collaborate with Interdisciplinary Team
Impaired wound healing	Wound leakage Purulent drainage Edge separation Redness Necrosis Dehiscence	Wound care Enzymatic debridement Antibiotics Hyperbaric oxygen treatments	Clinical provider Wound care nurse Nutritionist
Fluid and electrolyte imbalance	Poor skin turgor Changes in daily weight EKG rhythm disturbance Dry mucous membranes Decreased urine output Mental status changes Dyspnea Rales Edema Distended neck veins	Daily weights Replace urine output and nasogastric drainage with IV fluids. Replace electrolytes.	Nutritionist Clinical provider
Hypoglycemia	Cool and clammy skin Diaphoresis Mental status changes Palpitations	Perform capillary blood glucose measurements. Administer glucose. Offer carbohydrates.	Diabetes educator Nutritionist
Hyperglycemia	Polyuria, polydipsia Fatigue, blurred vision	Perform capillary blood glucose measurements. Administer insulin as prescribed.	Clinical provider Pharmacist Diabetes educator Nutritionist
Hypotension	Vital sign changes Orthostatic hypotension Dizziness	Fluid boluses Monitor I&O. Limit activities.	
Hypertension	Headaches	Administer vasoactive drugs as prescribed. Monitor I&O.	Physician Pharmacist
Altered bowel function	Abdominal pain Constipation Abdominal distention	GI stimulants Stool softeners, laxatives Suppositories Enemas Increase activity. Encourage adequate fluid and fiber intake. Ensure patient has a bowel movement at least every other day.	Clinical provider
Diarrhea	Diarrhea Amount and consistency of stools Stoma condition if applicable	Evaluate response to prescribed medications. Reinforce patient's knowledge regarding decreased GI motility and adverse effect of constipation on pancreas graft	Clinical provider

TABLE 15-3 Potential Complications and Appropriate Interventions (*Continued*)

Potential Complication	Report Signs and Symptoms	Intervene as Ordered by Provider and Evaluate Patient's Response	Collaborate with Interdisciplinary Team
Altered nutrition	Low serum albumin Changes in appetite Weight changes	Calorie counts Enteral and parenteral nutritional supplements	Nutritionist Ancillary nursing staff
Altered mobility/self-care deficit	Level of independence with activities of daily living and ambulation	Incentive spirometer volumes Encourage/assist with mobility Involve family or other caregiver	Physical therapist Respiratory therapist

EKG, electrocardiogram; GI, gastrointestinal; IV, intravenous; I&O, intake and output.

Data from Robertson PR. Benefits and Complications Associated with Kidney–Pancreas Transplantation in Diabetes Mellitus. Uptodate Online Version. Available at http://www.uptodate.com/application/topic.asp?file=renltran/14457&type=A&selectedTitle=2~6. Accessed January 2, 2015; Esterl RM, Abrahamian GA, Sutherland DE, et al. Care of the pancreas transplant recipient. In: Irwin RS, Rippe JM, eds. *Irwin and Rippe's Intensive Care Medicine*. 7th ed. Philadelphia, PA: Lippincott Williams & Wilkins; 2007:1857–1865; Gremizzi C, Vergani A, Paloschi V, et al. Impact of pancreas transplant on type 1 diabetes-related complications. *Curr Opin Organ Transplant*. 2010;15:119–123; James MM. Nursing care of the pancreas transplant recipient. *Crit Care Nurse Clin N Am*. 2011;23:425–441; Kaufman D, Koffron A. Pancreas Transplantation. *eMed J*. 2001. Available at http://www.emedicine.com/med/topic2605.htm. Accessed January 2, 2015; Troppmann C. Complications after pancreas transplantation. *Curr Opin Organ Transplant*. 2010;15(1):112–118; Humar A, Ramcharan T, Kandaswamy R, et al. Technical failures after pancreas transplants: why grafts fail and the risk factors—a multivariate analysis. *Transplantation*. 2004;78:1188–1192; Goodman J, Becker YT. Pancreas surgical complications. *Curr Opin Organ Transplant*. 2009;14(1):85–89.

D.   Anti-rejection medications[7,13]:

1. Most patients receiving pancreas transplants will receive triple therapy immunosuppression although regimens vary at individual transplant centers, including steroid-sparing protocols.

   a. Triple therapy includes

       i.   A calcineurin inhibitor: tacrolimus (Prograf) or cyclosporine (Neoral or Gengraf)

       ii. An antiproliferative agent: mycophenolate mofetil (CellCept) or mycophenolic acid (Myfortic)

       iii. A corticosteroid: methylprednisolone (Solu-Medrol) IV or oral prednisone

   b. Sirolimus (Rapamycin/Rapamune) is being used for some patients in lieu of a calcineurin inhibitor to minimize the nephrotoxic effects associated with calcineurin inhibitors.

   c. Most patients will remain on tacrolimus and mycophenolate long term but may taper off prednisone within the months following transplant (if they initially received prednisone).

2. Induction therapy is utilized by some pancreas transplant centers to minimize or avoid steroids due to the impact steroids have on blood glucose levels. These agents include

   a. Basiliximab (Simulect), monocolonal antibody

   b. Alemtuzumab (Campath), monoclonal antibody

   c. Antilymphocyte globulin (Thymoglobulin), polyclonal antibody

3. See the Chapter on Transplant Pharmacology for additional information regarding immunosuppression medications and their side effects.

E.   Other medications: See Table 15-4:

1. See Chapter on Noninfectious Diseases for additional information about posttransplant medications.

TABLE 15-4 Commonly Prescribed Nonimmunosuppressive Drugs

Antimicrobials	
Antibiotics	Trimethoprim-sulfamethoxazole against *Pneumocystis carinii* pneumonia and UTI; penicillins with beta lactamase inhibitor, quinolones, cephalosporins, aminoglycosides, linezolid
Antifungals	Anti *Candida albicans*: nystatin, clotrimazole; Broad spectrum: fluconazole, ketoconazole; Anti Streptomyces: amphotericin B
Antivirals	Anti herpes: acyclovir, valacyclovir, famciclovir Anti cytomegalovirus: ganciclovir, valgancyclovir, immunoglobulin, cytogam, foscarnet
Supplements	Sodium bicarbonate, magnesium oxide, potassium phosphate
Analgesics	Narcotics, non-narcotics, muscle relaxants
Cardiovascular	Beta blockers, angiotensin-converting enzyme inhibitors, calcium channel blockers cholesterol-lowering agents, diuretics
Acid reducers	Hydrogen ion (H2) blockers, proton pump inhibitors, antacids
Insulin and anti-hyperglycemic medications	Long-acting, regular insulin sliding scale, oral hypoglycemic agents

F. Activity:

  1. Patients should be out of bed postoperative day 1 and advance activity as tolerated.

G. Incisional care:

  1. Midline abdominal incision dressing should be changed daily or as needed.
  2. If staples or sutures were used, they will remain for approximately 3 weeks after surgery.

H. Psychosocial considerations:

  1. Transplantation is emotionally stressful and demanding.
  2. Most patients cope better when they have an understanding of the transplant process.
  3. It is important to assess patients' expectations.
     a. Transplantation is a treatment option, which, with improved surgical techniques and new drug therapies, has become a more desirable approach to treating diabetes while enhancing quality of life.
  4. Patients and caregivers are likely to need emotional support.
     a. They may be excited and hopeful that they are starting the transplant process and, at the same time, be anxious about what lies ahead.
     b. It is important to reassure patients and caregivers that these feelings are normal and encourage them to acknowledge and verbalize their feelings.
     c. Resources include the interdisciplinary transplant team, particularly psychologists and social workers, as well as support groups.

I. Patient/caregiver education:

  1. Names, purpose, and dose of medications using "teach-back" method.
  2. Provide the patient an opportunity to self-medicate under nursing supervision as a "rehearsal" for self-care following discharge.

VII. POSTTRANSPLANT ASSESSMENT AND MONITORING

A. A well-documented nursing assessment is essential to providing immediate and appropriate interventions during this critical phase of recovery.

B. The initial postoperative period necessitates close monitoring of
   1. Cardiovascular status
   2. Fluid and electrolyte balance
   3. Metabolic function
   4. Pancreatic graft function

C. Vital signs:
   1. Temperature:
      a. In pancreas transplant recipients, temperature elevations may indicate
         i. Infection
         ii. Pancreatitis
         iii. Acute rejection
   2. Heart rate: target range: 60 to 100 bpm
      a. Report heart rate below 60 or above 100 bpm
   3. Blood pressure:
      a. Assess and document supine and upright blood pressure readings:
         i. Orthostatic hypotension is common secondary to volume depletion.
      b. Parameters individualized to levels to maintain blood flow and graft patency.
      c. Report if readings beyond prescribed parameters (above or below).
      d. Diastolic blood pressure >100 mm Hg: consider antihypertensive agents.

D. Central venous pressure (CVP): acceptable range: 5 to 10 cm H_2O[14]

E. Weight:
   1. Review baseline weight that was obtained on admission.
   2. Record immediate postoperative weight.
   3. Record daily weight, preferably at the same time of day, using the same scale.
   4. Report weight gain or loss per program protocol.

F. Fluid and electrolyte balance:
   1. Postoperative nausea, vomiting, and ileus are common secondary to gastroparesis in diabetic patients.
      a. May contribute to fluid and electrolyte imbalance.
   2. An NG tube is commonly placed until bowel function improves to avoid problems associated with decreased motility.
   3. Strict hourly measurement of fluid intake and output is essential for the prompt detection of dehydration, which can occur rapidly.
      a. Output includes drainage from the NG tube, surgical drains, pancreatic drains, and incisional dressings.
      b. Notify the transplant team provider if urine output <50 and >200 mL/hour in the first 24 hours post transplant.
   4. Fluid imbalance is more common in bladder-drained pancreas recipients than in enteric-drained pancreas recipients due to the large amount of fluid loss.
      a. The transplanted pancreas excretes significant amounts of fluid rich in bicarbonate and pancreatic enzymes into the bladder.[15]

b. The pancreas graft is a "low blood flow" organ and has a higher potential for graft thrombosis. Therefore, adequate perfusion of the graft requires maintaining an appropriate intravascular volume.[7,10]

5. Promptly report indications of dehydration:
   a. Poor skin turgor
   b. Decrease in weight
   c. Negative fluid intake versus output ratio
   d. Dry mucous membranes
   e. Changes in vital signs
   f. Decreased urine output
   g. Increased blood urea nitrogen level and creatinine; decreased carbon dioxide[5]

G. Potential interventions to correct fluid and electrolyte imbalance may include

1. Administration of intravenous (IV) fluids to replace urine and NG tube output milliliter for milliliter (or per hospital protocol) in the first 24 hours following transplantation
2. Administration of albumin to restore plasma volume or to control for third spacing due to handling of the bowel
3. Administration of IV fluids containing bicarbonate to prevent dehydration and correct metabolic acidosis[7]
   a. For patients with BD pancreas transplants, dehydration and metabolic acidosis will remain potential posttransplant complications for the life of the pancreas graft.
4. IV or oral replacement of electrolytes

H. Patient/caregiver education:

1. Importance of adequate oral fluid intake to minimize the risk of hypotension and graft thrombosis
2. Frequent posttransplant dose adjustments in antihypertensive agents, particularly in the first 2 to 8 weeks following discharge

VIII. PANCREATIC GRAFT FUNCTION

A. Monitored by

1. Serum glucose levels
2. Serum amylase and serum lipase concentrations
3. Glycosylated hemoglobin
4. Fasting C-peptide

B. Serum glucose:

1. Glucose testing can be as frequent as every 1 to 2 hours.[7]
2. An acute spike in glucose level in the early postoperative period should be considered potentially indicative of vascular thrombosis of the graft.[7]
   a. Contact transplant surgical team immediately.[16]
   b. Ultrasound (urgent) is commonly ordered to rule out thrombosis.
   c. If thrombosis is detected via ultrasound, the patient may undergo emergent reoperation for thrombectomy.[7]
3. Mild hyperglycemia may also be due to the diabetogenic effect of high-dose corticosteroids and cyclosporine or tacrolimus.[6]

4. Management of hyperglycemia:
   a. An insulin drip may be ordered for the first 24 to 48 hours post transplantation.[7]
   b. As pancreas function improves, the need for insulin decreases.[7]
5. Patient education includes
   a. Blood glucose self-monitoring
   b. Use of short-acting insulin in a sliding scale for periods of hyperglycemia

C. Amylase concentrations
   1. Serum amylase levels
      a. May be elevated in the following settings:
         i. Within 48 to 96 hours posttransplantation[15] secondary to
            • Damage to the organ during cold ischemia preservation
            • Manipulation of the organ during surgery[7]
         ii. Subsequent to a transplant biopsy
         iii. Venous thrombosis
         iv. Anastomotic leak
   2. Amylase levels are also monitored in pancreatic (surgical) drain fluid in the early postoperative period (if drain is present).[7]
      a. The presence of high levels of amylase in surgical drain fluid is indicative of an anastomotic or parenchymal pancreatic leak.
      b. If amylase is present in surgical drain fluid, laparotomy is commonly performed to identify and correct the anastomotic leak.
   3. Urine amylase:
      a. In a bladder-drained pancreas transplant recipient, a pancreas exocrine product called amylase is excreted from the pancreas via the urine. Upon analyzing the amylase content of the urine, a decreased level can be indicative of graft rejection.
      b. An 8-hour urine collection is a way of monitoring for organ rejection in BD pancreas transplant recipients.[7]
      c. Daily 8-hour urine testing is conducted in the immediate posttransplant hospitalization, preferably from urine samples collected at the same hours of the day for better comparison of results.
         i. As the patient is further from the transplant, urine amylase specimens are collected less frequently based on protocols of the individual transplant center.
      d. Collection times and volume of collected urine must be accurately documented.
      e. A convenient collecting time period would be for 8 hours through the night.
         i. Specimens should be sent to the laboratory as soon as collection is completed the next morning.
      f. Baseline urine amylase levels between 1,500 and 7,000 IU/hour within a few days following transplantation indicate good initial graft function.[17]

D. Glycosylated hemoglobin (HbA$_1$C)
   1. HbA$_1$C should normalize to the levels of nondiabetic patients with a well-functioning pancreas graft.

E. Fasting C-peptide level
   1. Indicates function of the insulin-producing beta cells of the islet of Langerhans.

2. The absence of C-peptide indicates that there is no beta cell function or insulin production.[18]

3. Normal values are 0.8 to 3.1 ng/mL (conventional units) or 0.26 to 1.03 nmol/L (SI).

F. Serum bicarbonate

1. Levels should be watched closely in patients who have undergone BD pancreas transplantation
   a. The transplanted organ excretes large amounts of bicarbonate-rich pancreatic secretions into the bladder following transplantation.
   b. The may lead to dehydration, orthostatic hypotension, and acidosis.
   c. Supplemental sodium bicarbonate with doses as high as 100 to 150 mEq/day is administered to minimize the degree of metabolic acidosis for all BD transplant patients.[6]

2. In ED transplant procedures, the excreted pancreatic enzymes and bicarbonate drain into the intestine for reabsorption.[7] As a result:
   a. Dehydration is far less common than in BD transplant procedures.
   b. Electrolyte imbalances are rare.

G. Immunosuppression monitoring

1. Levels are monitored frequently, often daily, while the patient is in the hospital.

2. Trough levels of the previous dose are monitored to assure levels are at the target level:
   a. Trough levels are 12 hours after the previous dose.

3. Medications monitored with trough levels include
   a. Tacrolimus
   b. Cyclosporine
   c. Sirolimus
   d. Mycophenolic acid

4. Target therapeutic immunosuppression levels are determined for individual patients based on the length of time since transplantation.

5. Dosing is adjusted according to institutional guidelines and the patient's target level.

 IX. POSTOPERATIVE COMPLICATIONS

A. Primary graft nonfunction[19]

1. Absence of graft function as evidenced by minimal or no insulin production with no other explanation:
   a. Thrombosis and hyperacute rejection have been ruled out.

2. Rate: occurs in 0.5% to 1% of pancreas transplant cases.

3. Treatment is center specific.
   a. Treatment may include administration of insulin.

B. Technical complications

1. Overview
   a. The graft failure rate due to technical complications in all categories (i.e., PTA, PAK, and SPK) is 8% to 9%.[3]
   b. Over 50% of graft failures within the first six posttransplant months are due to technical failures.[8]
   c. Thrombosis is the major technical cause of graft failure. Other technical causes include pancreatitis, anastomotic leaks, infections, and bleeding.[8]

2. Vascular thrombosis
   a. One of several early complications following pancreas transplant.[3,7,19-21]
   b. Recent IPTR data indicate that the rate of graft thrombosis is slightly higher in solitary transplant recipients (PTA, PAK) (7%) than in SPK recipients (5%).[13]
   c. Thrombosis generally occurs within 24 to 48 hours after transplant and can be venous or arterial in origin; venous thrombosis is more common.[9]
   d. Many transplant centers use various anticoagulation therapies, either alone or in conjunction with antiplatelet options, to prevent graft thrombosis such as[7,9,15]
      i. Intravenous heparin
      ii. Enoxaparin (Lovenox)
      iii. Aspirin
   e. Clinical indications of vascular thrombosis may include the following[13,16,19,21]:
      i. An abrupt rise in glucose levels or continuously rising blood glucose levels in the immediate postoperative period.
      ii. Sharp rise in serum amylase and/or lipase levels.
      iii. Tenderness or pain over the graft site in some patients.
      iv. In the BD pancreas transplant recipient:
         • Massive hematuria
         • Decrease in, or absence of, urine amylase levels
   f. Potential interventions[9,19,21]:
      i. Exploratory surgery for possible thrombectomy is typically necessary.
      ii. If thrombectomy is unsuccessful, a pancreatectomy may be indicated.
   g. In addition to appropriate recipient selection, strategies to prevent vascular thrombosis include
      i. Appropriate donor selection
      ii. Minimizing cold ischemic time (<24 hours)
      iii. Cautious handling of the organ during procurement[3,9,11,15,19]
3. Pancreatitis
   a. Allograft pancreatitis is a relatively common postoperative occurrence.[6,12,18-21]
   b. Signs and symptoms of pancreatitis are similar to those of acute rejection or anastomotic leaks and may include[15,17,19,21]
      i. Low-grade fever
      ii. Elevated serum amylase and serum lipase levels:
         • Note: Serum amylase levels may be mildly elevated for the first 2 to 3 days after transplant.
         • This elevation may be related to the handling of the organ prior to transplant or ischemic injury prior to procurement and may not be clinically significant.[19]
      iii. Decreased urine amylase (with BD procedures)
      iv. Graft tenderness
      v. Abdominal pain
      vi. Nausea and vomiting
      vii. Endocrine secretory capacity (i.e., insulin secretion) often only mildly impaired
4. Reflux pancreatitis[11,12,15,19,21]
   a. Etiology:
      i. Occurs in BD pancreas transplant recipients when urinary retention causes resistance to the flow of pancreatic enzymes into the bladder.

        ii. As a result, urine and pancreatic enzymes flow back into and irritate the pancreas; serum amylase levels increase.

    b. Potential treatment options:

        i. Urinary catheter placement for 2 to 6 weeks to decompress the bladder.

        ii. Keep patient NPO; administer total parenteral nutrition.

        iii. Urologic assessment for any underlying problems such as neurogenic bladder.

        iv. In the setting of repetitive reflux pancreatitis: consider enteric conversion surgery.

  5. Anastomotic leaks

    a. Leaks can be one of the more serious complications postoperatively.

    b. Leaks occur most commonly in the first 3 months.[15]

    c. Anastomotic leaks are less common than pancreatitis or thrombosis of the pancreas allograft.[15]

    d. ED pancreas transplant anastomotic leak.

        i. Patients with an enteric anastomotic leak may present with[15,17,19,21]

- Fever
- Elevated white blood cell count
- Nausea and vomiting
- Abdominal pain
- Elevated serum amylase
- Elevated serum creatinine

        ii. Due to spillage of enteric content from intestines into peritoneum, ED pancreas transplant leaks carry significant morbidity risks.[11,19,21]

- Peritoneal fluid of the patient with an enteric leak often contains bacteria and fungi.

        iii. Potential treatment options:

- Administration of broad-spectrum antibiotics
- Return to the operating room for potential repair, irrigation, and debridement
- Allograft pancreatectomy

        iv. If treatment is inadequate, peritonitis can progress to sepsis, organ failure, and death.

    e. BD pancreas transplant anastomotic (urine) leaks[6,19,21]:

        i. This type of leak typically occurs in the first 3 months after pancreas transplantation.

        ii. Urine leaks typically originate from the deterioration of the duodenal segment, especially at the anastomotic site between this segment and the bladder.[11,15,19,21]

        iii. Clinical manifestations are similar to those seen with rejection or pancreatitis; patients experiencing urine leaks may present with

- Lower abdominal pain or tenderness over graft site
- Elevated serum amylase

        iv. Diagnosis: computed tomography (CT) scans.

        v. Treatment:

- Prolonged urinary catheter placement.[7,15,19,21]
- Recurring bladder leaks may require return to the operating room for leakage closure and/or enteric conversion.[11,19]

      6. Wound and intra-abdominal infections[7,19,21]

        a. More common post pancreas transplant than kidney transplant due to the associated contamination of opening the duodenal segment intraoperatively.

        b. Signs and symptoms of an intra-abdominal infection are similar to that of an anastomotic leak, from which the infection may have resulted.

        c. Intra-abdominal abscess: treatment options:

          i. Radiologically placed percutaneous catheter drains.

          ii. IV antimicrobial agents based on culture results.

            • Intra-abdominal infections tend to be caused by bacteria or fungi.

          iii. Return to the operating room and washout.

          iv. Graft pancreatectomy, depending on the type and severity of the complication.

  C. Infection/sepsis

      1. Types of infection[6–8,14]:

        a. UTIs

        b. Opportunistic infections

      2. UTIs[6,7,12]

        a. Pancreas transplant recipients, like many other postsurgical patients, are at risk for catheter-associated UTI.

        b. Pancreas transplant recipients are also at higher risk for UTIs secondary to urinary retention and inability to properly empty the bladder (neurogenic bladder related to diabetes mellitus).

        c. Recipients of BD pancreas transplants are particularly at risk for serious UTIs that can result in pyelonephritis or sepsis.

        d. In certain cases, the frequency of UTIs and sepsis may require BD recipients to undergo enteric conversion.[7]

      3. Opportunistic infections

        a. Opportunistic infections, particularly cytomegalovirus (CMV) infections, are common in all immunosuppressed patients.

        b. Risk factors for CMV infection:

          i. Recipient's pretransplant CMV serologic status (CMV positive)

          ii. CMV mismatch between donor and recipient

            • Donor is CMV seropositive and recipient is CMV seronegative.

          iii. Induction therapy[6]

        c. Most transplant programs utilize CMV prophylaxis regimens to address CMV risk such as

          i. Oral valganciclovir (Valcyte) or IV ganciclovir

        d. See Chapter on Infectious Diseases for additional information.

      4. Sepsis

        a. The aforementioned infections can progress to sepsis, a much more serious systemic infection and inflammatory response.

        b. If not promptly and adequately treated, sepsis can result in death.

  D. Other urologic complications

      1. Cystitis[11,19,21]

        a. Cystitis can occur in the pancreas transplant recipient who has a bladder-drained pancreas, secondary to the effect of pancreatic enzymes on the urinary tract.

        b. Cystitis can be treated with insertion of a Foley catheter, or in extreme cases, the patient may require enteric conversion.

2. Hematuria[11,19,21]
   a. Hematuria in BD pancreas transplant recipients:
      i. Hematuria may occur in the immediate posttransplant period and may resolve spontaneously without clinical significance.
      ii. However, of clinical significance, early hematuria might be related to anticoagulation agents to prevent graft thrombosis.
      iii. Treatment options for severe hematuria include
         • Discontinuation of anticoagulation
         • Continuous bladder irrigation until the bleeding stops
      iv. If hematuria persists, cystoscopy may be necessary.
   b. Late hematuria:
      i. In BD transplant recipients, late hematuria is often a sign of duodenal integrity issues. Continuous late hematuria may result in the need for enteric conversion.
      ii. Hematuria must never be disregarded, as it may be a symptom of rejection.

E. Posttransplant lymphoproliferative disorder (PTLD)[22]
   1. The risk of malignancy, specifically lymphoproliferative disorder, is increased following organ transplantation as a result of immunosuppressive therapy.
      a. The overall incidence of PTLD in pancreas transplant is 1% to 7% and appears to occur sooner in pancreas transplant recipients than in other solid organ transplant recipients.[22]

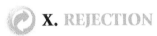

X. REJECTION

A. Overview
   1. Despite advances in transplant care, rejection remains a common cause of pancreas graft loss.[3,8,13,23]
   2. 1-year rates of immunological graft loss vary from 1.8% in SPK to 3.7% in PAK to 6.0% in PTA.[3]
   3. Graft loss due to acute rejection occurs most frequently between 3 and 12 months following all types of pancreas transplantation (SPK, PAK, and PTA); graft loss due to chronic rejection continues to increase over time post transplant.[13]

B. Types of rejection
   1. Acute rejection
      a. Rejection occurs earlier and more frequently in PTA recipients than in either PAK or SPK recipients.[13]
      b. Rejection may be difficult to detect and should be considered if patients experience[13,23]:
         i. Pain at the graft site
         ii. Increased serum amylase or lipase
         iii. Fever
         iv. Decreased urine amylase if the pancreas graft is bladder drained
         v. In the setting of SPK transplantation, elevated serum creatinine levels can serve as a surrogate marker of pancreas rejection as both organs share the same immunologic profile.[16,23]
         vi. Hyperglycemia:
            • Not an early sign of pancreas transplant rejection; in fact, in the initial stages of rejection, glucose levels remain normal[23]

* Is a much later sign, which develops when damage has occurred to islet cells
* Occurs in the more severe types of acute rejection, which are often irreversible[23]

2. Chronic rejection[23]
   a. Manifests as a progressive need for insulin.
   b. Risk of chronic rejection is greater with multiple episodes of acute rejection.

C. Diagnosis of rejection—pancreas allograft biopsy
   1. Patients with symptoms that may be indicative of graft rejection should have a CT- or US-guided percutaneous pancreas biopsy if possible.
   2. Purpose of biopsy[13,16,23,24]:
      a. Confirm diagnosis of rejection
      b. Grade the severity of the rejection
      c. Differentiate antibody-mediated rejection from acute cellular rejection
   3. In the setting of SPK transplantation, both organs reject simultaneously; kidney function markers and kidney biopsy can also serve as markers for pancreas rejection.[17,23]
   4. Postbiopsy nursing care:
      a. Bed rest for 4 to 6 hours for observation after the procedure.
      b. Monitor patient for
         i. External bleeding at the biopsy puncture site
         ii. Hematoma
         iii. Changes in vital signs including but not limited to hypotension and tachycardia
         iv. Pain
         v. Hematuria in the setting of BD pancreas transplant

D. Treatment options for rejection[7,17]
   1. The type and severity of rejection guide treatment
   2. Treatment options include
      a. Intravenous pulse steroids
      b. Antilymphocyte preparations
         i. Antithymocyte globulin (Thymoglobulin)
      c. Plasmapheresis
      d. IVIG
      e. Increasing maintenance dose of maintenance oral immunosuppressants[23]

E. Postbiopsy patient/caregiver education
   1. Biopsy results
   2. Potential complications of biopsy (e.g., bleeding at biopsy site; hematoma)
   3. Rejection treatment, if applicable
   4. Next biopsy, if applicable

 XI. PATIENT/CAREGIVER DISCHARGE EDUCATION

A. Key topics include, but are not limited to, the following:
   1. Posttransplant medications:
      a. Dose, frequency, medication schedule
      b. Target levels of immunosuppressants
      c. Dose adjustments
      d. Common and serious side effects

      e. What to do if a dosed is missed

      f. Proper storage of medications

      g. How to obtain refills

      h. Drug-drug or drug-food interactions

      i. Report medications ordered by other providers

2. Lab work:

      a. When to take immunosuppressants on day of labwork (e.g., withhold morning dose until blood is drawn)

3. Biopsies; follow-up in transplant clinic

4. Driving and weight-lifting restrictions (typically apply to first 1 to 2 months post transplant)

5. When to call the transplant center

XII. SUMMARY

A. Pancreas transplantation has become widely accepted as an effective therapeutic treatment for certain patients.

B. Potential complications include

    1. Vascular thrombosis

    2. Pancreatitis

    3. Anastomotic leaks

    4. Hematuria

    5. Infections/sepsis

    6. Cystitis

    7. Rejection

    8. PTLD

C. The increased use of the ED transplant technique, as opposed to the BD technique, has decreased the incidence of certain urologic and metabolic complications.[3]

D. Most patients tend to do very well following pancreas transplantation:

    1. Quality of life may be significantly enhanced by stable glucose control.[6,7]

    2. Progression of complications associated with diabetes may be arrested.[9]

      a. Diabetes is a hypercoagulable state and as such is prothrombotic.

      b. Micro- and macrovascular lesions are improved as a result of glucose level normalization.[8,9]

      c. These lesions include those associated with neuropathy, nephropathy, and retinopathy.[6-8]

        i. Neuropathy: Improvements in autonomic neuropathy have been reported following pancreas transplantation.

        ii. Nephropathy: If performed in early stages of kidney disease, pancreas transplantation may prevent kidney failure and need for kidney transplantation.

        iii. Retinopathy: Successful pancreas transplantation stabilizes the disease, thereby helping to prevent blindness.

E. Transplant clinicians must recognize the negative impact that posttransplant complications can have on survival and quality of life. Close posttransplant follow-up, including prophylactic measures to prevent complications, is imperative.

REFERENCES

1. World Health Organization. Diabetes Fact Sheet. Available at http://www.who.int/mediacentre/factsheets/fs312/en/. Accessed September 21, 2014.
2. Centers for Disease Control and Prevention. National Diabetes Statistics Report. 2014. Available at http://www.cdc.gov/diabetes/pubs/statsreport14/national-diabetes-report-web.pdf. Accessed September 21, 2014.
3. Gruessner AC. 2011 Update on pancreas transplantation: comprehensive trend analysis of 25,000 cases followed up over the course of twenty-four years at the International Pancreas Transplant Registry (IPTR). *Rev Diabet Stud.* 2011;8:6–16.
4. United States Renal Data System. *US Renal Data System Annual Report.* Available at http://www.usrds.org/atlas.aspx. Accessed September 30, 2014.
5. Cryer PE. Hypoglycemia. In: Braunwald E, Fauci AS, Kasper DL, et al., eds. *Harrison's 18th Ed Principles of Internal Medicine.* New York, NY: McGraw Hill; 2012:2139–2140.
6. Robertson PR. Benefits and Complications Associated with Kidney–Pancreas Transplantation in Diabetes Mellitus. Uptodate Online Version. Available at http://www.uptodate.com/application/topic.asp?file=renltran/14457&type=A&selectedTitle=2~6. Accessed January 2, 2015.
7. Esterl RM, Abrahamian GA, Sutherland DE, et al. Care of the pancreas transplant recipient. In: Irwin RS, Rippe JM, eds. *Irwin and Rippe's Intensive Care Medicine.* 7th ed. Philadelphia, PA: Lippincott Williams & Wilkins; 2007:1857–1865.
8. Gremizzi C, Vergani A, Paloschi V, et al. Impact of pancreas transplant on type 1 diabetes-related complications. *Curr Opin Organ Transplant.* 2010;15:119–123.
9. Muthusamy AS, Giangrande PL, Friend PJ. Pancreas allograft thrombosis. *Transplantation.* 2010;90(7):705–707.
10. Organ Procurement and Transplantation Network Policies, Policy 11. Available at http://optn.transplant.hrsa.gov/ContentDocuments/OPTN_Policies.pdf. Accessed September 30, 2014.
11. Boggi U, Amorese G, Marchetti P. Surgical techniques for pancreas transplantation. *Curr Opin Organ Transplant.* 2010;15:102–111.
12. Voskuil MD, Mittal S, Sharples EJ, et al. Improving monitoring after pancreas transplantation alone: fine-tuning of an old technique. *Clin Transplant.* 2014;28:1047–1053.
13. Gruessner AC, Sutherland DE, Gruessner RW. Pancreas transplantation in the United States: a review. *Curr Opin Organ Transplant.* 2010;15:93–101.
14. Wilkins RL, Stoller JK, Heuer AJ. *Egan's Fundamentals of Respiratory Care.* 10th ed. St. Louis, MO: Elsevier; 2012:1140.
15. Boggi U, Burke G, Belani K. Peri-operative management of the kidney–pancreas and pancreas transplant recipient. In: Pretto E Jr, Biancofiore G, DeWolf A, et al., eds. *Oxford Transplant Anaesthesia and Critical Care.* Oxford, UK: Oxford University Press; 2015:141–150.
16. James MM. Nursing care of the pancreas transplant recipient. *Crit Care Nurse Clin N Am.* 2011;23:425–441.
17. Robertson PR. Patient Selection For And Immunologic Issues Relating to Kidney–Pancreas Transplantation in Diabetes Mellitus. Uptodate Online Version 11.0. 2014. Available at http://www.uptodateonline.com/application/topic.asp?file=renltran/12278&type=A&selectedTitle=3~6. Accessed January 8, 2014.
18. Kaufman D, Koffron A. Pancreas Transplantation. *eMed J.* 2001. Available at http://www.emedicine.com/med/topic2605.htm. Accessed January 2, 2015.
19. Troppmann C. Complications after pancreas transplantation. *Curr Opin Organ Transplant.* 2010;15(1):112–118.
20. Humar A, Ramcharan T, Kandaswamy R, et al. Technical failures after pancreas transplants: why grafts fail and the risk factors—a multivariate analysis. *Transplantation.* 2004;78:1188–1192.
21. Goodman J, Becker YT. Pancreas surgical complications. *Curr Opin Organ Transplant.* 2009;14(1):85–89.
22. Jackson K, Ruppert K, Shapiro R. Post-transplant lymphoproliferative disorder after pancreas transplantation: a United Network for organ sharing database analysis. *Clin Transplant.* 2013;27:888–894.
23. Drachenberg CB, Odorico J, Demetris AJ, et al. Banff schema for grading pancreas allograft rejection: working proposal by a multi-disciplinary international consensus panel. *Am J Transplant.* 2008:1237–1249.
24. Redfield RR, Kaufman DB, Odorico JS. Diagnosis and treatment of pancreas rejection. *Curr Transplant Rep.* 2015;2:169–175.

SELF-ASSESSMENT QUESTIONS

1. The benefit of bladder drainage is that rejection episodes can be detected more readily by measuring which of the following in the urine?
   a. Sodium and potassium
   b. Solutes
   c. Amylase
   d. Glucose

2. In a bladder-drained pancreas recipient, what are the signs of rejection?
   a. Decreased urine amylase
   b. Increase blood (serum) amylase
   c. Increased urine amylase
   d. a and b
   e. b and c

3. Indications for pancreas or combined kidney/pancreas transplant include which of the following complications of type 1 diabetes?
   a. Hypoglycemic unawareness
   b. End-stage renal disease
   c. On insulin and C-peptide of ≤ 2 ng/mL
   d. All of the above

4. Bladder drainage of exocrine secretions may predispose the patient to which of the following complications?
   a. Dehydration
   b. Metabolic acidosis
   c. Volume overload
   d. Cystitis
   e. b, c, and d
   f. a, b, and d

5. Approximately 15% to 20% of BD recipients undergo a surgical procedure called "enteric conversion," which is best described as:
   a. sterilization of the bowel to minimize risk of posttransplant infections.
   b. the development of a postoperative ileus with nausea and vomiting.
   c. damage to the organ during cold ischemia preservation.
   d. movement of the duodenal segment from the bladder to the bowel.

6. Which of the following are benefits of pancreas transplantation?
   a. Insulin independence
   b. Reversal of end-stage renal disease
   c. Stabilize retinopathy
   d. Improved neuropathy
   e. a, b, and c
   f. a, b, and d

7. Postoperative ileus with nausea and vomiting is not uncommon following pancreas transplantation. These complications are attributed to which of the following pretransplant problems?
   a. Peripheral neuropathy
   b. End-stage renal disease
   c. Gastroparesis
   d. All of the above

8. A patient experiencing vascular thrombosis may present with which of the following symptoms?
   a. Elevated blood glucose levels
   b. Elevated serum amylase level
   c. Acute abdominal pain
   d. Acute thrombosis of the hepatic artery
   e. b, c, and d
   f. a, b, and c

9. Patients with an anastomotic leak may present with which of the following symptoms?
   a. Sharp increase in blood glucose levels
   b. Increase in white blood cells
   c. Abdominal pain
   d. Elevated serum creatinine
   e. a and c
   f. b, c, and d

10. Nursing management of a pancreas transplant recipient with sepsis includes which of the following interventions?
    a. Strict monitoring of blood glucose levels
    b. Management of drains
    c. Strict intake and output
    d. Strict hand-washing techniques
    e. a and d only
    f. All of the above

Correct Answers:
1.c   2.d   3.d   4.f   5.d   6.f   7.c   8.f   9.f   10.f

CHAPTER 16

Vascularized Composite Tissue Allotransplantation

T. Nicole Kelley, MS, ACNP, CCRN, CPSN, CANS, RNFA
Linda A. Evans, RN, PhD

I. INTRODUCTION

"Organ transplant" generally presumes the implantation of a kidney, heart, or other solid internal organ. In recent times, the concept of transplanting combination tissue grafts, which may include bone, skin, muscle, tendon, and nerve, has evolved.[1,2] Composite transplantations have been performed to replace body parts lost to disease,[3] trauma,[4–7] or congenital malformations.[8]

This chapter provides information for nurses caring for patients undergoing vascularized composite tissue allotransplantation (VCA), including historical perspectives, ethical considerations, government and agency oversight, patient evaluation criteria and preparation for surgery, novel surgical interventions, specialized considerations for perioperative care, VCA benefits and risks, and long-term patient monitoring care related to graft monitoring and immunosuppression. Specific focus is on facial and hand transplantation.

II. OVERVIEW

    A. Composite tissue allotransplantation (CTA)

        1. Definition: transplantation of histologically different tissues including skin, connective tissue, blood vessels, muscle, ligaments, cartilage, tendon, bone, nerve tissue, and tissue-based products.[9,10]

        2. CTA: early nomenclature for graft tissue regarding facial and hand transplants.[11]

        3. Viewed as a complex science during the conceptual phase with multiple clinical, ethical, and psychosocial considerations[12]:

            a. Determination of patient selection criteria

            b. Societal considerations

            c. Refining procurement techniques

            d. Limitations of obtaining a fully informed consent

            e. Immunological response and immunosuppressant requirements

            f. Ethical issues

            g. Donor family considerations

        4. An estimated 7 million people per year in the United States could benefit from CTA.[2,8,11]

B. Vascularized composite allotransplantation (VCA)
1. Definition: the simultaneous transplantation of multiple tissue types such as muscle, bone, nerve, and skin as a functional single unit (e.g., hand or face).[9,13,14]
2. Goal: restoration of sensory and motor functional status, anatomy, appearance, and psychosocial well-being including self-esteem and reintegration into family and social life.[15-18]
3. Surgical option when soft tissue and bone loss is accompanied by severe cosmetic, sensory, and functional deficiencies due to disease,[3] trauma,[4-6,19] or congenital malformations.[8]
4. VCA procedures are considered only after all conventional reconstructive methods, or prosthetics in the case of hand amputations, have failed.[8,14]
5. To date, more than 150 VCAs have been reported and include hand, abdominal wall, tongue, trachea, larynx, face,[2,20-23] esophagus, and a vascularized knee and femurs.[2,24]
6. No cases of pediatric facial transplantation have been reported to date.[24]
7. Current clinical trials:
   a. Facial allotransplantation: five trials actively recruiting[13]
   b. Hand allotransplantation: five trials actively recruiting[14]
8. Criteria for body parts defined as a VCA per the Department of Health and Human Services (DHHS).[4,25,26]
   a. Recovered from a human donor as an anatomical structural unit and contains multiple tissues.
   b. Transplanted into a human recipient as an anatomical structural unit.
   c. Vascularized tissue requiring blood flow by surgical connection of vessels to function following transplantation.
   d. Processing does not alter the original characteristics of the "organ graft."
   e. The donated graft performs the same basic functions in the recipient as in the donor.
   f. Not combined with another article or device.
   g. Susceptible to ischemia requiring rapid re-establishment of blood flow; thus can be stored only temporarily (cold storage with preservation medium with the intention of implantation within hours of recovery).
   h. Susceptible to allograft rejection requiring donor-recipient matching and generally requiring immunosuppression.
9. Short-term results of VCA transplantation have been positive.[12,27]
10. Long-term physical, emotional, and psychological effects on both VCA hand and face recipients as well as long-term (>10 years) consequences to the donor's family are unknown.[27]
11. Emotional and ethical impact on health care team members involved in facial transplant surgery and patient care has been positive.[28,29]

III. HISTORICAL PERSPECTIVE

A. Timeline: The development of VCA[4,10,12,22-24,29-32] (Table 16-1).

B. Approximately 35 facial transplant procedures have been reported.[31-36]

C. Facial transplant procedures 1st to 29th: 2005 to 2014[31,32] (Table 16-2).

TABLE 16-1 Timeline—Development of Vascular Composite Allograft Transplantation

Date	Event
348 AD	Legendary account of the transplantation of leg by Cosmos and Damian[12]
Late 16th century	Transplantation of a nose by Gaspare Tagliacozzi[12]
Early 20th century	Canine limb transplant by Carrel[12]
Early 20th century	Heterotopic allotransplantation of the heads of dogs by Guthrie[12]
1956	First successful human kidney transplant. Donor and recipient were identical twins mitigating risk of rejection.[12]
1963	Ecuador: first human hand transplant. Experienced acute rejection. Removed 3 wk after transplant[29]
1988	First successful laryngotracheal transplant[24]
1990s	Series of knee and femur transplantations with "long-term survival elusive"[23]
1994	Replantation of full facial tissue (autotransplant) in India[12]
1998	Second ever human unilateral hand transplant performed in France. First to survive more than 2 y. Eventually rejected and removed because of noncompliance[10]
1999–2013	>90 hand transplants in 46 patients. No mortality reported. Multiple episodes of rejection successfully reversed with medication management[30]
2000	World's first bilateral upper extremity transplant[23]
2005	First human facial transplantation in France[4]
2009	U.S. Department of Defense acknowledges facial transplant as a research priority in effort to care for wounded soldiers.[12]
2005–2014	>30 facial allotransplantation procedures have been reported as of May 2015.[22,31–33]

D. Five facial transplant deaths have been reported to date.[31,33–36]

1. First patient was noncompliant with immunosuppressive treatment.
2. Second patient developed recurrent squamous cell carcinoma of the hypopharynx.
3. Third patient developed multidrug-resistant *Pseudomonas aeruginosa* infection, graft failure, and cardiac arrest after a combined face and double-hand transplant.
4. The fourth and fifth deaths were related to tumor recurrence and self-inflicted injury.

 IV. ETHICAL CONSIDERATIONS

A. Innovative nature of VCA procedures lends themselves to increased scrutiny.[28]

B. Arguments in support of[20,36,37] and against[20,37–39] VCA were abundant during conceptual phase.

C. Concern that the innovative nature of the procedure precluded a fully informed consent.[28]

D. Most frequently discussed ethical issue during early discussions was concerned that the need for lifelong immunosuppressive therapy following transplantation did not warrant the cost or consequences of potential infections, malignancies, renal failure, diabetes, and death.[29]

TABLE 16-2 **Facial Transplant Procedures: 2005–2014**

	Date	Age/Gender	Location	Lead Surgeon	Mechanism of Injury
1	November 2005	38/female	Amiens, France	Devauchelle and Dubenard	Dog bite
2	April 2006	30/male	Xi'an, China	Guo	Bear attack
3	January 2007	29/male	Creteil, France	Lantieri	Neurofibromatosis
4	December 2008	46/female	Cleveland, OH, USA	Siemionow	Ballistic trauma
5	March 2009	27/male	Paris, France	Lantieri	Shooting accident
6	April 2009	30/male	Paris, France	Lantieri	Burn
7	April 2009	60/male	Boston, MA, USA	Pomahac	Electrical burn/traumatic injury
8	August 2009	33/male	Paris, France	Lantieri	Ballistic trauma
9	August 2009	42/male	Valencia, Spain	Cavadas	Cancer/radiation for tumor injury
10	November 2009	27/male	Amiens, France	Devauchelle and Dubenard	Ballistic trauma
11	January 2010	34/male	Seville, Spain	Gomez-Cia	Neurofibromatosis
12	March 2010	30/male	Barcelona, Spain	Barrett	Ballistic trauma/shooting victim
13	June 2010	35/male	Paris, France	Lantieri	Neurofibromatosis
14	March 2011	25/male	Boston, MA, USA	Pomahac	Electrical burn/traumatic injury
15	April 2011	30/male	Paris, France	Lantieri	Ballistic trauma
16	April 2011	41/male	Paris, France	Lantieri	Ballistic trauma
17	April 2011	30/male	Boston, MA, USA	Pomahac	Electrical burn
18	May 2011	57/female	Boston, MA, USA	Pomahac	Animal attack (chimpanzee)
19	January 2012	Unknown/male	Ghent, Belgium	Blondeel	Industrial accident
20	January 2012	45/male	Antalya, Turkey	Ozkan	Burn
21	February 2012	25/male	Ankara, Turkey	Nasir	Burn
22	March 2012	20/female	Antalya, Turkey	Ozkan	Ballistic trauma
23	March 2012	37/male	Baltimore, MD, USA	Rodriguez	Ballistic trauma, gunshot wound
24	May 2012	34/male	Antalya, Turkey	Ozkan	Burn
25	September 2012	Female	Amiens, France	Devauchelle and Dubenard	Vascular tumor
26	February 2013	44/female	Boston, MA, USA	Pomahac	Chemical burn
27	May 2013	33/male	Gliwice, Poland	Maciejewski	Blunt trauma
28	July 2013	27/male	Antalya, Turkey	Ozkan	Ballistic trauma
29	September 2014	Middle age/male	Ohio, USA	Papay	Motor vehicle crash

From Khalifian S, Brazio PS, Mohan R, et al. Facial transplantation: the first 9 years. *Lancet.* 2014;384(9960):2153–2163. Available at http://dx.doi.org/10.1016/S0140-6736(13)62632-X, www.TheLancet.com; Cleveland Clinic. *Face Transplant: Rebuilding Lives.* Available at http://www.clevelandclinic.org/lp/face/index.html?utm_campaign=facetransplant-url&utm_medium=offline&utm_source=redirect. Accessed January 15, 2015; Rodriguez E. State of the art: facial reconstruction and transplantation. *International Conference sponsored by AO North America, May 15–17, 2015, New York, NY.* Available at www.facerecon2015.org.

E. Financial burden is considerable, including lifelong immunosuppression.[20,29,36,37]

F. Level of disfigurement appropriate for transplant potentially has subjective quality.[28]

G. Unlike solid organ transplant, VCA grafts likely require immunosuppression in the treatment of *non*–life-threatening conditions versus life-threatening conditions of the solid organ transplant patient.[9]

H. Hand and facial transplantation is considered "life changing and/or life giving" not "lifesaving" and thus has been criticized for exposing otherwise healthy people to the risks of lifelong immunosuppression.[30,31]

I. Lifelong immunosuppressive therapy is known to increase the development of general metabolic derangements such as renal insufficiency and failure, hypertension, hyperglycemia, systemic infections, opportunistic infections, and malignancies.[29]

J. Complete facial graft loss, depending on the extensiveness of the donated tissue, could result in severe disfigurement, dysfunction, morbidity, and/or death.[10,23,29,40]

K. The "life-giving" nature of VCA procedures, by virtue of "normalizing" the patient's appearance, has been lauded as an ethical mandate for these procedures by proponents.[12,41]

L. Due to the innovative nature of these procedures and potential clinical and ethical concerns, full institutional review board (IRB) currently guides efforts.[28]

 V. PSYCHOSOCIAL CONSIDERATIONS

A. Understanding the "role of face" in social interactions.[20]

B. Interpreting how facial expression affects an individual's personal identity and societal roles.[41,42]

C. Quantifying the impact of an individual's facial disfigurement or loss of hands on their self-esteem, mood, independence, and social reintegration.[20]

D. Evaluating a patient's expectations regarding the outcome of facial and/or hand transplant surgery.[42]

E. Assessing the availability of appropriate social supports for the transplant recipient postoperatively.[3,20]

F. Assessing the patient's potential for adherence to the therapeutic regimen.

G. Procedures are only performed at select institutions, thus making the geographical considerations for follow-up care significant if the recipient is unable to easily access the VCA center.[12]

VI. U.S. FEDERAL GOVERNMENT OVERSIGHT VIA HEALTH RESOURCES AND SERVICES ADMINISTRATION (HRSA) FINAL RULE AND INSTITUTIONAL PREPAREDNESS[26]

A. VCAs were originally under the auspices of the Food and Drug Administration, which regulates human cells, tissues, and cellular tissue–based products.

B. VCAs were subsequently added to the definition of "organs" under the auspices of the Health Resources and Services Administration (HRSA), which oversees solid organ transplantation through the Organ Procurement and Transplantation Network (OPTN)—July 13, 2013.

   1. Purchase or sale of VCAs prohibited.
   2. Issues concerning allocation and recipient safety currently fall under the auspices of the OPTN.[26]

C. Final Rule effective July 3, 2014; OPTN now responsible for establishing policies pertaining to the procurement, allocation, and transplantation of VCAs.

D. The United Network for Organ Sharing (UNOS) establishes rules for allocation of solid organs but does not establish allocation regulations for potential VCA recipients.[10]

E. Facility criteria: VCA must be completed in an organized and synchronized health care delivery system; ideally, a center of excellence with experience in specializing in the treatment of complex craniofacial defects utilizing microsurgical techniques as well as medical science to manage vascularized composite transplants.[26,43]

   1. VCAs under a research protocol/IRB must have approval by IRB with consideration of posting to the National Institutes of Health Clinical Trials Web site (https://clinicaltrials.gov/).[26]
   2. Approval by the designated organ procurement organization, requiring hospitals to comply with the rules and requirements of the OPTN as a condition of participation in Medicare and Medicaid programs.[26]
   3. In order to perform VCAs, an institution must
      a. Be a designated organ-specific transplant center
      b. Become a member of the OPTN
      c. Comply with OPTN data submission requirements[26]
   4. Institutions failing to comply with OPTN policies are subject to sanctions and possible termination from Medicare and Medicaid programs.[26]

VII. CLINICAL INDICATIONS AND REQUIREMENTS MEETING THE AMERICAN SOCIETY FOR TRANSPLANTATION CRITERIA FOR VCA TRANSPLANTATION[9]

A. Facial VCA

   1. Facial Transplant Guiding Principles for Determining Medical Necessity[9,25]:
      a. Defects comprising 25% or more of the facial surface area and/or involving one or more central facial units such as the eyelids, lips, mouth, or nose.[9,25]

      b. Transplantation of **underlying** bone (maxilla/mandible/nose) or tongue is indicated.

      c. Defects are typically the result of trauma, burns, congenital conditions such as neurofibromatosis, or tumor resection resulting in severe irreversible aesthetic, sensory, and motor functions of the face.[29]

      d. Important functions of the face such as air humidification, nonverbal expression, intelligible speech, breathing, oral competence (ability to chew, swallow, kiss, and control drooling), facial sensation, and eyelid closure are absent.[9,43–45]

      e. Conventional reconstructive options have failed restoration and are deemed unsatisfactory.[9,43–45]

      f. Severe anatomical and functional abnormalities have resulted in detrimental effects on the patient's psyche, perception of body image, quality of life, and social interactions with loss of integration with family, friends, colleagues, and depression.[25]

  2. American Society for Reconstructive Transplantation (ASRT) Advisory Council medically necessary *Clinical Criteria*[9,25]:

      a. Comprehensive medical history and physical examinations conducted by a plastic and reconstructive surgeon, and/or a craniofacial surgeon, to evaluate the need for transplantation.

      b. Surgical treatment plan (which outlines the surgical approach and the prognosis for improvement of clinical signs/symptoms pertinent to the diagnosis) has been developed.

      c. Comprehensive medical history and physical examinations have been conducted by a transplant physician or surgeon to evaluate the physical ability of the patient to undergo transplantation.

      d. Comprehensive psychosocial and mental health examinations have been performed to evaluate the patient's motivation and ability to successfully manage a VCA allograft.

      e. The patient has had inadequate or failed functional recovery with conventional reconstructive surgical treatment and/or nonsurgical rehabilitation.

      f. The facial defect is accompanied by medical or functional complications and demonstrable loss of quality of life as determined by psychological evaluation.

  3. ASRT Advisory Council *Required Documentation* of medical necessity including[9,25]

      a. Primary and secondary diagnoses with clinical symptoms and comorbid conditions

      b. Complete history and physical, prior failed treatments and surgeries

      c. Photographic and radiologic studies confirming the facial defects and the planned surgical treatment

B. Hand VCA

  1. Hand Transplant Guiding Principles for Determining Medical Necessity[9,25]

      a. Amputation or irreversible traumatic functional loss.

      b. Failed use of prosthetic devices unless such devices were deemed medically contraindicated.

      c. Patients with congenital deficits should seek opportunities in other clinical trials until research demonstrates plasticity of neural networks.

  2. Eligibility determination is based on a combination of clinical data and indicators affecting the risks and benefits of the transplantation.

3. ASRT Advisory Council medically necessary *Clinical Criteria*[9,25]:
   a. Comprehensive medical history and physical examination conducted by a transplant physician or surgeon to evaluate the need for transplantation.
   b. Surgical treatment outlining the approach and prognosis for improvement of clinical findings pertinent to the diagnosis developed.
   c. Comprehensive medical history and physical examination conducted by a transplant physician or surgeon evaluating the health status of the patient to undergo transplantation.
   d. Comprehensive psychosocial and mental health examinations have been performed to evaluate the patient's motivation and ability to successfully manage a VCA allograft.
   e. Patient is generally over 18 years of age and has had inadequate functional recovery with previous conventional reconstructive surgical interventions and/or nonsurgical rehabilitation.
   f. The amputation or loss of function is accompanied by
      i. Medical or functional complications
      ii. Demonstrable loss of quality of life as determined by psychological evaluation
      iii. Tissue necrosis or ulcerations unresponsive to nonsurgical treatments
   g. Comorbid etiologies have been considered and ruled out.

VIII. EVALUATION/SCREENING OF POTENTIAL VCA CANDIDATES AND INFORMED CONSENT REQUIREMENTS[16–18,23,25,27,42,46,47]

A. "General" eligibility under current research protocols in the United States
   1. Currently, upper extremity and facial VCA procedures are considered "research protocols."[31,35,48,49]
   2. Inclusion and exclusion criteria vary between individual institutions including age limitations, infectious disease states, and US citizenship to name a few.[15,45,46,50–52]
   3. Inclusion criteria
      a. Face VCA
         i. Facial defect or injury requiring facial transplantation as determined by the treating plastic and reconstructive surgeon.
         ii. Autologous tissue options must be available in the event of facial graft failure.
      b. Upper extremity/hand VCA[23,46,47,51,52]
         i. Recent (<6 months) or remote unilateral or bilateral upper limb loss below the shoulder desiring limb transplantation.
         ii. Unilateral arm transplant may be considered at some institutions even if the transplanted arm is the nondominant arm.[23]
         iii. Single dominant hand or multiple-limb amputation.[46,50]
         iv. Patient consent to bone marrow transfusion as part of treatment regimen is institution specific.[46,52]
         v. Blind amputees may be considered poor candidates as sensory return in the hand may not provide sufficient protection; conversely, benefits to blind patients may outweigh this risk (K. Knott, *personal communication*, October 2nd, 2014. Johns Hopkins University, Transplant Nurse Practitioner).

      vi. Failed prosthetic trials.[46,47,49,51]

      vii. Upper extremity/hand transplant: clinical trials dictate that the patient must be cancer-free for 5 to 10 years.[46,47,49-51]

4. Exclusion criteria: face, upper extremity, and hand VCA[15-18,25,35,47,49,50,51]

  a. Preexisting diseases or medical conditions that would negatively impact success.

     i. Expose the patient to unacceptable risks under immunosuppressive treatments.

     ii. Unacceptable surgical risk to the recipient from transplantation.

     iii. Absolute and relative contraindications are determined by the specific institutional selection committees: diseases may include inherited coagulopathies, connective tissue or collagen diseases, amyloidosis, etc.

  b. Human immunodeficiency virus (HIV) positive (active or seropositive) (relative contraindication).

  c. Hepatitis B or C virus positive (relative contraindication).

  d. Active infection including, but not limited to, tuberculosis, toxoplasmosis, or viral encephalitis.

  e. Current malignancy.

  f. Malignancy history within the last 5 years[46,47,49,50] to 10 years.[16,51]

  g. Paralysis of ischemic or traumatic origin.[45]

  h. Inherited peripheral neuropathy or inflammatory axonal or demyelinating neuropathy.[50]

  i. Current pregnancy or breast-feeding.

  j. Cytomegalovirus virus (CMV) mismatch (relative contraindication).

  k. Lack of social support or care provider.

  l. History of persistent nonadherence.

  m. Active illicit drug use/abuse including alcoholism.

  n. Patients who do not meet psychosocial mental health eligibility criteria.

  o. Sensitized or elevated panel reactive antibodies (PRA) may exclude potential recipients at various centers.

     i. There is variability among VCA programs in terms of the percent of PRAs that would exclude a patient: for example, >50% at one institution and >70% at another institution.

  p. Severe or deforming rheumatoid or osteoarthritis in the limb.[50]

  q. Note: some VCA programs exclude male to female transplantation.[15,16,50]

B. Informed consent requirements

1. Signed written informed consents

  a. Screening consent:

     i. A screening consent should be obtained and include the risks and benefits for lab, diagnostic, and radiologic tests needed to be completed in order to initiate medical workup determining eligibility for a face or upper extremity/hand transplant.

  b. Research consent:

     i. A separate research consent for the face or upper extremity/hand transplantation is obtained after medical and surgical screening workup is completed, and the patient is deemed appropriate for the transplantation.

  c. The patient may choose to stop participation at any time without penalty or loss of benefits to which they are otherwise entitled.

2. Female recipients of childbearing age consent to use reliable contraception for at least 1 year following transplantation.

3. Willingness and ability to
   a. Complete psychiatric evaluations
   b. Complete all preoperative diagnostic tests
   c. Undergo review by a designated Patient Selection Committee[15]
   d. Adhere to all aspects of the posttransplant medical regimen, including immunosuppressant therapy
   e. Return for follow-up visits as described in the treatment plans/informed consents

 IX. ESTABLISHMENT OF A VCA TRANSPLANT PROGRAM

A. Given the fact that VCA is an innovative and "highly complex procedure that leaves little room for error"[43-45(p. 824)] and may present unique challenges to the interdisciplinary teams involved,[12,28,43,44,53] the establishment of a VCA program requires meticulous planning with consideration of the following:

1. Current efforts require protocol development and IRB approval.[44,45,53]
2. Extensive involvement and planning by all institutional and external stakeholders and VCA team members is essential, particularly with regard to training, equipment acquisition and preparation, environment of care considerations, and multidisciplinary coordination (internal) and collaboration with the regional organ procurement organization (OPO).[28,43-45]
3. Identification of a designated VCA coordinator with responsibilities for organizing all aspects of care including continuous communication of patient information to and from all members of the interdisciplinary VCA teams through appropriate and effective channels.[43-45]
4. Initiation of discussions with the institution's public relations, communication, and social media departments.
   a. Determine policies and procedures regarding anticipated timely release of facial and hand transplant events.[28,43-45]
   b. Maintain patients' and families' privacy of health care information and general protection from intrusions by reporters, other patients, the general public, and hospital staff not directly involved in the patient's care.[28,43-45]
5. Development and refinement of detailed communication due to large number of caregivers involved. Interdisciplinary teams may include members of the following teams and departments.[12,28,43-45]
   a. Skilled microvascular and reconstructive VCA surgical team
   b. Transplantation surgical team
   c. Transplant medicine team
   d. Specialized anesthesia team
   e. Immunology team and laboratory
   f. Otolaryngology team
   g. Infectious disease team
   h. Perioperative (pre-, intra-, and postoperative) nursing teams and surgical technologists
   i. General surgery department
   j. Ethicist
   k. Chaplain
   l. Nutritional support services/dieticians

    m. Social worker(s)

    n. Psychiatry department

    o. Speech pathology department

    p. Physical therapy department

    q. Occupational therapy department

    r. Integrative medicine/pain management service

    s. Wound-ostomy care nurse specialist

    t. OPO representative

6. Detailed protocols for preoperative and postoperative patient care order sets should address the following:

    a. Admission/diagnosis/condition

    b. Vital sign monitoring

    c. Flap/graft/perfusion monitoring for viability

    d. Cardiac and pulmonary status monitoring

    e. activity

    f. Wound/incision care

    g. Drains

    h. Fluid and electrolyte monitoring and balance:

        i. Continuous infusions

        ii. Electrolyte replacement protocols

    i. Dietary requirements

    j. Hyperglycemic management

    k. Medications including, but not limited to, the following:

        i. Induction/antibody therapy

        ii. Immunosuppressive therapy regimen

        iii. Infectious disease prophylaxis

        iv. Anticoagulation agents

        v. Analgesic agents

        vi. Neuropathic agents such as pregabalin (Lyrica) or gabapentin (Neurontin)

        vii. Anxiolytics

        viii. Gastrointestinal prophylaxis to prevent stress ulcers such as proton pump inhibitors or H_2 blockers

        ix. Antiemetics

    l. Laboratory tests and monitoring

        i. Basic laboratory tests

        ii. Immunosuppressant levels

    m. Other diagnostic tests

7. The immediate perioperative anesthesia and nursing staff should have broad knowledge of and experience in caring for patients undergoing extensive orthognathic and plastic surgery microsurgical procedures, complex craniofacial reconstruction, and organ procurement and transplantation protocols to thwart serious complications of hypothermia, blood loss, and microsurgical failure.[20,24,27,28,34]

8. Each patient's procedure is highly variable depending on the location and extent of the patient's structural defects and deficits, anticipated allograft size, and types of tissue to be transplanted.[52]

9. Previous multiple-staged surgical procedures to restore composite tissue defects and deficits result in extensive scarring and anatomical aberrancies that add to the intricate and difficult dissections of the recipient.[43]

a. Consider scheduled deceased donor dissection[43] that allows for
   i.   Practice, definitive planning, and refinement of both resection/removal of the recipient defect and anticipated donor VCA procurement utilizing computed tomography (CT)-guided virtual images and navigation or other essential surgical tools such as fluorescence angiography improve the efficacy of the surgical procedure and outcomes of VCA.[44]
b. Practice, definitive planning, and anticipated potential complications of VCA transplantation related to vessel anastomoses, bone osteotomies and reductions, VCA inset, and nerve coaptations.[44]
c. Consider "live" or "real-time" research procurement.[45]
   i.   Consent from the donor family is required.[45]
   ii. Meticulous consideration and care of the donor family must be assured.[12,28,45] A silicone facial mask of the donor is created prior to procurement.[45]
   iii. Research procurement offers both educational opportunities and essential real-time preparation in anticipation of VCA allograft transplantation for the surgical and anesthesia teams, the OPO, and the institution to better ensure allograft success.[45]

X. RECIPIENT PREOPEATIVE ORDERS AND TREATMENTS PER THE AMERICAN SOCIETY OF RECONSTRUCTIVE TRANSPLANTATION GUIDELINES[15,25,26]

A. Potential face and hand transplant recipient
   1. History and physical
     a. Comprehensive examination including review of all comorbidities, past medical and surgical history, medications, etc.[15,25,26]
     b. Includes photographs and videography of facial function.
     c. Documents should clearly show aesthetic, sensory, and motor defects limiting rudimentary function such as speaking, eating, drinking, and inability to complete activities of daily living (ADLs).
   2. Dental examination
   3. Ophthalmologic examination
   4. Diagnostic tests:
     a. Electrocardiogram
     b. Chest radiograph
     c. Functional magnetic resonance imaging (fMRI) to evaluate brain-muscular adaptation and reorganization of the transplanted tissues
     d. Electromyography (EMG) nerve conduction study
     e. Pressure-specified sensory device (PSSD) to quantify and record neurosensory pressure thresholds reflecting axonal degeneration and regeneration such as one- and two-point discrimination
     f. Tests similar to those required for solid organ transplantation, including, but not limited to, the following:
       i.   Complete blood cell count (CBC)
       ii. Complete metabolic panel (CMP)
       iii. Coagulation studies
       iv. Urinalysis
       v. Human leukocyte antigen (HLA)
       vi. Panel reactive antibody (PRA)

          vii. Infectious disease panel:
- Hepatitis B and C virus
- HIV
- Epstein-Barr virus (EBV)
- Cytomegalovirus (CMV)
- Human T-lymphotropic virus antibody (HTLV-1 and HTLV-2)
- Varicella-zoster virus (VZV; chicken pox)
- Herpes simplex virus (HSV)
- Toxoplasmosis
- Rapid plasma reagin (RPR)
- Purified protein derivative (PPD) skin test

5. Mental health/psychosocial evaluation:
   a. Standard Form-36 and Facial Disability Index.[3,15,31,35]
   b. Dual psychiatric evaluations may be done: one by the VCA team psychiatrist and one by an independent psychiatrist who is not a member of the VCA team.[3,15]
   c. Psychosocial evaluation by a social worker to assess patient's support system's potential for long-term commitment and involvement. This includes determining appropriate and reliable family, friend, and other social supports.[3,15,31,35]
   d. Evaluation of "current" compared to "expected" age-appropriate societal behaviors and community integration.[3,15,31,35]
   e. Determine with confidence anticipated patient compliance with the immunosuppressive and postoperative regimen.[3,15,31,35]
   f. Determine and document the patient's expectations regarding aesthetic, sensory, and functional outcomes.
   g. Patient selection is of paramount importance; specifically, "The best candidate is one who: fully understands the implications of the necessity of potentially lifelong immunosuppression and its serious morbidities, including infections, cancer, graft loss, and death"[31(p. 8)].
   h. The VCA team must be confident that the patient:
      i. "Is motivated, committed, with high likelihood of compliance with intense post-transplant rehabilitation, psychological treatment, and immunosuppression protocols…"[31(p. 8)].
      ii. "…Has a strong social support system that will help them address the many challenges, including media exposure, body image adaptation, and societal reintegration"[31(p. 9)].

B. Additional tests and examinations for face transplant recipient
1. CT angiogram of the face
   a. Determines current anatomy of blood supply to the face, particularly the branches off the carotid arteries
   b. Identifies potential recipient vessels of the face for possible anastomotic arterial and venous sites[43–45]
2. CT scan of facial bones (1-mm cuts)
   a. Creates virtual images of the patient's facial anatomy.
   b. Through web-based meetings with specialized medical device developers and the surgical team, locations of osteotomies are precisely determined based on bony defects. Surgical guides or "jigs" are then designed and manufactured.[43–45,52]

3. Speech therapist consultation to evaluate baseline function including[15]
   a. Dysphagia evaluation
      i.   12-cranial nerve motor and sensory examination
      ii. Vocal quality and cough strength
      iii. Oral competence (drooling, oral motor strength, use of tongue)
      iv. Swallowing evaluation with oral trials of various food bolus thicknesses
   b. Dysarthria evaluation
      i.   Vocal quality (hoarseness, wet, strained), resonance, phonation, and prosody
      ii. Speaking valve use if tracheostomy tube is present
      iii. Phonemic errors, intelligible sounds, words, use of sentences, and compensatory strategies
   c. Potential preoperative interventions prior to face transplantation
      i.   Gastrostomy feeding tube placement—open or percutaneous—ideally prior to admission for facial VCA[15]
      ii. Tracheostomy—ideally placed prior to admission for facial VCA transplantation[15]

XI. POTENTIAL DONOR IDENTIFICATION, AUTHORIZATION, EVALUATION, AND MATCHING CRITERIA

A. Identification
   1. Initial identification of a potential donor by the OPO[15,35,54]
      a. Representatives from OPO work to maintain integrity and quality of the donation process and provide emotional support to donor families to meet unique needs related to loss of a loved one.[12,28,43,45]

B. Authorization for donation: the OPO obtains authorization for facial VCA donation, completes the donor evaluation, and notifies the VCA transplant team of the potential donor.[15,26,43,45]

C. Donor evaluation: standard screening protocol is completed in accordance with the OPO standard of care[15,26,43] and may include
   1. Infectious disease tests (CMV, EBV, HCV HBV, and HIV).
   2. HLA compatibility, lymphocyte crossmatch, virtual crossmatch, and chimerism analysis/short tandem repeat (STR) prior to transfusions if possible to obtain a pretransplant phenotype DNA profile as well as help predict outcome for engraftment rejection.
   3. ABO typing.
   4. Donor tests similar to those for solid organ donors may include, for example, CBC, CMP, coagulation studies, and urinalysis.
   5. History and physical: comprehensive examination including all comorbidities, past medical and surgical history, and medications.[15,26,43,45]
   6. Exclusion criteria[15,26,43,45,50]
      a. Prior history of or current head, neck, or facial surgery or facial trauma
      b. Malignancy within the past 5 years[50] to 10 years
      c. Prior history of or current malignancy
      d. Positive HIV
      e. Positive hepatitis A, B, or C virus
      f. Active CMV or EBV
      g. Untreated sepsis
      h. Active tuberculosis

    i. Viral encephalitis

    j. Current intravenous (IV) drug use

    k. "Nonprofessional" tattoo within the last 6 months for both face and hand transplantations; presuming the tattoo was performed by a nonlicensed artist without regulation of needle sterility or contamination control

    l. Tattoos on arms for hand/upper extremity[50]

    m. Any inherited or metabolic peripheral neuropathy

    n. Infectious, postinfection, or inflammatory (axonal or demyelinating) neuropathy

    o. Systemic disease with associated neuropathy (diabetes, alcoholism, amyloidosis)

    p. Toxic neuropathy (i.e., heavy metal poisoning, drug toxicity, industrial agent exposure)

    q. Incarceration (jail or prison) >72-hour admission; donors who have been in lockup, jail, prison, or a juvenile correctional facility for more than 72 consecutive hours in the preceding 12 months are considered at increased risk for recent HIV, HBV, and HCV infection per the U.S. Public Health Service (PHS) Guidelines published July 2013. (K. Knott, *personal communication*, October 2014)

D. Matching criteria[15,26,43,45]

    1. ABO type

    2. HLA subtype sensitization of the recipient (evaluated in some centers) compatibility

    3. EBV and CMV serostatus (at some institutions)

    4. Negative crossmatch

    5. Skin tone

    6. Age, skin status

XII. DONOR PREOPERATIVE ORDERS AND TREATMENTS[15,22,26,42]

A. Donor is confirmed as an appropriate "match" based on matching and exclusion criteria, infectious disease markers, ABO typing, and HLA crossmatch.[15,43]

B. Lymph nodes (mesenteric or thoracic) for STR/chimerism, donor peripheral cells, 8 × 8 cm segment of skin, and a "wedge" of spleen will be obtained at the time of procurement to be utilized as an antigen source for immunologic monitoring. Tissues will be processed, frozen, and banked.[15,26,43]

C. CT scans to create images of donor's craniofacial bone anatomy and identify placement of osteotomies to match recipients by virtual overlay of the donor skull over recipient. In addition, a cephalometric analysis of anticipated facial symmetry and occlusion posttransplant is designed.[15,43,45,54]

D. Maxillary-mandibular fixation (jaws wired closed) performed to establish class I occlusion.[15,43,45]

E. Silicone mask of the donor's face is made by an anaplastologist to allow for coverage of the facial defect following procurement of the facial VCA and an open casket service if donor's family so desires.[15,43,45]

XIII. SURGICAL PROCEDURES

A. Environment of care[15,28,43,45]

1. Mobilization and coordination of the interdisciplinary VCA team by the designated VCA coordinator occur when a potential donor match is identified and authorization is obtained from the deceased donor family by the OPO.

2. Due to the heightened level of interest in VCA, a security detail or designated team member monitors and limits access to surgical suites to essential personnel.

3. Documentation of surgery via photographs and videography for evaluation and education is allowed; however, other photography is prohibited.

4. Scope and time of surgical procedures, team member involvement, and equipment are highly variable depending on the recipient's cosmetic and functional deficits.

5. Two surgical and anesthesia teams, donor team and recipient team, work simultaneously; donor team procures the donor VCA, while the recipient team prepares the recipient.

6. Multiple team members must be available to rotate due to lengthy nature of procedure.

7. Multiple sterile equipment tables and tray setups must be available, including two microscopes.

B. Anesthesia considerations (facial transplantation)[55]

1. No paralytic agents are administered during the facial motor nerve dissections due to the need to stimulate the motor nerves of both the donor and recipient.[15,43,45]

2. Time projections:
   a. Donor facial procurement: 4 to 6 hours
   b. Recipient facial resection and osteotomies, vessel and nerve dissection exposure and anastomoses, and inset facial "graft": 18 to 24 hours[15,35,43,50,55]

3. Donor considerations
   a. Hemodynamic management per transplant donor procurement protocols.
   b. Large-bore vascular access including triple-lumen central venous line and radial arterial line with numerous extensions for IVs and ventilator circuits.
   c. Resuscitative efforts aimed at homeostasis in anticipation of clinical deterioration including inflammatory/capillary leak states, progressing renal insufficiency, and diabetes insipidus.
   d. Type and cross 10 units of packed red blood cells (PRBC)/fresh frozen plasma (FFP)/platelets.
   e. Room logistics include body warmers with passive cooling, positioning with gel rolls, possible Trendelenburg, and lab draws including CBC, coagulation studies, and basic metabolic panel BMP every 90 minutes and as needed.

4. Recipient considerations[54]
   a. Dedicated anesthesiologist for 72 hours: during both the surgical procedure and the anticipated 72-hour admission to a postanesthesia care unit (PACU)/or intensive care unit (ICU) immediately following surgery.[16]
   b. Vascular access including large-bore venous catheters, triple-lumen central line, and radial arterial line with numerous extensions for IVs and ventilator circuits.[15,43,45]

    c. Other equipment may include placement of temperature-sensing Foley catheter, warming blanket, cell saver, continuous cardiac output monitoring, and table positioning.

    d. Infusions/medications[15,55]

      i. Administration of anesthetic induction agents: of note, tracheostomy placement prior to transplantation as stated above for facial transplantation with stoma enlarged to 8.0 ETT as appropriate.

      ii. Administration of steroid, antihistamine, and immunosuppression induction agents; infusion reactions may include, but are not limited to, the following:

- Pulmonary infiltrates
- Acute respiratory distress syndrome (ARDS)
- Respiratory arrest
- Cardiac arrhythmias
- Myocardial infarction
- Cardiac insufficiency
- Angioedema
- Anaphylactic shock
- Pyrexia
- Hypotension
- Urticaria
- Tachycardia

    e. Airway[15,43,45,55]

      i. Ventilatory management/pulmonary toilet per anesthesiologist with minute ventilation to maintain normocapnea, FiO_2 50%, with every 30-minute arterial blood gases (ABGs) during graft reperfusion and subsequent resuscitation

      ii. Plan extubation 72 hours postoperatively and wean to tracheostomy collar as appropriate

    f. Hemodynamic monitoring and goals[5,15]

      i. Potential for significant blood loss: type and cross 10 units of packed red cells (PRC)/FFP/platelets.

      ii. Potential systemic hyperkalemia from reperfusion: attenuate with furosemide (Lasix) and bicarbonate and/or calcium chloride.

      iii. Maintain hematocrit >25% to avoid inadequate O_2 delivery, ischemia, and tachycardia and <30% to avoid a "polycythemia state" to decrease risk of clot formation within the recipient-donor anastomosed vessels.

      iv. Autotransfusion as available.

      v. Maintain euvolemia.

      vi. Careful recording of intake and output.

      vii. Maintain mean arterial pressure (MAP): baseline +/-10 mm Hg

C. Donor procedures:

1. Facial allograft procurement is from brain-dead, heart-beating donors with facial graft dissection prior to cross-clamp; facial graft procurement is currently not performed after circulatory death secondary to high risk of graft failure related to ischemic intolerance and microscopic thrombus development.[34,43]

2. Facial allograft procurement is completed prior to most other organ procurement.[15,31,34,44,53]

3. Placement of custom silicone resin donor mask.[15,43,45]

D. Recipient perioperative procedures[15,43,45]

1. Admit to PACU/ICU on arrival to the hospital.
2. Obtain signed informed consent for surgical procedure confirming acceptability of the donor.
3. Aspirin 81 mg by mouth × one dose on the day of admission.
4. Heparin 5,000 units subcutaneous × one dose on call to the OR.
5. For facial transplant recipients: tracheostomy performed at start of procedure if not already performed during a prior surgery.
6. Antibiotic/antifungal medications 30 minutes prior to incision; for example[15,43,45,56]
   a. Cefazolin (Ancef) 2 g IV or piperacillin/tazobactam (Zosyn) 3.375 mg
   b. If penicillin allergic: clindamycin (Cleocin) 600 to 900 mg IV × one dose + ciprofloxacin (Cipro) 400 mg IV × one dose
   c. Fluconazole (Diflucan) 500 mg IV × one dose
7. Immunosuppression
   a. Per institution's specific IRB-approved research protocols.[10,15,39,43,45,56]
   b. VCA immunosuppression protocols are modifications of existing solid organ transplantation protocols.[10,45] For example:
      i. Antihistamine (diphenhydramine [Benadryl] 25 to 50 mg IV × one dose) and methylprednisolone (Solu-Medrol) 500 mg IV × single dose prior to immunosuppression induction.
      ii. Alemtuzumab (Campath) 30 mg IV over 2 hours.[15,43,45,56]
      iii. See section on Posttransplant Care for additional information.
   c. Conventional lympho-depleting induction therapies for both hand and facial VCA have included antithymocyte globulin (ATG), alemtuzumab (Campath), or basiliximab (Simulect) followed by high-dose tacrolimus (Prograf/FK506), mycophenolate mofetil (CellCept) and steroids[34] or rapamycin (Rapamune).[29,35]
8. Cold ischemic time goals
   a. Face graft: 4 hours with maximum of 8 hours for "cold ischemia" time; the graft placed on ice[53]
   b. Upper extremity: 10 to 12 hours depending on the level of the transplant and volume of muscle tissue subjective to ischemia in the respective graft[50] (K. Knott, *personal communication*, October 2014)
9. Surgical technique:
   a. Facial graft arterial and venous anastomoses, boney reductions, soft tissue insets and motor nerve coaptations are completed; sensory nerve coaptations may or may not be completed.
   b. Upper extremity arterial and venous anastomoses, boney reductions, soft tissue insets and nerve coaptations of both sensory and motor nerves are completed.
   c. Estimated intraoperative time is 12 to 16 hours for both unilateral and bilateral hand graft transplants as dual teams would operate simultaneously on each side.
   d. An additional "sentinel" flap, such as a free radial forearm flap from the donor to the recipient, may also be performed to utilize as a satellite site to monitor for rejection and take biopsies as indicated for both hand and facial grafts[23,35] (K. Knott, *personal communication*, October 2, 2014. Johns Hopkins Hospital, Transplant Nurse Practitioner).

e. Induction and immunotherapies may include, for example:

    i. Antihistamine (diphenhydramine [Benadryl] 25 to 50 mg IV × one dose) and Solu-Medrol 500 mg intravenous IV × single dose prior to immunosuppression induction and Campath 30 mg IV over 2 hours.[15,44,53,55]

10. Intraoperative patient points of care[15,55]

    a. Skin integrity

        i. Optimal surgical exposure and number of team members at surgical field must be considered.

        ii. Careful attention to positioning due to length of procedure and patient's risk factors.

        iii. Consider pressure redistribution surfaces.

        iv. Have multiple padding and positioning devices available.

    b. Infection control[15,55]

        i. Contact precautions are meticulously maintained.

        ii. Traffic pattern monitoring essential.

        iii. Hypervigilance regarding sterile technique intraoperatively.

            • Antibiotic administration per patient history of relevant prior infections and previous treatments as well as bacterial isolates and antibiograms specific to the institution.

    c. Thermoregulation[15,55]

        i. Length of surgical procedure potentiates risk of hypothermia.

        ii. Warming devices available and used to maintain "normothermia."

        iii. Safety: routine intraoperative safety protocols maintained.

        iv. DVT prophylaxis per hospital protocol

11. Facial graft preservation[15,23]

    a. University of Wisconsin solution infusion or other preservation solutions

XIV. POSTTRANSPLANT CARE

A. Postoperative management typically follows established institutional or research protocols.[15]

B. Admit to an ICU or PACU setting for immediate detection of early changes in declining hemodynamic status or graft viability related to perfusion.[15,55]

1. Continuous ECG, blood pressure, SpO_2, and ventilatory monitoring.

2. Monitor graft function for complications of arterial or venous obstruction

    a. Temperature

    b. Color—should look like the native tissue color of donor skin

        i. Hyperemia may indicate venous outflow obstruction.

        ii. Pale, blue, and purple colors indicate arterial inflow insufficiency or late sign of venous obstruction.

        iii. Capillary refill should be 2 to 6 seconds as this is typically the first bedside clinical sign of graft/flap blood flow compromise.

        iv. Capillary refill <2 and >6 seconds indicates venous outflow or arterial inflow abnormalities, respectively.

    c. Bedside Doppler signals of arterial and venous blood flow to monitor circulatory perfusion status of the graft

C. Special considerations to maximize perfusion of graft[15]

1. Avoid vasoactive medications, which may have significant vasoconstriction or vasodilatory effects.
2. Avoid nicotine patches and all food or drink products that may induce vasoconstriction (e.g., caffeine, chocolate)

D. Decubitus ulcer prophylaxis is essential due to inherent bed rest and restrictions on activity and range of motion (ROM).

1. Wound-ostomy nurse consultation
2. Use of a specialty bed or mattress[15]

E. DVT prophylaxis including lower extremity intermittent compression devices and medicinal therapies such as aspirin and enoxaparin sodium injection (Lovenox) per protocol.[15]

F. Gastrointestinal

1. Prophylaxis for gastritis with proton pump inhibitors or H_2 blockade
2. Agents to prevent or manage constipation[15]

G. Immunosuppression

1. VCAs are composed of multiple tissues and thus carry different immunogenic and functional properties.[9]
2. At present, there are no standard immunosuppression therapies; thus, protocols will vary from institution to institution.
3. Tacrolimus (Prograf) has been a cornerstone of nearly all VCA immunosuppression protocols with target trough levels of 10 to 15 ng/mL for the first 1 to 5 months followed by a subsequent dose reduction with a target trough level of 8 to 10 ng/mL for most patients.[30,31,35]
4. Steroids have been safely tapered after a few months, with complete withdrawal possible within a year in some cases, depending on patient response and the protocol immunosuppression regimen.[31]
5. Some institutions may use monotherapy therapy: a donor bone marrow cell–based treatment in which alemtuzumab (Campath) and steroids are combined with donor bone marrow infusion 10 ± 4 days post VCA, followed by tacrolimus (Prograf) monotherapy to exhaust and deplete host antidonor lymphocyte clones.[30,50]
6. Triple-therapy regimen of tacrolimus (Prograf), mycophenolate mofetil (CellCept), and steroids.[30,31,35]
   a. Tacrolimus 0.15 mg/kg/d in two divided doses BID, via percutaneous endoscopic gastrostomy (PEG) tube based on actual body weight (target trough level 10 to 12 ng/mL initial 3 months, then tapered to goal of 6 to 8 ng/mL)
   b. Mycophenolate mofetil 1 g BID, then tapered to 500 mg BID after 6 months
   c. Methylprednisolone (Solu-Medrol) 500 mg IV bolus intraoperatively, then 2-day taper to 125 mg IV
   d. Oral prednisone 21-day taper following IV steroid methylprednisolone
   e. Topical tacrolimus in a 0.1% ointment to transplanted skin BID during periods of rejection, until resolution of rash and rejection is confirmed by biopsy[15,30,31]
   f. Topical steroids, for example, clobetasol (Clobex), to transplanted skin BID during periods of rejection until resolution of rash and rejection is confirmed by biopsy[15,30,31]

    g. Investigational tolerance induction and immunosuppression—minimizing regimens include extracorporeal phototherapy and donor hematopoietic stem cell infusion[23,29]

H. Prevention of opportunistic infections[15,55]
  1. Contact precautions maintained meticulously
  2. Oral care with an antimicrobial oral rinse, soft foam swabs for oral mucosa, toothbrush, and paste
  3. Methicillin-resistant *Staphylococcus aureus* (MRSA) colonization prevention—mupirocin (Bactroban) 2% ointment to nares
  4. CMV prevention—valganciclovir (Valcyte) 450 mg daily × 3 months
  5. Antifungal prophylaxis—fluconazole (Diflucan) 200 mg daily for prevention of oral and esophageal candidiasis:
     a. Clotrimazole troches 10 mg BID for 3 months
     b. Nystatin swish and swallow 500,000 units, 5 mL orally QID while in maxillomandibular fixation (jaws are "wired shut")
  6. *Pneumocystis jiroveci* (formerly *Pneumocystis carinii*) pneumonia prevention
     a. Trimethoprim/sulfamethoxazole double strength (DS) (Bactrim DS) one tablet daily for 6 months.
     b. If the patient is allergic to Sulfa, then give dapsone 100 mg by mouth daily.
     c. If the patient has a G6pd deficiency, which is a contraindication with dapsone, then give pentamidine 300 mg nebulizer every 4 weeks.

I. VCA rejection
  1. In VCA, the skin is considered to be the most highly immunogenic tissue; thus, the skin is the target for monitoring alloimmune response and rejection by pathways of antigen-presenting cells, expression of MHC-II molecules by keratinocytes, secretion of proinflammatory cytokines, and attraction of lymphocytes.[35,57]
  2. Rejection monitoring involves clinical "bedside" skin assessment and confirmation with biopsies of the donor tissues.[58] (See Long-term Monitoring and Care below.)

J. Acute pain management service to monitor patient daily, prescribe IV analgesia, assist with patient control analgesia (PCA), and convert patient to oral analgesia as appropriate.[15]

K. Integrative medicine to provide alternative modalities to cope with pain and stress such as Reiki therapy, acupressure, music therapies, massage, and other relaxation techniques.

L. Rehabilitation—occupational and physical therapy consultations to assist with deconditioning and maximize mobility and independence with ADLs.

M. Speech and language pathology to address dysphagia and/or dysarthria with facial transplant patients by providing therapies and exercises focusing on
  1. Returning range of motion to oral structures
  2. Stimulating facial muscles and nerves
  3. Improving blood flow
  4. Regaining control of the tongue
  5. Forming basic oral sounds needed for fluent speech and mastication[15]

N. Mental health/psychiatric evaluations[15,23,31]

1. Acute admission phase includes orientation, behavior, mood, affect, coping mechanisms, assistance with anxiety and insomnia management or other negative or abnormal behaviors, thought processes, delusions, etc.

2. Frequency of visits are patient dependent and per IRB protocol; however, an example would be minimum of twice per week for first month, weekly for second and third months, and monthly for months 4 to 6.

XV. LONG-TERM MONITORING AND CARE

A. After 6 to 12 months, posttransplant care is focused on potential complications including acute and chronic graft rejection, sequelae of immunosuppressive therapies, and maximizing neurosensory and motor function, appearance, psychosocial well-being, and integration.

B. Acute and chronic graft rejection has been noted in hand transplant recipients, while only acute rejections have been reported in the facial VCA cohort.[30,31,35,40,57,58]

C. Acute graft rejection

1. Recent literature reviews indicate that acute rejections typically occur within the first few months of transplantation.

a. 85% of all hand transplant recipients had one rejection episode within the first year.[35,57]

b. 100% of facial transplants had at least one acute rejection episode within the first year.[31]

c. The rate of acute rejection in VCA patients is higher than solid organ transplant patients.[57]

2. Monitor via clinical examination.[23,24,26] Clinical manifestations include

a. Erythematous skin rash with swelling, itching, burning, and the presence of nodules and maculopapular lesions.[30,31,35,57]

b. Paresthesias and decreased sensitivity in hand transplantation have been reported.[30]

3. Biopsy of the donor and native tissues allows for histopathological (cellular and antibody) comparison and identification of cellular infiltrates and antibodies, which confirm rejection.[30,31,35,57,58]

4. Banff classification system standardizes histopathological findings on skin biopsy.[56] See Table 16-3 for the Banff 2007 working classification of skin-containing composite tissue allograft pathology.[59]

a. In hand transplant samples, infiltrates characteristically consisted of CD3-, CD4-, and CD68-positive T cells.[30,34]

b. Acute rejection first shows lymphocytic infiltration in the perivasculature of the dermis spreading to the dermis-epidermis junction as rejection progresses.[23,26,46]

c. Progression into the epidermis leads to keratinocyte necrosis with dermal-epidermal separation.[30,34,57]

d. Final stage of manifestation is irreversible cellular necrosis and epidermal loss.[23,26,50]

5. Skin changes in VCA patients may not necessarily represent rejection, but rather a simple pathology such as rosacea or localized erythema from trauma, insect bite, drug or allergic reactions, or other dermatological anomaly.[30,35,57,58]

TABLE 16-3 Banff 2007 Working Classification of Skin-Containing Composite Tissue Allograft Pathology

Grade 0	No or rare inflammatory infiltrates
Grade I mild	Mild perivascular infiltration. No involvement of the overlying epidermis
Grade II moderate	Moderate-to-severe perivascular inflammation with or without mild epidermal and/or adnexal involvement (limited to spongiosis and exocytosis). No epidermal dyskeratosis or apoptosis
Grade III severe	Severe dense inflammation and epidermal involvement with epithelial apoptosis, dyskeratosis, and/or keratinolysis
Grade IV necrotizing acute rejection	Frank necrosis of epidermis or other skin structures

Mundinger G, Drachenburg C. Chronic rejection in vascularized composite allografts. *Curr Opin Organ Transplant.* 2014;19: 309–314.

6. Although the skin is considered the most antigenic tissue, other tissues such as muscle, bone, blood vessels, adipose, and cartilage may also undergo rejection without manifestations in the skin. This is known as "split rejection" and may indicate an acute versus chronic rejection of deeper tissues independent of the skin.[57,58]

7. Standard skin biopsies alone may not reflect all the composite tissues of a VCA and require MRI, ultrasound biomicroscopy, or angiography to confirm vasculopathy as well as evaluate bone healing.[57]

D. Chronic graft rejection

1. Key features of chronic rejection in VCA appear to be transplant vasculopathy with intimal hyperplasia with less common findings of tertiary lymphoid follicles, graft fibrosis of skin, muscle and dermal adnexal structures, and edema.[35,59]

2. Chronic changes in the deep tissues may occur without obvious clinical changes in the skin; thus, symptoms lagging behind covert vascular changes, suggesting features of chronic rejection, may develop independent of acute rejection.[59]

3. VCA vasculopathy can occur without overt functional impairment of the VCA.[40,57-59]

4. Venous changes in VCA patients may be more pronounced than changes in solid organ transplant recipients.[57,59]

5. Table 16-4 lists immunologic and nonimmunologic factors that increase the risk of chronic rejection in VCA recipients.[58,59]

E. Treatment of acute rejection episodes

1. Acute rejection
   a. IV methylprednisolone (Solu-Medrol) boluses and/or thymoglobulin, daily steroid dosing, and increase of tacrolimus trough levels and/or triple-drug therapy[35,56,59]
   b. Resumption of opportunistic infection prophylaxis medications if immunosuppression therapy is increased[56]
   c. Follow-up for resolution of rejection episodes as evidenced by clinical evaluation and repeat biopsies and/or other diagnostic radiologic modalities[35,56]

2. VCA chronic rejection is ill defined with few treatments proposed.[59]

TABLE 16-4 Proposed Factors Contributing to the Development of Chronic Rejection in VCA[59]

Immunologic	NonImmunologic
Donor-recipient HLA disparities	Type of transplant
Number and degree of acute rejection episodes	Environmental/mechanical trauma—that is, thermal injury, sunburn—initiation of inflammatory and innate immune cytokine and chemokine responsive pathways leading to intimal hyperplasia
T-cell–mediated rejection	Degree of transplant vascular resistance to flow—presumably less in facial VCA
Antibody-mediated rejection	Degree of donor-recipient lymphatic channel regeneration
Transplant relative skin content	Graft denervation
Transplant relative–vascularized bone marrow content	Ischemia injury from arterial luminal occlusion
Donor and recipient CMV status	
Infection	

Mundinger G, Drachenburg C. Chronic rejection in vascularized composite allografts. *Curr Opin Organ Transplant.* 2014;19:309–314.

F. Complications of immunosuppressive therapies
   1. Similar to solid organ transplantation, complications include nephrotoxicity (renal failure), neurotoxicity, and cardiovascular disease including hypertension, hyperglycemia, hyperlipidemia, and hip osteonecrosis.[23,30,35,56]
      a. Routine blood urea nitrogen (BUN), creatinine, glucose, lipid, and electrolyte monitoring.
      b. Blood pressure monitoring.
      c. Hydrate as appropriate.
      d. Maximize nutrition/alter diet depending on degree of noted end-organ derangements.
      e. Alter immunosuppressive drug level goals versus changing immunosuppressive medicinal therapies simultaneously while monitoring for rejection episodes.
      f. Mitigate effects of immunosuppressive therapy by reducing target trough levels or changing immunosuppressive agents while monitoring for rejection.
   2. Pancytopenia—routine CBC with differential monitoring
   3. Neoplasias
      a. Patients on immunosuppressant therapy for solid organ transplant have a fivefold higher incidence of developing a malignancy.[30,35]
      b. Skin cancers, viral cancers, and posttransplant lymphoproliferative disease are the most prevalent malignancies documented.[30,35]
      c. Reported cases of neoplasia include basal cell carcinoma in a hand transplant recipient and aggressive recurrent squamous cell carcinoma of the tongue and HIV infection.[30,35]

G. Prevention of opportunistic infections
   1. Monitor signs and symptoms of development of local and systemic infection.
   2. Consider continuing prophylaxis of both PCP and CMV × 6-month course depending on individual patient.[56]
   3. Routine CBC and drug level monitoring.
   4. Scheduled serologic PCR infection surveillance including EBV and CMV titers.[15,30,56]

H. Chronic pain management—referral to pain specialist.

I. Neurosensory and neuromotor function

1. Nerve regeneration: functionality of VCAs is dependent on the rate and growth of recipient nerves into the grafted donor tissue.[9]

2. The mechanism by which the central nervous system accommodates and organizes new nerve growth is not completely understood.[9]

3. Tacrolimus (Prograf) has a beneficial side effect of acceleration of axonal regeneration.[24,29,57,59]

4. Documentation with routine photographs and videography demonstrating an improving or a plateauing neuromotor function is essential.

5. Documentation with functional MRIs may assist in defining the incompletely understood central nervous system role in organized new nerve growth.[9,15]

6. Electromyography (EMG) nerve conduction studies and PSSD to elucidate neuromotor and sensory progression and improvement or plateau.[15]

7. Utilization of the standardized "Hand Transplantation Scoring System" and the "Disabilities of the Arm, Shoulder, and Hand" scores to compare pre- to posttransplant functional outcomes.[29]

8. Hand transplantation recipients may be required to participate in physical therapy 8 hours per day/5 days per week[45] (K. Knott, *Personal communication/interview*, October 2014. Johns Hopkins Hospital, Transplant Nurse Practitioner).

J. Physical appearance

1. Documentation with routine photographs and routine, planned videography

2. Documentation of patient's perception of physical appearance

K. Psychological evaluations and interventions

1. Mental status examination including orientation, general appearance, attitude, behavior, speech, language, mood, affect, thought processes, abstractions, associations, sensorium, thought content, perceptions, delusions, ability to concentrate, insight, and judgment.

2. Frequency of psychiatric visits varies between institutions, and patient and can be IRB protocol driven; visits may be held at 12, 24, and 48 months and more frequently if clinically indicated.[15,31]

3. Societal reintegration—renewed social interactions including attending public events such as major league baseball games, shopping in grocery stores, dating, and attending schools.

4. Supportive psychotherapy.

5. Sleep hygiene.

6. Relaxation techniques.

7. Substance abuse consultation and therapy as indicated.

8. Evaluation of patient-reported outcomes of depression, social function, and well-being and other outcomes as stated above.[25,31,43]

XVI. FINANCIAL ASPECTS

A. In 2014, the estimated cost for a facial transplant procedure was $300,000 (in US dollars). This does not include the cost of life-long immunosuppressive therapy after discharge.[31]

B. Funding must be assured prior to any VCA transplant to guarantee financial coverage for posttransplant immunosuppressive medications.

1. In one country, almost all early hand VCA recipients lost their grafts when government authorities ceased immunosuppressive treatment support.[23]

C. Potential funding sources at this time include research grants, donations, and private and public insurance.

1. At this time, the Centers for Medicare and Medicaid cover VCAs under certain circumstances.[60]
2. In various states within the United States, VCAs are considered investigational and do not meet medical criteria for coverage.[60]

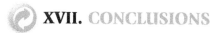

XVII. CONCLUSIONS

A. VCA benefits and positive findings

1. Potential to render superb cosmetic and functional outcomes such as basic facial functions of smell, smile, kiss, chew, use tongue to swallow and phonate, and control drooling.
2. Potential to return basic hand-and-arm functional outcomes including protective sensation, grip, pinching activities, picking up objects, feed one's self, communicate and interact through touch and gestures, and return to independent living.[10,29]
3. Potential to avoid multiple, lengthy, and possibly morbid conventional surgical operations that utilize the patient's own tissues, create significant donor site morbidity, and do not fully achieve acceptable aesthetic results or return patients to premorbid "normal" functions of craniofacial or hand sensory and motor skills.[3,10,29,31,35,43]
4. Clinical outcomes of improved and/or restored neuromotor sensory and motor function as early as 12 weeks posttransplantation have been noted; facial appearance and general quality of life and psychosocial outcomes have been positive for both hand and facial transplantation.[35]
5. No surgical failures of facial transplantation have been reported despite meticulous and highly skilled microsurgical techniques required.[35]
6. Although acute episodes of rejection have occurred with both facial and hand transplant recipients to date, they have been controlled with thymoglobulin; conventional IV; oral and topical immunosuppressant therapies, such as prednisone; and/or augmentation of maintenance immunotherapy.
7. To date, there have been no documented reports of chronic rejection (original estimation incidence of 30% to 50%) or graft versus host disease among facial transplant recipients.

B. Future research

1. Continue research in new pharmacological agents and/or mesenchymal stem cell utilization, bone marrow engraftment, or other novel therapies to achieve minimization of immunosuppression therapies and improvement of transplant tolerance to decrease toxic side effects of immunosuppression, ultimately eliminating lifelong suppression completely.[24,41]
2. Donor bone marrow engraftment may be effective at minimizing immunosuppression therapy needed by providing a supply of stem cells that maintain peripheral blood chimerism and facilitate donor graft tolerance by suppressing developing T cells in the thymus and thus thwart the rejection cascade.[10,24,35]
3. Compare the short- and long-term results of VCA relative to other therapeutic options (e.g., prostheses, extensive reconstructive surgery) in terms of quality-of-life measures including functionality, pain, psychological well-being, and social integration.

4. Long-term results of clinical, immunological, and psychological outcomes at 10 to 30+ years posttransplant.

5. Development of comprehensive, worldwide registry for tracking VCA procedures.[29]

6. Develop standardized guidelines and protocols for hand and facial transplantation based on shared or "pooled" reporting of outcomes from international sources to optimize neurosensory and motor function, craniofacial oral occlusion, symmetry, and aesthetics, as well as psychosocial behaviors and coping.[29]

7. Continue ongoing research to look at definitive genetic and cellular markers for rejection and patient-specific gene profiles in addition to alternative therapies for immunosuppression, achieving donor-antibody tolerance to mitigate and/or resolve the complications of infection, organ and tissue metabolic derangements, and neoplasias.[23,30,31,35,40,57]

8. Evaluate immediate- and long-term impact of VCA on donor families.[28]

9. Continue to elicit support and funding through various channels including private donations, grants, and insurance coverage by governmental and third-party payers. The US Department of Defense has funded some investigatory and procedural efforts as a means to providing care to wounded warriors.[15,39]

REFERENCES

1. The University of Texas MD Anderson Cancer Center 2011. *Composite Tissue Allotransplantation.* Available at http://www.mdanderson.org/education-and-research/departments-programs-and-labs/departments-and-divisions/plastic-surgery/composite-tissue-allotransplantation/index.html. Accessed September 30, 2014.

2. Wu D, Xu K, Ravinda K, et al. Composite tissue allotransplantation: past, present, and future—the history and expanding applications of CTA as a new frontier in transplantation. *Transplant Proc.* 2009;41:463–465.

3. Hui-Chou H, Nam A, Rodriguez E. Clinical facial composite tissue allotransplantation: a review of the first four global experiences and future implications. *Plast Reconstr Surg.* 2010;125(2):538–546

4. Devauchelle B, Badet L, Lengele B, et al. First human face allograft: early report. *Lancet.* 2006;368:203–209.

5. Ravinda K, Wu S, McKinney M, et al. Composite tissue allotransplantation: current challenges. *Transplant Proc.* 2009;41:3519–3528.

6. Pomahac B, Pribaz J, Eriksson E, et al. Restoration of facial form and function after severe disfigurement from burn injury by a composite facial allograft. *Am J Transplant.* 2011;10:1–8.

7. Siemionow M, Zor F, Gordon C. Face, upper extremity, and concomitant transplantation: potential concerns and challenges ahead. *Plast Reconstr Surg.* 2010;126(1):308–315.

8. Barker J, Stamos N, Furr A, et al. Research and events leading to facial transplantation. *Clin Plast Surg.* 2007;34:233–250.

9. American Society for Transplantation. *Vascularized Composite Allotransplantation (VCA) Research, the Emerging Field. Approved by the AST Executive Committee on June 1, 2011.* Available at http://www.myast.org/public-policy/vascularized-composite-allotransplantation-vca-research. Accessed September 30, 2014.

10. Weissenbacher A, Hautz T, Pratschke J, et al. Vascularized composite allografts and solid organ transplants: similarities and differences. *Curr Opin Organ Transplant.* 2013;18(6):640–644.

11. Gander B, Brown C, Vasilic D, et al. Composite tissue allotransplantation of the hand and face: a new frontier in transplant and reconstructive surgery. *Transpl Int.* 2006;19:868–880.

12. Evans L. A historical, clinical, and ethical overview of the emerging science of facial transplantation. *Plast Surg Nurs.* 2011;31(4):151–157.

13. ClinicalTrial.gov. *A Service of the US National Institutes of Health.* Available at http://clinicaltrials.gov/ct2/results?term=facial+allotransplantation. Accessed June 24, 2015.

14. ClinicalTrial.gov. *A Service of the US National Institutes of Health.* Available at http://clinicaltrials.gov/ct2/results?term=hand+allotransplantation. Accessed June 24, 2015.

15. University of Maryland, Department of Defense, University of Maryland: The Founding Campus, Maxillofacial Composite Tissue Allograft Transplantation: Face Transplant, Protocol Study No HP-00040219. *Maxillofacial Composite Tissue Allograft Transplantation: Face Transplant.* Available at http://clinicalstrials.gov/ct2/show/NCT011140087. Accessed October 31, 2014.

16. New York University of School of Medicine. *Face Transplantation.* Available at http://clinicaltrials.gov/ct2/show/ NCT02158793?term=facial+allotransplantation&rank=3. Accessed October 31, 2014.

17. Johns Hopkins University. *Human Craniomaxillofacial Allotransplantation.* Available at http://clinicaltrials.gov/ ct2/show/NCT01889381?term=facial+allotransplantation&rank=5. Accessed October 31, 2014.

18. Brigham and Women's Hospital. *Face Transplantation for Treatment of Severe Facial Deformity.* Available at http://clinicaltrials.gov/ct2/show/NCT01281267?term=facial+allotransplantation&rank=8. Accessed October 10, 2014.

19. Siemionow M, Papay F, Alam D, et al. Near-total human face transplantation for a severely disfigured patient in the USA. *Lancet.* 2009;374:203–209.

20. Morris P, Bradley J, Doyal L, et al. Face transplantation: a review of the technical, immunological, psychological, and clinical issues with recommendations for good practice. *Transplantation.* 2007;83(2):109–128.

21. Swearingen B, Ravindra K, Xu H, et al. Science of composite tissue allotransplantation. *Transplantation.* 2008;86(5):627–635. doi: 10.1097/TP.0b013e318184ca6a.

22. Wikipedia. *The Free Encyclopedia.* Available at https://en.wikipedia.org/wiki/Face_transplant. Accessed June 24, 2015.

23. Diaz-Siso J, Bueno E, Sisk G, et al. Vascularized composite tissue allotransplantation—state of the art. *Clin Transplant.* 2013;27(3):330–337. doi: 10.1111/ctr.12117.

24. Leonard D, Gordaon C, Sachs D, et al. Immunobiology of face transplantation. *J Craniofac Surg.* 2012;23(1): 268–271.

25. American Society for Reconstructive Transplantation. *Guidelines for Medical Necessity for Determination for Partial or Full Transplantation of the Face.* Available at http://www.a-s-r-t.com/education/education.html. Accessed September 30, 2014.

26. Department of Health and Human Services. Organ procurement final rule adding VCAs to the definition of organs covered by the OPTN. *Fed Regist.* 78(128) Wednesday, July 3, 2013/*Rules and Regulations*:40034–40042.

27. Siemionow M, Gordan C. Overview of guidelines for establishing a face transplant program: a work in progress. *Am J Transplant.* 2010;10:1290–1296.

28. Evans L. Experiences of healthcare team members involved in facial transplant surgery and patient care. *Nurs Res.* 2014;62(6):372–382.

29. Murphy B, Zuker R, Borschel G. Vascularized composite allotransplantation: an update on medical and surgical progress and remaining challenges. *J Plast Reconstr Aesthet Surg.* 2013;66:1449–1455.

30. Schneeberger S, Khalifian BA, Brandacher G. Immunosuppression and monitoring of rejection in hand transplantation. *Tech Hand Up Extrem Surg.* 2013;17(4):208–214.

31. Khalifian S, Brazio PS, Mohan R, et al. Facial transplantation: the first 9 years. *Lancet.* 2014;384(9960): 2153–2163. Available at http://dx.doi.org/10.1016/S0140-6736(13)62632-X, www.TheLancet.com

32. Cleveland Clinic. *Face Transplant: Rebuilding Lives.* Available at http://www.clevelandclinic.org/lp/face/index. html?utm_campaign=facetransplant-url&utm_medium=offline&utm_source=redirect. Accessed January 15, 2015.

33. Rodriguez E. State of the art: facial reconstruction and transplantation. International Conference sponsored by AO North America. May 15–17, 2015. New York, NY. Available at www.facerecon2015.org

34. Siemionow M, Gharb BB, Rampazzo A. Successes and lessons learned after more than a decade of upper extremity and face transplantation. *Curr Opin Organ Transplant.* 2013;18(6):633–639.

35. Smeets R, Rendenbach C, Birkelbach M. Face transplantation: on the verge of becoming clinical routine? *Biomed Res Int.* 2014:2014;907272:1–9. Available at http://dx.doi.org/10.1155/2014/907272

36. Alexander A, Alam D, Gullane P, et al. Arguing the ethics of facial transplantation. *Arch Facial Plast Surg.* 2010;12(1):60–63.

37. Kalliainen L. Supporting facial transplantation with the pillars of bioethics. *J Reconstr Microsurg.* 2010;26(8): 547–554.

38. Morris P, Bradley J, Doyal L, et al. Facial transplantation: a working party report from the Royal College of Surgeons of England. *Transplantation.* 2004;77(3):330–338.

39. Strong C. An ongoing issue concerning facial transplantation. *Am J Transplant.* 2010;10:1115–1116.

40. Kauffman C, Ouseph R, Marvin M, et al. Monitoring and long-term outcomes in vascularized composite allotransplantation. *Curr Opin Organ Transplant.* 2013;18(6):652–658.

41. Fitchett J. Facial reconstruction: the impact of facial allograft transplantation on surgery. *Int J Surg.* 2008;6: 439–440.

42. Furr L, Wiggins O, Cunningham M, et al. Psychological implications of disfigurement and the future of human face transplantation. *Plast Reconstr Surg.* 2006;120(2):559–565.

43. Dorafshar A, Bojovic B, Christy M, et al. Total face, double jaw, and tongue transplantation: an evolutionary concept. *Plast Reconstr Surg.* 2012;131(2):1–11. PMID: 23076416. Available at www.PRSJournal.com

44. Brown E, Dorafshar AH, Bojovic B, et al. Total face, double jaw, and tongue transplant simulation: a cadaveric study employing computer-assisted techniques. *Plast Reconstr Surg.* 2012;130(4):815–823. PMID: 22691839. Available at www.PRSJournal.com

45. Bojovic B, Dorafshar AH, Brown EN, et al. Total face, double jaw, and tongue transplant research procurement: an educational model. *Plast Reconstr Surg*. 2012;130(4):824–834. PMID: 22691842. Available at www.PRSJournal.com

46. Brigham and Women's Hospital. *Vascularized Composite Allotransplantation for Multiple Extremity Amputations*. Available at http://clinicaltrials.gov/ct2/show/NCT01293214?term=hand+allotransplantation&rank=2. Accessed October 29, 2014.

47. Southern Illinois University. *Upper Extremity/Hand Transplant in Hand Amputees*. Available at http://clinicaltrials.gov/ct2/show/NCT02165865?term=hand+allotransplantation&rank=1. Accessed October 29, 2014.

48. Rooney R. Future of facial transplants defined: hope, courage, and medical triumph. *Univ Maryland Med Bull*. 2012;97(1):6–10.

49. Louisville KY. *Allogeneic Hand Transplantation Composite Tissue Allotransplantation (Hand CTA)*. Available at http://clinicaltrials.gov/ct2/show/NCT00711373?term=hand+allotransplantation&rank=3. Accessed October 29, 2014.

50. Johns Hopkins University. *Human Upper Extremity Allotransplantation*. Available at http://clinicaltrials.gov/ct2/show/NCT01459107?term=hand+transplant&rank=2. Accessed October 29, 2014.

51. University of Pittsburgh. *Human Upper Extremity (Hand and Forearm) Allotransplantation*. Available at http://clinicaltrials.gov/ct2/show/NCT00722280?term=hand+allotransplantation&rank=5. Accessed October 29, 2014.

52. Brigham and Women's Hospital. *U.S. Department of Defense Studies*. Available at http://www.brighamandwomens.org/departments_and_services/surgery/services/plasticsur g/reconstructive/facetransplantsurgery/dodstudy.aspx. Accessed September 30, 2014.

53. Barker J, Furr A, McGuire S, et al. Patient expectations in facial transplantation. *Ann Plast Surg*. 2008;61(1):68–72.

54. Comprehensive Facial Transplant. Using Synthes Proplan CMF, Matrixmidface and Matrixmandible Plating systems: a case report, J11702-A. *Synthes, CMF* 2012;1–9.

55. Fox M, Sliwkowski J. Total face, double-jaw and tongue transplantation: anesthetic considerations and the STC experience. Presentation at the Maryland Association of Nurse Anesthetists Spring Conference. March 2013. Annapolis, MD.

56. Barth R, Klassen D, Bojovic B, et al. Immunologic and clinical outcomes 20 months after full face transplant. Poster of distinction. Presentation at World Transplant Congress, July 2014: San Francisco, USA. *Am J Transplant*. 2014;14(53):412.

57. Sinha I, Pomahac B. Split rejection in vascularized composite allotransplantion. *Eplasty*. 2013;461–465. Available at www.eplasty.com

58. Cendales LC, Kanitakis J, Schneeberger S, et al. The Banff 2007 working classification of skin-containing composite tissue allograft pathology. *Am J Transplant*. 2008;8:1396–1400.

59. Mundinger G, Drachenburg C. Chronic rejection in vascularized composite allografts. *Curr Opin Organ Transplant*. 2014;19:309–314.

60. Composite Tissue Allotransplantation (CTA) of the Hand and Face. *Blue Cross/Blue Shield of Alabama, Policy #: 521 Latest Review Date: February 2014*. Available at https://www.bcbsal.org/providers/policies/final/521.pdf. Accessed September 1, 2014.

SELF-ASSESSMENT QUESTIONS

1. Which of the following are criteria for facial transplant candidacy established by the American Society for Reconstructive Transplantation (ASRT)?
    1. Defects comprising 25% or more of the facial surface area and/or involving one or more central facial units such as the eyelids, lips, mouth, or nose.
    2. Severe irreversible aesthetic, sensory, and motor dysfunctions of the face including loss of air humidification, verbal expression, intelligible speech, comfortable breathing, oral competence (ability to chew, swallow, kiss, control drooling), facial sensation, and complete eyelid closure.
    3. Failed restoration of aesthetic, sensory, and motor function through conventional surgical means.
    4. Anatomical and functional abnormalities have resulted in detrimental effects on the patient's psyche, perception of body image, quality of life, and social interactions with loss of integration with family, friends, colleagues, and depression.
    5. Comprehensive psychosocial and mental health examinations have been performed demonstrating a patient's motivation and ability to successfully manage a vascular composite allograft (VCA).
    a. 1, 3, and 4
    b. 2, 4, and 5
    c. 1, 3, and 5
    d. All of the above

2. Which of the following are criteria for hand transplant candidacy established by the ASRT?
    1. Demonstrable loss of quality of life as determined by psychological evaluation.
    2. Amputation or irreversible traumatic functional loss.
    3. Failed use of prosthetic devices, unless such devices were deemed medically contraindicated.
    4. Comprehensive psychosocial and mental health examinations have been performed to demonstrate a patient's motivation and ability to successfully manage a VCA.
    5. Patients with congenital hand defects.
    a. 1, 2, and 3
    b. 1, 3, and 4
    c. 2, 3, and 5
    d. All except number 5

3. In order to perform VCAs, an institution must:
    1. be a designated organ-specific transplant center.
    2. become a member of the Organ Procurement and Transplantation Network (OPTN).
    3. comply with OPTN data submission requirements and policies pertaining to the procurement, allocation, and transplantation of VCAs.
    4. None of the above. The health care institution would follow requirements and policies established by the United Network for Organ Sharing (UNOS).
    a. 1 and 2 only
    b. 2 and 3 only
    c. 1, 2, and 3 only
    d. 4 only

4. VCAs are considered investigational. Funding sources in the United States include the following:
    1. Research, grants, and donations
    2. Private insurance
    3. Public insurance (Medicare and some state Medicaid programs, provided that criteria are met)
    a. 1 only
    b. 1 and 2 only
    c. 1 and 3 only
    d. All of the above

5. The potential benefits of facial VCA include which of the following:
    1. Cosmetic and functional outcomes such as basic facial functions of smell, smile, kiss, chew, use tongue to swallow and phonate, and control drooling
    2. Improved self-esteem, mood, social reintegration, and return to independent living
    3. Less risk of complications than solid organ transplant from immunosuppressive medications such as infection, malignancies, renal failure, and death
    a. 1 and 2
    b. 2 and 3
    c. 1 and 3
    d. All of the above

6. The potential benefits of hand VCA include which of the following:
    1. Return basic hand-and-arm functional outcomes including protective sensation, grip, pinching activities, picking up objects, feed one's self, and communicate and interact through touch and gestures
    2. Improved self-esteem, mood, social reintegration, and return to independent living
    3. Less risk of complications than solid organ transplant from immunosuppressive medications such as infection, malignancies, renal failure, and death
    a. 1 and 2
    b. 2 and 3
    c. 1 and 3
    d. 1, 2, and 3

7. Which of the following statements regarding the clinical signs of transplant rejection of a facial or hand transplant are **TRUE**?
    1. Clinical signs may include erythema, swelling, and pruritus of the skin of the transplanted tissue.
    2. Clinical signs may include paresthesias and decreased sensitivity of the transplanted tissue.
    3. There are no reliable "bedside" physical clinical signs.
    4. Routine biopsies or MRI, biomicroscopy, or angiography imaging of the deeper tissues such as the bone or muscle demonstrating lymphocytic infiltration of the vascular tissue is the only way to determine active rejection.
    a. 1 only
    b. 2 only
    c. 1 and 2 only
    d. 3 only
    e. 4 only

8. VCA matching criteria of the recipient and donor *may* include all of the following **EXCEPT**:
   a. ABO.
   b. human leukocyte antigen subtype sensitization.
   c. cytomegalovirus, Epstein-Barr virus.
   d. positive crossmatch.
   e. skin tone.
   f. age.
   g. gender.

9. Which of the following statements regarding the procurement of a donor facial allograft is **TRUE**?
   1. Procurement can occur following circulatory death.
   2. A facial allograft may be procured from brain-dead, heart-beating donors with facial graft dissection prior to cross-clamp.
   a. 1 only
   b. 2 only
   c. Both 1 and 2

10. While monitoring a VCA graft in the immediate postoperative phase, positive signs of VCA arterial and venous perfusion through the graft include all of the following **EXCEPT**:
    a. warm temperature to touch.
    b. color is consistent with the native tissue of the donor skin (devoid of hyperemia, pale, blue coloring).
    c. capillary refill that is <2 seconds or >6 seconds.
    d. audible Doppler signals of venous and arterial blood flow.

11. Clinical, ethical, and psychosocial implications may have an impact on short-term outcomes of facial transplantation procedures. Which of the following considerations is **LEAST LIKELY** to challenge the health care team?
    a. Impact of procedure on the patient's psychological well-being
    b. Societal considerations including financial implications
    c. Surgical skills required to perform VCA transplants
    d. Ethical issues
    e. Donor family considerations

12. The advent of facial transplant surgery encompassed multiple ethical discussions on which of the following topics:
    a. Level of disfigurement appropriate for transplantation
    b. Potential effects of long-term use of immunosuppressant medications
    c. High emotional burden on family members being approached for facial graft donation
    d. Difficulty in obtaining fully informed consent given the innovative nature of VCA procedures
    e. All of the above

13. Perioperative nursing interventions that may have a direct impact on a VCA patient's immediate postoperative course include:
    a. careful calculations of blood loss.
    b. techniques that ensure normothermia.
    c. attention to detail when positioning for lengthy procedure and padding of bony prominences.
    d. impeccable attention to infection control measures.
    e. all of the above.

Correct Answers:
1.d 2.d 3.c 4.d 5.a 6.a 7.c 8.d 9.b 10.c 11.c 12.e 13.e

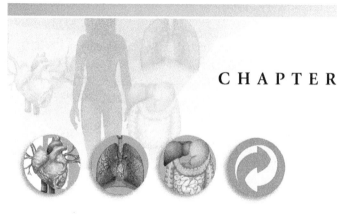

CHAPTER 17

Pediatric Solid Organ Transplantation

Stacee Lerret, RN, PhD, CPNP-AC/PC, CCTC
Gail Stendahl, RN, DNP, CPNP-AC/PC, CCTC

 ## I. INTRODUCTION

Organ transplantation for end-stage disease in children is the treatment of choice.

A. Longer waiting times for organs are a result of
    1. Critical shortage of potential donor organs
    2. Expansion of acceptable diagnoses for transplantation
    3. Increase in the number of children on the waiting list[1]

B. Improving graft and patient outcomes has led the transplant community to focus on the quality of life of pediatric recipients.[2]

C. This chapter will focus on pediatric kidney, liver, heart, and lung transplantation. Small-bowel transplantation is covered in the chapter on Intestine Transplantation.

 ## II. GENERAL PRINCIPLES ACROSS ALL ORGAN TYPES

A. Pretransplant evaluation
    1. The child is evaluated by the interdisciplinary transplant team.
        a. Transplant surgeon, organ-specific physician, social worker, psychologist, dietician, pharmacist, transplant coordinator, and other specialists as indicated based on patient disease
    2. Psychosocial evaluation:
        a. Psychosocial screening is performed by the transplant social worker and/ or psychologist to identify family or financial problems that may affect transplant outcomes.
        b. The child should be prepared physically, psychologically, and socially.
        c. Specific cultural and religious beliefs are identified and addressed on an individual basis and include issues such as
            i.   Dietary requirements
            ii. Use of blood products
            iii. Beliefs surrounding transplantation

3. Medical evaluation typically consists of
   a. Laboratory tests (e.g., complete blood cell count, complete metabolic profile)
   b. Infectious disease screening
   c. Review of immunization records
   d. ABO
   e. Human leukocyte antigen (HLA)
   f. Organ-specific diagnostic tests
4. Indications and contraindications to transplant:
   a. Organ-specific indications for transplant will be discussed in each section.
   b. Contraindications to transplant are similar across all organ types and include the following:
      i. Active infection
      ii. Active substance abuse specifically for adolescents
      iii. Active refractory seizure disorder
      iv. Active malignancy
      v. Irreversible multisystem organ failure
   c. Relative contraindications will vary across centers but may include the following:
      i. Psychiatric illness
      ii. Nonadherence with medical regimen in the pre-evaluation phase
      iii. History of substance abuse
      iv. Profound neurological devastation

B. Psychosocial support
   1. Emotional support, reassurance, and education are important for patients and families throughout the transplant continuum.
   2. Patients/families must be given ample time to verbalize their concerns and ask questions.

C. Education for patient/family awaiting transplantation, including, but not limited to
   1. Evaluation process
   2. Placement on waiting list
   3. Monitoring while on waiting list
   4. Organ matching
   5. Perioperative events:
      a. Preoperative tests/procedures
      b. Insertion of lines, tubes, etc
   6. Postoperative course
   7. Care of incision
   8. Pain management
   9. Physical activity
   10. Posttransplant regimen (medications, side effects, biopsies, etc.)
   11. Postdischarge follow-up
   12. Complications

D. Pretransplant immunizations
   1. Significant morbidity and mortality can result from preventable diseases. When possible, children should be fully immunized prior to transplantation based on age.
   2. Vaccination protocols depend on transplant program guidelines.

3. Many diseases are prevented by using "live" vaccines.
   a. Live vaccines are contraindicated in immunocompromised individuals; therefore, they should be given before transplantation.
   b. If the child has no antibodies to specific diseases, appropriate vaccination will be administered during the evaluation period.

E. Pretransplant optimization of dental health
   1. A dental examination is an important component of the pretransplant evaluation.
   2. Poor dental hygiene and caries are a potential source of infection in the immunocompromised patient.
   3. It is essential to optimize dental health prior to transplantation.

F. Placement on waiting list
   1. Once the transplant evaluation has been completed, the child will be presented to the interdisciplinary transplant team.
   2. Assessments by members of the interdisciplinary transplant team are reviewed. These members include, but are not limited to, organ-specific surgeons and other physicians (e.g., nephrologist, hepatologist, cardiologist, pulmonologist), transplant coordinators, nurse practitioners, social workers, psychologists, dietitians, pharmacists, anesthesiologists, and other pediatric specialists based on patient need.
   3. Children who meet eligibility criteria can be placed on the deceased donor waitlist in their respective countries, for example:
      a. United States: United Network for Organ Sharing (UNOS)
      b. Europe: Eurotransplant
   4. Children in need of a liver, kidney, or lung transplant may have the option of living donation.

G. Immediate preoperative care
   1. This period can be challenging, particularly when families have been called in for a transplant from a deceased donor.
   2. It is essential that the transplant team explain what will happen in the perioperative and immediate postoperative periods, such as
      a. Preoperative procedures:
         i. Insertion of tubes, lines, wires, etc
      b. Anticipated length of surgery
      c. Operating room (OR) waiting room; periodic updates by member of surgical team
      d. Transfer from the operating room to the postanesthesia care unit (PACU) or intensive care unit (ICU)
      e. Postoperative pain management

H. Postoperative pain assessment and management
   1. Pain assessment and management
      a. Assessment is patient centered, ongoing, and dependent on the child's stage of development.
         i. Infants and toddlers:
            * Monitor vital signs.
            * Observe for change in behavior:
               ◦ Characteristics of child's cry
               ◦ Body movement
               ◦ Facial expression

      ii. Preschoolers may be able to use a FACES scale or simple Likert scale indicating 0 (no pain) to 10 (worst pain in their life).

      iii. Although school-age children and adolescents can use a self-report visual analog scale, it is important to monitor them for physiologic and behavioral indicators of pain.

  b. Explain all procedures using age-appropriate language.

  c. Patient-controlled analgesia (PCA):

      i. Allows the patient or nurse to administer small doses of opioids in addition to a continuous infusion

      ii. Appropriate with guidance from the pain management team

      iii. Common side effects to observe for when opioids are administered via the epidural/IV route include

- Respiratory depression
- Facial pruritus
- Urinary retention
- Nausea and vomiting

III. PEDIATRIC KIDNEY TRANSPLANTATION

  A. Overview: Renal transplant in children

    1. According to current United Network for Organ Sharing (UNOS) data[3]:

      a. 718 children 0 to 17 years old underwent kidney transplantation in 2015 in the United States.

      b. More than 1,000 children continue to wait for a new kidney on the waiting list.[3]

  B. Indications and contraindications

    1. Causes of renal failure in children are different than those of adulthood.[4]

    2. Diagnoses leading to end-stage renal disease include (Table 17-1):

      a. Glomerulonephritis

TABLE 17-1 Diagnoses Leading to End-Stage Organ Disease in Children

Lung Diseases	Kidney Diseases
Alveolar proteinosis	Renal dysplasia/hypoplasia/aplasia
Bronchiectasis	Obstructive uropathy
Bronchopulmonary dysplasia	Focal segmental glomerulosclerosis
Cystic fibrosis	Reflux pyelonephritis
Interstitial lung disease	Henoch-Schönlein purpura
Pulmonary hypertension	Bilateral Wilms' tumor
Liver Diseases	**Heart Disease**
Biliary atresia	Congenital heart disease such as hypoplastic left heart syndrome
Alpha-1 antitrypsin deficiency	
Wilson's disease	Cardiomyopathies
Alagille's syndrome	Cardiac tumors
Acute liver failure	
Viral hepatitis	
Glycogen storage disease	
Liver tumor (hepatoblastoma)	

    b. Focal segmental glomerulosclerosis (FSGS)
    c. Polycystic kidney disease
    d. Pyelonephritis
    e. Rarely, metabolic disease such as cystinosis
    f. Bilateral Wilms' tumor
3. Incidence is age dependent:
    a. In the younger child, the cause is more commonly congenital.
    b. In the older child, glomerulonephritis or FSGS is more frequently the cause.
4. Contraindications to kidney transplantation are listed above in the "all organ section."
5. Timing of kidney transplantation:
    a. Transplantation may be considered when the glomerular filtration rate (GFR) is approximately 30 mL/min per 1.73 m[2].[5]
    b. Internationally, there are differences in practice:
        i. Some countries promote preemptive transplantation.
        ii. Some countries do not promote living donor transplantation.

C. Pretransplant evaluation
1. Blood tests:
    a. ABO (blood type)
    b. Human lymphocyte antigen (HLA) typing
    c. Panel of reactive antibodies (PRA)
        i. See the Basics in Transplant Immunology chapter for an explanation of HLA typing and PRA.
    d. Complete metabolic profile
    e. Complete blood cell count (CBC) with differential
    f. Coagulation studies:
        i. Prothrombin time (PT) and partial thromboplastin time (PTT)
        ii. Consider thrombophilia screen:
            • Arterial or venous thrombosis can cause graft failure in the immediate postoperative period, usually within the first 2 to 3 days.[2]
            • Screening includes[2]
                ○ Anticardiolipin antibodies
                ○ Factor V Leiden
                ○ Antilupus coagulant
                ○ Protein C
                ○ Protein S
                ○ The genetic component methylenetetrahydrofolate reductase (MTHFR)
            • Patients found to have a clotting tendency or genetic predisposition to coagulation are treated with anticoagulants immediately after the transplant surgery.
            • Treatment may continue for approximately 6 months thereafter depending on the transplant center protocol.
    g. Lipid profile
    h. Infectious disease screening to include
        i. Cytomegalovirus (CMV)
        ii. Epstein-Barr virus (EBV)
        iii. Hepatitis B virus (HBV) and hepatitis C virus (HCV)
        iv. Tuberculosis (TB) skin test:
            • Purified protein derivative (PPD) skin test

   v. Measles, mumps, rubella (MMR) titers
   vi. Varicella-zoster virus (VZV) titers
   vii. Human immunodeficiency virus (HIV)
   viii. Toxoplasmosis[5]
   ix. Syphilis by testing rapid plasma reagin (RPR) or venereal disease research laboratory (VDRL)

 2. Urinalysis and urine culture
 3. Renal ultrasound
 4. Additional tests: Potential recipients also may be screened with the following:
  a. Audiologic examination
  b. Bone age films
  c. Ophthalmologic examination
  d. Chest radiograph
  e. Electrocardiogram (ECG)
  f. Echocardiogram
 5. Children with bladder problems require additional evaluation prior to transplantation:
  a. Poor bladder function can cause kidney damage to the newly transplanted kidney; therefore, the nature and extent of bladder abnormalities must be determined.
  b. This evaluation can include ultrasound, voiding cystourethrogram (VCUG), and/or urodynamics.
  c. Bladder function tests must be carried out with the patient awake because sedatives will affect the bladder and confound the test results.
  d. Renal failure secondary to reflux nephropathy, obstructive uropathy, or neuropathic bladder may demonstrate abnormalities that affect continence and bladder capacity.
  e. Corrective action may include
   i. Double voiding. This is a method that can be used to help with urinary retention. Double voiding consists of an initial urination and then a second attempt within 5 minutes.
   ii. Initiating self-catheterization.
   iii. Bladder augmentation. This is done when a piece of the bowel or stomach is added to the bladder in order to increase the volume of the bladder.
  f. Treatment, including surgical correction, is done prior to transplantation to ensure the bladder function is optimized.
  g. Occasionally, the surgical procedure is performed after transplantation.

D. Placement on the waiting list
 1. Time is the main factor in waiting for a kidney transplant as kidneys are allocated based on recipient length of time on waitlist.
 2. Patients are either active or inactive on the waitlist.
 3. Pediatric candidates accrue waiting time upon listing and receive additional time if dialysis was started prior to listing.
 4. There is no GFR requirement with children in order to place on waitlist.

E. Pediatric organ allocation
 1. Refer to adult kidney transplant chapter.
 2. The Kidney Donor Profile Index (KDPI) score can help predict how a particular kidney is expected to function.

F. Waitlist management

1. While on the waitlist, children receive dialysis as indicated and are seen by the transplant team as dictated by disease severity.

G. Care of the pediatric transplant candidate

1. Scheduled appointments with dialysis and transplant teams to assure optimal health
2. Routine monitoring of nutritional status and risk for infection

H. Immediate preoperative care or perioperative management

1. If the child has been dialysis dependent, a dialysis session may be necessary immediately prior to transplantation to optimize fluid and electrolyte balance.
2. Baseline vital signs: temperature, blood pressure, and heart and respiratory rates
3. Preoperative tests may include
   a. ECG
   b. Chest radiograph
   c. Blood tests (chemical profile, clotting screen, complete blood cell count)
   d. Urinalysis and microscopy
   e. Type and cross for blood
4. Calculation of a child's body surface area (BSA) is essential for accurate prescribing and administration of medication.
   a. BSA = height × weight/3,600
5. Administration of preoperative medications per program-specific protocols, such as
   a. Induction immunosuppressive agents
   b. Monoclonal antibody, steroids, calcineurin inhibitors, or antiproliferative agents

I. Surgical Procedure

1. The main blood vessels used in kidney transplantation are
   a. Inferior vena cava (IVC)
   b. Aorta
   c. Iliac arteries and veins
2. Placement of kidney:
   a. Older children (typically >3 years) will have the donor kidney implanted in an extraperitoneal position.
      i. Donor vessels are anastomosed to the iliac vessels.
   b. Infants or small children have the kidney placed intraperitoneally.
      i. Donor blood vessels are anastomosed directly to the aorta and the IVC.
      ii. Following reperfusion, the donor ureter is anastomosed to the bladder.
3. Native kidneys usually are not removed prior to renal transplantation because removing the native kidneys has been noted to increase the rate of surgical-related morbidity.
   a. Clinical situations that may involve removing native kidneys in a child include
      i. Severe or poorly controlled hypertension to prevent damage to the new kidney
      ii. Polycystic kidney disease owing to space issues

J. Posttransplant care
1. In the immediate postoperative period, emphasis will be on monitoring for posttransplant complications.
    a. Regular recording of vital signs (Table 17-2).
    b. Frequency is determined by program-specific protocols.
    c. Observations include
        i.   Blood pressure
        ii.   Heart and respiratory rates
        iii. Core/peripheral temperature
        iv.   Pulse oximetry
        v.   Central venous pressure (CVP) monitoring
        vi.   Intake and output initially recorded hourly including
            • Intravenous (IV) infusions
            • Blood loss from drains and surgical incision
            • Output via urinary catheter and/or emesis
2. Perfusion of the kidney is evaluated immediately postoperatively using Doppler ultrasound depending on the center specific transplant protocol.
3. Hemodynamic stability is a priority and is monitored closely.
4. Fluid balance:
    a. If the child is polyuric, hypovolemia may occur rapidly.
    b. If the child is oliguric, hypervolemia may develop.
        i.   Oliguria is defined as a urine output <1 mL/kg/h in infants and <0.5 mL/kg/h in children.
        ii.   Initially, the IV fluid regimen includes 100% replacement of urine output with 0.45% normal saline.
        iii. Close observation of respiratory rate and effort is necessary to monitor for pulmonary edema, especially in the oliguric patient.

TABLE 17-2 **Typical Postoperative Observations**

	Kidney	Liver	Heart-Lung
General observation	Y	Y	Y
Temperature (core +/− peripheral)	Y	Y	Y
Blood pressure	Y	Y	Y
Heart rate	Y	Y	Y
Respiratory rate	Y	Y	Y
CVP	Y	Y	Y
Pulse oximetry	Y	Y	Y
Pulmonary artery catheter measurement	N	N	Y
Telemetry/epicardial pacemaker	N	N	Y
Fluid balance	Y	Y	Y
Wound site	Y	Y	Y
Daily weights	Y	Y	Y

c. If the child is hyponatremic or has a urinary sodium >100 mmol/L:
  i. Urinary replacement fluid should be alternated between 0.45% and 0.9% normal saline.
  ii. Urinary sodium, potassium, and creatinine levels can assist with fluid management and should be assessed regularly based on individual center guidelines.

5. CVP measurement is continuous.
  a. Maintain in the range of + 4 to + 8 cm H_2O with IV infusion of either 4.5% albumin or 0.9% saline.
  b. Low CVP can be indicative of hypovolemia, which can lead to poor graft perfusion.
    i. Hypovolemia may be presumed if
      • There is a gap of >2°C between the core and peripheral temperature.
      • The child is hypertensive and has a low CVP.
  c. Hypovolemia can be corrected by
    i. Administering 5 to 10 mL/kg of 0.45% albumin over 0.5 to 1 hour with close monitoring of CVP changes.
    ii. Repeating albumin infusion as clinically necessary.
    iii. Dopamine may be administered to maintain cardiac output and increase allograft perfusion.

6. Observation for excessive bleeding via the wound site, catheter, or abdominal drain is vital.
  a. The abdominal drain remains in place for the first few days postoperatively until minimal drainage is observed.
  b. The bladder urinary catheter remains on gravity drainage for a time period determined by center protocols, but usually for 4 days.
    i. If the patient suddenly becomes oliguric, assess for a blocked catheter.
  c. Observe the patient for pallor, hypotension, and tachycardia.

7. Monitor laboratory data at the frequency determined by transplant program protocols.
  a. Chemistry profile:
    i. Hypocalcemia may occur in the very early postoperative period in children with
      • A long history of dialysis therapy
      • Poorly controlled hyperparathyroidism
  b. CBC and differential
  c. Venous blood gas
  d. Immunosuppressant trough levels

K. Organ-specific posttransplant complications
  1. Complications after renal transplant can be divided into immediate, early, and late complications.
  2. Immediate complications relate to the intraoperative period and include
    a. Hyperacute rejection
    b. Obstruction
    c. Thrombus
    d. Delayed graft function
    e. Acute tubular necrosis (ATN):
      i. Major cause of delayed or primary nonfunction in kidney transplant recipients.
      ii. Results from damage to the proximal tubular membranes.

iii. May last for variable periods from hours up to several weeks.

iv. Long cold ischemic times in the donor kidney are considered a predisposing factor for ATN.

v. Children with ATN present with oliguria prior to becoming anuric.

- Close observation of serum potassium levels is vital as an anuric patient will quickly become hyperkalemic.
- Dialysis therapy is required.

vi. During prolonged periods of ATN, serial renal biopsies are performed to assess kidney function and monitor for rejection.

vii. Management of ATN includes avoiding nephrotoxic drugs and conservative fluid replacement to prevent hypervolemia.

3. Early complications—often related to surgical issues:

a. Bleeding:

i. Bleeding can occur at the site of the vascular anastomosis or arterial branches.

ii. Bleeding is manifested clinically as

- Tachycardia
- Hypotension
- Falling CVP
- Abdominal distension
- Pain
- Oliguria

iii. Replacement of blood volume and surgical intervention are necessary to control the bleeding.

b. Thrombus:

i. Children younger than 5 years are at highest risk for vascular thrombosis secondary to low flow states.

ii. Arterial thrombosis presents with sudden anuria and is often irreversible resulting in graft loss.

c. Renal artery stenosis:

i. Diagnosed when the Doppler ultrasound demonstrates turbulent flow

ii. Clinical symptoms are

- Hypertension that is difficult to control with or without erythrocytosis
- Deteriorating renal function

d. Renal vein thrombosis:

i. More common in young recipients

ii. Can often be treated with heparin

iii. Clinical presentation includes

- Gross hematuria
- Graft swelling
- Deterioration of graft function

e. Wound dehiscence

f. Lymphocele:

i. Lymphoceles are collections of lymph that occur when the lymphatic system is cut intraoperatively.

ii. Majority are asymptomatic.

iii. Larger lymphoceles can cause obstruction and hydronephrosis.

iv. Diagnosis is made by Doppler ultrasound or nuclear medicine renal scan examination.

v. Treatment depends on whether the lymphocele is causing obstruction or dysfunction.

vi. Treatment is by percutaneous aspiration.

- May be drained on a single occasion.
- May require an indwelling drainage system.
- Drainage that continues long-term may require surgical fenestration.

g. Infection:

i. Predisposing factors:

- Immunosuppressive agents
- Hypoalbuminemia

ii. Prevention—prophylactic antibiotics:

- Administered at the time of surgery.
- Prophylactic antibiotics are typically discontinued after 3 doses.

iii. Signs of infection and/or impaired wound healing include, but are not limited to

- Redness
- Purulent discharge
- Dehiscence
- Pyrexia

iv. Diagnosis: swab for microscopy, culture, and sensitivities

v. Treatment:

- Initially broad-spectrum coverage is provided for both aerobic and anaerobic organisms.
- Once a specific organism is identified, the appropriate agent is ordered (antiviral, antifungal, or antibacterial).

h. Urinary leak:

i. Another potential complication after renal transplantation is a urinary leak at the ureterovesical anastomosis.

ii. Clinical signs include

- Unexplained fever
- Abdominal pain
- Decreased urinary output
- Elevated creatinine
- Wound drainage

iii. Treatment

- Urine leaks are treated with long-term indwelling urinary catheters, or surgical intervention for minor leaks.

i. Obstruction at the anastomotic site:

- Can occur any time after transplantation
- Presents as oliguria or elevation of BUN and/or creatinine
- Treatment requires surgery:

j. Acute rejection (See section on Rejection below)

4. Late complications:

a. Chronic rejection (See section on Rejection below).

b. Refer to the chapter on Transplant Complications: Noninfectious Diseases for additional information.

L. Rejection
1. Types of rejection:
   a. Acute cellular rejection:
      i. Children with rejection present with
         * Decreased urine output
         * Increased weight
         * Hypertension
         * Increased creatinine levels
         * Pain over the graft area
         * Other clinical signs of acute rejection include
            ○ Proteinuria or hematuria
   b. Antibody-mediated (humoral) rejection:
      i.   Frequently referred to as "vascular" rejection
      ii. Always involves blood vessels
   c. Chronic rejection:
      i.   Characterized by slow and progressive increase in creatinine
      ii. Frequently associated with hypertension and proteinuria
      iii. Causes may include
         * Inadequate immunosuppression
         * Nonadherence to immunosuppression regimen
      iv. Associated with recipients who have had multiple episodes of acute rejection
      v.   Treatment typically includes
         * Increasing the primary immunosuppressive agent dose to achieve a higher drug level
         * Adjuvant immunosuppressive agents in addition to increase in primary immunosuppressive agent
      vi. As renal function continues to deteriorate, the child experiences symptoms of chronic renal failure.
         * May require phosphate binders, vitamin D administration, and erythropoietin to manage anemia
2. Diagnosis of rejection:
   a. A definitive diagnosis of rejection can only be made by histopathologic examination of renal tissue following a biopsy (See section on Biopsy and postbiopsy monitoring below)
3. Grading of rejection:
   a. Banff criteria allow standardization of the diagnosis and rejection grade.
   b. See Table 17-3 for specific Banff criteria.[6]
4. Treatment of rejection:
   a. Acute cellular rejection:
      i.   Acute cellular rejection is typically treated with methylprednisolone according to individual center protocol.
      ii. Additional immunosuppression agents such as antithymoctye globulin (Thymoglobulin; Atgam) may be used for rejection unresponsive to methylprednisolone.
   b. Antibody-mediated rejection:
      i.   Choice of therapy depends on program-specific protocols as well as patient-specific considerations based on pretransplant induction therapy.
      ii. Treatment may include IVIG and/or plasmapheresis antibody therapy, depending on program-specific protocols.

TABLE 17-3 Banff Criteria Grading of Rejection in Renal Transplant Recipients

Grade	Nomenclature
1	Normal
2	Antibody-mediated rejection (coincides with grades 3, 4, 5)
	ATN
	Capillary
	Arterial
3	Borderline changes—mild tubulitis
4	T-cell–mediated rejection
5	Interstitial fibrosis and tubular atrophy
6	Other

M. Biopsy and postbiopsy monitoring
   1. Indications for biopsy include
      a. Primary nonfunction of the kidney.
      b. A >10% rise over the previous day's creatinine level.
      c. Individual center protocols may include surveillance or routine biopsies.
   2. Preparation for biopsy:
      a. Explain procedure to parents and child.
      b. Ensure that informed consent is signed by parents.
      c. Obtain laboratory tests as ordered.
         i. Clotting screen including prothrombin time (PT)/international normalized ratio (INR)
         ii. Type and cross of blood:
            • At least one unit of blood should be available in case of bleeding after biopsy.
   3. Anesthesia options:
      a. Renal biopsy can be performed under general anesthesia, conscious sedation, or local anesthesia depending on the age of the child and transplant program protocol.
   4. Procedure:
      a. Usually performed under ultrasonic guidance
   5. Complications:
      a. The nurse should monitor for bleeding from the biopsy site as well as routine postanesthesia complications including nausea and vomiting.
   6. Biopsy results:
      a. May demonstrate any of the following:
         i. Healthy kidney tissue
         ii. Resolving ATN
         iii. Calcineurin inhibitor (CNI) toxicity
         iv. Rejection

N. Summary
   1. Kidney transplantation is
      a. A treatment for end-stage kidney disease where the patient and family trade a life-threatening illness for a posttransplant chronic illness:
         i. Lifelong medication to suppress the immune system
         ii. Long-term clinical follow-up

b. Internationally accepted as the best option for children with end-stage renal failure[7]

2. A successful kidney transplant is measured by both patient and graft survival rates.
   a. Current US data:
      i. 1-year patient survival: 96%
      ii. 1-year graft survival: 92%.[8]
   b. Current UK data:
      i. 1-year patient survival: 99%
      ii. 1-year graft survival: 97%[9]

IV. PEDIATRIC LIVER TRANSPLANTATION

A. Overview

1. Liver transplantation is the accepted treatment for end-stage liver disease in children.
2. According to the UNOS database, 580 children 0 to 17 years of age underwent liver transplantation in 2015.[3]
3. More than 450 children continue to await liver transplantation.[3]
4. Until the mid-1990s, survival rates for children had been limited by the lack of available size-matched donors.
5. Long waiting periods for an appropriate donor resulted in high mortality rates for patients on the transplant waiting list.
6. Reduced-size liver transplantation using the right lobe, left lobe, or left lateral segment from a deceased donor was recommended.
   a. Purpose:
      i. To address the issues of small intra-abdominal space
      ii. To alleviate the high rates of mortality
   b. Initially, this procedure was used in critically ill children who required immediate transplantation.
   c. Improved survival rates on the liver transplant waitlist were demonstrated as more patients were undergoing transplantation.
7. Today, multiple procedures exist for transplantation of the smallest recipients including
   a. Living related donor transplants:
      i. Living donors are evaluated by a separate adult transplant team.
      ii. Centers that offer this option must consider the ethical dilemma of subjecting a healthy donor to surgery.
   b. Split liver grafts:
      i. Division of a liver graft into two sections resulting in liver transplantation of two individuals
   c. Reduced-size liver grafts:
      i. Surgically modified graft to fit participant
   d. Whole liver grafts

B. Indications and contraindications

1. Children referred for liver transplantation have end-stage liver disease; see Table 17-1.
2. Contraindications to liver transplantation are listed above in the "all organ section."

C. Pretransplant liver evaluation
  1. The child is evaluated by the interdisciplinary transplant team.
     a. Transplant surgeon, hepatologist or gastroenterologist with expertise in liver disease, social worker, psychologist, dietician, pharmacist, transplant coordinator, and other specialists as indicated based on patient disease[10]
  2. Laboratory tests:
     a. ABO
     b. PT/INR and partial thromboplastin time (PTT)
     c. Comprehensive metabolic panel that typically includes albumin, blood urea nitrogen, calcium, carbon dioxide, chloride, creatinine, glucose, potassium, sodium, total bilirubin, total protein, liver enzymes (alanine aminotransferase [ALT], alkaline phosphatase [ALP], aspartate aminotransferase [AST])
     d. CBC
     e. Lipid panel
     f. Ammonia
     g. Amylase
     h. Lipase
     i. Alpha fetoprotein
     j. Vitamin A, D 25-hydroxy, and E levels
  3. Infectious disease screening:
     a. Herpes simplex virus (HSV)
     b. CMV
     c. Hepatitis viruses A, B, and C
     d. VZV titer
     e. EBV
     f. Syphilis by testing rapid plasma reagin (RPR) or venereal disease research laboratory (VDRL)
     g. Toxoplasmosis antibody
     h. HIV
     i. MMR titers
  4. Diagnostic tests:
     a. EKG and/or echocardiogram
     b. Chest radiograph
     c. Doppler ultrasound of the liver
     d. Computerized tomography (CT) scan or magnetic resonance imaging (MRI) of the liver[11]
  5. Review of immunization records

D. Placement on waiting list
  1. In the United States, potential recipients are listed by blood type, weight, and labs according to age on the UNOS waiting list.[12]
  2. The pediatric end-stage liver disease (PELD) score was developed simultaneously with the adult model for end-stage liver disease (MELD) score to create an effective system for donor liver allocation in the United States.
     a. PELD score lists children <12 years of age according to the probability of death within 3 months of listing.
     b. Developed from data derived from a sample of children enrolled in the Studies of Pediatric Liver Transplantation (SPLIT).
     c. Factors included in the PELD score include
        i. INR
        ii. Total bilirubin (mg/dL)

   iii. Serum albumin (g/dL)
   iv. Age at listing, <1 year
   v. Growth failure (based on gender, height, and weight)[12]
  d. MELD score lists children >12 years of age:
   i. Please refer to Liver Transplantation chapter for details regarding MELD score.

 3. Other variables include the following:
  a. Although the maximum adult MELD score is 40, there is no minimum or maximum to the PELD score.
  b. Status 1A and 1B listing for children with acute or chronic liver disease meeting certain criteria.
  c. Pediatric donors maintain priority for allocation to pediatric patients.
  d. Regional boards maintain discretion to upgrade patients to higher PELD score or status 1 if the PELD score does not reflect the urgency for transplantation.[13]

E. Pediatric organ allocation

 1. Organs are allocated to the patients highest on the list indicative of being the sickest patients.
  a. Status 1A, Status 1B, MELD/PELD scoring system

F. Waitlist management

 1. Patients maintain their active status on the waitlist by confirming the MELD/PELD parameters as documented above and outlined in Liver Transplantation chapter on a periodic basis as directed by UNOS guidelines.

G. Care of the pediatric transplant candidate

 1. Children with end-stage liver disease are at risk for several other problems that require management in the pretransplant period.
 2. Reduced caloric intake:
  a. Nutritional support is required in the pretransplant period.
   i. Cholestasis associated with malabsorption deprives the infant/child of essential fat-soluble vitamins (A, D, E, and K).
   ii. Other factors that affect caloric intake include
    • Anorexia that occurs with chronic disease
    • Increased abdominal pressures associated with organomegaly, ascites, and varices resulting in
     ○ Early satiety
     ○ Increased incidence of emesis
   iii. Management includes the use of increased caloric density formulas with medium chain triglycerides and night time drip feedings via nasogastric or nasojejunal tubes.[10]
  b. Aggressive nutritional support before transplant improves patient and graft survival.[14]
 3. Portal hypertension:
  a. Results from:
   i. Increased portal resistance and/or increased portal blood flow
  b. Therapy is directed at management of the major complication, variceal hemorrhage.
   i. Sclerotherapy or banding may be necessary to minimize risk of variceal bleeding.

4. Encephalopathy:
   a. Elevated ammonia levels play a central role in the development of encephalopathy.
   b. Manifestations:
      i.   Altered mental status
      ii. Complaints of increased sleeping
      iii. Poor school performance
   c. Treatment:
      i. Lactulose is commonly used although it lacks evidence of efficacy.
      ii. Bowel decontamination with rifaximin or neomycin.[15]

H. Immediate preoperative care or perioperative management
   1. Once a donor organ is available, the child is brought to the hospital and preoperative laboratory tests are obtained.
   2. The child is brought into the operating room and intubated.
   3. One to two large-bore catheters and/or central lines are placed.

I. Surgical procedure
   1. The liver transplant procedure takes approximately 8 to 12 hours.
   2. Procurement of the donor liver occurs according to the standard procedure for whole liver transplantation.
      a. The donor liver is prepared at the back table simultaneously with hepatectomy of the native liver by a second surgical team.
      b. In a reduced-size liver transplant, the liver is reduced by lobectomy (right or left) or trisegmentectomy for left lateral segment implants, with ligation of the main vessels and ducts.
      c. The biliary and vascular structures along the cut edge are ligated and the remaining vascular structures are flushed with preservation solution.
   3. Surgical incision
      a. A bilateral subcostal incision is made to visualize major structures
         i. Known as the Mercedes incision
         ii. May be an extension of the previous incision if the child underwent a Kasai portoenterostomy for management of biliary atresia
   4. Explantation of the native liver
      a. The vena cava, portal vein, and hepatic artery are crossed clamped prior to hepatectomy.
      b. Hemodynamic instability is a risk during the anhepatic phase secondary to
         i.   Decreased intravascular volume
         ii. Ongoing fluid and blood losses
         iii. Decreased venous return to the heart
   5. Implantation of the allograft
      a. Orthotopic
         i. Vascular anastomoses are generally performed in the following order:
            • Suprahepatic inferior vena cava
            • Intrahepatic inferior vena cava
            • Portal vein
            • Hepatic artery
         ii. Reperfusion of the graft occurs after the portal vein anastomosis.
            • During reperfusion, massive fluid shifts can result in intestinal edema, third spacing, and renal compromise.
            • Children generally tolerate the caval clamping and reperfusion well because of collateral circulation

       iii. Bile duct reconstruction is performed with an end-to-side roux-en-Y limb of the jejunum.

       iv. Two or three Jackson-Pratt drains may be inserted.

       v. Duct-to-duct biliary reconstruction is often performed in children with an adequate biliary tree (recipients diagnosed with metabolic disorders or fulminant hepatic failure).

  b. Other surgical options

    i. Split liver transplantation

- Split liver grafts differ from reduced sized grafts in the approach to separating the vascular and biliary structures.
- Produce two viable grafts for separate recipients
- The goal with this procedure had been to address donor shortages by providing a two-for-one application.
- Carries a higher incidence of postoperative complications such as biliary leaks and bleeding

    ii. Living related donor transplants

- The arterial reconstruction necessary in a living donor liver transplant presents a surgical challenge because of the many normal variants found in the hepatic arterial system.

J. Posttransplant care

  1. In the immediate postoperative period, emphasis will be on monitoring for posttransplant complications.

    a. Monitoring vital signs (see Table 17-2).

    b. Program-specific protocols should be followed.

K. Organ-specific posttransplant complications

  1. The child is taken to the pediatric intensive care unit (PICU), intubated, and monitored for

    a. Hemorrhage:

      i. May occur as a result of preexisting coagulopathy or bleeding at the anastomoses.

      ii. Children who have undergone previous abdominal procedures are at higher risk for bleeding and adhesions.

      iii. Frequent monitoring of output from the Jackson-Pratt drains is necessary.

      iv. Indications of bleeding include

- Increasing abdominal girth
- Oozing from the suture line

      v. Managing of coagulopathies:

- Blood products are used per discretion of the transplant team.

    b. Fluid and electrolyte balance:

      i. Hemodynamic instability may occur in the postoperative period, related to altered renal function and volume losses.

      ii. Fluids are administered

- On the basis of fluid status, vital signs, CVP, and weight compared to preoperative baseline values
- To provide necessary intravascular volume and assure adequate perfusion to the allograft and other vital organs

      iii. Adjustments of electrolytes and acid-base balance are made to assure appropriate fluid status.

       iv. Patients at risk for cerebral edema require a careful balance between maintaining adequate intravascular volume and avoiding increasing intracranial pressure.

       v. Hyperkalemia and metabolic acidosis are two early signs of vascular graft insufficiency or dysfunction.

       vi. Decreased urine output (<1 mL/kg/h) may indicate early graft dysfunction.

  c. Neurologic status: monitor for

       i. Mental status changes

       ii. Hepatic coma/encephalopathy

       iii. Seizures:

           • Seizures are rare although they may be result of calcineurin inhibitor toxicity.

  d. Gastrointestinal (GI) status:

       i. A nasogastric tube will be placed to decompress the stomach.

       ii. Monitor for nausea, vomiting, and presence of bowel sounds.

  e. Hepatic artery thrombosis (HAT):

       i. Complication occurring in 4% to 6% of pediatric recipients.

       ii. A duplex ultrasound of the liver is obtained in the first 12 hours to assess vessel patency.

       iii. Diagnosis of HAT in the first 1 to 6 postoperative days is possible with a duplex ultrasound.

           • If collateral vessels have developed, angiography may be the most definitive test.

       iv. Clinical signs of HAT:

           • Elevated transaminases and bilirubin

           • Change in mental status

           • Biliary leak, which may present as abdominal pain, jaundice, or bilious drainage from incision sites/drains

           • Sepsis

       v. Heparin may be administered in the immediate postoperative period to prevent thromboses.

       vi. Management of HAT:

           • Thrombectomy to restore blood flow

           • Retransplantation

  f. Portal vein (PV) thrombosis:

       i. May present with enlarging liver or spleen and decreasing platelet counts

       ii. May initially be diagnosed by daily liver ultrasound

  g. Biliary complications:

       i. In the immediate postoperative period, a change may be noted in the color of fluid in the Jackson-Pratt drain.

       ii. Bacterial contamination is possible if the leak occurs at the roux-en-Y anastomosis.

       iii. Diagnosis is made by ultrasound or percutaneous transhepatic cholangiogram.

       iv. Treatment involves surgical revision with insertion of a transhepatic biliary stent and broad-spectrum antibiotics.

L. Rejection
   1. Signs of rejection may include
      a. Low-grade fever.
      b. Increased liver enzymes and bilirubin.
      c. There may not be any physical signs or symptoms.
   2. Diagnosis: confirmed with a percutaneous liver biopsy
   3. Types of rejection:
      a. Acute rejection:
         i. Can occur as early as the first week posttransplant; risk of rejection continues lifelong
         ii. Treatment:
            • Majority of episodes respond to bolus doses of steroids and/or increased levels of calcineurin inhibitors, and/or other immunosuppressants including mycophenolate mofetil (CellCept) and mammalian target of rapamycin (Rapamune) mTOR inhibitors.[16,17]
      b. Chronic rejection:
         i. Frequent cause of graft loss
         ii. Underlying causes may be multifactorial including
            • Multiple episodes of acute rejection
            • CMV infection
            • Inconsistent immunosuppressant levels
         iii. Biopsy demonstrates bile duct loss with fibrosis and cirrhosis.
         iv. Treatment:
            • Treatment is similar to acute rejection utilizing, increasing immunosuppression per transplant program guidelines.[17]

M. Liver biopsy and postbiopsy monitoring
   1. Performed under conscious sedation with local anesthesia
   2. Preparation:
      a. Type and cross the child for blood.
      b. Obtain PT and PTT.
   3. Postbiopsy monitoring:
      a. Hemoglobin level should be obtained 4 to 6 hours after the procedure.
      b. The child should remain flat in bed for 4 to 6 hours.

N. Summary
   1. Liver transplantation is
      a. A treatment for end-stage liver disease where the patient and family trade a life-threatening illness for a posttransplant chronic illness
         i. Lifelong medication to suppress the immune system
         ii. Long-term clinical follow-up
   2. Future directions focus on immunosuppression withdrawal and continuing to expand the donor pool.[18,19]

V. PEDIATRIC HEART TRANSPLANTATION

A. Overview
   1. The first pediatric heart transplant was performed in 1985 at Loma Linda Hospital in an infant diagnosed with hypoplastic left heart syndrome.[16]

2. The number of children and adolescents worldwide undergoing heart transplantation has increased to approximately 550 per year.[17]
3. According to the United Network for Organ Sharing database, 456 children 0 to 17 years old underwent heart transplantation in 2016.[3]
   a. Survival rates have steadily increased with 5-year survival ranging between 75% and 80% based on age, diagnosis, and clinical characteristics.[17]
   b. Advancement in heart transplantation has occurred as a result of
      i.   Improved procurement procedures increasing the number of available donors
      ii. Virtual crossmatching, which is used in management of the sensitized recipient or patient with antibodies[20-22]
      iii. Development of a consistent grading system to diagnose rejection[23]
      iv. Improved immunosuppressive agents[24]

B. Indications and contraindications
   1. Indications:
      a. Heart transplantation is considered a viable option for children with end-stage heart disease, resulting from congenital heart defects or cardiomyopathy not responsive to medical or surgical treatment.[16] See Table 17-1.
   2. Contraindications[25]:
      a. Heart transplant-specific absolute contraindications include
         i. Significant perivascular disease
         ii. Active myocarditis
      b. Relative contraindications:
         i.   Pulmonary hypertension
         ii.   Complex cardiopulmonary anatomy
         iii. HLA antibody sensitization
         iv.   Poor nutrition and impaired wound healing
         v.   Renal and/or hepatic insufficiency
         vi.   Chronic protein-losing enteropathy (PLE) and/or aortopulmonary (AP) collaterals
         vii. Mitochondrial or muscular dystrophies

C. Pretransplant evaluation
   1. Purpose:
      a. Evaluate possibility of medical or surgical alternatives to transplantation
      b. Determine suitability of the candidate
   2. Diagnostic evaluation includes
      a. Echocardiogram.
      b. Cardiac catheterization (as indicated).
      c. Chest radiograph.
      d. Exercise stress test, if patient is able.
      e. Head computed tomography (CT) scan or ultrasound may be used to rule out intracranial bleed if patient is at risk for bleed based on disease.
      f. Abdominal ultrasound.
      g. Cardiac MRI.
   3. Laboratory evaluation includes
      a. ABO typing
      b. Chemistry panel
      c. Thyroid function tests

      d. Lipid profile

      e. CBC

      f. Human lymphocyte antibody (HLA) recipient typing as well as identification and detection (recipient's PRA along with antibody specificities)

      g. Isohemagglutinin titers (blood test done in infants to see if infant is able to accept an ABO incompatible heart)

      h. Viral screening:

         i. CMV

         ii. EBV

         iii. Herpes virus

         iv. Hepatitis A, B, and C viruses

         v. HIV

         vi. Toxoplasmosis

         vii. Syphilis by testing rapid plasma reagin (RPR) or venereal disease research laboratory (VDRL)

         viii. VZV titer

         ix. MMR titers[26]

4. Pretransplant evaluation as discussed above include meeting with each of the following:

      a. Social worker or psychologist for a psychosocial assessment, dietician, pharmacist, and financial counselor

      b. Purpose of these interviews is to identify

         i. Family coping skills

         ii. Stressors

         iii. Readiness for transplantation process

         iv. Financial needs

D. Placement on the waiting list

1. The interdisciplinary transplant team reaches consensus about the child's candidacy by transplant team committee review.

2. The child is placed on the United Network for Organ Sharing (UNOS) waiting list.

      a. Listed according to height, weight, and blood type:

         i. Donor organ may be two times above the recipient's actual weight.

           • Highly variable listing range depending on recipient heart size. Typical pediatric listing range is 10% below and two to three times above recipient's weight.

           • MRI echocardiographic technique to measure total cardiac volume is a validated tool for donor-recipient size matching in pediatric heart transplant patients.[26]

E. Pediatric organ allocation

1. Organ allocation is determined according to urgency.

      a. Children listed as 1A are the sickest and often in the ICU.[27] Clinical criteria include a minimum of one of the following:

         i. Use of continuous mechanical ventilation and admitted to the hospital

         ii. Assistance of a mechanical circulatory support device

         iii. Assistance of an intra-aortic balloon pump and admitted to the hospital

        iv. Ductal dependent pulmonary or systemic circulation with ductal patency maintained by stent or prostaglandin infusion and admitted to the hospital

        v. Congenital heart disease requiring multiple inotropes or a single high-dose inotrope and admitted to the hospital

   b. Status 1B signifies a child who is hospitalized but not in the ICU with any one of the following clinical criteria:

        i. Infusion of one or more inotropes but does not qualify for pediatric status 1A

        ii. Less than 1 year of age at the time of the candidate's initial listing and has a diagnosis of hypertrophic or restrictive cardiomyopathy

   c. Status 2 patients do not meet 1A or 1B criteria.[28]

   d. Exception: candidates can be listed in a higher category than their standard criteria would allow if there are higher risk elements to their disease. Listing by exception is subject to review by the UNOS Regional Review Committee.

   e. Utilization of the virtual crossmatch as a listing strategy can lead to shorter wait times and better outcomes for sensitized children waiting for heart transplantiont.[20]

F. Waitlist management

   1. While on the waitlist, children are seen by the transplant team as dictated by disease severity.

     a. Medical management: maintain optimal hemodynamics through use of medications

     b. Surgical management: maintain optimal hemodynamics through mechanical circulatory support including, but not limited to, ECMO and LVAD

G. Care of the Pediatric Transplant Candidate

   1. Children and families should focus on maintaining the child's normal/ideal weight.

     a. Referral to a dietician may be necessary to review caloric intake.

     b. Supplemental feedings may be required to provide for adequate growth.

   2. Monitor height and weight every 2 to 3 months in children younger than 3 years

   3. Children should be scheduled for visits to maintain their immunization status.

   4. Some children may require evaluation by physical therapy.

   5. School-age children and adolescents may need hospital- or home-based educational tutoring by certified teachers.

   6. During hospital visits, the interdisciplinary transplant team (nurses, nurse practitioners, social workers, and physicians) should evaluate

     a. Child's emotional adjustment to waiting for transplantation

     b. Progress toward developmental milestones

     c. Plan for the appropriate intervention such as a consult with psychology, physical or occupational therapy, and nutrition

   7. Child life specialists play an important role in preparing children for painful or invasive procedures and helping children cope.[29]

H. Immediate preoperative care and perioperative management
1. Once a donor organ is available, the child is brought to the hospital and preoperative laboratory testing is obtained.
2. The child is brought into the operating room, anesthesia is administered, lines are placed, and the child is intubated for surgery.

I. Surgical procedure
1. Special surgical options must be carefully considered and tailored for children with all forms of congenital heart disease, such as hypoplastic left heart syndrome, transposition of the great vessels, and dextrocardia.
2. The transplant procedure replaces diseased or absent vascular structures that have been previously treated surgically.[25]
3. Sequence:[25]
   a. A median sternotomy incision is made.
   b. Patient is placed on cardiopulmonary bypass.
   c. Body temperature is cooled to a nasopharyngeal temperature of 18°C to 32°C.
   d. Circulatory arrest is established.
   e. Intracardiac lines are placed for pressure monitoring and vascular access.
   f. Cardiectomy is performed.
   g. The donor heart is prepared and implanted in an orthotopic position
      i. The most common technique is known as the bicaval technique.
         • Heart is implanted in a more anatomical position avoiding enlarged atria.
         • Separate end-to-end anastomoses of the caval veins are performed.
         • Bicaval anastomosis of donor and recipient inferior vena cava (IVC) and superior vena cava (SVC).
         • The bicaval technique has been further refined by the addition of a bipulmonary vein technique whereby common cuffs of the pulmonary veins are left in place.
      ii. The biatrial technique is an older and less frequently performed procedure.
         • The left and right atria are sutured in situ.
         • This is followed by reanastomosis of the aorta and main pulmonary arteries to the respective vessels.
         • Technical problems with atrial arrhythmias are more common with this procedure.[25]

J. Posttransplant care
1. Child is transferred from the operating room to the ICU or PACU.
2. Invasive lines and temporary pacer lines are maintained according to hospital policy.
3. Mediastinal chest tube is connected to a closed sterile chest tube drainage system.
   a. Maintained at −20 cm H_2O suction.
   b. Mediastinal dressing is removed in 24 to 48 hours.
   c. Monitor insertion site for signs for infection.
4. Foley catheter is removed as soon as possible to prevent urinary tract infections.
5. Patients are suctioned on an as-needed basis until weaned from mechanical ventilation.

6. Once weaned from mechanical ventilation, use of incentive spirometry is encouraged to prevent pulmonary infection.[30]
7. In the immediate postoperative period, emphasis will be on monitoring for posttransplant complications.
   a. Monitoring vital signs (see Table 17-2).
   b. Program-specific protocols should be followed.

K. Organ-specific posttransplant complications
1. Etiology of early graft failure:
   a. Hyperacute rejection due to ABO incompatibility or circulating donor-specific HLA antibodies associated with a positive crossmatch.
   b. Primary graft dysfunction may be related to pretransplant injury, prolonged ischemic time, or failure of preservation.
   c. Failure due to residual lesions more common in congenital heart disease, chronic pulmonary disease, aortopulmonary collaterals, pulmonary vein stenosis, arteriovenous malformations (AVM).[31]
2. Manifests clinically as pulmonary hypertension (right heart failure)
3. Medical management includes
   a. Initiation of vasodilators prior to weaning bypass:
      i.   Nitrous oxide inhalation (5 to 20 ppm)
      ii. Milrinone (Primacor) (0.5 to 1.0 µg/kg/min)
      iii. Isoproterenol (Isuprel) (1 to 5 µg/kg/min)
      iv. Nitroglycerine (5 to 15 µg/kg/min)
   b. Maintain a systolic pulmonary pressure between 30 and 40 mm Hg.
   c. Patients should remain sedated and on mechanical ventilation until the systolic pulmonary pressure normalizes.
   d. Serial measurement of pulmonary pressure with left arterial pressure or pulmonary capillary wedge pressures (PCWP).[31]
4. If graft failure is suspected, it may be necessary to intervene with either extracorporeal life support (ECMO) or pulsatile assist devices as a bridge to recovery in the immediate transplant period.[25]
5. Potential complications include
   a. Hemorrhage
   b. Arrhythmias
   c. Seizures
   d. Rejection (discussed in detail below)
   e. Infection (discussed in detail below)
6. Common posttransplant medications:
   a. Lifelong immunosuppression therapy[31]
   b. Antihypertensive agents to treat hypertension associated with calcineurin inhibitors, denervation of the heart due to transplant so the patient does not feel chest pain, and size mismatch:
      i.   Calcium channel blockers
      ii. Angiotensin-converting enzyme (ACE) inhibitors
      iii. Angiotensin-receptor blockers (ARB)
      iv. Beta-blockers
   c. Statins: may lower cholesterol, have anti-inflammatory properties, and prevent coronary artery disease
   d. Supplementation as needed:
      i.   Magnesium oxide
      ii. Ferrous sulfate[30]

    e. Prophylactic treatment posttransplant varies among institutions[32]

      i. Opportunistic infections:

- *Pneumocystis carinii* pneumonia prophylaxis: sulfamethoxazole and trimethoprim (Bactrim) required for 6 months posttransplantation.
- An alternative for sulfa-sensitive patients is inhaled pentamidine.

      ii. Viral infections:

- Prophylactic regimens for high-risk patients (CMV/EBV donor positive/recipient negative) with valganciclovir (Valcyte) for 3 to 6 months posttransplant

      iii. Fungal infections:

- Nystatin or fluconazole (Diflucan)[30]

      iv. See the chapter on Transplant Complications: Infectious Diseases for additional information on posttransplant infections.

7. Cardiac-specific long-term complications:

    a. Cardiac allograft vasculopathy (CAV):

      i. Diffuse and progressive narrowing of the coronary arteries

      ii. Major cause of late mortality following cardiac transplantation

      iii. Risk factors associated with the development of CAV include

- Older age
- Donor-recipient race mismatch
- Immunosuppressant regimen

      iv. Clinical manifestations:

- Manifestations may include arrhythmias, congestive heart failure, myocardial infarct, or sudden death.

      v. However, the patient with CAV is often asymptomatic[30]

- Transplanted heart is denervated; therefore, the patient may not experience chest pain.

      vi. Diagnosis of CAV:

- Most commonly confirmed by stenosis of 50% on coronary angiography.
- CAV stenosis is graded utilizing the International Society for Heart and Lung Transplantation (ISHLT) Cardiac Allograft Vasculopathy Report.[33]
- Alternative screening for CAV includes
  - CT angiography
  - Dobutamine stress test
- The routine use of statins has been shown to reduce cholesterol levels and the associated risk of CAV.[30]
- mTOR inhibitors (sirolimus [Rapamune]) have been found to be effective in preventing CAV or the progression of CAV.[30]

L. Rejection

1. Diagnosis of rejection:

    a. Noninvasive methods to diagnose acute cellular rejection continue to be explored (e.g., gene expression testing, proteomics, and donor-specific cell–free DNA).[34,35]

    b. Endomyocardial biopsy remains the gold standard for diagnosing cellular rejection in heart transplant recipients.[36]

      i. The biopsy of the right apex is performed through a right internal jugular vein or a right femoral approach.

    c. Although rare, potential complications of endomyocardial biopsy include
       i.   Cardiac perforation
       ii. Tamponade
       iii. Pneumothorax
       iv. Arrhythmias
       v.   Tricuspid valve damage
       vi. Loss of peripheral vascular access
       vii. Formation of scar tissue that does not permit an accurate reading of the state of rejection[36]
    d. Surveillance biopsy schedules vary from institution to institution.
       i.   A typical biopsy schedule might consist of biopsies performed at the following times[30]:
- 1 to 2 weeks posttransplant
- 1 month posttransplant
- 3 months posttransplant
- 6 months posttransplant
- Yearly thereafter

       ii. Some institutions are recommending fewer surveillance biopsies with close clinical follow-up and biopsy for symptomatic patients only.

2. Signs and symptoms of heart rejection may include
    a. Arrhythmias.
    b. Unexplained, persistently elevated resting heart rate (HR).
    c. Decreased CO.
    d. Fatigue.
    e. Elevated CVP.
    f. Cool extremities.
    g. Tachypnea.
    h. Diaphoresis.
    i. Decreased ventricular compliance.
    j. Hepatosplenomegaly.
    k. Presence of a third heart sound.
    l. Rejection may also present as fever, irritability, or a change in feeding or sleeping patterns.

3. Clinical signs and symptoms are not well correlated with the diagnosis of rejection, therefore emphasizing the importance of obtaining a biopsy.

4. Types of rejection:
    a. Acute cellular rejection:
       i.   Cellular rejection is graded according to the revised (ISHLT) grading system. See Table 17-4 for ISHLT grading of cardiac rejection.

TABLE 17-4 International Society of Heart and Lung Transplantation Standard Grading for Cellular Rejection

Grade	Nomenclature
0R	No rejection
1R	Mild- or low-grade rejection
2R	Moderate, intermediate-grade acute rejection
3R	Severe, high-grade acute cellular rejection

Stewart S, Winters G, Fishbein M, Tazelaar H, Billingham M. Revision of the 1990 working formulation for the standardization of nomenclature in the diagnosis of heart transplantation. *J Heart Lung Transplant.* 2005;24(11):1710–1720. Reference 37.

    ii. Treatment is recommended for grade 2R and 3R rejection.
- Treatment for acute cellular rejection includes administration of methylprednisolone 10 mg/kg daily for 3 days.
- Cytolytic therapy: For example, antithymocyte globulin [Thymoglobulin] may be necessary in the setting of hemodynamic compromise.

    iii. Repeat biopsy is typically planned in 2 to 3 weeks to ensure resolution of rejection.

    iv. Additional treatment strategies include
- Total lymphoid irradiation (TLI)
- Photopheresis
- Alemtuzumab (Campath)[30]

  b. Antibody-mediated rejection (AMR) is diagnosed based on histologic and immunopathologic biopsy results.[38]

    i. Diagnosis of AMR (ISHLT grading scale):
- pAMR0—negative for pathologic AMR; histologic and immunopathologic studies are both negative.
- pAMR1—suspicious for pathologic AMR (either the histologic or immunologic study is positive)
- pAMR2—positive pathologic AMR; both histologic and immunopathologic findings are present.
- pAMR3—severe pathologic AMR; interstitial hemorrhage capillary fragmentation, mixed inflammatory infiltrates, endothelial cell pyknosis, and/or karyorrhexis and marked edema.[38]

    ii. Treatment of AMR:
- Plasmapheresis
- Intravenous immunoglobulin (IVIG)
- Rituximab (Rituxan)
- Bortezomib (Velcade)
- Cyclophosphamide (Cytoxan)[30]

M. Postbiopsy monitoring
1. May be performed under conscious sedation with local anesthesia in the cath lab
2. Preparation:
   a. May need type and cross for blood
3. Postbiopsy monitoring:
   a. May require echocardiogram following biopsy to monitor for pericardial effusion.
   b. Child should remain flat in bed for 4 to 6 hours.

N. Summary
1. Heart transplantation is
   a. A treatment for heart failure where the patient and family trade a life-threatening illness for a posttransplant chronic illness.
      i. Lifelong medication to suppress the immune system
      ii. Long-term clinical follow-up
2. Continued improvement in mechanical circulatory support options for children[39]
3. Improved desensitization and virtual crossmatching techniques[20]
4. Expansion of ABO incompatible transplantation in infants[40]
5. Advances in immunosuppression[24]
6. Stem cell replacement therapies[24]

VI. PEDIATRIC LUNG TRANSPLANTATION

  A. Overview

    1. Survival benefits in lung transplantation have lagged behind other solid organs because of anatomic differences of the bronchial anastomoses and increased risk for bacterial and viral infections.

    2. Denton Cooley performed the first heart-lung transplant on a 2-month-old child in 1968; the patient survived for 14 hours.

    3. In 1987, the first successful lung transplant was performed on a 16-year-old with familial pulmonary fibrosis.

    4. Statistics about lung transplantation:

      a. According to the ISHLT registry, there have been 1,875 pediatric lung transplants and 667 pediatric heart-lung transplants performed worldwide since 1986.[35]

      b. On average, between 110 and 125 pediatric lungs transplants are performed worldwide annually.[35]

      c. Survival after pediatric lung transplant is generally comparable to that reported in adults with a median survival of 4.9 versus 5.4 years, respectively, in recipients undergoing transplant between January 1990 and June 2010.

      d. Bronchiolitis obliterans is

        i. The leading cause of death (50%) ≥5 years after transplantation

        ii. The most common form of chronic lung allograft dysfunction (CLAD)

        iii. The leading reason why long-term survival rates after pediatric lung transplant are lower than survival rates following heart or other types of solid organ transplantation in children.[35]

  B. Indications and contraindications

    1. Most common indications for lung transplantation are (dependent on age)[1]

      a. Cystic fibrosis (CF) (54% to 70%)

      b. Primary pulmonary hypertension (22%)

      c. Congenital heart disease (8%)

      d. Pulmonary hypertension (7%)

    2. Contraindications to pediatric lung transplantation[41]:

      a. Absolute contraindications:

        i. Active malignancy

        ii. Sepsis

        iii. Severe tracheomegaly or tracheomalacia

        iv. Severe transpleural systemic to bronchial artery collateral arteries

        v. Active tuberculosis

        vi. Lower respiratory infection (carries approximately 50% mortality)

        vii. Severe neuromuscular disease

        viii. Active infection (including HIV)

        ix. Documented, refractory nonadherence

        x. Multiorgan dysfunction

        xi. Hepatitis C with liver disease

      b. Relative contraindications:

        i. Pleurodesis

        ii. Renal insufficiency

        iii. Osteoporosis

        iv. Markedly abnormal BMI

v.   Mechanical ventilation

vi.   Poorly controlled diabetes mellitus

vii.   Chronic airway infections, multiple-resistant organisms

C. Pretransplant evaluation

1. Each child is evaluated by the pediatric pulmonologist.
2. Diagnostic tests include
   a. Pulmonary function tests (PFTs)
   b. Arterial blood gas
   c. Chest radiograph
   d. Ventilation perfusion scan
   e. CT scan of the thoracic cavity
3. Children with cystic fibrosis also undergo an evaluation of the sinuses.
4. Consults:
   a. A cardiology consult is obtained to assess anatomic problems such as a patent foramen ovale.
      i.   Possible studies include
         • EKG
         • Echocardiogram
         • Cardiac catheterization
      ii.   If a cardiac defect is diagnosed, it will be repaired at the time of transplantation.
   b. Mental health clinician (social worker, psychologist)
   c. Dietician
   d. Pharmacist
   e. Financial counselor
   f. Infectious disease specialist (typically consulted in lung transplantation) due to pretransplant infections specific to the cystic fibrosis population
5. Laboratory tests:
   a. ABO
   b. HLA typing
   c. HLA antibodies (PRA with antibody specificities)
   d. Chemistry panel
   e. CBC with differential
   f. Fasting lipid panel
   g. Infectious disease:
      i.   Hepatitis virus B and C
      ii.   HIV
      iii.   CMV
      iv.   EBV
      v.   VZV
      vi.   Tuberculosis
      vii.   Syphilis by testing rapid plasma reagin (RPR) or venereal disease research laboratory (VDRL)
      viii.   Toxoplasmosis[42]

D. Placement on the waiting list

1. The UNOS lung allocation score (LAS) ranges from 0 to 100 with higher scores indicating the child is more likely to benefit from a lung transplant. The LAS is for children older than 12 years utilizing the following medical information:
   a. Age
   b. Height

      c. Weight

      d. Blood type

      e. O_2 requirements

      f. Forced vital capacity (FVC)

      g. 6-minute walk test results

      h. New York Heart Association (NYHA) class

  2. Children younger than 12 years are listed according to blood type.

E. Pediatric organ allocation[41]

  1. For patients <12 years of age, waiting time is used for organ allocation.

  2. For patients 12 years of age and older who have a LAS score, waiting time is used to break a tie between two candidates with a similar LAS.

  3. Size matching of donor lungs is based on height and weight parameters.

      a. This may not be the most accurate method of estimating intrathoracic volume.

      b. Calculating the predicted total donor lung capacity compared to the recipient's predicted and actual lung capacity may provide a more accurate estimate of recipient intrathoracic volume.

      c. Size mismatch can lead to complications in the postoperative period including

         i. Atelectasis

         ii. Altered bronchial anatomy leading to retention of secretions

         iii. Anastomotic airway complications

         iv. Increased risk of infection if the lung is oversized

      d. Undersized lungs can lead to

         i. Persistent pneumothorax

         ii. Hyperexpansion of the lung resulting in increased work of breathing

         iii. Limited exercise tolerance

  4. An alternative to deceased donor lung transplantation is living-related or unrelated lung donation.

      a. This procedure was first used in patients with cystic fibrosis.

      b. Criteria for living-related lobar lung transplant include

         i. Rapid progression of disease, which precludes waiting for deceased donor

         ii. Low priority for deceased donor lung transplantation indicated by a low LAS score

         iii. Rare ABO

         iv. High PRA level

         v. Retransplantation

      c. In living donor transplantation, the recipient undergoes bilateral pneumonectomy.

         i. The lower lobes from two separate healthy donors are implanted into the recipient.

         ii. With two living lung donors and a recipient, three simultaneous surgical procedures are carried out requiring a maximum utilization of resources.

         iii. Children younger than 6 years are not good candidates as the healthy adult donor lobe is too large.

F. Waitlist Management

  1. While on the waitlist children, age 12 and older must have the following tests at least twice a year to maintain their status on the waitlist:

      a. Age

      b. Height

      c. Weight

      d. Blood type

      e. O_2 requirements

      f. Forced vital capacity (FVC)

      g. 6-minute walk test results

      h. New York Heart Association (NYHA) class

  2. While on the waitlist, children <12 years of age are seen by the transplant team as dictated by disease severity.

G. **Care of the pediatric transplant candidate**

  1. Nutrition:

      a. During the waiting period, nutrition must be maximized to prevent muscle wasting.

      b. Dietary supplementation may be necessary to optimize nutrition.

      c. If the patient is unable to consume enough calories orally, tube feedings or insertion of a feeding gastrostomy should be considered.[42]

      d. Physical endurance and respiratory requirements:

         i. Patients are referred to physical therapy for endurance and strength training to optimize oxygenation.

         ii. Prior to transplant, many children require supplemental oxygen through a nasal cannula or mask.

         iii. As the lung disease progresses or during sleep, children may require noninvasive positive pressure ventilation with continuous positive airway pressure (CPAP) or bilevel positive airway pressure (BiPAP).[42]

         iv. If the child requires additional assistance with breathing, mechanical ventilation is discussed with the family.

            • Mechanical ventilation prior to transplantation is associated with a poor outcome posttransplant and is a relative contraindication to transplantation.

H. **Immediate preoperative care or perioperative management**

  1. Once a donor organ is available, the child is brought to the hospital and preoperative laboratory and radiological tests are obtained per hospital protocol.

  2. The child is brought into the operating room and intubated.

  3. Operative lines are placed.

I. **Surgical procedure**[41]

  1. Typical surgical procedure:

      a. Removal of donor lungs:

         i. Lungs are removed at the same time.

         ii. Lungs are perfused with a high-molecular, low-potassium dextran solution and epoprostenol (Flolan).

      b. Surgical incision:

         i. An isolated bilateral segmental lung transplantation is performed through a bilateral anterolateral thoracotomy or bilateral transsternal thoracotomy.

         ii. A "clamshell" incision is then made at the fourth intercostal space.

      c. Cardiopulmonary support during surgical procedure:

         i. In a small child, a double-lumen endotracheal tube may not be an option, and thus, cardiopulmonary bypass (CPB) is often used.

            • The advantages of CPB include

               ○ The ability to deflate the native lungs permitting easier dissection

○ The ability to clamp and cleanse the proximal tracheobronchial airway
  • The disadvantages of CPB are
    ○ Associated coagulopathy and capillary leak syndrome
  ii. If ECMO support was required prior to transplantation, it is maintained intraoperatively instead of CPB.
  iii. In some institutions, ECMO has replaced the use of CPB.
d. Removal of recipient's lungs and implantation of allograft:
  i. After placing the child on CPB, the lungs are removed and implanted in a sequential manner.
  ii. An end-to-end bronchial anastomosis is performed by connecting the donor bronchus with the recipient's bronchus.
  iii. Additional suture lines are placed at the pulmonary arterial and venous sites.
e. Weaning from CPB or ECMO:
  i. The recipient is weaned from CPB or ECMO at the conclusion of the procedure.
  ii. If the child is hemodynamically unstable, inotropic support such as epinephrine and milrinone infusions may be required.
f. Transesophageal echocardiogram and bronchoscopy:
  i. A transesophageal echocardiogram and bronchoscopy may be performed to ensure adequate vascular and bronchial anastomoses.
  ii. Repeat bronchoscopies may be required for airway clearance and anastomosis checks.
g. Chest tubes:
  i. Anterior and posterior bilateral chest tubes are inserted to evacuate chest secretions and obtain accurate measurement of pleural drainage.
2. Alternative surgical techniques:
  a. Numerous alternative operative techniques to whole-lung transplantation have been developed to meet the increasing need for donor lungs.
  b. Downsizing of lungs is achieved by
    i. Split lung/lobar transplantation
       • Left donor lung is separated at the back table.
       • The choice of lobes is determined by chest radiograph.
       • All lobes are usually suitable for transplantation.
       • Advantage: Ability to estimate the best match of the size of the inflated donor lung and the recipient's chest cavity.
    ii. Peripheral wedge section:
       • Performed after implantation and full inflation of the lung.
       • Careful estimation of the amount of lung resection required is determined prior to stapling of the suture line.
  c. Use of single lobes is warranted if the recipient's chest cavity is small or localized pathology is present in one or multiple donor lobes.
  d. If necessary, these techniques may be combined at the time of transplantation.[43]

J. Posttransplant care
1. In the immediate postoperative period, emphasis will be on monitoring for posttransplant complications.
  a. Monitoring vital signs (see Table 17-2).
  b. Program-specific protocols should be followed.

K.   Organ-specific posttransplant complications
    1. Pulmonary function:
        a. Postoperative care focuses on maintaining pulmonary function.
        b. The lungs are denervated during surgery and therefore
            i.   The cough reflex is absent from the suture line downward.
            ii. The patient must be assisted to mobilize and expel mucus.
                • This is accomplished by gentle chest physiotherapy or a bed that provides gentle vibration.
            iii. Frequent suctioning is required while the patient remains intubated.
        c. Patients are weaned from ventilatory support as quickly as possible, usually within 72 hours.
        d. Frequent assessment of chest tube function is necessary to prevent air leaks or pleural effusions.
            i.   Initially, the suction is kept at low levels (5 to 10 mm Hg) to prevent hemodynamic instability.
            ii. Chest tubes are removed when fluid drainage is minimal.
            iii. Adjustment in caloric intake may be necessary if a pleural or chylous effusion persists.[44]
    2. Prevention of infection:
        a. CF transplant recipients:
            i.   May require antipseudomonal antibiotics based on recent cultures.
            ii. Antifungal agents are added if the patient has a history of *Aspergillus* infection.[45]
        b. Non-CF patients can be prophylaxed with a first-generation cephalosporin such as cefazolin (Ancef).
        c. CMV:
            i.   If the recipient or donor is positive for CMV, the recipient is treated with
                • IV ganciclovir (Cytovene) for at least 1 week followed by oral valganciclovir (Valcyte) for 6 months
        d. Pneumocystis pneumonia:
            i.   Trimethoprim-sulfamethoxazole (Bactrim):
                • Started postoperative week 1 and given daily for 4 to 6 months to prevent pneumocystis pneumonia
                • Followed by same dose three times a week indefinitely with a typical dose of 80 mg of sulfamethoxazole.
        e. Other recommended prevention therapies include
            i.   Oral nystatin or fluconazole to prevent *Candida*
            ii. Oral acyclovir (Zovirax) to prevent herpes simplex infection[45]
    3. Incidence: 2013 ISHLT registry data indicate the following:
        a. The most common complication at 1 year after transplant was hypertension (>40% of patients), followed by diabetes mellitus (23%).
        b. Within 5 years posttransplant, hypertension had developed in almost 70% of recipients, followed by chronic kidney disease and diabetes.
        c. The incidence of renal dysfunction within 5 years after transplant was 32%, and 3% of these recipients required dialysis or a renal transplant.[35]

L.   Rejection
    1. Description:
        a. Acute Rejection:
            i.   Characterized by lymphocytic infiltration of the vessels
            ii. Generally reversible with treatment

b. Chronic Rejection:
   i. Obliterative bronchiolitis (OB) is a chronic form of rejection and diagnosed by biopsy.
      * A patient is at increased risk for OB after multiple episodes of acute cellular rejection or one episode of severe acute cellular rejection.[46]
      * OB is diagnosed by biopsy.
   ii. Bronchiolitis obliterans syndrome (BOS) is used to describe patients with progressive airflow obstruction without histologic evidence of rejection.
      * BOS is an inflammatory process of the small airways that results in
) Narrowing
) Distortion
) Plugging with granulation tissue
2. Symptoms of acute or chronic rejection in the lung transplant recipient are vague and may include
   a. Crackles on auscultation
   b. Tachypnea
   c. Wheezing
   d. Decreased breath sounds
   e. Shortness of breath
   f. Activity intolerance
   g. Decreased oxygenation (93% to 100% oxygen saturation)
   h. Decreased pulmonary function documented by a change of >10% of FEV1 with spirometer[44]
3. Diagnosis of obliterative bronchiolitis (OB) or chronic rejection:
   a. Diagnosis is confirmed with bronchoalveolar lavage or transbronchial biopsy (TBB).
      i. Bronchoalveolar lavage is less sensitive than TBB in the diagnosis of BOS.
   b. TBB is the "gold standard" for diagnosing rejection with high sensitivity and specificity.
      i. TBB is obtained through a flexible bronchoscope.
      ii. Biopsy forceps are passed through the suction channel.
      iii. Several samples are obtained from the lower lobe.
   c. Potential complications of TBB:
      i. Bleeding, particularly if platelet count <50,000 mm^3
      ii. Pneumothorax
   d. Alternative noninvasive testing in the diagnosis of BOS:
      i. PFTs
      ii. FeNO: exhaled nitric oxide
4. Management of chronic rejection (OB and BOS):
   a. Prevention or early diagnosis is crucial in the management of chronic rejection.
   b. Management includes
      i. Frequent clinic visits.
      ii. Prevention/management of gastroesophageal reflux due to risk of acid or alkaline aspiration is related to a decrease in graft survival.[1]
      iii. Home monitoring of lung function with a handheld spirometer.
   c. Diagnostic testing:
      i. Frequent, comprehensive PFTs; may be done routinely at every clinic visit
      ii. High-resolution CT scan of the lungs to rule out complications

iii. Ventilation/perfusion scans to rule out complications

iv. Gas-exhaled measurements[46]

d. Similar to heart transplantation, the use of surveillance versus clinical biopsy remains controversial and differs from center to center.

5. Treatment of acute rejection:

a. Treatment of acute rejection consists of IV methylprednisolone 10 mg/kg for 3 consecutive days.

b. Repeat episodes of acute rejection are managed with an antilymphocyte preparation such as (Thymoglobulin)[47]

M. Postbiopsy monitoring

1. May be performed under conscious sedation with local anesthesia in the interventional radiology department

2. Preparation:

a. May need type and cross for blood

3. Postbiopsy monitoring:

a. Check hemoglobin and hematocrit 4 hours post biopsy to monitor for bleeding.

b. Child should remain flat in bed for 4 to 6 hours.

N. Summary

1. Lung transplantation is

a. A treatment for severe lung disease where the patient and family trade a life-threatening illness for a posttransplant chronic illness.

i. Lifelong medication to suppress the immune system

ii. Long-term clinical follow-up

2. Future directions include advancing the care of organ donors to expand the donor pool.

3. Research and collaborative efforts among pediatric lung transplant centers for continued advancements for use of immunosuppression and medical management.

VII. IMMUNOSUPPRESSION AFTER PEDIATRIC TRANSPLANTATION

A. The goal of immunosuppressant therapy is to balance the risk of rejection and infection.

1. The risk of acute rejection is greatest during the first 1 to 2 months after transplantation.

B. The approach is slightly different for each type of organ transplant; however, most recipients receive a combination of immunosuppressant medications.

C. Children metabolize medications at substantially different rates than adults; therefore, children require special formulations and schedules.

D. Initially, patients may receive a combination of the following types of immunosuppressive agents based on the type of organ transplanted and individual transplant center guidelines.

1. Calcineurin inhibitor designed to block T-cell cytokine gene expression:

a. Tacrolimus (Prograf) 0.1 to 0.15 mg/kg/d divided every 12 hours:

i. Initial target tacrolimus trough levels range from 10 to 15 ng/mL.

      b. Cyclosporine (Neoral, Gengraf) 5 to 10 mg/kg/d every 12 hours:
         i. Typically, initial target cyclosporine trough levels are maintained between 300 and 400 ng/mL.
  2. Corticosteroids:
      a. Inhibit leukotrienes and prostaglandins that are part of the inflammatory process.
      b. Dosage is usually high in the immediate posttransplant period and then tapers over time, depending on type of organ transplant.
  3. Cell toxins that inhibit purine biosynthesis:
      a. Mycophenolate mofetil (CellCept) 500 mg/m^2 or azathioprine (Imuran) 1 to 2 mg/kg/d

E. Lung transplant recipients routinely receive induction therapy with antilymphocyte globulin (Thymoglobulin), antithymocyte globulin (ATG), or an interleukin-2 receptor (basiliximab [Simulect]).

F. Several additional immunosuppressant management strategies include
  1. Induction therapy:
      a. Thymoglobulin 1.5 mg/kg for 1 to 2 weeks posttransplant.
      b. Dose is dependent on age at transplant and lymphocyte count.
  2. Steroid-free maintenance regimens:
      a. The goal is to avoid the morbidity associated with corticosteroids.
      b. Providers must carefully identify patients who are suited to steroid withdrawal or avoidance.
      c. During steroid weaning, it is essential that children be carefully monitored because acute rejection can occur at any time.
  3. mTOR inhibitor:
      a. Sirolimus (Rapamune) (1 to 5 mg daily)
      b. Note: Sirolimus is contraindicated in the immediate postoperative period following liver transplantation because of the increased risk of thrombotic events and prolonged wound healing.[48]

VIII. POSTTRANSPLANT INFECTIONS

A. Due to lifelong immunosuppression, infection is a common complication and a significant cause of posttransplant morbidity and mortality.

B. Several factors affect the incidence and timing of infection including
  1. The type of transplant procedure:
      a. For example, lung transplant recipients are at increased risk for infection due to an impaired cough reflex.
  2. The immunosuppressant regimen (dose, duration, and timing)
  3. Drug-related neutropenia
  4. Presence of invasive objects (e.g., catheters) that disrupt cutaneous barriers.
  5. Metabolic abnormalities such as
      a. Malnutrition
      b. Low albumin levels
  6. Exposures:
      a. Viral exposures pre- and posttransplant
      b. Preexisting infection such as mediastinitis or pneumonia[45]

C. Timing of infection:
  1. In the first 30 days posttransplant:
     a. Infection is associated with preexisting conditions or complications of surgery.
     b. Bacteria or yeast are the most frequent pathogens.
     c. Superficial or deep surgical wounds are the most common sites of infections.
  2. The major infections observed from 1 to 6 months posttransplant include
     a. Organisms acquired from the donor or opportunistic infections:
        i. Viruses (donor or recipient-derived viruses)
           • EBV and/or CMV
        ii. Adenovirus
        iii. *Pneumocystis jiroveci*
        iv. *Toxoplasma gondii*
        v. *Aspergillus fumigatus*[45]
  3. Late infections:
     a. Rates and severity of late infections are similar to those observed in otherwise healthy children.
     b. Chronic or recurrent infections are dependent on the level of immunosuppression and presence of uncorrected anatomic or functional abnormalities.[45]

D. Types of infections: viral:
  1. CMV:
     a. CMV is the most commonly occurring infection in the early posttransplant period, particularly in the recipient CMV negative/donor CMV positive group. However, all recipients are potentially at risk.
     b. There is an association between CMV infection and rejection.[49]
     c. Periodic CMV surveillance and use of prophylactic therapy are dependent on center protocols.
     d. CMV disease:
        i. Primary CMV infection occurs secondary to direct exposure to bodily fluids such as saliva, tears, urine, stool, or breast milk.
        ii. Can present as fever, hepatitis, enteritis, pneumonia, or a viral syndrome with neutropenia and thrombocytopenia.
        iii. Polymerase chain reaction (PCR) tests are sensitive indicators of CMV disease in solid organ transplant recipients.[49]
        iv. CMV may accelerate the development of rejection and increase the risk of other serious infections such as PCP or aspergillosis.
        v. The highest rate of active transmission is toddlers.[49]
        vi. Prevention of CMV disease is divided into universal prophylaxis versus preemptive therapy.
           • Universal prophylaxis:
             ○ Involves the administration of antiviral agents with or without an immunologic agent to all transplant recipients regardless of CMV risk
             ○ Delays the onset of symptoms for several months following solid organ transplant
             ○ No consensus among experts regarding the best route of administration of antivirals (oral vs. IV) or the use of immunoglobulin prophylaxis

- Preemptive therapy:
  - Involves a short course of therapy only for high-risk recipients such as recipient CMV seronegative and donor CMV seropositive
  - Requires the ability to detect changes in the viral load with tests that have sufficient sensitivity and specificity to differentiate latent from active replicating virus

vii. Treatment of CMV disease:
- Historically treated with IV ganciclovir (Cytovene).
- Cost and safety concerns associated with the long-term administration of ganciclovir led to other effective management strategies.[49]
- Transition to oral valganciclovir (Valcyte) can be used when enteral function is normal and the patient is improving.[45]
- Foscarnet (Foscavir):
  - Limited to cases of ganciclovir resistance
  - Is comparable to IV ganciclovir for CMV resistance
  - Significant side effects, including nephrotoxicity and neurotoxicity, are associated with its administration.[45]

2. EBV:
   a. Epstein-Barr virus is a common viral infection that can lead to posttransplant lymphoproliferative disease (PTLD).
   b. EBV manifests as a spectrum of diseases ranging from asymptomatic viremia through infectious mononucleosis to PTLD.[50]
   c. PTLD:
      i. Risk factors for PTLD include
         - Lifelong immunosuppression
         - Recipient is EBV seronegative
         - Young age at time of transplantation
      ii. The incidence of PTLD is reported between 1% and 16%, with lung and heart-lung transplant recipients having the highest incidence.[50]
      iii. Mortality rates are variable and children do better than adults.
         - 1-year survival after diagnosis (includes pediatric and adults) ranges between 56% and 73% with 5-year survival estimates between 40% and 61%.[50]
      iv. Presentation:
         - PTLD that presents with polyclonal features typically responds well to a reduction in immunosuppression.
         - Children who present with monoclonal features with a diffuse large B-cell lymphoma, such as a Burkitt's lymphoma, have no response to reduction in immunosuppression.
         - Clinical presentation includes
           - Fever
           - Malaise
           - Sore throat
           - Abdominal pain
           - Diarrhea with protein or blood loss in the stool
           - Generalized malaise
           - Headache
           - Graft dysfunction
      v. Common sites are the tonsils, adenoids, cervical lymph nodes, lung, abdomen, and allograft.

      vi. Management strategies may include
- Reduction or withdrawal of immunosuppression
- Antiviral therapy (acyclovir [Zovirax] or ganciclovir [Cytovene])
  - Continues to be controversial.
  - Efficacy of these agents has not been established and their role in treatment has been questioned.
- IV immune globulin
- Rituximab (Rituxan)
- Chemotherapy
- Surgery (removal of node or mass)

      vii. Serial monitoring of EBV PCR loads has been proposed as a method to reduce the incidence of PTLD.
- Every 2 to 4 weeks in the first 3 months post transplant
- Every 1 to 3 months >3 months post transplant
- Patients with significant increase in viral load (quartile or log) or EBV biopsy-proven infection undergo weaning of immunosuppression, radiological monitoring with CT scan and ongoing assessment of EBV viral loads.[45]

3. Adenovirus:
   a. Third most important viral infection following liver transplant.
   b. Symptoms range from self-limited fever and gastroenteritis to necrotizing hepatitis or pneumonia.
   c. Can be latent or can reactivate.[45]

4. VZV:
   a. Aggressive response to varicella exposure and disease is warranted.
   b. VZV immunoglobulin should be administered within 72 hours of a varicella exposure in nonimmune patients.
   c. Because the production of varicella-zoster immune globulin (VZIG) has been halted, it has been recommended that oral acyclovir (Zovirax) be started at day 7 post exposure. If lesions develop, hospitalize the patient and administer acyclovir IV until fever abates, no new lesions erupt, and existing lesions begin to crust.[45]

E. Types of infections: bacterial:
1. Bacterial infections tend to occur at or near the transplanted organ.[45]
   a. Infections that occur during the first 30 days post transplant are more frequently associated with death in the first year after transplant.
2. Tuberculosis:
   a. Etiologic agent: *Mycobacterium tuberculosis*.
   b. Patients with a history of tuberculosis or a positive purified protein derivative (PPD) test should have a chest x-ray and receive isoniazid for at least 9 months post transplant.
3. Common bacterial infections in specific pediatric transplant populations:
   a. Renal transplant recipients:
      i. Urinary tract infection, especially pyelonephritis, is the most common (gram-negative organisms).
      ii. Lower respiratory tract infections (such as pneumonia).
   b. Liver transplant recipients:
      i. Abdominal or surgical wound infection (gram-negative organisms)
      ii. Ascending cholangitis associated with biliary tract abnormalities

c. Heart transplant recipients:
   i.   Lower respiratory tract infections (pneumonia and lung abscess)
   ii. Mediastinitis (*Staphylococcus aureus* and gram-negative organisms)
d. Lung transplant recipients:
   i.   Lower respiratory tract infections (pneumonia: *Staphylococcus aureus* or *Pseudomonas*)[45]

F. Types of infections: fungal:
   1. PCP:
      a. Caused by fungus: *Pneumocystis jirovecii*
      b. Typically occurs after the first month following transplantation; however, use of trimethoprim-sulfamethoxazole (Bactrim; Cotrim) prophylaxis has essentially eliminated this problem.
   2. If diseases, including cryptococcosis, coccidioidomycosis, or histoplasmosis are identified pretransplant, a minimum of 4 months of antifungal therapy is recommended with antifungal agents such as fluconazole (Diflucan).

G. Types of infections: parasitic:
   1. Toxoplasmosis is caused by *Toxoplasma gondii*—a parasitic protozoan.
   2. Toxoplasmosis is rare. Trimethoprim-sulfamethoxazole (Bactrim) is used to prevent reactivation of toxoplasmosis.

H. Community-acquired infections:
   1. Community-acquired infections can be more severe in young children, especially if they occur soon after transplantation and during highly immunosuppressed periods.
   2. Types:
      a. Parainfluenza
      b. Influenza
      c. Respiratory syncytial virus[45]

IX. INFECTIONS IN PEDIATRIC POPULATIONS: GENERAL PRINCIPLES

A. Solid organ recipients are at risk for common childhood illnesses.

B. Evaluation of fever should include a thorough history and physical examination.

C. If no source of fever is immediately identified, a septic workup is required, including
   1. CBC with differential
   2. Blood and urine cultures
   3. Complete metabolic panel
   4. Assessment for latent viruses (CMV, EBV)

D. Acetaminophen is recommended for temperature elevations as nonsteroidal anti-inflammatory medications may impair compromised hepatic/renal function.[51]

E. The "common cold" and gastroenteritis occur frequently in the fall and winter months.
   1. If pneumonia is suspected, a chest radiograph should be obtained.

2. Symptoms of a cough, cold, and GI illness are likely to last longer in transplant recipients than in well children.
3. Patients should avoid the use of over-the-counter cold medications, unless they are approved for use by the transplant team.
4. Supportive care to prevent dehydration and keep secretions thin is important.
   a. If the child is unable to orally hydrate, IV fluids should be given to prevent abnormally elevated calcineurin levels in the setting of dehydration.
5. Lung transplant recipients who present with a cough should be referred to the transplant center for evaluation of potential bronchiolitis obliterans.

F. Influenza:
1. An acute illness characterized by
   a. Coryza (rhinitis)
   b. Cough
   c. Fever
   d. Pharyngitis
   e. Headache
   f. Myalgia
   g. Malaise
2. Transplant recipients may experience more complications related to influenza than the general population.
   a. The immunologic response may result in acute allograft rejection.
   b. Recipients are candidates for early antiviral therapy with oseltamivir (Tamiflu).[51]
3. Prevention of influenza:
   a. Enhanced by encouraging immunization of all household contacts and health care providers on transplant units with the inactivated influenza vaccine.
      i. Further study is needed to determine if organ transplant recipients can mount a protective immune response to the live attenuated influenza vaccine.
   b. Antiviral medications (oseltamivir [Tamiflu]), in addition to vaccines, may be required to prevent or treat influenza.
      i. Recommend injectable inactivated influenza vaccine.
      ii. Nasal spray is contraindicated in transplant recipients.
   c. Infected transplant patients require isolation or should be cohorted to prevent the transmission of virus.
   d. Bronchiolitis obliterans has been reported as a long-term complication of influenza in lung transplant recipients.[51]

G. Live virus vaccines are contraindicated after transplantation.[52]
1. Live vaccines are generally not administered after transplantation.
   a. Recipients should avoid the live oral polio, MMR, varicella, and intranasal influenza vaccine.
2. Timing of vaccine administration is variable.
   a. Most centers restart vaccination at 3 to 6 months post transplant when baseline immunosuppression is reached.[52]
3. See Table 17-5 for a summary of recommendations for immunizations post transplant.

H. Antibiotics:
1. Care should be taken when prescribing antibiotics.

TABLE 17-5 **Vaccinations Posttransplant**

Vaccine	Kidney	Liver	Heart-Lung
Polio (inactivated)	Y	Y	Y
Pertussis	Y	Y	Y
Diphtheria	Y	Y	Y
Tetanus	Y	Y	Y
Meningitis (adolescents or splenectomized patients)	Y	Y	Y
Haemophilus influenzae type B	Y	Y	N
Measles, mumps, rubella	N	N	N
Hepatitis A	N	Y	Y
Hepatitis B	Y	Y	Y
Human papillomavirus (HPV)	Y	Y	Y
Bacillus Calmette-Guérin (BCG)	N	N	N
Pneumococcal (2–23 mo)	N	Y	Y
Annual influenza (inactivated)	Y	Y	Y
Varicella	N	N	N

For additional information, see Danziger-Isakov L, Kumar D; AST Infectious Diseases Community of Practice. Vaccination in solid organ transplantation. *Am J Transplant*. 2013;13:311–317.

2. Macrolide antibiotics (erythromycin, clarithromycin [Biaxin], and azithromycin [Zithromax]) are avoided because they
   a. Interact with calcineurin inhibitors and can raise serum blood levels of tacrolimus (Prograf) and cyclosporine (Neoral, Gengraf)
   b. Elevated blood levels of tacrolimus and cyclosporine can result in renal insufficiency and electrolyte imbalance. Please see chapter on Transplant Pharmacology for more detail regarding immunosuppression medication.
3. Indiscriminate use of antibiotics in the transplant recipient increases the risk of developing a secondary fungal infection.

I. Herbal supplements and over-the-counter medications:
   1. Avoid the use of herbal supplements and over-the-counter medications because of potential interactions with immunosuppressant medications.[51]

 X. LONG-TERM COMPLICATIONS

A. Endocrine and bone issues post transplant
   1. Bone disease in transplant recipients is the sum of preexisting bone disease before transplant and posttransplant bone loss due to the effects of immunosuppressive medications.
   2. Transplant recipients are at increased risk for bone loss compared to the general population.[53]

3. Transplant recipients with bone disease are also at risk for
   a. Slipped femoral epiphysis
   b. Rickets
   c. Valgus and vargus deformities of the knee
   d. Avascular necrosis of the femoral head, talus, and humerus
   e. Poor growth
4. Exposure to diuretics which affects calcium reabsorption.
5. Immobilization secondary to disease severity, which impacts on osseous complications.[53]

B. Growth following transplant
   1. The child's height at the time of transplant is certainly an important consideration, with more severe growth retardation at transplant leading to the need for greater catch-up growth following transplant.
      a. A normal target height at transplant has the potential to result in normal final adult height.
   2. Factors that impact growth:
      a. Age at transplant: younger recipients tend to have more growth retardation at transplant; therefore, these patients may exhibit greater catch-up growth.
      b. Graft dysfunction: the number of acute rejection episodes, number and length of hospitalizations, and retransplantation all have adverse effects on growth.
      c. Renal dysfunction, whether in renal allograft recipients or in recipients of other solid organ transplants:
         i. In renal allograft recipients, primary renal dysfunction has been associated with an adverse effect on growth.
         ii. In recipients of other types of allografts, renal dysfunction may be secondary to drug toxicity (due to calcineurin inhibitors, antibiotics, and antivirals).
      d. Corticosteroid therapy:
         i. Steroid use can affect growth; thus, minimizing steroid exposure is idea. Steroid-free regimens are optimal, with steroid withdrawal being a secondary option.
      e. Abnormal growth hormone, gonadotropin, and sex hormone secretion have been noted following transplantation.[54]
      f. In the posttransplant period, careful monitoring of growth and development is helpful by obtaining hand films for bone age.
   3. Prevention of bone loss:
      a. Therapies that may prevent bone loss related to steroids include
         i. Combined calcium and vitamin D (400 IU ergocalciferol and 500 to 1,000 mg calcium) in low daily doses
         ii. Age-appropriate physical activity
      b. Periodic measurement of serum 25-hydroxyvitamin D, 1,25-dihydroxyvitamin D, and parathyroid hormone (PTH) may be helpful in monitoring for renal insufficiency in solid organ recipients. Supplementation can be initiated when indicated to aid in bone growth.
      c. Administration of growth hormone may be appropriate in some patients.[54]

 XI. LIVING WITH A SOLID ORGAN TRANSPLANT

A. Psychosocial adjustment
   1. Posttransplant challenges for the child can include poor academic performance, low self-esteem, depression, and anxiety.

2. Wray and Radley-Smith[55] reported on the incidence of depression and depressive symptoms in children before and 1 year after heart and heart-lung transplantation.
   a. Children reported more depressive symptoms than their parents reported for them.
   b. One proposed explanation was the change in physical appearance related to immunosuppressive agents that contribute to lower self-esteem and poor body image.

B. Psychological distress
1. Increased psychological distress can lead to behavior problems and anxiety.
2. Early identification of children and families at risk and referral to a psychologist or psychiatrist may help with adjustment in the posttransplant period.[56]

C. Quality of life (QOL)
1. Several studies have examined posttransplant QOL among pediatric recipients:
   a. Pediatric liver transplant recipients: QOL improves following transplantation but, overall, is lower than that of healthy children.[57,58]
   b. Pediatric kidney transplant recipients: QOL reportedly increased or improved following pediatric kidney transplant in comparison to children on dialysis and those diagnosed with other chronic kidney diseases.[59]

D. Return to school
1. Encourage children to return to school approximately 3 months after transplantation.
2. Partnerships should be developed with the school to promote successful return of students.

E. Neurocognitive delays
1. A large longitudinal multicenter study of pediatric liver transplant recipients reported that cognitive delay could be identified as early as 5 to 7 years of age for children who received a transplant when they were younger than 5 years of age.[60]

F. High-risk behaviors
1. The interdisciplinary transplant team should discuss risk-taking behaviors with transplant recipients, including alcohol and tobacco use as well as sexual activity.
2. Poor decisions made by teens regarding sexual behavior and drug and alcohol use can have serious consequences.[61]

G. Nonadherence
1. While a transplant can dramatically improve a young person's QOL, it is not without its own set of challenges.
2. Adherence to the medication regimen should be discussed at each clinic appointment.
   a. The developmental stage of each child should be considered when discussing adherence to the medication regimen.
   b. Adolescents are at increased risk of medication nonadherence due to their developmental stage and their desire to be independent despite inexperience.[61]

      c. Nonadherence with immunosuppressive therapy is problematic and places patients at higher risk for acute and chronic rejection.[62–65]

        i. Nonadherence to the medication regimen places patients at higher risk for acute and chronic rejection.[66,67]

        ii. Nonadherent patients may present with symptoms of end-stage disease representative of organ transplanted:

- Jaundice (liver)
- Elevated creatinine (kidney)
- Decreased pulmonary function studies (lung)
- Arrhythmias, poor functional capacity (heart)

      d. Assessing medication adherence:

        i. Clinicians must be vigilant in assessing children for risk factors. O'Grady[68] reported barriers to medication adherence:

- Side effects and drug regimen complexity
- Lack of support from the medical team
- Lack of patient education
- Mixed messages from the medical team

H. Transition from pediatric to adult care

1. Transition from pediatric to adult care is considered a vulnerable time period as patients transfer their medical care to the adult transplant program.
2. Pediatric and adult transplant coordinators play a critical role in the transition process.

    a. Individual patient education and communication between the adult and pediatric transplant nurse coordinator have been identified as ways to improve the transition process.[61,69]

    b. Recent consensus statements provide further insight to addressing the needs of patients, families, and providers during this vulnerable transition time period including addressing needs of both the patient and the parents.[70,71]

XII. CONCLUSION

A. Pediatric solid organ transplant is a viable option for infants, children, and adolescents with end-stage organ disease.

B. Surgical advances and improving immunosuppressant agents and regimens have increased the number of long-term survivors.

C. Addressing the acute and chronic care needs of the children and their families requires a coordinated effort among all interdisciplinary transplant professionals.

D. Nurses play a pivotal role in providing continuity of care for the patient and family from initial diagnosis through the transplant procedure to living with transplantation.

REFERENCES

1. Fine RN, Webber SA, Olthoff KM, et al. *Pediatric Solid Organ Transplantation.* 2nd ed. Malden, MA: Blackwell Publishing; 2007.
2. Tong A, Chapman JR, Israni A, et al. Qualitative research in organ transplantation: recent contributions to clinical care and policy. *Am J Transplant.* 2013;13:1390–1399.
3. United Network for Organ Sharing. 2016. Available at http://www.unos.org
4. Bartosh SM. Recipient characteristics. In: Fine RN, Webber SA, Olthoff KM, et al., eds. *Pediatric Solid Organ Transplantation.* 2nd ed. Malden, MA: Blackwell Publishing; 2007.
5. Patel UD, Thomas SE. Evaluation of the candidate. In: Fine RN, et al., eds. *Pediatric Solid Organ Transplantation.* 2nd ed. Malden, MA: Blackwell Publishing; 2007:153–160.
6. Solez K, Colvin RB, Racusen LC, et al. Banff 07 classification of renal allograft pathology: updates and future directions. *Am J Transplant.* 2008;8:753–760.
7. Tsai EW, Ettenger RB. Kidney transplantation in children. In: Danovitch GM, ed. *Handbook of Kidney Transplantation.* 5th ed. Philadelphia, PA: Lippincott Williams & Wilkins; 2010.
8. Organ Procurement and Transplantation Network. *Kidney Patient and Graft Survival Rates for Transplants Performed: 1997–2004.* 2014. Available at optn.transplant.hrsa/gov
9. Transplant UK. Survival Rates Following Transplantation. Available at http://www.organdonation.nhs.uk/statistics/transplant_activity_repot/current_activity_reports/ukt/survival_rates.pdf
10. Squires RH, Ng V, Romero R, et al. Evaluation of the pediatric patient for liver transplantation: 2014 practice guideline by the American association for the study of liver diseases, American society of transplantation and the North American society for pediatric gastroenterology, hepatology and nutrition. *Hepatology.* 2014;60(1):362–387.
11. Kamath BM, Rand EB. Evaluation of the candidate: liver transplantation. In: Fine RN, Webber SA, Olthoff KM, et al., eds. *Pediatric Solid Organ Transplantation.* 2nd ed. Malden, MA: Blackwell Publishing; 2007.
12. United Network for Organ Sharing. *Talking About Transplantation: Questions and Answers for Transplant Candidates About Liver Allocation Policy.* Richmond, VA: Sharing UNfO; 2013.
13. Organ Procurement and Transplantation Network. Policies. In: Organ Procurement and Transplantation Network, ed. Available at: http://optn.transplant.hrsa.gov/governance/policies; 2015.
14. Sultan MI, Leon CD, Biank VF. Role of nutrition on pediatric chronic liver disease. *Nutr Clin Pract.* 2011;26:401–408.
15. Suchy FJ, Sokol RJ, Balistreri WF. *Liver Diseases in Children.* 4th ed. New York, NY: Cambridge University Press; 2014.
16. Bailey LL. The evolution of infant heart transplant. *J Heart Lung Transplant.* 2009;28(12):1241–1245.
17. Dipchand A, Kirk R, Edwards LB, et al. The registry of the international society for heart and lung transplantation: sixteenth official pediatric heart transplantation report-2013: focus theme: age. *J Heart Lung Transplant.* 2013;32(10):979–988.
18. Feng S, Ekong UD, Lobrito SJ, et al. Complete immunosuppression withdrawal and subsequent allograft function among pediatric recipients of parental living donor liver transplants. *JAMA.* 2012;307(3):283–293.
19. Zarrinpar A, Bucuttil RW. Liver transplantation: past, present and future. *Nat Rev Gastroenterol Hepatol.* 2013;10:434–440.
20. Zangwill S, Ellis T, Stendahl G, et al. Practical application of the virtual crossmatch. *Pediatr Transplant.* 2007;11(6):650–654.
21. Zangwill S, Ellis T, Zlotocha J, et al. The virtual crossmatch—a screening tool for sensitized heart transplant recipients. *Pediatr Heart Transplant.* 2006;10(1):38–41.
22. Castleberry C, Ryan RD, Chin C. Transplantation in the highly sensitized pediatric patient. *Circulation.* 2014;129:2313–2319.
23. Berry GJ, Angelini A, Burke M, et al. The ISHLT working formulation for pathologic diagnosis of antibody mediated rejection in heart transplantation: evolution and current status 2005–2011. *J Heart Lung Transplant.* 2011;30(6):601–611.
24. Kitteson MM, Kobashigawa J. Long term care of the heart transplant recipient. *Curr Opin Organ Transplant.* 2014;19(5):515–524.
25. Pigula FA, Webber SA. Donor evaluation, surgical technique and perioperative management. In: Fine RN, Webber SA, Olthoff KM, et al., eds. *Pediatric Solid Organ Transplantation.* 2nd ed. Malden, MA: Blackwell Publishing; 2007.
26. Camarda J, Saudek D, Tweddel J, et al. MRI validated echocardiographic technique to measure total cardiac volume: a tool for donor recipient size matching in pediatric heart transplantation. *Pediatr Transplant.* 2013;17(3):300–306.
27. United Network for Organ Sharing. Allocation of Hearts and Heart-Lungs. In: Organ Procurement and Transplantation Network, ed. 6.1.D. OPTN; April 14, 2016. Avaliable at https://optn.transplant.hrsa.gov/governance/policies/

28. United Network for Organ Sharing. Allocation of Hearts and Heart-Lungs. In: Organ Procurement and Transplantation Network, ed. *6.1.F.* OPTN; April 14, 2016. Avaliable at https://optn.transplant.hrsa.gov/governance/policies/

29. Boyle GJ. Evaluation of the candidate: heart transplantation. In: Fine RN, Webber SA, Olthoff KM, et al., eds. *Pediatric Solid Organ Transplantation.* 2nd ed. Malden, MA: Blackwell Publishing; 2007.

30. Miyamoto SD, Pietra BA. Post-transplant management: cardiac transplantation. In: Fine RN, Webber SA, Olthoff KM, et al., eds. *Pediatric Solid Organ Transplantation.* 2nd ed. Malden, MA: Blackwell Publishing; 2007.

31. Kohen B, Raflei M, Yu Z, et al. Characteristics of primary graft dysfunction. *Experimental Clin Cardiol.* 2014;20(1):2890–2896.

32. Stendahl G, Bobay K, Berger S, et al. Organizational structure and processes in pediatric heart transplantation: a survey of practices in pediatric transplantation. *Pediatr Transplant.* 2012;16(3):257–264.

33. Mehra M, Crespo-Leiro MG, Dipchand A, et al. International Society for Heart and Lung Transplantation working formulation of a standardized nomenclature for cardiac allograft vasculopathy. *J Heart Lung Transplant.* 2010;29(7):717–727.

34. Hidestrand M, Tomita-itchell A, Hidestrand PM, et al. Highly sensitive noninvasive cardiac transplant rejection monitoring using targeted quantification of donor specific cell free deoxyribonucleic acid. *J Am Coll Cardiol.* 2014;63(12):1224–1226.

35. Benden C, Edwards LB, Kucheryavaya AY, et al. The registry of the International Society for Heart and Lung Transplantation: sixteenth official pediatric lung and heart-lung transplantation report –2013: focus theme: age. *J Heart Lung Transplant.* 2013;32(10):989–997.

36. Parizhskaya M. Pathology of the cardiac allograft. In: Fine RN, Webber SA, Olthoff KM, et al., eds. *Pediatric Solid Organ Transplantation.* 2nd ed. Malden, MA: Blackwell Publishing; 2007.

37. Stewart S, Winters G, Fishbein M, et al. Revision of the 1990 working formulation for the standardization of nomenclature in the diagnosis of heart transplantation. *J Heart Lung Transplant.* 2005;24(11):1710–1720.

38. Kobashigawa J, Crespo-Leiro MG, Ensminger SM, et al. Report from a consensus conference on antibody-mediated rejection in heart transplantation. *J Heart Lung Transplant.* 2011;30(3):252–269.

39. Neibler RA, Ghanayem N, Bobke A, et al. Use of the HeartWare ventricular assist device in a patient with failed fontan circulation. *Ann Thorac Surg.* 2014;97(4):E115–E116.

40. West LJ. ABO incompatible hearts for infant transplantation. *Curr Opin Organ Transplant.* 2011;16(5):548–554.

41. Faro A, Sweet SC. Textbook of organ transplantation. In: Kirk A, Knechtle SJ, Larsen CP, et al., eds. *Textbook of Organ Transplantation.* Hoboken, NJ: Jon Wiley and Sons; 2014:1420–1430.

42. HIrche TO, Knoop C, Kebestreit H, et al. Practical guidelines: lung transplantation in patients with cystic fibrosis. *J Pulm Med.* 2014;22.

43. Deuse T, Sill B, von Samson P, et al. Surgical technique of lower lobe lung transplantation. *Ann Thorac Surg.* 2011;92(2):e39–e42.

44. Woo MS. Post-transplant management: lung transplantation. In: Fine RN, Webber SA, Olthoff KM, et al., eds. *Pediatric Solid Organ Transplantation.* 2nd ed. Malden, MA: Blackwell Publishing; 2007.

45. Green M, Michaels MG. Infections in solid organ transplant recipients. In: Long S, ed. *Principles and Practice of Pediatric Infectious Diseases: Expert Consult.* 4th ed. Philadelphia, PA: Elsevier Inc.; 2012.

46. Hayes D. A review of bronchiolitis obliterans syndrome and therapeutic strategies. *J Cardiothorac Surg.* 2011;6(1):92.

47. Krisl JC, Alloway RR, Woodle S. Off label use of immunosuppressive agents in solid organ transplant. In: Kirk A, Knechtle SJ, Larsen CP, et al., eds. *Textbook of Organ Transplantation.* Hoboken, NJ: John Wiley and Sons; 2014:1236–1242.

48. Harmon WE. Induction and maintenance immunosuppression. In: Fine RN, Webber SA, Olthoff KM, et al., eds. *Pediatric Solid Organ Transplantation.* 2nd ed. Malden, MA: Blackwell Publishing; 2007.

49. Kotton CM, Kumar D, Caliendo AM, et al. Updated international consensus guidelines on the management of cytomegalovirus in solid organ transplantation. *Transplantation.* 2013;96(4):333–359.

50. Green M, Michaels MG. Epstein-Barr virus infection and posttransplant lymphoproliferative disease. *Am J Transplant.* 2013;13:41–54.

51. Green M, Michaels MG. Infections post transplant. In: Fine RN, Webber SA, Olthoff KM, et al., eds. *Pediatric Solid Organ Transplantation.* 2nd ed. Malden, MA: Blackwell Publishing; 2007.

52. Danziger-Isakov L, Kumar D; AST Infectious Diseases Community of Practice. Special article: vaccination of solid organ transplantation. *Am J Transplant.* 2013;13:311–317.

53. Chauhan V, Ranganna KM, Chauhan N, et al. Bone disease in organ transplant patients: pathogenesis and management. *Postgrad Med.* 2012;124(3):80–90.

54. Fine RN. Growth following solid organ transplantation in childhood. *Clinics.* 2014;69(S1):3–7.

55. Wray J, Radley SR. Depression in pediatric patients before and 1 year after heart or heart-lung transplantation. *J Heart Lung Transplant.* 2004;23(9):1103–1110.

56. Shemesh E. Psychosocial adaptation and adherence. In: Fine RN, Webber SA, Olthoff KM, et al., eds. *Pediatric Solid Organ Transplantation.* 2nd ed. Malden, MA: Blackwell Publishing; 2007:418–424.

57. Alonso EA, Neighbors K, Barton FB. Health related quality of life and family function following pediatric liver transplantation. *Liver Transpl.* 2008;14(4):460–468.
58. Limbers CA, Neighbors K, Martz K, et al. Health related quality of life in pediatric liver transplant recipients compared with other chronic disease groups. *Pediatr Transplant.* 2011;15(3):245–253.
59. Kul M, Cengel KE, Senses DG, et al. Quality of life in children and adolescents with chronic kidney disease: a comparative study between different disease stages and treatment modalities. *Turkish J Pediatr.* 2013;55(5):493–499.
60. Sorenson LG, Neighbors K, Martz K, et al. Cognitive and academic outcomes after pediatric liver transplantation: functional outcomes group (FOG). *Am J Transplant.* 2011;11:303–311.
61. Lerret SM, Stendahl G. Working together as a team: adolescent transplant recipients and nurse practitioners. *Prog Transplant.* 2011;21(4):288–298.
62. Dobbels F, Decorte A, Roskams A, et al. Health related quality of life, treatment adherence, symptom experience and depression in adolescent renal transplant patients. *Pediatr Transplant.* 2010;14(2):216–223.
63. Dobbels R, Ruppar T, DeGeest S, et al. Adherence to the immunosuppressive regimen in pediatric kidney transplant recipients: a systematic review. *Pediatr Transplant.* 2010;14(5):606–616.
64. Connelly J, Pilch N, Oliver M, et al. Prediction of medication non-adherence and associated outcomes in pediatric kidney transplant recipients. *Pediatr Transplant.* 2015;19:555–562.
65. Oliva M, Singh RP, Gauvreau K, et al. Impact of medication non-adherence on survival after pediatric heart transplantation in the USA. *J Heart Lung Transplant.* 2013;32(9):881–888.
66. Butler JA, Roderick P, Mullee M, et al. Frequency and impact of nonadherence to immunosuppressants after renal transplantation: a systematic review. *Transplantation.* 2004;77:769–776.
67. Fredericks EM, Lopez MJ, Magee JC, et al. Psychological functioning, nonadherence and health outcomes after pediatric liver transplantation. *Am J Transplant.* 2007;7:1974–1983.
68. O'Grady JGM, Asderakis A, Bradley R, et al. Multidisciplinary insights into optimizing adherence after solid organ transplantation. *Transplantation.* 2010;89(5):627–6632.
69. Lerret SM, Menendez J, Weckwerth J, et al. Essential components of transition to adult transplant services: the transplant coordinators' perspective. *Prog Transplant.* 2012;22(3):252–258.
70. Bell LE, Bartosh SM, Davis CL, et al. Adolescent transition to adult care in solid organ transplantation: a consensus conference report. *Am J Transplant.* 2008;8:2230–2242.
71. Webb N, Harden P, Lewis C, et al. Building consensus on transition of transplant patients from paediatric to adult healthcare. *Arch Dis Child.* 2010;95(8):606–611.

SELF-ASSESSMENT QUESTIONS

1. Signs of rejection following pediatric kidney transplantation may include which of the following symptoms?
   a. Increased heart rate, jaundice, and shortness of breath
   b. Hypertension, pain over graft site, and hematuria
   c. Proteinuria and increase in weight
   d. b and c
   e. All of the above

2. You are assigned to care for a 12-year-old recipient of a renal transplant that took place 8 days ago. In evaluating your patient's laboratory work results, you note that the serum creatinine today is 3.4 but was recorded as 1.8, 2.0, and 2.1 on previous days. Which of the following tests would be most important today to evaluate for rejection?
   a. Urine for electrolytes
   b. Renal ultrasound
   c. Spiral CT scan
   d. Renal biopsy
   e. Urine culture for BK viral inclusion cells

3. You are assigned to a 4-year-old female heart transplant recipient. Her transplant was performed 4 days ago, and she has been quite unstable with variable vital signs, fever, and alterations in hemodynamics. In your initial assessment of the child, you find her cardiac output to be 2.4 and central venous pressure to be 14. She is slightly febrile with a temperature of 38.1°C at 8 AM. Her heart rate is 124 and blood pressure is 88/60. You report your findings to the intensivist and deduce from your knowledge of transplantation that this child may have which of the following problems?
   a. Hyperacute rejection
   b. Chronic rejection
   c. Acute rejection
   d. Bacterial endocarditis

4. In evaluating a heart transplant recipient for rejection, the most accurate way to determine rejection is:
   a. an elevation in the amplitude of the EKG tracing.
   b. an endomyocardial biopsy.
   c. an echocardiogram to assess left and right ventricular ejection fractions.
   d. a MUGA scan to assess left ventricular ejection fraction.

5. Your assignment today includes a 6-year-old child who had a liver transplant 3 days ago. She has been reported to be responsive to verbal commands. On your morning assessment, the child is somnolent and difficult to arouse. You check her bilirubin and note a rise from yesterday's findings. Her transaminase is also three times greater than yesterday. She is febrile. You know that these signs are most likely indicative of:
   a. hyperacute liver rejection.
   b. portal vein thrombosis.
   c. hepatic artery thrombosis.
   d. posttransplant sepsis.

6. A liver biopsy has been ordered on a 2-year-old recipient of a living liver transplant from her mother. In preparing the child for a liver biopsy, which of the following tests would be most important?
   a. Liver enzymes
   b. PT/PTT
   c. Hemoglobin level
   d. Protein S

7. In the immediate postoperative care of a child with a lung transplant, you know that suctioning is important because:
   a. lungs are denervated after transplantation.
   b. lung recipients lack a cough reflex below the site of anastomosis.
   c. secretions can lead to a severe pulmonary infection.
   d. b and c.
   e. All of the above.

8. Following lung transplantation, an inflammatory process of the small airways that results in narrowing and scarring of the bronchioles is called:
   a. hyperacute rejection.
   b. acute rejection.
   c. bronchiolitis obliterans or obliterative bronchitis.
   d. cellular rejection of the alveoli.

9. Infections are a major cause of morbidity and mortality in transplant recipients. Factors associated with the development of infections in the immediate postoperative period include which of the following?
   a. Neutropenia secondary to immunosuppression
   b. Invasive monitoring
   c. Malnutrition
   d. b and c
   e. All of the above

10. Posttransplant lymphoproliferative disorder (PTLD) is most commonly diagnosed in children following thoracic transplants. Risk factors for the development of PTLD include which of the following?
    a. Young age at the time of transplantation.
    b. Higher doses of immunosuppression.
    c. Recipient is EBV negative at the time of transplant.
    d. b and c.
    e. All of the above.

Correct Answers:
1.d   2.d   3.c   4.b   5.c   6.b   7.e   8.c   9.e   10.e

CHAPTER 18

Psychosocial Issues in Transplantation

Kay Kendall, MSW, LISW-S, ACSW, CCTSW

Kim Ansley, MSW, LSW

Melissa Skillman, MSW, LISW-S

I. INTRODUCTION

A. Psychosocial assessments have been an integral component of evaluations of patients for solid organ transplantation since the inception of these programs over 30 years ago.

   1. Despite evolution of the medical and psychosocial criteria for listing patients for transplant, no universal criteria have been adopted across programs and substantial variability remains, especially with respect to psychosocial contraindications to transplant.

   2. Research has identified factors that predict survival and quality of life posttransplant.

     a. These findings can help to determine which patients would benefit most from this scarce resource.

     b. Transplant programs do not consistently apply existing knowledge in making decisions regarding individual candidates.

     c. Programs are challenged with the need to balance this knowledge with ethical considerations and a desire to serve patients in immediate need.

   3. Evaluation of patients' psychosocial status is part of this decision-making process and is critical in caring for patients and families pre- and posttransplant.

   4. This chapter includes a review of the literature pertaining to

     a. Psychosocial contraindications to listing

     b. Predictors of patient outcomes

     c. Difficulties patients and families face before and after transplant

     d. Strategies that are useful in promoting better medical management and patient/family coping.

II. PSYCHOSOCIAL EVALUATION

A. US Requirements

   1. Transplant centers in the United States require that patients undergoing transplant evaluations complete psychosocial assessments with qualified social workers.

2. In some circumstances, other mental health professionals, such as psychologists or psychiatrists, may be consulted.[1]
3. In the United States, an assessment with a social worker is required by Medicare and state Medicaid programs.
4. Private insurance companies may also request information from such an assessment before they will approve coverage for transplantation.

B. Purpose
   1. Pretransplant psychosocial evaluation:
      a. Is conducted primarily to provide the team with information to assist them in distinguishing those patients likely to benefit from transplantation from those whose risk levels may be too high.[2-7]
      b. Alerts the interdisciplinary transplant team to patients who may likely experience individual or family problems during the course of the transplant process.
      c. Reveals need for interventions by other members of the transplant team as they work to prepare the individual for listing, eventual surgery, and reintegration into society.[6]
      d. Provides an opportunity for educating and counseling patients and their support systems about the transplant process.
      e. Helps to ensure that candidate selection is appropriate, that patients are fully prepared for transplantation, and that the team is addressing the patient's psychosocial needs.[3]
      f. This initial assessment between the social worker and patients and their support system serves to establish what may be an ongoing relationship.
         i. The detailed information gathered in this assessment is helpful as these patients may be followed for many years by the same clinician and transplant team members.
   2. Posttransplant psychosocial evaluations
      a. Attention is paid to specific presenting concerns, appropriate treatments, and interventions.
      b. The assessment:
         i. Usually focuses on a specific area of patient need that may be
            • Disclosed or initiated by the patient
            • Identified during a hospital admission or an outpatient clinic visit
         ii. Tends to focus on the patient's adjustment to transplantation or needs during a particular phase of care
         iii. Evaluates the patient's overall functioning and perceived quality of life, which are viewed as primary indicators of a successful transplantation[1]

C. Format
   1. Pretransplant psychosocial evaluation
      a. Although the timing, format, manner of obtaining information and its use vary among programs and across centers, the content of the assessment is fairly uniform.[2-7]
      b. Generally takes the form of a structured assessment.
         i. The assessment follows an outline specific to the requirements and preferences of the particular assessor and program.
      c. The assessment occurs in tandem with the medical workup.

  d. The social worker typically meets with the patient for 90 minutes to 2 hours.
   i. Some programs may require that a support person be present for all or part of the session.[7]
  e. Professional interpreters are recommended for interviews with patients not proficient in English, as patient responses may not be accurately conveyed by members of the patient's support system.
  f. Transplant programs may require that transplant patients sign a separate psychosocial consent form acknowledging their understanding that the psychosocial assessment will be part of the deciding factors regarding their potential transplant candidacy.
  g. The assessment is documented in a structured format.
   i. Findings are shared with the team via the written report and during the team "selection" meeting.
   ii. A copy of the evaluation is placed in the patient's medical record.
 2. Posttransplant psychosocial evaluations
  a. May not include all areas addressed in the pretransplant evaluation.
  b. Documentation placed in patient's medical record.
  c. Findings are discussed with the team; intervention is instituted; and outcomes are recorded as previously described.

D. Process
 1. Because information must be understandable to patients and presented at an appropriate level of complexity, the patient's and his/her support system's level of attained education and language proficiency must be ascertained.
 2. Patient education information is often too difficult for patients to understand. It is estimated that more than one third of individuals don't have the knowledge to make medical decisions. This can lead to missed appointments, delayed recovery, and frequent emergency department visits.[8]
 3. It is imperative to determine health literacy of the patient and his/her support system and assess how well the information that has been provided is understood. Lack of understanding can significantly compromise a patient's ability to give informed consent for the transplant procedure itself as well as make sound self-care decisions following transplantation.
  a. Health literacy
   i. Health literacy is the degree to which individuals have the capacity to obtain, process, and understand basic health information and services needed to make appropriate health decisions.[8]
   ii. It involves more than simply asking patients and members of their support systems if they can read and write. How well patients read does not determine how well they understand what they are told about health care.
   iii. Factors that affect health literacy include
    • Age
    • Education
    • Language
    • Culture
    • Access to resources
    • Experience with the health care system
    • Emotional responses

iv. Measures to assess health literacy include the following:
- Short Assessment of Health Literacy (SAHL–S and E)[9]
- Rapid Estimate of Adult Literacy in Medicine–Short Form (REALM-SF)[10]

v. Identifying how the patient learns can strengthen the care partnership between the patient and the interdisciplinary transplant team. Transplant programs can offer patient education in a number of different formats that are appropriate to the patient's level of health literacy.

b. Teach back
i. A common method in hospital settings to assess if a patient is comprehending information is the "teach back" method.
ii. This method asks patients to repeat and summarize the medical information and instructions they have received.

 III. COMPONENTS OF THE PRETRANSPLANT PSYCHOSOCIAL ASSESSMENT

A. The content of the evaluation is rooted in the literature.[1-7] Basic elements include assessment of the following:
1. Demographic data/identifying information
2. Family/relationship history
3. Support system
4. Financial resources
5. Advanced directives
6. History of adherence
7. Motivation for treatment
8. Mental health and psychiatric history
9. History of use of alcohol, substances, and nicotine products.

B. Demographic data/identifying information
1. Information on the patient's identity and background is obtained early in the assessment interview.
2. Full name, marital status, age, and gender are included as factual information.
3. Additional information:
a. Persons with whom the patient resides
b. If married, number of marriages
c. Number of children and their ages
d. Status of parents and siblings of patient
i. Alive or deceased
ii. If deceased, cause of death

C. Family/Relationship History
1. A family/relationship history gives a snapshot of the patient's family of origin, current family and living arrangements, friendships, and community and religious networks.
2. This history includes information regarding family members and friends who are positive factors in the patient's life, as well as persons with whom the patient has conflicts or from whom the patient receives little support.
3. Awareness of any difficult or unstable relationships is useful to the interdisciplinary transplant team, as these relationships could create concerns

for the patient or become barriers to medical care or patient adherence. Discussion with other care providers and nursing staff can yield helpful information.

4. Patients may discuss important past events, quality of relationships, and histories of abuse and losses, all of which are significant to the interdisciplinary transplant team in helping them understand patient concerns and stressors.

D. Assessment of support systems

1. Definition of social support: "the network of relationships that provide concrete, emotional and informational assistance to meet the perceived subjective or objective needs of the patient"[11(p. 262)]

2. This assessment includes the identification of

a. Sources of support

i. One important assessment goal is to identify specific individuals or organizations that will be able to offer emotional support and practical help such as in-home support and transportation.

b. Intended roles of support persons and organizations

i. Members of the patient's support system are educated during the pretransplant process regarding their roles.

ii. In the pre- and posttransplant period, support persons or organizations may be required to

- Provide transportation
- Obtain the patient's prescriptions
- Monitor the patient's adherence to the medical regimen with regard to medications, dietary restrictions, etc.
- Attend medical appointments with the patient to ensure understanding of information
- Help the patient with meal preparation, keeping track of medical appointments, etc.
- Provide ongoing emotional support to minimize psychological distress.

iii. Transplant centers may require members of the patient's support system to sign a document acknowledging the expectations of their role as a support person(s) during the pre- and posttransplant phases.

c. Potential gaps in the plan that could become barriers to pre- or posttransplant care.

i. Where there is insufficient support, the social worker helps the patient/support system to assess the available alternatives and recommends agencies to fill in the gaps when support is limited.

ii. Often, patients are educated on benefits of home health care, transportation assistance, support groups, and/or mentoring programs. The social worker counsels patients and their support system about these options and eligibility criteria as they prepare for surgery.

E. Assessment of financial resources

1. Questions regarding employment status, sources of income, and monthly income may reveal areas of potential financial concern.

2. Insurance coverage for medications, oxygen, hospital admissions, clinic visits, and other potential surgical and medical expenses must be determined and any additional financial needs clarified prior to listing.

      a. Patients are advised about procedures for obtaining these necessary resources.

      b. Additional expenses faced by patients may include costs associated with

          i. Relocation, travel, parking, and meals away from home

          ii. Loss of income for patient and family members

          iii. Care for dependent members of the family

3. Patients and their families need to be aware of the financial implications of the transplant process so they are able to plan appropriately.

4. Because transplantation necessitates a commitment to lifelong treatment, many transplant centers require patients to meet with a financial counselor for education on

      a. Potential costs of immunosuppressive medications

      b. Possible loss of funding resources posttransplant

      c. Insurance benefits

      d. Development of a financial plan prior to listing.

5. Social workers are able to advocate on their behalf with institutions and community agencies when requested to do so by patients.

F. Advanced Directives

1. During the evaluation process, patients are asked if they have completed a durable power of attorney for health care and a living will.

      a. If completed, a copy is requested so that it can be scanned into the patient's electronic medical record.

          i. It is essential to document the names and contact information for the next of kin and any designated substitute decision maker.

          ii. For patients with dependent children or dependent adults, plans for care of these children/adults should be discussed and families counseled regarding the needs of the children for emotional support, planning, and resources.

      b. If not completed, patients are asked if they would like to complete these documents. Patients are

          i. Educated on the importance of completing an advanced directive to identify a health care decision maker and the patient's end-of-life wishes.

          ii. Informed of the benefits of completing these documents, which can

             • Potentially avoid additional stress for their support system

             • Ensure that the patient's end-of-life wishes are followed.

          iii. Encouraged to discuss their preferences regarding life support and their decisions related to end-of-life care in the event of a poor transplant outcome and their inability to make their own health care choices.

G. Adherence history

1. Patients' past and current adherence to medical regimens and response to their current illness are assessed.[12]

2. Learning about patients' ability to care for themselves and follow medical recommendations is important in determining their ability to care for themselves posttransplant. This assessment includes

      a. Identifying any physical or cognitive deficits that may prevent the patient from being self-directed with his/her own care

          i. The social worker can help the patient and the patient's support system identify such barriers and potential ways of overcoming them through either education or resources.

      b. Asking who sets out the patient's medications helps the social worker determine if the patient is independent with this task or if the patient relies on a family member to do this.

         i. If the patient does not manage this task independently, it is important to explore why the patient relies on others. Is it because of illiteracy or does it reflect a dependence on a family member because of an established familial role?

      c. Assessing the patient's knowledge about and compliance with his/her medications. Does the patient

         i. Know the name, purpose, and dose of each of medication?

         ii. Consistently take medications at the prescribed dose and time?

         iii. Keep track of medications by using a pillbox?

      d. Determining how the patient keeps track of medical appointments (e.g., by using an electronic calendar, appointment book, etc.).

         i. This is an opportunity for the social worker to suggest and encourage patients to use tools that can help them manage their self-care.

      e. Additional important assessment questions include the following:

         i. Does the patient keep scheduled medical appointments?

         ii. Was there ever an extended time when the patient did not receive medical care and what were the reasons for that gap in care?

         iii. In the past, has the patient ever left the hospital against medical advice?

         iv. Does the patient alert his/her care provider of changes in condition? Or, does the patient rely on a family member or other support person to notify care providers of changes in the patient's condition?

         v. Is the patient compliant with other aspects of self-care such as daily weights, blood pressure monitoring, glucose testing, personal hygiene, etc.?

         vi. Does the patient have a history of multiple hospital admissions due to medical nonadherence?

         vii. Is the patient able to identify his/her medical diagnosis or the cause of his/her organ failure?

H. Motivation for transplantation and comprehension of illness and risks associated with transplantation

    1. This component of the psychosocial evaluation involves assessment of the following:

      a. The patient's motivation and readiness to proceed with the transplant process

         i. Some patients may

- Perceive that their current health status does not yet warrant transplantation
- Experience difficulty in resolving conflicting feelings, beliefs, or values, which may lead to ambivalence about transplantation
- Be responding to pressure from others or be extremely fearful

         ii. Ambivalence and/or lack of motivation require further assessment.

      b. The patient's understanding of transplant risks and possible complications

         i. Patients need to have realistic expectations of transplantation.

         ii. Transplant teams must make efforts to ensure that potential recipients fully understand the risks of transplantation.

- Transplant recipients need to be aware that the organ they receive may not function optimally or insure them a determined period of survival.

          iii. Surgical and medical risk factors should be discussed, as well as the possible side effects and complications associated with immunosuppressive medications.
     c. The patient's religious beliefs regarding such issues as
       i. Accepting blood products
       ii. Having a living donor versus a deceased donor
  2. A finding that a patient's expectations of transplantation are not realistic indicates the need for intervention and additional education.

I. Mental health and psychiatric history and current status
  1. In this component of the psychosocial evaluation, the social worker obtains information regarding the patient's
    a. Current or history of mental health symptoms
    b. Current or history of psychiatric diagnosis
    c. Current or history of suicidal ideation or attempts
    d. Current or history of homicidal attempts or ideation
    e. Current or history of mental health counseling and/or history of psychiatric hospitalization
    f. Current or history of use of psychotropic medications
  2. In addition, the social worker
    a. Determines if the patient is fully oriented, has appropriate insight, and displays sound judgment
    b. Identifies areas of concern requiring immediate or possible future intervention
  3. Mental health status also affects patients' abilities to understand the transplant process, appreciate their own responsibilities for self-care, and give informed consent.
  4. Cognitive status may be affected by such factors as preexisting conditions or the end-stage organ disease itself.
    a. Impaired cognitive function that interferes with the patient's daily functioning requires further assessment (such as a formal neuropsychological evaluation).
  5. Patients experiencing common somatic complaints as panic attacks, depression, or serious sleep disturbances will require further evaluation and possible psychiatric treatment to better prepare them to cope with the stressors associated with the transplant process.
  6. Those with serious psychological instability or dysfunction may be considered too high risk for transplantation.

J. Substance use history and current status
  1. A history is taken of the patient's past and current use of alcohol, tobacco, over-the-counter drugs, prescription medications, and illegal drugs.
  2. A history of or current substance use disorder may be a contraindication to transplantation in some programs, as it may have caused or contributed to the organ failure and it may become a source of potential damage to the transplanted organ.[2]
  3. Most lung and heart transplant programs require patients to be abstinent from smoking for a specified time prior to listing for transplant. Most commonly, this is a minimum of 6 months of documented abstinence.
  4. Transplant programs may defer listing patients with a diagnosis of alcohol dependence until they have ceased alcohol consumption for a prescribed time and completed a treatment program.[13]

K. The ultimate goal of the pretransplant psychosocial evaluation is to permit the interdisciplinary transplant team to enter into informed decision making regarding patient selection.

    a. Identification of potential patient vulnerabilities allows monitoring and/or intervention by the team throughout the complex and demanding transplant process.

    b. Identification of any gaps in the patient's plan enables the team to assist the patient in overcoming potential barriers to treatment.

 IV. ASSESSMENT INSTRUMENTS

A. When solid organ transplant programs began in the early 1980s, a variety of assessment methods were used to evaluate patients' psychosocial status.

    1. An assessment was completed by a social worker and a psychiatrist.[14]

    2. It was not unusual for patients to be evaluated by a psychologist or a neuropsychologist or to undergo an evaluation with a chemical dependency counselor.

B. As transplant teams gained more experience with the evaluation process, the assessment process was streamlined to avoid redundancies and other disciplines were consulted based on information obtained in the psychosocial evaluation.

C. Today, at most transplant centers in the United States, a master's level social worker at the highest level of licensure in his/her state of practice completes an initial assessment and then determines which other professionals need to be consulted to complete the evaluation process.

    1. All patients may not need a chemical dependency evaluation, nor do all patients require a battery of psychological/neuropsychological tests.

    2. Standardized assessments of psychosocial status are useful in evaluating some patients and in conducting research on quality of life and outcomes pre- and posttransplant.

D. Standardizing psychosocial evaluations—transplant-specific scales

    1. Psychosocial Assessment of Candidates for Transplantation (PACT) scale

        a. The seminal work in standardizing psychosocial evaluations was done by Olbrisch and Levenson who developed the Psychosocial Assessment of Candidates for Transplantation (PACT) scale in the late 1980s with the goal of standardizing psychosocial criteria.[15]

        b. This PACT scale:

            i. Was developed to identify psychosocial criteria and to assess how centers viewed the importance of these criteria in the selection process

            ii. Has also been used to measure pre- and posttransplant quality of life

            iii. Has been used by a number of centers to study the clinical decision-making process and to help with consistent interpretation of criteria[16]

        c. Characteristics of the PACT scale

            i. This tool consists of eight items with an initial rating and a final rating score. The eight items measure aspects of psychosocial functioning including support, lifestyle factors, compliance, psychological health, and substance abuse.

    ii.   The initial and final ratings are on a scale of 0 to 4 with a lower number indicating more problematic or concerning behavior.

- The information to rate candidates is obtained in the psychosocial evaluation.
- After the interview is complete, one general rating is made before considering each of the individual ratings. This is followed by a final rating.

    iii. The scale has been shown to have a high degree of interrater reliability.

2. Transplant Evaluation Rating Scale (TERS)[17]
   a. Developed in the early 1990s, the TERS is a standardized measure that rates the following psychosocial characteristics on a 3-point scale:
      i.   Prior psychiatric history DSM-III-R Axis I
      ii.   Prior psychiatric disorder DSM-III-R Axis II
      iii. Substance use/abuse
      iv. Compliance
      v.   Health behaviors
      vi. Quality of family/social support
      vii. Prior history of coping
      viii. Coping with disease and treatment
      ix. Quality of affect
      x.   Mental status (past and present)

3. Stanford Integrated Psychosocial Assessment for Transplantation (SIPAT)[18]
   a. This 18-item standardized scale is based on a comprehensive literature review of the psychosocial factors that influence transplant outcomes.
   b. The SIPAT is used to rate the following:
      i.   Patient's Readiness Level
      - Knowledge and understanding of medical illness process
      - Knowledge and understanding of the transplant process
      - Willingness/desire for transplantation
      - Treatment compliance/adherence
      - Lifestyle factors (e.g., diet, exercise)

      ii.   Social Support System Level of Readiness
      - Availability of social support system
      - Functionality of social support system
      - Appropriateness of physical living space and environment

      iii. Psychological Stability and Psychopathology
      - Presence of psychopathology
      - History of organic psychopathology or neurocognitive impairment
      - Influence of personality traits versus disorder
      - Effect of truthfulness versus deceptive behavior in presentation
      - Overall risk for psychopathology

      iv. Lifestyle and Effect of Substance Use
      - Alcohol use/abuse/dependence
      - Alcohol use/abuse/dependence: risk for recidivism
      - Substance use/abuse/dependence (including prescribed and illicit substances)
      - Substance use/abuse/dependence: risk for recidivism
      - Nicotine use/abuse/dependence

   c. The SIPAT is highly correlated with the PACT scale and is highly predictive of transplantation psychosocial outcomes.

E. Several other established instruments commonly used with the general population are frequently used to evaluate patients prior to transplant and to assess posttransplant outcomes.

1. The Beck Depression Inventory (BDI) is a self-rating instrument used widely in both medical and psychiatric settings.[19]
2. The Millon Behavioral Health Inventory (MBHI), a self-report instrument designed to assess psychological adjustment, has been used to predict posttransplant outcome.[20]
3. The Health Status Questionnaire (HSQ) is a measure of physical health and the impact of the patient's physical condition on social functioning, mental health, fatigue, and pain.[21]
4. The Psychosocial Adjustment to Illness Scale (PAIS) rates patients' orientation to health care, functioning at work and home, and sexual and social functioning.[22]
5. The Short Form 36 (SF-36) is a widely used instrument designed to evaluate health-related quality of life.[23]
    a. This self-administered assessment of health status measures several health-related domains, such as physical status, social functioning, pain, and role limitations due to physical problems.
6. Another commonly used psychiatric diagnostic measure is the Symptoms Checklist 90 (SCL-90), a self-report instrument that assesses multiple types of psychological distress.[24]

 V. PSYCHOSOCIAL CRITERIA FOR TRANSPLANTATION

A. Background

1. Psychosocial assessments have been a component of transplant evaluations since the inception of solid organ transplant programs.[25]
2. Initially, transplant team members were unclear how the information obtained from these assessments would be applied to the decision-making process and how the assessment findings could impact posttransplant survival.
3. Transplant teams felt that it was important to know about patients' support systems, how they coped and took care of themselves, and about past or present behaviors that might lead to medical management problems after transplant.
4. However, these assessments also raised ethical dilemmas such as
    a. Concerns that transplant programs were making judgments about individual worth
    b. Inconsistencies among programs[25]
    c. Variable views on contraindications to transplant
        i.   Variations in experiences in following patients after transplantation have led to differing perspectives on candidacy.
    d. Denying transplant on the basis of psychosocial concerns alone
        i.   Most transplant teams have been uncomfortable with denying a physiological need based on psychosocial concerns.
        ii. Clinical experience supports the need to consider some patients as being at high risk for complications or death following transplant, though few studies have formally researched the criteria used to make these judgments.
        iii. As morbidity and mortality rates have changed over the years and as transplant programs established medical and psychosocial eligibility criteria, patients who did not meet these criteria were not placed on the transplant waiting list.

B. Relative and Absolute Psychosocial Contraindications

1. In their landmark 1991 article, Olbrisch and Levenson described absolute, relative, and irrelevant psychosocial contraindications. Today, each transplant program establishes its own medical and psychosocial eligibility criteria for transplantation. This information is available for public view.

2. Contraindications may be categorized as "social" or "psychopathological."

3. Potential relative psychosocial contraindications[26]:
   a. Patient has no or limited social support.
   b. Patient has experienced a recent death or loss.
   c. Patient is currently a felony prisoner.
   d. Patient has a history of significant criminal behavior.
   e. Family history of mental illness.
   f. Controlled schizophrenia.
   g. History of or current affective disorder.
   h. History of suicide attempt (distant).
   i. Personality disorder.
   j. Mental retardation: intelligence quotient <70.
   k. Mental retardation: intelligence quotient <50.

4. Potential absolute psychosocial contraindications[26]
   a. Active schizophrenia/active psychosis
   b. Current suicidal ideation
   c. Multiple suicide attempts
   d. Recent suicide attempt
   e. Dementia

5. Individual transplant programs may consider these contraindications to be absolute, relevant, or irrelevant.[14]

C. Research on psychosocial criteria (selected studies)

1. Olbrisch and Levenson
   a. In commenting on the responsibility to fairly evaluate patients and to predict outcome, Olbrisch and Levenson noted that "the science of prediction cannot be divorced from philosophical questions"[25(p. 239)].
   b. These authors began researching the psychosocial evaluation process in the early 1980s[26] and noted that psychosocial screening was a component of patient evaluation at most transplant centers, but that criteria for determining candidacy for transplant were informal, unpublished, and likely varied from center to center.
   c. In the early 1990s, they surveyed the evaluation methods used at 204 heart transplant programs.[26]
      i. They asked these programs to identify psychosocial criteria and to rate each criterion as a relative or absolute contraindication to transplantation.
      ii. Examples of the psychosocial criteria identified by these programs were a psychiatric diagnosis, smoking, substance use, obesity, and nonadherence with medical recommendations.
      iii. These researchers found agreement among the centers on several *absolute contraindications* including
         • Active schizophrenia
         • Current suicidal ideation
         • History of multiple suicide attempts
         • Dementia
         • Current substance abuse

       iv. The centers disagreed, however, with respect to the use of criteria such as smoking, controlled schizophrenia, or affective disorders.

    d. In a second study, Olbrisch and Levenson[14] expanded the groups surveyed to include liver and kidney transplant teams along with heart programs and found that

       i. Heart transplant programs applied the most stringent psychosocial selection criteria and that kidney programs were the least restrictive.

       ii. Significant variations existed across all programs.

2. As the number of solid organ transplants increased in the 1980s, researchers began to examine pre- and posttransplant behaviors as predictors of posttransplant outcomes.

    a. Researchers investigated questions such as

       i. Would a patient who did not take medications and follow through with physician recommendations prior to transplantation do the same posttransplant?

       ii. Would the lack of a support system affect a patient's survival?

       iii. Would a certain psychiatric diagnosis lead to more medical management problems posttransplant?

    b. The results of these early studies were mixed:

       i. Some researchers failed to find an association between pretransplant psychological distress and mortality, graft rejection, or infections[27]

       ii. Other studies demonstrated that some patients are at higher risk for poor outcomes than others.

         • In a prospective study of 125 adult patients undergoing heart transplantation, Shapiro and colleagues reviewed psychosocial evaluation data and reported the following:

           ○ There were significant associations between personality disorder, living arrangements, global psychosocial risk, and history of substance abuse and posttransplant compliance problems.

           ○ Substance abuse and global psychosocial risk were significant predictors of compliance. Of note, patients with known substance abuse histories who had short remission periods and had only stopped using substances when their conditions declined were particularly at high risk for poor compliance.

       iii. Paris and colleagues[28] examined the incidence of psychosocial factors before and after heart transplantation and the influence of posttransplant psychosocial factors on clinical outcomes. These researchers concluded that

         • Psychosocial difficulties prior to heart transplantation (nonadherence, psychiatric problems, excessive weight) were likely to continue posttransplant.

         • Recipients with posttransplant psychiatric problems had a significantly higher risk of infection during the first posttransplant year.

         • Posttransplant nonadherence and psychiatric problems were related to more frequent hospital readmissions and higher medical costs.

3. Chacko and colleagues—1996[29]

    a. This study examined the correlation between pretransplant Axis I and II diagnoses and psychosocial adjustment and health status in heart ($n = 148$), kidney ($n = 109$), liver ($n = 22$), and lung/heart-lung ($n = 31$) candidates.

b. Candidates completed in-depth pretransplant psychosocial evaluation and psychometric testing.
c. Over 60% of the candidates met criteria for a DSM-III-R Axis I diagnosis.
   i. There was a significant difference in the overall frequency of current Axis I diagnoses among organ types.
   ii. Axis I diagnoses were most common in liver transplant candidates (83%) followed in decreasing order by lung (68%), heart (62%), and kidney (51%) transplant candidates.
d. Although 32% of candidates met criteria for a current Axis II disorder, there was no significant difference in the overall frequency of Axis II diagnoses across organ types.
   i. Axis II diagnoses were most common in liver transplant candidates (50%) followed in decreasing order by kidney (34%), heart (29%), and lung (23%) transplant candidates.
e. Approximately 25% of candidates had dual Axis I/Axis II diagnoses.
f. Relationship between Axis diagnosis and outcomes:
   i. An Axis I diagnosis was significantly associated with poorer psychosocial adjustment and poorer health status.
   ii. An Axis II diagnosis was significantly related to both global nonadherence and specific lack of adherence regarding diet, appointment keeping, medications, and avoiding smoking and drug misuse.
   iii. A combined Axis I/Axis II diagnosis was not significantly associated with poorer psychosocial adjustment or health status. However, these candidates were an important subgroup in that they had the poorest social support and coping ability and could potentially strain transplant team resources.
g. Although Axis I disorders were related to measures of psychosocial adjustment and health status and Axis II disorders were associated with nonadherence, these researchers concluded that there were no psychiatric diagnoses that would definitively preclude transplantation and highlighted the need for pretransplant interventions with these high-risk groups.

4. Dew and colleagues (1996)[30]
   a. This prospective study investigated the rates, characteristics, and risk factors for depression (DSM-III-R Major Depression), anxiety (Generalized Anxiety Disorder), adjustment disorders, and posttraumatic stress disorder related to the transplant (PTSD-T) in a sample of 154 patients during the first year after heart transplantation.
   b. Key findings included the following:
      i. The 1-year rates of the most prevalent disorders following heart transplantation were
         • Major depression (17.3%)
         • PTSD-T (13.7%)
         • Adjustment disorders (10.0%)
      ii. The specific pretransplant and perioperative factors that increased recipients' risk of posttransplant psychiatric disorder included
         • A history of pretransplant psychiatric disorder
         • Poor social support
         • Use of avoidant coping strategies
         • Early posttransplant low self-esteem

      iii. Recipients with the highest relative risk for posttransplant anxiety were those who had
- A shorter wait for a donor heart
- A family history of psychiatric disorder
- The poorest social support
- The poorest coping skills
- A poor sense of mastery

5. Dew and colleagues—1999[31]
   a. In a sample of 145 participants, these researchers prospectively examined whether compliance and psychiatric problems during the first posttransplant year predicted mortality and morbidity (acute rejection, cardiac allograft disease [CAD]) through the 3 years following heart transplantation.
   b. Controlling for known transplant-related predictors of morbidity and mortality (e.g., donor age, race, and gender, mechanical circulatory support before transplantation, recipient age, diabetes, cytomegalovirus status), these researchers reported that
      i. Recipients who were not compliant with medications during the first year posttransplant had a 4.17 times greater risk of rejection.
      ii. Recipients' risk of CAD was increased by
      - Persistent depressive symptoms (odds ratio [OR] = 4.67)
      - Persistent symptoms of anger/hostility (OR = 8.00)
      - Nonadherence with medications (OR = 6.91)
      - Obesity (OR = 9.92) during the first year posttransplant

      iii. Recipients who met criteria for posttraumatic stress disorder during the first year posttransplant had an increased risk of mortality (OR = 13.74).
   c. These investigators concluded that interventions to maximize transplant recipients' psychosocial status in these particular areas may improve their long-term posttransplant outcomes.
6. Owen and colleagues—2006[32]
   a. Using a retrospective chart review of pretransplant psychiatric evaluations in a sample of 108 heart transplant candidates, Owen and colleagues evaluated the ability of these evaluations to predict posttransplant outcomes (time to rehospitalization, infection, and survival).
   b. Past suicide attempt, medical nonadherence, history of drug or alcohol rehabilitation, and depression were significant predictors of shortened survival.
   c. Previous suicide attempt predicted time to infection.
7. Havik and colleagues—2007[33]
   a. In this cross-sectional study, these investigators prospectively examined the influence of depression on posttransplant survival in a sample of 147 heart transplant recipients who had a minimum of 5 years posttransplant follow-up.
   b. Mild to severe depressive symptoms on the BDI were noted at baseline in 25% of the sample and increased the risk of mortality during the 6-year follow-up period.
   c. BDI scores >10 indicated higher symptomatology and were associated with an approximately threefold risk of mortality (unadjusted relative risk).
      i. After controlling for medical (e.g., weight, BMI, glomerular filtration rate) and lifestyle (e.g., smoking) variables, depressive symptoms predicted all-cause mortality independent of these risk factors.

    d. Based on these findings, Havik and colleagues recommended
       i. Continuous attention to the potential for depressive symptomatology
       ii. Systematic screening for depression
       iii. Prompt initiation of pharmacological and/or psychological treatment.
8. Dobbels and colleagues—2009[34]
    a. In a sample of 141 heart (28), liver (61), and lung (52) transplant patients, these researchers prospectively examined pretransplant psychosocial and behavioral factors that predicted self-reported nonadherence with the immunosuppression regimen and clinical outcomes (late acute rejection, graft loss, number of hospitalizations and hospitalization days) at 1 year posttransplant.
    b. Predictors of nonadherence with immunosuppressant regimen:
       i. Independent predictors of self-reported posttransplant medication nonadherence included pretransplant medication nonadherence, higher level of education, less received social support with medication taking, and a lower score on the personality trait of "conscientiousness."
         • Regarding level of education, these investigators posited that a higher level of education might be associated with higher employment status and a subsequent busier lifestyle or increased decisiveness and an ensuing preference for independent decision making.
    c. Predictors of graft loss: The only significant predictors of graft loss (within 6 to 12 months posttransplant) were not being married and not living in a stable relationship.
    d. Predictors of late acute rejection: Self-reported medication nonadherence prior to transplant was the only significant predictor of late acute rejection.
    e. This study confirmed that patients who are nonadherent prior to transplantation have an eightfold greater risk of posttransplant nonadherence.
    f. This was the first prospective study to
       i. Demonstrate that transplant psychosocial factors predict nonadherence and poor posttransplant clinical outcomes.
       ii. Substantiate transplant guideline recommendations regarding pretransplant screening for psychosocial factors.
9. Farmer and colleagues—2013[35]
    a. In a nonrandom sample of 555 heart transplant recipients, these researchers prospectively examined demographic, psychosocial, behavioral, and clinical predictors of mortality 5 to 10 years following heart transplantation.
    b. Predictors of improved survival:
       i. Educational level (having at least a high school education)
       ii. Higher levels of social and economic satisfaction relative to home, neighborhood, community, employment, and finances
    c. Predictors of worse survival:
       i. Married status
       ii. More cumulative posttransplant infections
       iii. Posttransplant hematologic disorders
       iv. Worse New York Heart Association class
       v. Poor adherence to the medical regimen
    d. These researchers noted that the findings have important implications not only for patient selection but also for posttransplant care.

10. Summary
   a. Despite progress in identifying psychosocial factors that may impact posttransplant quality of life and survival, centers continue to differ in the medical and psychosocial criteria they apply to determine candidacy for transplantation.[36]
   b. This cross-site variation likely reflects the philosophy of the transplant program director and members of the team, program-specific statistics such as transplant volume and survival rates, and the impact of recent controversial high-profile cases.
   c. Factors previously considered absolute contraindications may no longer be viewed in that manner. For example:
      i.   Body mass index may be ignored if the program has been successful in transplanting obese patients.
      ii. A program that has transplanted a number of individuals with histories of recurrent depression may alter this practice if these patients have poor transplant outcomes.
   d. The current dilemma regarding psychosocial criteria for transplantation substantiates the need for additional prospective research in this area and the use of psychosocial rating scales. Selection of patients who stand to benefit most from these scarce resources remains a fundamental responsibility of the interdisciplinary transplant team.

VI. PATIENT AND SUPPORT PERSON STRESSORS ACROSS THE TRANSPLANT CONTINUUM

A. Although transplant patients must cope with the waiting period, surgery, and posttransplant recovery, the lives of their families and/or other members of their support system are also significantly impacted.
   1. Patients often comment that they feel that transplantation is more difficult for their families than for themselves.

B. Each phase of the transplant process presents unique challenges to patients and their support persons.[37]

C. Evaluation phase
   1. Potential patient stressors
      a. During this phase, patients wonder if transplantation will be the recommended treatment or if they will have to make end-of-life decisions.[30,38]
      b. Stress of the evaluation itself.
      c. Patients report relief after treatment plans have been determined but then face new uncertainties. While on the waiting list, patients may experience
         i.   Uncertainty that a donor organ will become available in time
         ii.   Deterioration of health and quality of life
         iii. Increasing disabilities
         iv.   Feelings of being a burden to others
         v.   Worries over finances[39]
         vi.   Fear of dying
         vii. Distress from seeing fellow patients suffer and perhaps die
         viii. Disappointment from missed opportunities for transplant (i.e., patient is notified of potential donor organ that subsequently is not acceptable)
         ix.   Guilt about the fact that someone must die for the patient to receive an organ[30]

     d. Patients are called upon to cope with the prospect of dying while at the same time hoping and fighting for extended life.

  2. Potential support person stressors

     a. Spousal support has a beneficial effect on health and quality of life[40] and spousal relationships can be a stabilizing factor for pre- and posttransplant patients.[41]

     b. Spouses and other support persons may be required to

       i. Provide ongoing emotional and physical care to a loved one who is slowly dying, often with little help or respite.[42]

       ii. Put their own lives on hold and ignore their personal needs.

       iii. Defer going forward with their own lives until the transplant takes place.

       iv. Relinquish social activities in order to care for the patient.

  3. Stress and coping during the evaluation phase

     a. The strength of a relationship may be tested as couples have to deal with time apart and the lack of privacy and intimacy associated with the hospital setting.

     b. As the patient's condition worsens, family responsibilities shift. A spouse may be required to return to work and children may have to assume more household duties.[39,40]

     c. Patients may question their role in the family and their ability to contribute meaningfully to family well-being.

     d. It is essential that the interdisciplinary transplant team monitor family coping throughout the entire transplant process.[43]

D. Pretransplant hospitalization

  1. Most transplant candidates wait at home until they are notified of a potential donor organ. However, there are times when heart and other transplant candidates must either wait in the hospital for a donor organ to become available or be hospitalized for episodic care.

  2. Potential patient stressors

     a. Separation from support persons

     b. Noise

     c. Lack of privacy

     d. Interrupted sleep

     e. Uncertainty about length of hospital stay

     f. Uncertainty that a donor organ will become available in time

  3. Potential support person stressors:

     a. Separation from patient

     b. Assumption of the patient's responsibilities

     c. Caregiver burden

     d. Belief that they have to "protect" the patient from family issues/concerns

  4. While hospitalized:

     a. Transplant candidates often develop relationships with other transplant patients and they may become sources of support for one another.

       i. Other sources of support during this time may include the nursing staff, the interdisciplinary transplant team, and hospital volunteers.

     b. Patients may assume many aspects of their care, such as taking medications, daily recording of weight, and monitoring intake and output.

E. Immediate posttransplant phase:

  1. Recovery may be highly variable in duration

2. Potential patient stressors:
   a. Receiving complex, highly technical care in an unfamiliar hospital unit.
   b. Worry about the success of the transplant procedure
      i.   Despite the relief of receiving a transplant, patients and their support persons remain apprehensive and may wonder when they can feel assured that the transplant has been successful.[43]
      ii.   Uncertainty with regard to the recovery may be particularly difficult for recipients of organs where treatments, such as dialysis, are not available should the transplant fail.
   c. Discomfort related to incisional pain, consequences of confinement in the intensive care unit (ICU), complications, and side effects of posttransplant medications, particularly mood lability associated with corticosteroid therapy
      i.   Mood lability may be manifested by tearfulness, irritability, increased anxiety, and sleep disturbance.[44]
      ii.   Severe reactions, however, such as a steroid-induced psychosis are rare.
   d. Concerns regarding their condition during the early postoperative period
   e. Potential for serious complications, including infection and rejection
   f. Transfer from the smaller nurse/patient staffing ratio in the ICU to an intermediate care unit with a larger nurse/patient staffing ratio
3. Potential support person stressors:
   a. Similar to those experienced by the patient
   b. In addition, support persons may feel that they can do little for the patient at this time, as the interdisciplinary transplant team manages acute care issues.

F. Discharge from hospital
1. The return home will be quite different for patients who waited at home for transplant than for those who had extended pretransplant hospital stays.
2. Potential patient stressors:
   a. Patients hospitalized for extended periods following the transplant surgery may experience heightened anxiety as they contemplate leaving the security of the hospital environment.
   b. Concerns about ability to follow the complex posttransplant regimen
   c. Worries about development of medical complications
3. Potential support person stressors:
   a. Family adjustment; changing family dynamics
      i.   As a patient's family commented: "We got used to him not being home, now we have to figure out what to do when he is back."
      ii.   Often, patients and families must re-establish a new "normal" life. Patients are no longer sick in the way they were prior to transplantation but are now required to manage a chronic medical condition.[43]

G. First posttransplant year
1. Patients often describe recovery from transplant as a multistage process, with dramatic improvements 4 to 6 weeks posttransplant, and then again 3, 6, 9, and 12 months after transplant.
2. Outcomes for patients who survive the first year vary widely with some patients experiencing an excellent quality of life and others hampered by ongoing problems.[45]
   a. Many patients state that it is a full year before the worst is behind them and they have attained their recovery goals.
3. Although transplantation extends life and offers the possibility of improved functional ability, caring for a transplanted organ can be a burdensome task.

4. Patients and families must learn to handle ongoing psychological stress and face continuing uncertainty about health outcomes.[40]

5. During this phase, patients are adapting both physically and psychologically to having a new and functioning organ.

6. Potential patient stressors:
   a. The origin and condition of the organ
   b. The possibility of rejection and infection
   c. Adherence to new and complex medical regimens
   d. The physical and emotional side effects of immunosuppressive medications
   e. An altered body image
   f. Changes in family and personal relationships.[41]
   g. Disappointment regarding pace of functional improvement (slower than expected)
   h. Fear of new health problems
   i. Inability to return to work
   j. Hospital readmission
      i. Readmissions are a common occurrence after transplantation, especially in the first year posttransplant.
      ii. It is important to note that patients may delay reporting symptoms to the transplant team because they are afraid of being readmitted to the hospital or because they worry about ever returning home if they are rehospitalized for serious complications
   k. Frequent follow-up visits
      i. Frequent posttransplant follow-up visits are scheduled immediately after discharge from the hospital. These visits gradually decline in frequency over time.
      ii. Some patients may resent continuing to have to spend so much time at the hospital for transplant clinic visits.
         • However, this frequent contact can also be comforting to patients, particularly the knowledge that a cadre of interdisciplinary professionals is available for any problems that may arise.

7. Potential support person stressors:
   a. Patient's delay in reporting symptoms
   b. Patient's rehospitalization
   c. Resumption of patient's responsibilities
   d. Caregiver burden, especially in early posttransplant months.

8. In addition to providing medical management, routine follow-up visits with the interdisciplinary transplant team can facilitate adjustment of patients and their support persons.
   a. Monitoring how patients and their support persons are coping at home is an important component of these visits.
      i. Patients and support persons are sometimes surprised that day-to-day issues and problems resurface as posttransplant life becomes more routine.[43]
      ii. These problems may have seemed unimportant while the patient was awaiting transplant, but they come to the forefront again when the patient returns home.[40]
      iii. A spouse, other family member, or support person may
         • Harbor hopes that transplantation would transform the patient's personality or adjustment

- Become discouraged with the resurgence of prior conflicts
- Express frustration that the recipient is not as grateful as would be expected about the transplant
- Be concerned about how the recipient is caring for him/herself.

9. Ongoing transplant support groups may also help patients and their support persons realize that others are experiencing similar problems and may reinforce positive coping strategies

H. Long-Term Years

1. A number of investigators have studied stressors in transplant recipients 5 to 15 years posttransplant.[37,45,46]
2. Potential patient stressors[46,47]
   a. Symptom management (weight control; medication side effects)
   b. Feeling worn out
   c. Medication costs
   d. Participating in sexual activity
   e. Continued biopsies; continued threat of rejection
   f. Sequelae of long-term immunosuppressant therapy
   g. Learning that a fellow transplant recipient was sick or had died
3. Potential support person stressors:
   a. Threat of rejection
   b. Recipient's decline to pretransplant state
4. The fact that stressors persist into the long-term posttransplant period underscores the need for continued psychosocial monitoring and interventions for both patients and support persons.

VII. DISCHARGE PLANNING AND EDUCATION

A. The process of education and discharge planning begins at the time of the pretransplant evaluation. The days preparing for hospital discharge include activities related to

1. Medical management (e.g., medication adjustment, biopsies, etc.)
2. Building the patient's strength
3. Educating patients and support persons about medications, self-monitoring, and other aspects of home care.

B. The goal at hospital discharge is for patients to be medically stable, ambulating, and knowledgeable about their medications and self-care responsibilities.

C. Regulatory requirements

1. In the United States, the Centers for Medicare and Medicaid Services (CMS) Conditions of Participation require that weekly multidisciplinary rounds are held to discuss the care and management of posttransplant patients. These rounds are held in whatever unit the patient is in (ICU, intermediate care unit, regular nursing floor).
2. Interdisciplinary team members who attend these rounds include, but are not limited to, the following:
   a. Nurses caring for the patient at the bedside
   b. Nurse transplant coordinators and nurse managers
   c. Providers (physicians, advanced practice nurses)

        d. Social workers
        e. Physical and occupational therapists
        f. Pharmacologists
        g. Dieticians
    3. The goals of these interdisciplinary rounds are to
        a. Discuss the care of these patients
        b. Update the interdisciplinary team regarding any changes in the posttransplant protocol
        c. Coordinate discharge education for patients and their support persons.

VIII. RETURN TO WORK

A. As they progress through the first posttransplant year, many patients are required to return to work for financial reasons.[48]

B. Some patients relish their return to work, view it as a sign of good posttransplant recovery and a return to a "normal" life, and welcome the opportunity to begin contributing again to the financial well-being of their families.

    1. There is some evidence that returning to work positively influences health-related quality of life among long-term (>15 years) liver transplant recipients, particularly with regard to physical functioning.[49]

C. Re-entry into the workforce is often easiest for individuals who have been unemployed for only a brief time pretransplant and those who are able to return to previously held positions.

D. Potential concerns regarding returning to work include

    1. Physical demands of the job
    2. Risk of infection from exposure to groups of people
    3. Inability to perform a job well
    4. The need for retraining
    5. Potential loss of disability insurance and Medicaid/Medicare benefits

IX. SUPPORT GROUPS

A. Meeting the needs of patients and their support persons may involve

    1. Developing support groups that allow for concurrent monitoring of patients
    2. Creating mentoring programs that offer local assistance
    3. Establishing a network of health care professionals with transplant experience in the patient's own community

B. Data indicate that ignoring pretransplant candidates' psychosocial needs leaves them in distress and poses risks for nonadherence and graft loss after transplant.[50]

C. Patients and members of their support system often find it extremely helpful to meet with others who have had similar transplant experiences.

D. A number of transplant centers have found support groups useful in meeting patients' needs.[51,52]

E.   An international support group, the Transplant Recipient International Organization, has chapters in many communities.

  1. Volunteers from this group often visit pre- and posttransplant patients in the hospital.

  2. Some chapters have regular meetings in the community that are open to patients and family members.

X. MENTORING PROGRAMS

A.   Because transplantation is a relatively uncommon medical treatment, few candidates have firsthand knowledge of transplantation.

B.   A number of transplant centers have developed formal or informal mentoring programs.

C.   Mentors are typically transplant recipients or members of the transplant recipient's support system. They volunteer to offer support to transplant candidates and/or members of their support system. A mentor can provide insight from the perspective of someone who has lived through the transplant experience.

D.   Training for mentors varies. Transplant knowledge, communication skills, and an ability to offer emotional support are important qualities.[53]

E.   Mentoring programs are also offered online. For example, the National Kidney Foundation provides a national, telephone-based, online program that offers support and education (https://www.kidney.org/professional/peers)

F.   Primary goals of mentoring programs:

  1. Provide social and emotional support.

  2. Educate patients about the transplant process.[53,54]

  3. Encourage adherence with medications and other aspects of the therapeutic regimen.

G.   Providing a mentor to transplant candidates and members of their support system gives them the chance to discuss the prospect of transplantation with someone who has already coped successfully with it. Conversations with mentors can help prepare patients for what often is a complicated, highly demanding, and stressful process.

XI. NONADHERENCE

A.   "Adherence" versus "compliance"

  1. These words are often considered to be synonyms. However, there is a subtle difference in their meanings.[55]

    a. The term "adherence" implies that there is a therapeutic relationship between the patient and the provider.

    b. The term "compliance" implies that the patient is following the provider's orders.

B. Definition of "nonadherence"
   1. World Health Organization definition: "the extent to which a person's behavior—taking medication, following a diet, and/or executing lifestyle changes—corresponds with agreed recommendations from a health care provider"[56(p. 18)].
   2. Nonadherence for a transplant patient includes failure to adhere to all aspects of the therapeutic regimen including failure to
      a. Take medications as prescribed
      b. Keep follow-up appointments
      c. Get required follow-up tests
      d. Avoid tobacco, alcohol, and substance use
      e. Promptly report symptoms[53]

C. Consequences of nonadherence
   1. The goal is for patients to preserve their transplanted organ so that their lives can be extended and their quality of life improved.[57]
   2. Nonadherent behaviors:
      a. Threaten the patient's longevity
      b. Compromise graft function
      c. Increase the risk of comorbidities
      d. Decrease quality of life
      e. Increase health care costs

D. Nonadherence in the pediatric population
   1. Nonadherence rates:
      a. Rates of nonadherence reported in the literature are as low as 3% and as high as 71%.[58]
         i. Adolescent kidney transplant recipients have the highest reported incidence of nonadherence.
      b. A 2009 meta-analysis of the published literature pertaining to medical regimen adherence among pediatric heart, liver, and kidney recipients indicated the following average rates of nonadherence with[59]:
         i. Keeping clinic appointments and getting required tests: 13 cases per 100 patients per year (PPY)
            • This means that the transplant team would expect to see 13 pediatric recipients per 100 recipients per year who are nonadherent with clinic appointments and tests
            • This nonadherence rate was twice as high in liver and kidney transplant recipients than in heart transplant recipients.
         ii. Taking immunosuppression medications: 6 cases per 100 patients per year (PPY)
         iii. Following diet and exercise recommendations: 5 cases per 100 PPY
         iv. Avoiding alcohol and illicit drugs: 0.6 cases per 100 PPY
         v. Avoiding tobacco use: 0.7 case per 100 PPY
   2. Associations with sociodemographic and psychosocial variables:
      a. Among pediatric heart, liver, and kidney transplant recipients, nonadherence has been shown to be significantly correlated with the following[59]:
         i. Sociodemographic characteristics:
            • Older age of child
              ◦ The rate of nonadherence with immunosuppression was more than twice as high in adolescents than in younger recipients.
            • Nonintact parental marriage

    ii. Psychosocial variables
- Lower family cohesion and support
- Child's greater psychological distress
- Longer time since transplant
- Greater parental distress or burdens
- Child's poorer behavioral functioning

  b. Results of studies from the kidney transplant literature suggest that pediatric recipients are at greater risk of nonadherence if they[58]

    i. Have greater perceived adversity related to their medical regimen

    ii. Identify barriers such as difficulty in swallowing pills or maintaining a consistent schedule

    iii. Encounter inconsistency regarding whether the adolescent recipient or the parent has primary responsibility for tasks associated with medications (e.g., filling the medication pillbox, obtaining refills, etc.).

3. Recommendations[58,59]

  a. The interdisciplinary transplant team should

    i. Routinely and consistently monitor adherence in all areas (medications, appointments, diet, exercise, etc.)

    ii. Use multiple sources to assess adherence (e.g., the recipient, the family, clinical data)

    iii. Routinely question recipients and/or family about factors associated with nonadherence (e.g., parental and/or child distress, family support)

    iv. Address this issue promptly as nonadherence rates increase with age and may continue into adulthood if ignored

    v. Given that family and child functioning variables affect adherence, recognize that adherence in children is actually "family adherence" and therefore

- Consider family context, dynamics, and relationships.
- Recognize the need for multifaceted interventions.

  b. The time when the pediatric recipient transitions to an adult transplant program is a particularly vulnerable period with regard to adherence. Strategies to improve adherence during this critical time include close interdisciplinary collaboration, routine monitoring of adherence, and identifying and addressing barriers to adherence.[60]

  c. Strategies to improve adherence in the adolescent population should include multifaceted, developmentally appropriate, and tailored interventions that focus on[60,61]

    i. Health-related education

    ii. Motivational techniques

    iii. Behavioral skills

E. Nonadherence in the adult population

1. Nonadherence rates:

  a. In their meta-analysis of 147 studies involving more than 29,000 kidney, heart, and liver transplant recipients, Dew and colleagues reported the following rates of nonadherence with[62]

    i. Following dietary recommendations: 25 cases per 100 PPY

    ii. Taking immunosuppressant medications: 23 cases per 100 PPY

    iii. Monitoring vital signs: 21 cases per 100 PPY

    iv. Exercising: 19 cases per 100 PPY

    v. Getting blood work and other tests: 12 cases per 100 PPY

vi. Attending clinic appointments: 6 cases per 100 PPY
vii. Avoiding alcohol use: 4 cases per 100 PPY
viii. Avoiding tobacco products: 3 cases per 100 PPY
ix. Avoiding illicit drug use: 1 case per 100 PPY
b. Differences between types of transplant recipients:
i. Kidney transplant recipients had a significantly higher rate of nonadherence with immunosuppressant medications (36 cases per 100 PPY) than heart recipients (15 cases per 100 PPY) or liver recipients (7 cases per 100 PPY)
ii. Heart recipients had the highest rate of nonadherence with exercise (38 cases per 100 PPY)
c. Association with psychosocial variables
i. There was little correlation between nonadherence and
   - Demographic variables
   - Social support
   - Perceived health
ii. Pretransplant substance use was a strong predictor of posttransplant substance use.
2. Costs: In the United States, the estimated cost of nonadherence among adult transplant recipients that results in acute rejection and graft failure is between $15 to $100 million annually.[55]
3. Interventions
a. General interventions
i. Nonadherence may be viewed by health care professionals as irrational, delusional, and willful self-destructive behavior.[63] However, patients usually have a reason for their nonadherence.
   - It is important to talk with patients and members of their support systems in order to determine the reason for nonadherence. In many instances, problems associated with nonadherence can be resolved.
ii. One of the purposes of the pretransplant psychosocial assessment is to gather information about patients' prior follow-through with medical recommendations.
iii. Support persons' perceptions regarding the patient's adherence and feedback from other health care professionals who have cared for the patient are also useful in assessing adherence.[64,65]
iv. The transplant team also has a special opportunity to evaluate adherence in patients who are hospitalized at the time of the pretransplant evaluation, through monitoring of patients' response to instructions and their follow-through with recommendations.
v. In addition, the interdisciplinary team should[66]
   - Listen to patients' stories and try to understand their perspectives
   - Ascertain patients' goals for therapy
   - Allow patients to assume control and responsibility for their treatment by educating them so that they can make informed decisions
   - Involve the patient in the treatment plan as much as possible
   - When necessary, consult with a psychiatrist or psychologist for assistance in determining patients' decision-making abilities or in managing nonadherent patients
   - Remain patient and persistent

b. Interventions to increase medication adherence[67]

   i. Recommended interventions for which efficacy has been demonstrated by strong evidence from rigorously designed studies:

   - Reduce medication dosing frequency

   ii. Interventions with less well-established evidence but are likely to be effective:

   - Use of medication calendars
   - Timing medications with routine activities
   - Using a pillbox with an alarm
   - Setting alarms on a watch, cell phone, etc.
   - Using email or text reminders
   - Receiving regular prescription reminders by mail
   - Receiving written medication instructions
   - Using packaging options such as time-specific blister packs
   - Teaching patients to self-monitor vital signs, side effects, etc.
   - Using electronic medication packaging/feedback
   - Assessing/treating depression related to medication taking

   iii. Interventions for which there is currently no evidence but are suggested based on clinical practice and expert consensus

   - Review how to take medication with patient; discuss potential alternate medications or dose adjustment with prescriber.
   - Involve support persons who can encourage medication adherence.
   - Place medications in visible location.
   - Keep spare medications at work, at home, in car, etc.
   - Obtain financial assistance for medication or switch to less expensive medication.
   - Use pillbox with an alarm.
   - Take pills one by one or swallow with meals or beverages.
   - Institute self-medication program for pre- and posttransplant patients.

   iv. Interventions that do not have proven efficacy and should only be used in combination with the above interventions

   - Providing education that explains why medications should be taken

XII. STRATEGIES FOR PATIENT EDUCATION

A. In providing education for the patient and members of the patient's support system, it is important for the interdisciplinary transplant team to

1. Assess preferred learning style, level of health literacy, degree of interest,[68] and readiness to learn.

   a. Critically ill pretransplant patients typically have difficulty understanding and retaining information, though their abilities may improve significantly posttransplant.

2. Identify barriers to learning and potential solutions.

   a. Some patients may need additional instruction or alternative approaches, such as a written outline of procedures or step-by-step instructions.

3. Offer a variety of educational resources such as

   a. Videos, CD-ROMs, brochures

   b. Opportunities for transplant candidates to meet transplant recipients

   c. Support groups or mentoring programs

4. Utilize the "teach back" method to assess the effectiveness of education.
   a. Do not assume that patients have absorbed or will recall all information presented to them.[69]
   b. Ask patients to summarize the information they have received.
5. Obtain a neuropsychological consult for patients with cognitive dysfunction.
   a. Neuropsychological testing is also helpful in identifying problems that could hinder patients' abilities to care for themselves independently posttransplant.
6. Consider a self-medication program during the posttransplant hospitalization that can
   a. Help patients become more comfortable with their medication routines, work out their own cueing systems, and learn how to manage problematic dosing times before discharge home
   b. Discourage reliance on family members and health care staff to provide medications
   c. Provide patients an opportunity to demonstrate independence with this task

B. See chapter on Education for Transplant Patients and Caregivers for additional information.

XIII. FINANCIAL RESOURCES FOR TRANSPLANT PATIENTS

A. Medical costs associated with transplantation include the following:
   1. Hospitalization costs.
   2. Medications.
      a. Posttransplant maintenance medications can cost in excess of $6,000 a month if the patient had no health care coverage.
   3. Outpatient clinic visits.
   4. Monitoring procedures (e.g., biopsies).
   5. These costs may diminish over time as follow-up visits become less frequent and fewer medications are required.
   6. Table 18-1 lists 2014 Estimated Average Billed Charges per Transplant by Organ. These charges include
      a. Medical costs during the 30 days prior to the transplant admission
      b. Organ procurement costs

TABLE 18-1 2014 Estimated Average Billed Charges per Transplant by Organ

Organ	Total
Heart	$ 1,242,200
Intestine	$ 1,547,200
Kidney	$ 334,300
Liver	$ 739,100
Lung—Single	$ 785,000
Lung—Double	$ 1,037,700
Pancreas	$ 317,500

From Milliman Research Report. *2014 U.S. Organ and Tissue Transplant Cost Estimates and Discussion.* Available at http://us.milliman.com/uploadedFiles/insight/Research/health-rr/1938HDP_20141230.pdf. Accessed June 3, 2015.

    c. Hospital admission facility charges

    d. Professional nonfacility services

    e. Postdischarge facility and professional nonfacility services including hospital readmissions

    f. Outpatient immunosuppressants and other prescriptions during 180 days following transplant discharge.[70]

B. Nonmedical costs associated with transplantation

  1. In addition to medical expenses, patients requiring transplant are faced with other associated expenses, including

    a. Additional housing costs when relocation to the transplant center is required

    b. Loss of income for both patients and support persons

    c. Transportation

    d. Costly equipment such as a microspirometer for lung transplant recipients

C. Insurance coverage

  1. Private insurance

    a. The cost of transplantation is covered by most private insurance programs in the United States.

    b. Most private US health insurances require patient co-payments.

      i. With increases over the last 5 years, the total patient co-payment responsibility may be several hundred dollars a month.

  2. Medicare

    a. Individuals qualify for Medicare if they are over age 65 or if they have been receiving Social Security Disability benefits for 2 years.

    b. Medicare covers 80% to 100% of in- and outpatient charges.

    c. For eligible patients, Medicare covers 80% of costs for antirejection medications.[71]

    d. End-Stage Renal Disease (ESRD) Program

      i. Depending on their work credits, individuals diagnosed with ESRD are eligible for Medicare:

        • The beginning of the fourth month after starting hemodialysis

        • The first month of peritoneal dialysis

        • The first month of home hemodialysis

        • The month they have the kidney transplant if they never received dialysis

      ii. Medicare coverage is effective for 3 years posttransplant.

      iii. For patients who receive Social Security Disability benefits, the coverage will change from the ESRD Program to the Social Security Disability program.

      iv. If an individual has a private insurance, the ESRD Program coverage is secondary for 30 months.[71]

  3. State Medical Assistance Programs (Medicaid)

    a. State Medicaid programs typically cover all prescriptions at 100%, but some programs have a small patient co-payment.

D. Changes in insurance coverage

  1. The patient's insurance coverage for transplant charges may vary over time posttransplant.

  2. Medicare

    a. Patients may no longer qualify for disability or Medicare benefits after they have recovered and returned to work.

   b. Individuals, however, can continue to receive Social Security Disability benefits and Medicare and earn a monthly income.[71]
    i. Annual guidelines determine the amount of monthly income allowed.
   c. Patients who have worked in organizations with comprehensive benefit packages may receive disability incomes for the duration of their illness.
  3. State Medical Assistance Programs
   a. Many state Medicaid programs have work incentive plans that encourage individuals with disabilities to return to work following transplantation.
   b. These programs allow individuals to earn a defined income and continue to qualify for Medicaid benefits.
  4. Given the importance of having an uninterrupted source of medications, patients are urged to notify their coordinator or social worker if they are not able to obtain medications or if they are aware of a change in their medication coverage.
  5. Educating patients before transplant about potential costs of posttransplant medications may help with planning and budgeting for these expenses.

E. Pharmaceutical assistance programs
  1. Most pharmaceutical companies have drug assistance programs to help defray medication expenses.
  2. Eligibility for these programs is typically need-based.
  3. However, many of these programs will not offer assistance if patients have private insurance, Medicaid, or Medicare.
  4. For the Medicare patient, drug assistance programs will not typically assist with the 20% cost of medications not covered by Medicare.
  5. Some private assistance programs cover patient co-payments that are not covered by Medicare or private insurance (e.g., the HealthWell Foundation)
   a. The posttransplant coordinator and social worker assist patients in applying for these programs. However, with the increased use of the Internet, some patients are able to research assistance programs more independently.

F. Fundraising resources
  1. There are several US-based fundraising foundations for transplant patients.
  2. The funds raised by these programs help offset the cost of transplantation and related expenses for medications and travel not covered by the patient's insurance.
  3. Pediatric
   a. The Children's Organ Transplant Association (COTA) was founded in 1986 and primarily assists children in need of transplantation and their families.[72]
  4. Adult
   a. Funded 30 years ago, the Help, Hope, Live nonprofit organization and the National Foundation for Transplants provide similar assistance to adults.[72]

XIV. END-OF-LIFE ISSUES

A. Mortality is always of concern, even for patients who undergo successful transplant procedures.
  1. Transplant programs assist transplant candidates to recognize the possibility that their transplant might fail, in which case they might die.
  2. Patients' acknowledgement of this possibility is required as part of the process of obtaining informed consent to insure that patients are aware of potential risks.

3. Thus, the pretransplant assessment period is a critical time for most patients and members of their support system, many of whom are learning for the first time about the uncertainties and limitations of transplantation.

4. The extent to which individuals are able to prepare themselves for dying is highly variable and is related to such factors as personal philosophies and experience, religious beliefs, individual fear of death, age, and the involvement of dependents and other loved ones.[73]

5. Because transplantation offers the possibility of extended life, many patients and members of their support systems focus on a positive outcome, an outlook that can be viewed as a successful coping strategy.[43]

   a. In some cases, however, there is also a conscious or unconscious decision to avoid contemplating mortality issues, which are considered too painful and frightening.

   b. Furthermore, an individual's age and stage in the life cycle may affect his/her ability to consider or come to terms with the possible end of life.[73]

      i. For the very young, having to face death often seems both untimely and unimaginable both to them and their families.

      ii. Older patients, who have themselves experienced losses, may more readily accept their own mortality.

6. The inability to come to terms with one's mortality when in the midst of the dying process may lead to increased anxiety and stress for patients and members of their support system.[73]

7. From the time of the initial assessment, the social worker and other interdisciplinary transplant team members have the responsibility to broach issues of mortality at appropriate times and help prepare patients and members of their support system for this possibility.

B. Substitute decision maker

1. On a practical level, patients must choose a substitute decision maker with whom they can discuss their wishes in the event of their death. This is discussed in the initial psychosocial evaluation.

2. Patients are advised to prepare wills and make any other necessary financial arrangements to insure that their wishes are fulfilled should they become incapacitated. It is also important to have discussions with family members regarding how finances will be managed while the patient is hospitalized.

C. Patients with dependent children

1. Care of dependent children

   a. The need for preparatory arrangements is especially acute when the patient is also the parent of dependent children.[74]

   b. Integral to the parental role is the responsibility to be present in a nurturing capacity and to protect the child until the child becomes independent.[75]

   c. Facing possible death inevitably plunges parents into projections about a future in which they no longer exist.

2. Separation from dependent children

   a. Parents who must be separated from their children for lengthy periods to obtain medical care may have concerns about the children's present situation and the possibility of not being with them at the end of life.[76]

   b. Parents frequently express concerns about not being able to meet role expectations, fear and panic about the future, and guilt related to letting their children down.

   c. The transplant team must be cognizant of the fact that separated parents may be forced to envision uncomfortable, stressful scenarios with their spouses or other family members.

   d. Single parents may be especially vulnerable to these concerns, particularly those without an engaged and supportive extended family.

3. Discussions with dependent children

   a. Providing emotional support for the child and disclosing the truth about the parent's illness is often problematic for the family.

   b. Many patients seek to protect family members by misleading them or by failing to fully disclose the risks.

4. Role of the interdisciplinary transplant team

   a. At the initial contact, the transplant social worker collects information about the patient's support system and ascertains and documents what has been planned for the children in the event of the patient's death.

      i. The plan for the future of the children is discussed, including the children's feelings about this plan.

   b. Parents are encouraged to

      i. Tell children that they are loved and valued and that the ill parent wants very much to be with them.

         • Even quite ill or disabled patients can be caring and capable parents despite the severity of their illness.

      ii. Be forthright with children.[74]

      iii. Include children in an age-appropriate manner that reduces feelings of isolation and anger.

      iv. Assure children that they are not responsible for the parent's health problem.

      v. Acknowledge that children have an important role in the parent's life, both pre- and posttransplant.

         • Should the parent die, the children become the principal mourners.

         • Excluding children from family meetings and age-appropriate health care discussions denies them the status they deserve as important and integral members of the family.

      vi. Seek additional counseling if they are concerned about the children's coping.

   c. The interdisciplinary transplant team supports parents by

      i. Helping them deal effectively with planning for their dependent children

      ii. Strategizing ways to minimize the children's confusion or pain

      iii. Assuring children that the transplant team will do all it can to help the patient but that even if things do not work out, the children will be looked after.

XV. PALLIATIVE CARE

   A. The World Health Organization defines palliative care as an "approach that improves the quality of life of patients and their families facing the problem associated with life-threatening illness, through the prevention and relief of suffering by means of early identification and impeccable assessment and treatment of pain and other problems, physical, psychosocial and spiritual"[77(p. 6)]

B. Historical perspective:
1. For many years, clinicians were somewhat reluctant to refer patients to the palliative care service because they thought that
   a. The only role for palliative care was at the end of life.
   b. A palliative care consult meant they had given up on the patient.
   c. The involvement of this discipline precluded aggressive treatment.
2. However, the role of palliative care in transplantation has expanded over the past 5 years as clinicians' knowledge of and comfort with this concept have increased.

C. The role of palliative care in transplantation
1. Transplant team members, including social workers, nurse practitioners, and physicians may suggest that a palliative care consult be placed.
2. It is important to explain to patients and members of their support system[78]:
   a. That members of the palliative care service are part of the interdisciplinary team
      i. In many transplant programs, a specific palliative care physician may be assigned to the interdisciplinary transplant team.
   b. The role of the palliative care service in assisting with
      i. Symptom and pain management
         • With improved symptom management, patients may be better able to tolerate medical treatments.
      ii. Clarification of treatment goals
      iii. Advanced care planning
      iv. Maximizing quality of life for the patient and members of the support system
   c. In addition, the palliative care team, in concert with the transplant team, may suggest the following:
      i. Patients with spiritual or religious backgrounds may gain psychological and emotional support from their beliefs and religious communities.
      ii. Chaplains and other spiritual advisors, as well as persons familiar with therapies such as meditation, visualization, and Reiki, can offer unique assistance during hospitalization and upon the patient's return home.[73]

D. Who can benefit from palliative care?
1. Transplant candidates whose conditions deteriorate to the point that transplant is no longer an option
2. Transplant patients with complex care needs, particularly for coordination of care and pain management
3. Transplant recipients with graft failure
4. Transplant recipients with serious posttransplant comorbidities (e.g., malignancy)

E. Expert palliative care is essential when death is imminent.[73]
1. As noted above, transplant recipients face the prospect of death due to organ failure at any time following surgery.
2. The interdisciplinary palliative care team can
   a. Help patients cope with fears about suffering during the dying process.
   b. Reassure patients that care will be provided in accordance with their wishes, using all available treatments to relieve discomfort and anxiety.
   c. Assure patients that the palliative care team:
      i. Affirms life and regards dying as a normal process
      ii. Intends to neither hasten nor postpone death
   d. Offer assistance to help the patient's support system cope during the patient's illness and their own bereavement process.

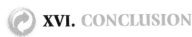

XVI. CONCLUSION

A. The field of transplantation has advanced significantly since the first successful solid organ transplant procedure was performed in 1954.

B. Numerous research studies have led to best practices for improving pre- and posttransplant survival.

C. In addition, more evidence-based data are now available about the psychosocial aspects of transplantation, such as
   1. The manner in which transplant candidates and recipients cope with changes in their lives
   2. The types of adjustment and compliance problems patients encounter.
   3. Pre- and posttransplant quality of life of patients and their support systems
   4. The types of information that is most critical in evaluating potential transplant candidates.

D. There is substantial consensus about
   1. The importance of assessing psychosocial factors
   2. The components of a comprehensive psychosocial evaluation
   3. The influence of patient characteristics and psychosocial support on transplant outcomes

E. Further studies are needed to identify more effective methods of preparing patients and members of their support system for transplantation and promoting successful adaptation to life after transplant.

REFERENCES

1. Dew MA, Switzer GE, DiMartini AF, et al. Psychosocial assessments and outcomes in organ transplantation. *Prog Transplant.* 2000;10:239–259.
2. Dobbels F, De Geest S, Cleemput L, et al. Psychosocial and behavioral selection criteria for solid organ transplantation. *Prog Transplant.* 2001;11:121–132.
3. Olbrisch ME, Benedict SM, Ashe K, et al. Psychological assessment and care of organ transplant patients. *J Consult Clin Psychol.* 2002;70:771–783.
4. Hillerman WL, Russell CL, Barry D, et al. Evaluation guidelines for adult and pediatric kidney transplant programs: the Missouri experience. *Prog Transplant.* 2002;12:30–35.
5. Phipps L. Psychiatric evaluation and outcomes in candidates for heart transplantation. *Clin Invest Med.* 1997;20: 388–395.
6. Favaloro RR, Perrone SV, Moscoloni SE, et al. Value of pre-heart-transplant psychological evaluation. Long-term follow up. *Transplant Proc.* 1993;31:3000–3001.
7. Bright MJ, Craven JL, Paul JK, et al. Assessment and management of psychological stress in lung transplant candidates. *Health Soc Work.* 1990;15(2):125–131.
8. U. S. Department of Health and Human Services. *Healthy People 2010. Washington DC: U.S. Government Printing Office. Publication number CMB 2000–1.* Bethesda, MD: National Institutes of Health and Human Services; 2000.
9. Health Literacy Measurement Tools (Revised): Fact Sheet. Rockville, MD: Agency for Healthcare Research and Quality; November 2014. Available at http://wwwahrqgov/professionals/quality-patient-safety/quality-resources/tools/literacy/indexhtml. Accessed June 1, 2015.
10. Arozullah AM, Yarnold PR, Bennett, CL, et al. Development and validation of a short form rapid assessment of adult literacy in medicine. *Med Care.* 2007;45(11):1026–1033.
11. Lewis K, Winsett RP, Cetingok M, et al. Social network mapping with transplant recipients. *Prog Transplant.* 2000;10:262–266.
12. Burker EJ, Evon DM, Sedway JA, et al. Appraisal and coping as predictors of psychological distress and self-reported physical disability before lung transplantation. *Prog Transplant.* 2004;14:222–234.
13. Tringali RA, Trzepacz PT, DiMartine A, et al. Assessment and follow-up of alcohol-dependent liver transplantation patients. *Gen Hosp Psychiatry.* 1996;18:70S–77S.

14. Levenson JA, Olbrisch ME. Psychosocial evaluation of organ transplant candidates. A comparative survey of process, criteria, and outcomes in heart, liver, and kidney transplantation. *Psychosomatics.* 1993;34(4):314–323.
15. Olbrisch ME, Levenson JL, Hamer R. The PACT: a rating scale for the study of clinical decision-making in psychosocial screening of organ transplant candidates. *Clin Transplant.* 1989;3:164–169.
16. Skotzko CE, Rudis R, Kobashigawa JA, et al. Psychiatric disorders and outcome following cardiac transplantation. *J Heart Lung Transplant.* 1999;18:952–956.
17. Twillman RK, Manetto C, Wellisch DK, et al. The transplant evaluation rating scale: a revision of the psychosocial levels system for evaluating organ transplant candidates. *Psychosomatics.* 1993;34(2):144–153.
18. Maldonado JR, Dubois H, David, E, et al. The Stanford Integrated Psychosocial Assessment for Transplantation (SIPAT): a new tool for the psychosocial evaluation of pre-transplant candidates. *Psychosomatics.* 2012;53(2):123–32.
19. Beck AT, Ward CH, Mendelson M, et al. An inventory for measuring depression. *Arch Gen Psychiatry.* 1961;4:561–571.
20. Bradwin M, Coffman KL. The Millon Behavioral Health Inventory Life Threat Reactivity Scale as a predictor of mortality in patients awaiting heart transplantation. *Psychosomatics.* 1999;40:44–49.
21. Maercker A, Schutzwohl M. Assessment of post-traumatic stress reactions. *Diagnostica.* 1998;44:130.
22. Spitzer RL, Williams JBW. Structured clinical interview for DSM-III-R *(non-patient version and personality disorders).* New York, NY: Biometrics Research, NY State Psychiatric Institute, NY; 1985.
23. Rector TS, Ormaza SM, Kubo SH. Health status of heart transplant recipients versus patients awaiting heart transplantation: a preliminary evaluation of the SF-36 Questionnaire. *J Heart Lung Transplant.* 1993;12:983–986.
24. Deragotis LF. *SCL-90 Administration, Scoring and Procedures Manual-II—Revised.* Baltimore, MD: Clinical Psychometric Research; 1983.
25. Olbrisch ME, Levenson JL. Psychosocial assessment of organ transplant candidates. Current status of methodological and philosophical issues. *Psychosomatics.* 1995;36:236–243.
26. Olbrisch ME, Levenson JL. Psychosocial evaluation of heart transplant candidates: an international survey of process, criteria and outcomes. *J Heart Lung Transplant.* 1991;10(6):948–955.
27. Maricle RA, Hosenpud JD, Norman DJ, et al. The lack of predictive value of pre-operative psychologic distress for post-operative medical outcome in heart transplant recipients. *J Heart Lung Transplant.* 1991;10:942–947.
28. Paris W, Muchmore J, Pribil A, et al. Study of the relative incidences of psychosocial factors before and after heart transplantation and the influence of post-transplantation psychosocial factors on heart transplantation outcome. *J Heart Lung Transplant.* 1994;13:424–432.
29. Chacko RC, Harper RG, Kunik M, et al. Relationship of psychiatric morbidity and psychosocial factors in organ transplant candidates. *Psychosomatics.* 1996;37:100–107.
30. Dew MA, Roth LH, Schulberg HC, et al. Prevalence and predictors of depression and anxiety-related disorders during the year after heart transplantation. *Gen Hosp Psychiatry.* 1996;18:48S–61S.
31. Dew MA, Kormos RL, Roth LH, et al. Early post-transplant medical compliance and mental health predict physical morbidity and mortality one to three years after heart transplantation. *J Heart Lung Transplant.* 1999;18(6):549–562.
32. Owen JE, Bonds CL, Wellisch DK. Psychiatric evaluation of heart transplant candidates: Predicting Post-transplant hospitalizations, rejection episodes, and survival. *Psychosomatics.* 2006;47(3):213–222.
33. Havik EI, Sivertsen B, Relbo A, et al. Depressive symptoms and all-cause mortality after heart transplantation. *Transplantation.* 2007;84(1):97–103.
34. Dobbels F, Vanhaecke J, Dupont L, et al. Pretransplant predictors of posttransplant adherence and clinical outcome: an evidence base for pretransplant psychosocial screening. *Transplantation.* 2009;87(10):1497–1504.
35. Farmer SA, Grady KL, Wang E, et al. Demographic, psychosocial and behavioral factors associated with survival after heart transplantation. *Ann Thorac Surg.* 2013;95:876–883.
36. Cimato TR, Jessup M. Recipient selection in cardiac transplantation: contraindications and risk factors for mortality. *J Heart Lung Transplant.* 2002;22:1161–1173.
37. Rosenberger EM, Dew MA, DiMartini AF, et al. Psychosocial issues facing lung transplant candidates, recipients, and family members. *Thorac Surg Clin.* 2012;22(4):517–529.
38. Deshields TL, McDonough EM, Mannen K, et al. Psychological and cognitive status before and after heart transplantation. *Gen Hosp Psychiatry.* 1996;8:62S–69S.
39. Buse McS, Pieper B. Impact of cardiac transplantation on the spouse's life. *J Heart Lung Transplant.* 1990;16(6):641–648.
40. Nolan MT, Cupples SA, Brown MM, et al. Perceived stress and coping strategies among families of cardiac transplant candidates during the organ waiting period. *J Heart Lung Transplant.* 1992;21(6):540–547.
41. Gier MD, Levick MD, Blazina PJ. Stress reduction with heart transplant patients and their families: a multidisciplinary approach. *J Heart Lung Transplant.* 1988;7:342–347.
42. Rogers KR. Nature of spousal supportive behaviors that influence heart transplant patient compliance. *J Heart Lung Transplant.* 1987;6(2):90–95.
43. Mishel MH, Murdaugh CL. Family adjustment to heart transplantation: redesigning the dream. *Nurs Res.* 1987;36(6):332–338.
44. Shapiro PA, Kornfeld DS. Psychiatric outcome of heart transplantation. *Gen Hosp Psychiatry.* 1989;11:352–357.

45. Grady KL, Jalowiec A, White-Williams C. Predictors of quality of life in patients at one year after heart transplantation. *J Heart Lung Transplant.* 1999;18:202–210.

46. Grady KL, Wang E, White-Williams C, et al. Factors associated with stress and coping at 5 and 10 years after heart transplantation. *J Heart Lung Transplant.* 2013;2(4):437–446.

47. Song MK, DeVito Dabbs A, Studer SM, et al. Exploring the meaning of chronic rejection after lung transplantation and its impact on clinical management and caregiving. *J Pain Symptom Manage.* 2010;40(2):246–255.

48. Bohachick P, Anton BB, Wooldridge, RL, et al. Psychosocial outcome six months after heart transplant surgery: a preliminary report. *Res Nurs Health.* 1992;15:165–173.

49. Kousoulas L, Neipp M, Barg-Hock H, et al. Health-related quality of life in adult transplant recipients more than 15 years after orthotopic liver transplantation. *Transpl Int.* 2008;21(11):1052–1058.

50. Campbell B, Etringer G. Post-transplant quality of life issues: depression-related nonadherence in cardiac transplant patients. *Transplant Proc.* 1999;31(suppl 4A):59S–60S.

51. Skotzko CE, Stowe JA, Wright C, et al. Approaching a consensus: psychosocial support services for solid organ transplant programs. *Prog Transplant.* 2001;11:163–168.

52. Suszycki LH. Social work groups in a heart transplant program. *Heart Transplant.* 1988;5:66–170.

53. Wright L. Mentorship programs for transplant patients. *Prog Transplant.* 2000;10:267–272.

54. Gardner A. Mentoring in the 1990s: a new look at an old idea. *Maturity.* 1993;13(5):6–8.

55. Su GC, Greanya ED, Partovi N, et al. Assessing medication adherence in solid organ transplant recipients. *Exp Clin Transplant.* 2013;11(6):475–481.

56. World Health Organization. 2003. *Adherence to Long-Term Therapies: Evidence for Action.* Available at http://www.who.int/chp/knowledge/publications/adherence_full_report.pdf. Accessed June 8, 2015.

57. Littlefield C, Abbey S, Fiducia D, et al. Quality of life following transplantation of the heart, liver and lungs. *Gen Hosp Psychiatry.* 1996;18:36S–47S.

58. Shellmer DA, DeVito Dabbs A, Dew MA. Medical adherence in pediatric organ transplantation: what are the next steps? *Curr Opin Organ Transplant.* 2011;16(5):509–514.

59. Dew MA, DeVito Dabbs A, Myaskovsky L, et al. Meta-analysis of medical regimen adherence outcomes in pediatric solid organ transplantation. *Transplantation.* 2009;88(5):736–746.

60. Shemesh E, Annunziato RA, Arnon R, et al. Adherence to medical recommendations and transition to adult services in pediatric transplant recipients. *Curr Opin Organ Transplant.* 2010;15(3):288–292.

61. Fredericks EM, Dore-Stites D. Adherence to immunosuppressants: how can it be improved in adolescent organ transplant recipients? *Curr Opin Organ Transplant.* 2010;15(5):614–620.

62. Dew MA, DiMartini AF, DeVito Dabbs, et al. Rates and risk factors for nonadherence to the medical regimen after adult solid organ transplantation. *Transplantation.* 2007;83(7):858–873.

63. Sherry DC, Simmons B, Wung SF, et al. Nonadherence in heart transplantation: a role for the advanced practice nurse. *Prog Cardiovasc Nurs.* 2003;18:141.

64. Hathaway DK, Combs C, De Geest S, et al. Patient compliance in transplantation: a report on the perceptions of transplant clinicians. *Transplant Proc.* 1991;31(suppl 4A):10S–13S.

65. Collins DC, Wicks MN, Hathaway DK. Health-care professional perceptions of compliance behaviors in the pre-renal and post-renal transplant patient. *Transplant Proc.* 1999;31(suppl 4A):16S–17S.

66. Edwards SS. The "noncompliant" transplant patient: a persistent ethical dilemma". *Prog Transplant.* 1999;9(4):202–208.

67. Transplant360. *Pocket Guide: Interventions to Common Medication Adherence Barriers.* Available at www.transplant360.com. Accessed March 30, 2015.

68. Cramer JA. Practical issues in medication compliance. *Transplant Proc.* 1999;31(suppl 4A):7S–9S.

69. Robbins ML. Medication adherence and the transplant recipient helping patients at each stage of change. *Transplant Proc.* 1999;31(suppl 14A):29S–30S.

70. Milliman Research Report. *2014 U.S. Organ and Tissue Transplant Cost Estimates and Discussion.* Available at http://us.milliman.com/uploadedFiles/insight/Research/health-rr/1938HDP_20141230.pdf. Accessed June 3, 2015.

71. Centers for Medicare and Medicaid Services. *What Medicare Covers.* Available at www.medicare.gov. Accessed June 1, 2015.

72. United Network of Organ Sharing. *Financial Resources Directory.* Available at www.transplantliving.org/before-the-transplant/financing-a-transplant/directory/. Accessed June 8, 2015.

73. Roberson H. *Meeting Death: In Hospital, Hospice, and at Home.* Toronto, Canada: McLeeland & Stewart Ltd.; 2000.

74. Muirhead J, Meyerowitz BE, Leedham B, et al. Quality of life and coping in patients awaiting heart transplantation. *J Heart Lung Transplant.* 1992;11:265–272.

75. Harris M. *The Loss That Is Forever: The Lifelong Impact of the Early Death of a Mother or Father.* New York: Plume;1996.

76. Silverman PR. *Never Too Young to Know: Death in Children's Lives.* New York: Oxford University Press; 2000.

77. Hall S, Petkova H, Tsouros AD, et al., eds. *Palliative Care for Older People: Better Practices.* Denmark: World Health Organization; 2011.

78. Goldstein N, Kalman J. Palliative Care and the Heart Failure Patient. American Heart Association presentation, January 10; 2012.

SELF-ASSESSMENT QUESTIONS

1. A psychosocial evaluation should include questions pertaining to the patient's history of psychiatric disturbances. This should include which of the following problems?
   a. Serious sleep disorders
   b. Suicide attempts
   c. History of hospitalizations for mental health reasons
   d. Panic attacks
   e. b and c
   f. All of the above

2. The ultimate goals of the psychosocial evaluation are to:
   a. provide education to the patient on pain management related to posttransplant care.
   b. provide the transplant team with information on the candidate's support system.
   c. identify gaps in the patient's insurance plan.
   d. identify potential compliance issues.
   e. b, c, and d.
   f. all of the above.

3. Once the social worker has assessed a patient for transplantation, the determination may be made for referral to which of the following services?
   a. Chemical dependency consult
   b. Neuropsychiatry
   c. Endocrinology
   d. Cardiac surgery
   e. a and b
   f. All of the above

4. Research on heart transplant recipients has demonstrated that individuals with consistently elevated levels of depression, anger, and hostility have a four to eight times greater likelihood for developing which of the following?
   a. Primary graft failure
   b. Alcoholism
   c. Coronary artery disease
   d. Chronic graft rejection
   e. Chronic renal failure

5. Research has demonstrated that patients with posttraumatic stress disorders (PTSD) were 13 times more likely to:
   a. have chronic rejection episodes.
   b. die within 3 years posttransplantation.
   c. require a retransplant within 3 years.
   d. develop chronic renal failure.

6. While awaiting transplantation, patients have reported concerns about which of the following?
   a. Becoming a burden to friends and family
   b. Financial issues
   c. Dying while awaiting a suitable donor organ
   d. a and c
   e. All of the above

7. Family burden may increase as the patient's health deteriorates while awaiting a suitable organ for transplantation. Spouses may experience which of the following during the waiting period?
   a. Anxiety related to separation from the individual hospitalized while awaiting transplantation
   b. A need to return to work to support the family
   c. Difficulty coping with added responsibilities that were once shared
   d. All of the above

8. Heart transplant candidates may often be hospitalized while awaiting a suitable donor heart. Social workers and nurses help to create a supportive environment with interventions such as which of the following?
   a. Educational programs for patients and families
   b. Support groups with other patients awaiting transplantation
   c. Weekly dinners together with other patients on the unit
   d. Weekly excursions to the shopping mall with their IV inotropes
   e. a, b, and c
   f. All of the above

9. Patients who are hospitalized for several months pre- and posttransplant may experience which of the following upon discharge from the hospital?
   a. Heightened anxiety about leaving the hospital environment
   b. Insecurity related to fear of complications
   c. Fear about changes in personal relationships with family members during the extended absence
   d. Role confusion
   e. a, b, and d
   f. All of the above

10. Upon returning to a routine home environment, patients and families are often surprised to find which of the following?
    a. Day-to-day pretransplant problems resurface and begin to cause conflict.
    b. The excitement of a new life overcomes all fears.
    c. Transplantation has fixed all the pretransplant family problems.
    d. The personality change in the recipient has made life more tolerable.

Correct Answers:
1.f   2.e   3.e   4.c   5.b   6.e   7.d   8.e   9.f   10.a

CHAPTER 19

Quality Assurance and Performance Improvement (QAPI) and Regulatory Issues in Transplantation: A New Focus in Transplantation

Linda Ohler, RN, MSN, CCTC, FAAN

Samira Scalso de Almeida, RN, MS

Karina Dal Sasso Mendes, RN, PhD

Luciana Carvalho Moura, RN, MS, MBA(c)

I. INTRODUCTION[1]

A. Since the first successful kidney transplant by Dr. Joseph Murray in Boston in 1954, advances in solid organ transplantation have resulted in lifesaving procedures for individuals with end-organ diseases.[1]

B. Historical perspective:

1. Starzl and colleagues performed the first successful liver transplant in the United States in 1967.
2. The heart transplant procedure was developed by Shumway and Lower in the mid-1960s. These initial heart transplants were in dogs, and interestingly, some of the transplant dogs went on to have puppies.
   a. However, the first successful human heart transplant was performed by Dr. Christian Barnard in 1967 who studied under Lower and Shumway. Barnard had spent time with Dr. Lower in 1967 and learned the surgical technique for this procedure. He is credited with the first successful heart transplant, which he performed upon his return to South Africa.
3. Cooper and colleagues performed the first successful lung transplant in Toronto, Canada, in 1983.
4. During these early years, there was very little oversight of the allocation of organs.

C. The foundations for transplantation in the United States were established when Congress passed the National Organ Transplant Act (NOTA) in 1984.[2]

1. This act established the Organ Procurement Transplantation Network (OPTN), which required
   a. A national registry for organ matching, which would be operated by a private, not-for-profit organization:
      i. The United Network for Organ Sharing (UNOS) has been awarded the OPTN contract for organ allocation and waiting list registry since 1986.
   b. Public release of program-specific information regarding the performance of transplant programs:
      i. This requirement is accomplished through an OPTN contract with the Scientific Registry of Transplant Recipients (SRTR) that was established in 1987.[3]
2. Each transplant program in the United States submits required data on transplant candidates and recipients to UNOS through a secure portal.
   a. These data are aggregated and sent to the SRTR for analysis.
   b. Following analysis, SRTR releases the data publicly via their Web site: www.srtr.org.[3] These data include applicable program-specific, local, and national data relative to:
      i. Waitlist information such as
         • Characteristics of waitlisted patients
         • Transplant and mortality of waitlisted patients
         • Percent transplanted, waitlisted patients
         • Time to transplant, waitlisted patients
      ii. Recipient characteristics: deceased and living donors
      iii. Donor characteristics: deceased and living donors
      iv. Transplant operation characteristics
      v. Patient survival
      vi. Graft survival

II. EVOLUTION OF REGULATORY OVERSIGHT

A. Oversight for performance of transplant programs based on outcomes and quality was not fully established in the United States until 2007 when the Centers for Medicare and Medicaid Services (CMS) issued the Conditions of Participation (CoPs) for transplant programs.[4]

B. With the release of the CoPs, every transplant program in the United States was required to submit a letter to CMS indicating the program's commitment to follow the new CoPs. This was the beginning of the linkage of Medicare payment to data-driven outcomes as well as standardized regulations in transplantation.

C. Initially, there were doubts in the transplant community that these new regulations and outcome expectations would or could be upheld by CMS.

D. As the SRTR began to release data twice annually, patient and graft survival outcomes were being scrutinized by public (CMS) as well as private insurers.

E. CMS began site surveys of transplant programs in 2007 to evaluate adherence to the newly released CoPs.
   1. Regulatory on-site surveys from CMS occur every 3 to 5 years without notification to transplant programs, much like The Joint Commission hospital surveys.

2. Transplant programs must be ready at all times for a site survey that may continue for 2 to 5 days, depending on the size of the transplant program.

3. If deficiencies are identified, the transplant program must develop a corrective action plan to improve program compliance with CMS standards.

4. Additionally, data reflecting program changes stipulated in the corrective action plan must be tracked and reported to demonstrate positive results and sustainability of processes or outcomes.

F. Implementation of the CMS CoPs has resulted in most transplant programs adding personnel such as quality and regulatory managers, clinicians, and data managers to ensure adherence to the structured oversight.

G. In addition to the structure and personnel necessary to meet expectations, the CoPs stipulate organ-specific volume requirements as well as expectations regarding patient and graft survival outcomes.

1. Programs that report statistically lower than expected outcomes in two of the last five SRTR releases are likely to receive a notification from CMS that they are at risk of losing Medicare reimbursement unless they can demonstrate improvements in their outcomes.

2. If the progress toward better outcomes is not satisfactory to CMS, a transplant program may enter into a probationary period with a systems improvement agreement (SIA) issued by CMS.

3. SIA process:
   a. An independent peer review team consisting of an interdisciplinary group of transplant professionals is directed by CMS to conduct on-site survey of the transplant program.
   b. A report of recommended corrective actions is submitted to the transplant program and conveyed verbally to CMS.
   c. Transplant programs are given 8 to 12 months to make the required improvements to meet expected outcomes.
   d. During an SIA, a transplant program is required to hire consultants to assist with implementation of a corrective action plan that has been reviewed and approved by CMS officials.
   e. Monthly calls are conducted with the consultants, CMS (national and regional), and the transplant program on probation.
   f. Updates on progress are assessed through a review of the transplant program's performance improvement projects and data.
   g. Programs are released from the SIA based on demonstration of improvements and completion of their corrective action plans.

H. UNOS surveys of regulatory requirements:
1. UNOS began site surveys to evaluate transplant programs for compliance with UNOS policies and data integrity in 2006.

2. In 2009, UNOS began to survey transplant programs with living donor programs to ensure all national living donor policies are being upheld.

3. UNOS schedules 2-day site surveys and provides transplant programs with a list of patient charts they review while on site.

4. It is possible for a transplant program to have three to four on-site surveys in 1 year.
   a. CMS site survey
   b. CMS focused QAPI survey
   c. UNOS site survey
   d. UNOS living donor survey

III. EVOLUTION OF DATA-DRIVEN QUALITY IN TRANSPLANT PROGRAMS

A. Medicare is a federally funded insurance program administered through CMS.

B. If Medicare does not pay for a transplant in a specific transplant program, most private insurers will not pay for the transplant either.

1. CMS CoP requirements for transplant programs are similar to a private insurer's requirements for a transplant program to become a center of excellence (CoE).

C. Prior to 2007, there was very little enforcement of transplant outcomes.

1. Once enforcement began, transplant programs became more focused on data-driven outcomes.
2. Data were submitted and analyzed but outcomes were not initially tied to payment.

D. Although the initial CoPs required transplant programs to begin implementing quality assessment and performance improvement (QAPI) programs, at first, the surveys did not delve deeply into the QAPI programs.

1. In August 2013, CMS issued more focused quality standards for transplant programs.[5]
2. CMS surveys on Focused QAPI began in 2014.
3. Because most clinicians and administrations were not formally trained in QAPI processes, initially, there were concerns about the new focus on quality, the SRTR's analytic methodologies, and potential additional staffing requirements for transplant programs.
4. At the same time, however, clinicians and administrators began to examine the quality and accuracy of data being collected by their own transplant programs and submitted to UNOS.
    a. Problems associated with data collection/submission and opportunities for improvement were identified, for example:
        i.   Lack of staff trained in data collection and submission process
        ii. Data entry by busy clinicians who already had a full patient care workload and for whom patient care was their first priority
        iii. Failure to submit data in a timely manner
5. Transplant programs began to take note of the seriousness of failure to meet UNOS and CMS data submission deadlines.
    a. Timeliness of data submission is monitored.
    b. Metrics regarding the timeliness of data submission are reported for each organ-specific transplant program.
6. Initiatives to improve data collection and submission were implemented.
    a. Programs began to train additional staff whose sole job was to enter data into the secure UNOS portal.
    b. Representatives of the SRTR began presenting at transplant conferences to help clinicians understand the importance of data integrity.
    c. Various agencies offered webinars to help transplant programs understand the importance of integrity of the data entered for analysis.

d. Today, many data coordinators receive a comprehensive orientation with regard to
   i. Key components of data management
   ii. SRTR data submission processes and reports
   iii. Risk adjustment profiles

 IV. FOCUS ON QUALITY IN TRANSPLANTATION

A. Quality in health care is a complex process and reflects the degree to which health services increase the probability of desired health outcomes and are reliable with current professional knowledge.[6]

B. The Institute of Medicine has identified six dimensions of quality in health care: health care must be safe, effective, patient centered, timely, efficient, and equitable.[7]

C. The publication of three reports, "The Urgent Need to Improve Health Care Quality,"[8] "To Err Is Human,"[5] and "Crossing the Quality Chasm"[6] provided evidence regarding quality deficiency in health care and directed clinicians to develop improvements.
   1. Most United States programs have hired a quality manager or quality team, depending on the size of the program.
   2. This new focus on quality has resulted in a better understanding of the need for data accuracy and methods used by the SRTR to determine outcomes.
   3. An example of the emerging global emphasis on quality in transplantation is discussed below.

D. Elements of a QAPI plan
   1. CMS surveyors spend several days focused on the quality aspects of a transplant programs starting with the quality assessment and performance improvement (QAPI) plan.
   2. The QAPI plan serves as a guidance document for a transplant program's QAPI program.
   3. According to CMS, a quality plan for transplantation includes five elements that must be addressed in a QAPI plan:
      a. Element 1: Design and scope
         i. The design and scope must describe:
            • How the transplant QAPI plan is integrated with the hospital QAPI plan
            • A bidirectional flow of communication between the hospital quality department and transplantation
            • How outcomes are communicated to transplant staff
            • Activities of all three phases across the continuum of care of transplantation
            • Activities of all three phases of living donation
            • Contracted services in terms of reporting their outcomes on a regular basis
            • The frequency of quality meetings
            • Members of the steering (or QAPI leadership) committee and each organ committee
            • The roles of individual(s) responsible for each meeting

- How the transplant program addresses adverse events for inpatients and ambulatory care patients
- How adverse events are analyzed, including a time frame and staff involved
- Roles and responsibilities of transplant personnel in overseeing the quality and safety of patient care across the continuum of pretransplant care, perioperative care, and posttransplant follow-up care

b. Element 2: Executive responsibilities/governance and leadership
   i. Leadership involvement must be described in the transplant QAPI plan.
      - This refers to hospital leadership as well as transplant leadership.
      - It is important for hospital leadership to be aware of the outcomes and quality in a transplant program.
      - The transplant QAPI plan should be reviewed and approved by the hospital's governing body. This should be addressed in the QAPI plan.
   ii. Resources available to the transplant QAPI should be described to ensure quality and outcomes are effectively covered.

c. Element 3: Feedback and data systems
   i. This section of the QAPI plan should describe
      - How data are collected for each measure
      - Resources available for timely collection of data
      - How staff is trained and communicates any concerns about processes to leadership
      - How leadership responds to staff
      - How communication flows from the program to front line staff
      - How data are maintained and reported

d. Element 4: Analyses
   i. The QAPI plan should address
      - How data are collected and analyzed
      - Tools used for analyzing data
      - How data are tracked and used to make meaningful improvements that are sustainable

e. Element 5: Performance improvement interventions
   i. The plan should describe
      - How decisions are made to focus performance improvement on high risk, high volume, or problem areas
      - How performance improvement projects are organized, led, tracked, analyzed, and reported

V. MANAGING DATA WITH SCORECARDS

A. Goals of scorecards
1. The demand to improve patient safety, quality of the processes, and information in transplantation is increasing as it is within all health care organizations.[9]
2. In 1998, the IOM made recommendations to improve performance measures through the collection and evaluation of reliable data.[10]

     a. In transplantation, we have seen an increase in the amount of data that are being collected by health information systems.

  3. One way to improve the quality of the processes and information is to utilize a scorecard approach.

  4. This method provides clinicians with a visualization of the transplant program's information.

     a. Analysis of data captured in the scorecard allows clinicians to develop specific interventions to improve their organizational processes or clinical practice.[1]

B. Advantages of scorecards[11-13]

  1. Help health care clinicians to

     a. Define strategies

     b. Monitor and evaluate performance

     c. Set targets for performance measures

     d. Track process improvement efforts

     e. Provide information on clinical practice

     f. Construct indicators

     g. Offer evidence for action needed

     h. Identify gaps and potential hazards

     i. Benchmark against national data

     j. Visualize financial results

     k. Focus on measurement and accountability

     l. Enhance communication with key stakeholders

C. Risks associated with scorecards[13]

  1. A few negative factors have been associated with the use of scorecards such as

     a. Tracking indicators that not useful or feasible

     b. Tracking metrics that are not valid or reliable

     c. Assigning indicators that do not align with the organization

     d. Lack of timely access to integrate performance data

  2. However, scorecards are useful in many ways as discussed below.

D. Implementing scorecards in transplantation

  1. Each organ system should have a scorecard that monitors data specific to pretransplant, perioperative, and posttransplant periods.

     a. This includes scorecards specific to living donors in the predonation, donation, and postdonation phases.

  2. It is important to create and utilize scorecards that ensure patient safety and excellent outcomes.

  3. To develop the most effective scorecards, it is important to

     a. Determine what performance measures or metrics are important to each organ system in the transplant program.

     b. Identify metrics that measure process/activities and outcomes for each phase of transplantation and living donation.

     c. Describe measures in terms of clinical quality or operational effectiveness.

     d. Identify appropriate standard metrics.

     e. Establish a methodology for the metrics.

     f. Define each performance measure (metric).

     g. Benchmark performance measures using evidence from published literature, SRTR outcomes, and database outcomes or with other transplant programs with similar volumes.

h. In some cases, such as length of stay or return to the operating room or time from referral to listing candidates for transplantation, programs may benchmark metrics against their own data to demonstrate and track improvement.

i. Utilize a color-coded system that indicates the level of performance in a particular metric. Identifying the parameters for the color coding helps staff to determine where processes and outcomes are doing well and where interventions are needed.

j. Once a performance measure has reached expected or green for an entire year, it may be "retired" and audited just quarterly rather than monthly.

k. With continued expected (green) results, a program may decide to discontinue monitoring a specific performance measure.

l. Yellow or amber colored areas in a scorecard indicate caution. The program should look at a potential problem in the area before it becomes serious.

m. Red indicates a performance measure that is out of compliance and needs a corrective action.

E. Scorecard tips
1. Scorecards are a visual resource for guiding and managing quality in your program.
2. By creating a separate scorecard for each organ system for each adult and pediatric organ system and for living donors, transplant programs can make data-driven decisions for each system based on analysis of the collected data.
3. By dividing scorecards into the phases of transplantation, we can measure our practice across the continuum of care.
4. Most scorecards are developed using excel spreadsheets. Columns on the left provide performance measures.
5. Benchmark data are included for most performance measures to provide a score against which a program can measure itself.
6. Using tabs at the bottom of each organ-specific spreadsheet to identify each year of data collection allows programs to visualize data over time in a single scorecard.
   a. Tabs keep data in one place for each organ system or living donors.

F. Determining performance measures
1. Performance measures are usually decided upon by transplant quality leadership teams in collaboration with the organ-specific transplant team.
2. Performance measures should be used in each of the three phases of transplantation for each organ system in your program, including living donors.
   a. Preoperative phase:
      i. Many of the initial preoperative performance measures are based on regulations such as ABO and UNOS ID verifications and documenting patient selection criteria in the patient's chart.
      ii. Tracking the number of inactive patients on the list for each organ system is a good way to measure program effectiveness in patient selection.
         • All waitlisted patients should be monitored to ensure they continue to meet selection criteria. This includes inactive patients.
      iii. Tracking the number of days from referral to first appointment and to listing also evaluates a program's efficiency in the evaluation process.
   b. Perioperative phase:
      i. This section can be divided into medical and surgical issues that can affect transplant recipients in the intraoperative phase of care.

      ii. The perioperative phase can identify medical or surgical problems.

      iii. Surgical complications specific to each organ system.

- Return to the operating room prior to discharge.
- Bleeding may be another surgical complication to track as evidenced by blood transfusions required.

      iv. Medical complications may include the following:

- Need for reintubation
- Requirement for dialysis in the postoperative phase
- Seizures in the immediate posttransplant phase
- Fever and chills in the immediate postoperative phase
- Rejection in the immediate postoperative phase

      v. Discharge processes followed.

      vi. Length of stay.

  c. Postoperative phase:

      i. Readmission within 30 or 90 days of discharge

      ii. Development of infection in the first 90 days

      iii. Death of recipient with first year of transplant

      iv. Loss of graft within first year posttransplant

G. Evidence-based benchmarking

1. Benchmarking performance measures requires reviewing literature especially systematic reviews, meta-analyses, and multicenter prospective studies.
2. Data such as this provides evidence by which to measure outcomes for performance such as length of stay, readmission rates, etc.
3. Benchmarking should not just involve comparing your hospital with national averages; it should involve looking at best practice hospitals and evaluating clinical practice/processes at that facility that can be implemented in your program.
4. Benchmarking resources:
   a. PubMed searches: articles that provide data based on single-center or multicenter studies (www.pubmed.gov).[14]
   b. The Agency for Healthcare Research and Quality: evidence-based clinical practice guidelines (www.ahrq.gov)[15]:
      i. This site also has meta-analyses that may provide benchmarking resources.
   c. Transplant organizations that have published organ-specific guidelines for the care of patients with end-stage disease and transplant candidates and recipients. This evidence-based information may be a useful resource for benchmarking purposes.
      i. The International Society of Heart and Lung Transplantation (www.ISHLT.org)[16]
      ii. The American Association for the Study of Liver Diseases (www.aasld.org)[17]
      iii. Kidney Disease Improving Global Outcomes: www.kdigo.org[18]

H. Tracking data

1. Collecting, organizing, and disseminating data for analysis involve tremendous effort from professionals at transplant centers.
2. The main goal of tracking data is to obtain numbers and information to develop indicators.

3. Indicators or performance measures are essential to the planning and control processes of transplant programs, thereby enabling the establishment and achievement of goals:
   a. The results are essential for critical analysis of performance, for decision making, and for the new planning cycle.[19]
   b. The purpose of indicators is to measure qualitative and quantitative aspects of variables such as the environment, structure, processes, and outcomes.
   c. Indicators cannot be construed as direct measurements of quality.
   d. Instead, they point to what requires the attention of the assessed health care organization.[19]
4. Monitoring the indicator data may also help to evaluate specific quality improvement initiatives such as educational programs and development of protocols in transplant.

I. Policies
1. Transplant policies should reference hospital policies whenever possible.
   a. All protocols, procedures, and policies should be readily available and accessible to all transplant clinicians.
   b. Having policies available on an intranet allows for easy access.
   c. Some transplant programs have implemented a grassroots policy whereby each clinician partners with a member of leadership to ensure a policy or policies are followed correctly. This process increases policy compliance.
   d. QAPI policies, procedures, and protocols define the processes and criteria; these policies can be definitions and/or descriptions of[20,21]:
      i. The process
      ii. Areas of responsibility
      iii. Resources (structural/professional/services)
      iv. Activities (candidate evaluation, waitlist management, surgical procedure, postoperative management, follow-up)
      v. Processes for entering data and information into registries
      vi. Indicators
      vii. Frequency of data collection
      viii. Treatment algorithms
   e. All data must be recorded in a standard manner such as Teidi, UNOS' client-server application.
   f. Data coordinators should be provided with information to ensure accuracy of data to be entered into registries and scorecards.
   g. Developing a data dictionary for the data coordinator may increase the accuracy of data entered and provides a resource for data coordinators.
   h. The individuals responsible for tracking information must have some clinical training for understanding transplantation.
   i. Data must be submitted within 90 days of the due date stipulated by UNOS.
      i. Both CMS and UNOS monitor compliance with data submission deadlines.

J. Analyzing data
1. By examining the sources, quality, and organization of the different types of transplant data available, we hope to improve the understanding and utility of existing results while ensuring excellent outcomes that meet and surpass CMS-expected requirements.

2. Evidence suggests that audits and feedback based on indicator data can be effective in changing health care professional practice.

3. Table 19-1 lists examples of QAPI tools that may be useful for data collection and analysis.

4. QAPI regulations do not specify which particular tools/instruments a transplant program must use, but rather expects whatever tool/instrument is chosen meets the needs of the transplant program. It is best to determine what tool the hospital uses.

K. Adverse events

1. The first report concerning the topic of patient safety was published in 1999 by the IOM.[6] *To Err is Human* included a review of the literature on adverse events and injuries resulting from medical care.[6]

2. CMS defines the term "adverse event" as "an untoward, undesirable, and usually unanticipated event that causes death or serious injury, or the risk thereof. As applied to transplant centers, examples of adverse events include but are not limited to serious medical complications or death caused by living donation; unintentional transplantation of organs of mismatched blood types, transplantation of organs to unintended recipients; and unintended transmission of infectious disease from a donor to a recipient"[22(p. 11)].

TABLE 19-1 Quality Assessment Process Improvement Methods

Name of Method	Notes
Plan-do-study-act (PDSA)	Continuous quality improvement method
Focus, analyze, develop, and execute (FADE)	Continuous quality improvement method Similar to PDSA
Six Sigma	Focuses on improving quality by reducing the number of errors/incidents Includes two methodologies: DMAIC and DMADV Inspired by PDSA
Define measure analyze improve control (DMAIC)	Six Sigma method used to improve an existing process
Define measure analyze design verify (DMADV)	Six Sigma method used to create a new process, also known as DFSS
Design for Six Sigma (DFSS)	Six Sigma method used to create a new process, also known as DMADV
Failure mode and effects analysis (FMEA)	Method of analysis of failures and the consequences within a system Related method is health care failure mode and effects analysis (HFMEA) which combines hazard analysis and critical control points (FMEA and HACCP), a food safety method
Total quality management (TQM)	Focuses on improving quality by ensuring conformance with requirements
Wills-ideas-execution (WIE)	Framework for system-level improvement in health care
Whole system measures (WSM)	System used to measure overall quality of a health system and to align improvement to work across a hospital or large health care system

a. Many hospitals follow The Joint Commission standards and use the term "sentinel event." The Joint Commission does not use the term adverse event.

b. A near miss is an unplanned incident or event that did not cause harm (also known as a close call).[23]

3. Transplant-related adverse events:

a. The scientific literature and media have reported cases where organ recipients had serious injuries or death as a result of errors during the donation and transplant process.[24,25]

b. Despite the formal protocols for assessing donor suitability and guidelines to prevent injuries and transmission of diseases, adverse events continue to be reported.

4. Transplant programs should have an adverse events policy that is specific for transplantation.

a. The adverse events policy should reference and reflect elements of the hospital adverse events policy.

b. Examples of transplant adverse events may include issues such as

i.   Immediate graft dysfunction requiring mechanical support

ii.   Graft loss in the first year post transplantation

iii. Patient death within the year after transplantation

iv.   Serious injury or death to a living donor

5. Reporting an adverse event is a crucial step in the assessment of safety in transplantation.

a. Many hospitals use an electronic system to report an adverse event.

b. These reports go directly to the hospital risk manager or to the hospital quality department.

c. All adverse events associated with the care of transplant candidates or recipients while hospitalized must be attended to by transplant team members involved in the event. This includes patient falls, medication errors, and device malfunction causing harm to the patient.

• Identified adverse events during inpatient stays are the responsibility of the hospital and transplant quality teams as well as risk management.

d. The root cause or other thorough analytic methodology can be evaluated collaboratively with leadership from the hospital risk management or quality departments and the transplant quality leadership.

e. The transplant program assists with coordination of the analysis by providing data, establishing meetings with involved team members and providing patient information.

f. The hospital risk management or quality department will ensure a legally protected and confidential approach to a root cause or thorough analysis.

g. It is important to define the time period in which the root cause must be analyzed in the adverse events policy and in the transplant QAPI plan.

h. This process should be reflected in the transplant adverse event policy.

i. A log of adverse events must be maintained and provided to the hospital's risk management department.

• This log must also be available to site surveyors upon request.

j. An adverse events analysis should be addressed in a separate meeting with all clinicians who were involved in the event in attendance.

• Minutes from the meetings should be marked "confidential" and available only within the hospital and to site surveyors.

6. Root cause/thorough analysis:
   a. All investigations for adverse or sentinel events consist of a series of steps to be followed systematically.
   b. Most hospital adverse events policies describe methods used to analyze an adverse event.
   c. A root cause analysis is conducted by professionals with specific training and in conjunction with the risk manager or hospital quality manager, depending on hospital policy.
   d. Process:
      i.   Start by completing an initial summary with all the circumstances and a list of individuals involved in the incident.
      ii.   Prepare a time line of the event; the time line should start with the pretransplant phase and cover each phase involved in the process.
      iii. Identify the problems involved.
      iv.   Interview the staff and ask questions about how the treatment was conducted and reasons for each problem identified.
         * If new problems appear in the middle of the investigation, new interviews can be arranged as needed.
      v.   Compile reports of the event, listing causes of care management problems.
      vi.   Develop a corrective action plan to correct the problem and prevent recurrence.
      vii. Submit report to senior clinicians and management according to local arrangements.
      viii. Implement actions arising from report.
         * Track and monitor progress of changes in corrective action plan.
         * Report the progress at QAPI meetings.
         * Document and demonstrate sustainability of changes.
7. The CMS survey on adverse events:
   a. Surveyors will want to see a report showing resolution of each adverse event as well as a corrective action plan.
   b. CMS surveyors will ask
      i.   How you know your action plan is making a difference and is sustainable.
      ii.   If the event analysis led to a performance improvement project, surveyors will want to see the results of that project.
   c. It is important to monitor all corrective actions resulting from performance improvement projects, root cause analysis, and any survey deficiencies.
   d. Analyzing the data from these projects helps to demonstrate the sustainability of changes made in the corrective action plans.
8. Near miss: An event or situation that did not produce injury, but only because of chance.[22]
   a. An analysis should be completed on near misses.
   b. A thorough analysis describes the key facts of the event and includes
      i.   What occurred
      ii.   Severity of the event
      iii. What affect it may have had on a patient
   c. A root cause analysis must be reported within the hospital quality and risk system.
   d. A thorough analysis may be kept in minutes within the transplant program.

    e. Both analytic methodologies provide staff with an opportunity to learn from incidents.

    f. It is important that these analyses look at *systems problems* and *not* be punitive to individuals.

    g. Programs should focus on making systems changes to prevent human errors.

 VI. THE BRAZILIAN EXPERIENCE WITH QAPI

The Brazilian transplant nurses have begun to learn about QAPI from the US experience. The Brazilian nurses who coauthored this chapter have taken classes and begun to use scorecards, benchmarking, developing performance measures, analyzing data, and performing a root cause analysis. While their government does not require transplant programs to monitor and report data, they are collecting and analyzing data for their programs. They are being proactive.

REFERENCES

1. McRae D. *Every Second Counts: The Race to the First Human Heart Transplant, 2006.* New York, NY: G.P. Putnam's Sons; 2006.
2. Legislation and Policy. The Organ Procurement and Transplantation Network Policies and Reports. Available at http://www.organdonor.gov/legislation/. Accessed June 20, 2015.
3. The Scientific Registry for Transplant Recipients (SRTR). Available at www.srtr.org. Accessed September 30, 2015.
4. CMS Conditions of Participation for Transplant Programs. Available at http://www.cms.gov/Regulations-and-Guidance/Legislation/CFCsAndCoPs/downloads/trancenterreg2007.pdf. Accessed June 20, 2015.
5. Centers for Medicare and Medicaid Services. Focused Quality Assessment and Performance Improvement (F-QAPI) Surveys for Organ Transplant Programs. Available at http://www.cms.gov/Medicare/Provider-Enrollment-and-Certification/SurveyCertificationGenInfo/Policy-and-Memos-to-States-and-Regions-Items/Survey-and-Cert-Letter-13-51.html. Accessed June 20, 2015.
6. Institute of Medicine. *To Err is Human: Building a Safe Health System.* Washington, DC: National Academy Press; 2000.
7. Institute of Medicine. *Crossing the Quality Chasm: A New Health System for the 21st Century.* Washington, DC: National Academy Press; 2001.
8. Chassin MR, Galvin RW. The urgent need to improve health care quality. Institute of Medicine National Roundtable on Health Care Quality. *JAMA.* 1998;280(11):1000–1005.
9. Pronovost PJ, Berenholtz SM, Needham DM. A framework for health care organizations to develop and evaluate a safety scorecard. *JAMA.* 2007;298(17):2063–2065.
10. Institute of Medicine. *Organ Procurement and Transplantation: Assessing Current Policies and the Potential Impact of the DHHS Final Rule.* Washington, DC: The National Academies Press; 1999.
11. Kaplan RS, Norton DP. *The Balanced Scorecard: Translating Strategy into Action.* Boston, MA: Harvard Business School Press; 1996.
12. Ransom ER, Joshi MS, Nash DB, et al. *The Healthcare Quality Book: Vision, Strategy, and Tools.* Chicago, IL: Health Administration Press; 2011.
13. Wyatt J. Scorecards, dashboards, and KPIs keys to integrated performance measurement. *Healthc Financ Manage.* 2004;58(2):76–80.
14. Outcomes for Prior Living Donors. Available at http://www.ncbi.nlm.nih.gov/pubmed/?term=kidney+transplant+outcomes+for+prior+living+organ+donors. Accessed September 12, 2015.
15. AHRQ Systematic Reviews. Available at http://effectivehealthcare.ahrq.gov/index.cfm/search-for-guides-reviews-and-reports/?productid=1984&pageaction=displayproduct. Accessed September 12, 2015.
16. ISHLT Standards and Guidelines. Available at http://www.ishlt.org/guidelines/. Accessed September 12, 2015.
17. Evaluation for Liver Transplantation in Adults: 2013. Practice Guidelines. Available at https://www.aasld.org/sites/default/files/guideline_documents/evaluationadultltenhanced.pdf. Accessed September 12, 2015.
18. Clinical Practice Guidelines: KDIGO. Available at http://kdigo.org/home/guidelines/. Accessed September 12, 2015.
19. de Vos M, Graafmans W, Kooistra M, et al. Using quality indicators to improve hospital care: a review of the literature. *Int J Qual Health Care.* 2009;21(2):119–129.

20. Ferraz AS, Santos LG, Roza Bde A, et al. Integrative review: indicators of result process of organ donation and transplants. *J Bras Nefrol.* 2013;35(3):220–228.

21. Varona MA, Soriano A, Aguirre-Jaime A, et al. Statistical quality control charts for liver transplant process indicators: evaluation of a single-center experience. *Transplant Proc.* 2012;44(6):1517–1522.

22. Quality Assessment and Performance Improvement Programs: a Resource Guide for Transplant surveyors. Available at http://www.cms.gov/Outreach-and-Education/Outreach/OpenDoorForums/downloads/QAPI ResourceGuide090810.pdf. Accessed June 20, 2015.

23. Near Miss Reporting Systems. Available at http://www.nsc.org/WorkplaceTrainingDocuments/Near-Miss-Reporting-Systems.pdf. Accessed July 4, 2015.

24. Bellandi T, Albolino S, Tartaglia R, et al. Unintended transplantation of three organs from an HIV-positive donor: report of the analysis of an adverse event in a regional health care service in Italy. *Transplant Proc.* 2010;42(6):2187–2189.

25. Tugwell BD, Patel PR, Williams IT, et al. Transmission of hepatitis C virus to several organ and tissue recipients from an antibody-negative donor. *Ann Intern Med.* 2005;143(9):648–654.

SELF-ASSESSMENT QUESTIONS

1. The regulations from Medicare require transplant programs to develop a Quality Program. This includes which of the following?
   a. Monitoring adverse events on transplant candidates and recipients who are inpatients
   b. Developing a data-driven program to monitor performance measures
   c. Ensuring a bidirectional flow of information with hospital QAPI
   d. All the above

2. The SRTR reports data to the public on each transplant program in the United States every _____.
   a. Year
   b. 2 years
   c. 6 months
   d. 3 months

3. The Conditions of Participation for transplant were developed by which of the following insurance companies?
   a. Blue Cross
   b. Anthem
   c. Medicare
   d. Kaiser

4. Participation in a root cause or thorough analysis includes which of the following?
   a. All clinicians involved in the adverse events
   b. Only the risk manager and the transplant QAPI manager
   c. Physicians who transplanted the patient
   d. All transplant coordinators

5. The purpose of benchmarking performance measures is to:
   a. balance the spreadsheet between months.
   b. provide a score against which the program's data can be measured.
   c. determine if there is an adverse event.
   d. demonstrate how data are collected and analyzed.

6. Transplant scorecards are divided in which of the following ways?
   a. According to high risk
   b. According to high cost
   c. According to volumes of transplants performed each month
   d. According to the three phases of transplantation: preoperative, perioperative, and postoperative

7. Advantages of maintaining scorecards includes which of the following?
   a. Scorecards identify potential safety concerns and hazards
   b. Allows programs to identify strategies to ensure safe care for patients
   c. Provides a tool for tracking performance improvement
   d. All the above

8. Which of the following are included in the five elements of a QAPI plan as defined by CMS?
   a. Design and scope
   b. Governance and leadership
   c. Feedback and data systems
   d. All the above

9. Which of the following are negative factors identified in the use of scorecards?
   a. Tracking indicators that are not useful or feasible
   b. Tracking metrics that are not valid or reliable
   c. Assigning indicators that do not align with the organization
   d. All the above

10. Per the Institute of Medicine, there are six dimensions of quality in health care including the following: patient centered, efficient, cost effective, safe, equitable, and _____.
    a. Data driven
    b. Outcomes oriented
    c. Timely
    d. Process oriented

Index

(Note: Page number in "f" indicates figures, followed by "t" indicates tables and followed by "b" indicates boxes)

A

A1AT. *See* Alpha-1 antitrypsin deficiency (A1AT)
Abdominal infections
   liver transplant recipients, 184–185
   pancreas transplant recipients, 679
ABO antigens, 37
ABO blood typing, 3
ABO incompatibility, rejection due to, 42
ACR. *See* Acute cellular rejection (ACR)
Acute cellular rejection (ACR)
   heart transplantation
     asymptomatic, 365
     EMB grading, 357, 358f, 358t
     pediatric solid organ transplantation, 729
     recurrence/resistance, 365
     treatment options, 352, 364–365
     types, 352, 364–365
   ISHLT, 744–745, 744t
   patient education, 77–78
   pediatric solid organ transplantation, 729
Acute rejection. *See also* Cardiac allograft rejection
   heart transplantation
     Allomap testing, 360
     asymptomatic, 365
     complications, 357–358
     diagnosis of, 354–355
     factors, 362
     gene expression profiling, 360
     immunosuppressive therapy, types of, 362, 363t
     patient education, 359
     postrejection follow-up, 359
     prevention, 360–362
     recurrence/resistance, 365
     rejection therapy, 365, 366t–368t
     signs and symptoms, 353–354, 354b
     treatment options, 352, 364–365
     types, 352, 364–365
   immune response, 42
   immunosuppression therapy, 91
   kidney transplant recipients, 92
   lung transplantation
     clinical findings, 493
     diagnosis, 493–494

facts, 493
     grading, 494
     postoperative complications, 487, 494t, 498t
     risk factors, 493
     treatment, 494–495
     types, 492–493
   pancreas transplantation, 680–681
   pediatric transplant recipients, 737, 751
   by T-cell activation, 653
Acute tubular necrosis (ATN)
   clinical manifestations, 651
   contributing factors, 651
   etiology, 651
   patient monitoring, 651–652
   treatment options, 651
Acyclovir (Zovirax), 93, 111t, 255t
Adjuvant pharmacotherapy
   analgesics, 115
   antimicrobials
     antibacterial therapy, 108–109, 110t
     antifungal therapy, 109, 113t–114t
     antiviral therapy, 109, 111t–112t
     infections, 108
     predicting infectious complications, 108, 108f
   medications
     to manage cardiovascular complications, 119, 120t–122t
     to manage DM, 115, 116t–117t
     to manage GI symptoms, 115, 118t
Alcoholic liver disease, 513
Alemtuzumab (Campath-1H), 89, 90t
Allograft. *See also* Cardiac allograft rejection
   bacterial infections, 169t–173t
   CMV, risk of, 159, 159t
   EBV infection, incidence of, 159, 159t
Allopurinol (Zyloprim), 245
Allotransplantation, 36
Alpha-1 antitrypsin deficiency (A1AT), 514
Altered mobility and self-care deficit, 403
Altered nutrition, 401–403
American cancer society routine cancer screening guidelines, 232, 232t
American Nurses Association Code of Ethics, 297